The Equine Veterinary Nursing Manual

The Equine Veterinary Nursing Manual

EDITED BY

Karen M Coumbe

MA VetMB CertEP MRCVS
Bell Equine Veterinary Clinic
Mereworth
Near Maidstone
Kent ME18 5GS
UK

For the BRITISH EQUINE VETERINARY ASSOCIATION

**Blackwell
Science**

© 2001 by
Blackwell Science Ltd
© 2001 by Vicki Martin for some line illustrations

Editorial Offices:
Osney Mead, Oxford OX2 0EL
25 John Street, London WC1N 2BS
23 Ainslie Place, Edinburgh EH3 6AJ
350 Main Street, Malden
  MA 02148 5018, USA
54 University Street, Carlton
  Victoria 3053, Australia
10, rue Casimir Delavigne
  75006 Paris, France

Other Editorial Offices:

Blackwell Wissenschafts-Verlag GmbH
Kurfürstendamm 57
10707 Berlin, Germany

Blackwell Science KK
MG Kodenmacho Building
7-10 Kodenmacho Nihombashi
Chuo-ku, Tokyo 104, Japan

Iowa State University Press
A Blackwell Science Company
2121 S. State Avenue
Ames, Iowa 50014-8300, USA

First published 2001

Set in 9/12 Palatino
by Best-set Typesetter Ltd., Hong Kong
Printed and bound in Great Britain
at the Alden Press Ltd, Oxford and Northampton

The Blackwell Science logo is a trade mark of Blackwell Science Ltd, registered at the United Kingdom Trade Marks Registry

DISTRIBUTORS

Marston Book Services Ltd
PO Box 269
Abingdon
Oxon OX14 4YN
(*Orders*: Tel: 01235 465500
            Fax: 01235 465555)

USA and Canada
Iowa State University Press
A Blackwell Science Company
2121 S. State Avenue
Ames, Iowa 50014-8300
(*Orders*: Tel: 800-862-6657
            Fax: 515-292-3348
            Web   www.isupress.com
            email: orders@isupress.com

Australia
Blackwell Science Pty Ltd
54 University Street
Carlton, Victoria 3053
(*Orders*: Tel: 03 9347 0300
            Fax: 03 9347 5001)

A catalogue record for this title
is available from the British Library

ISBN 0-632-05727-0

Library of Congress
Cataloging-in-Publication Data

The equine veterinary nursing manual / [edited by] Karen Coumbe.
      p. cm.
   Includes bibliographical references.
   ISBN 0-632-05727-0 (alk. paper)
   1. Horses—Diseases. 2. Veterinary nursing.
 I. Coumbe, Karen.

 SF951 .E68 2001
 636.1'089073—dc21

                              2001025149

For further information on
Blackwell Science, visit our website:
www.blackwell-science.com

Contents

List of Contributors

R. J. Baxter
MA, VetMB, MRCVS
The Old Golfhouse Veterinary Group
Brandon Road
Thetford
Norfolk IP24 3ND

C. L. Blake
BVSc, CertES, MRCVS
Division of Equine Studies
Department of Veterinary Clinical Science and Animal Husbandry
University of Liverpool
South Wirral CH64 7TE

J. C. Boswell
MA, VetMB, CertVA, CertES (Orth), MRCVS, DipECVS
The Liphook Equine Hospital
Forest Mere
Liphook
Hampshire GU30 7JG

E. R. J. Cauvin
DVM, MVM, CertVR, CertES (Orth), DipECVS, MRCVS
Clinique Vétérinaire Equine
SCE Stockwell
L'Attache
14700 Falaise
France

P. D. Clegg
MA, VetMB ,CertEO, DipECVS, PhD, MRCVS
Division of Equine Studies
Department of Veterinary Clinical Science and Animal Husbandry
University of Liverpool
South Wirral CH64 7TE

R. C. Conwell
BVetMed, MRCVS
Division of Equine Studies
Department of Veterinary Clinical Science and Animal Husbandry
University of Liverpool
South Wirral CH64 7TE

E. Hainisch
MRCVS
Klinik für Chirurgie und Augenheilkunde
Veterinärmedizinische Universisität Wien
Veterinärplatz 1
1210 Wien
Austria

N. E. Haizelden
BSc, BVetMed, MRCVS
The Ridgeway Veterinary Group
Valley Equine Hospital
Upper Lambourn Road
Lambourn
Berkshire RG16 7QG

H. J. Hangartner
VN
Homelea
Great Waldingfield
Sudbury
Suffolk CO10 0RY

P. A. Harris
MA, VetMB, PhD, MRCVS
Waltham Centre for Pet Nutrition
Freeby Lane
Waltham on the Wolds
Melton Mowbray
Leicestershire LE14 4RT

L. L. Hillyer
BVSc, CertEM (IntMed), MRCVS
Division of Companion Animals
Department of Clinical Veterinary Science
University of Bristol
Langford House
Langford
Bristol BS40 5DU

M. H. Hillyer
BVSc, CertEP, CertEM (IntMed), CertES (Soft tissue), MRCVS
Division of Companion Animals
Department of Clinical Veterinary Science
University of Bristol
Langford House
Langford
Bristol BS40 5DU

C. B. Johnson
BVSc, PhD, DVA, DipECVA, MRCA, MRCVS
Institute of Veterinary, Animal and Biomedical Sciences
Massey University
Private Bag 11-222
Palmerston North
New Zealand

A. Jones
BSc
Division of Companion Animals
Department of Clinical Veterinary Science
University of Bristol
Langford House
Langford
Bristol BS40 5DU

E. Jones
MA, VetMB, MRCVS
Department of Veterinary Clinical Studies
Royal (Dick) School of Veterinary Studies
The University of Edinburgh
Large Animal Hospital
Easter Bush
Roslin
Lothian EH25 9RG

R. D. Jones
MA, VetMB, CertEP, MRCVS
Bell Equine Veterinary Clinic
Mereworth
Near Maidstone
Kent ME18 5GS

D. C. Knottenbelt
BVM&S, DVM, MRCVS
Division of Equine Studies
Department of Veterinary Clinical Science and Animal Husbandry
University of Liverpool
South Wirral CH64 7TE

D. Lloyd
BVMS, MRCVS
Rossdale & Partners
Beaufort Cottage Equine Hospital
Cotton End Road
Exning
Newmarket CB8 7NN

L. C. Marlborough
BVM&S, MRCVS
The Coach House Veterinary Clinic
Burlyns
East Woodhay
Newbury
Berkshire RG20 0NU

J. Masters
VN
Vetlink School of Veterinary Nursing
Administrative Office
Cats Drove House
Ashcott
Near Bridgwater
Somerset TA7 9QP

D. P. McHugh
DipAVN (Surg), EVN, VN
Greenwood, Ellis & Partners
Reynolds House
166 High Street
Newmarket CB8 9QA

B. M. Millar
CVT(USA), EVN, VN
Rossdale & Partners
Beaufort Cottage Equine Hospital
Cotton End Road
Exning
Newmarket CB8 7NN

G. A. Munroe
BVSc, PhD, CertEO, DESM, DipECVS FRCVS
Flanders Veterinary Services
Cowrig Cottage
Greenlaw
Duns
Berwickshire TD10 6UN

J. C. Murrell
BVSc, PhD, CVA, MRCVS
University of Utrecht
Faculty of Veterinary Medicine
Department of Clinical Sciences of Companion Animals
PO Box 80154
3508 TD Utrecht
The Netherlands

J. M. Naylor
BVSc, PhD, BSc, DipACIVM, DipACVN, MRCVS
Department of Vet Internal Medicine
Western College of Vet Medicine
University of Saskatchewan
52 Campus Drive
Saskatoon
Saskatchewan S7N 5B4
Canada

S. A. Newton
BVSc, CertEM, MRCVS
Division of Equine Studies
Department of Veterinary Clinical Science and Animal Husbandry
University of Liverpool
South Wirral CH64 7TE

T. J. Phillips
BVetMed, CertEP, CertEO, DESTS, DipECVS, MRCVS
The Liphook Equine Hospital
Forest Mere
Liphook
Hampshire GU30 7JG

E. M. Post
DVM, MRCVS
Division of Equine Studies
Department of Veterinary Clinical Science and Animal Husbandry
University of Liverpool
South Wirral CH64 7TE

J. F. Pycock
BVetMed, PhD, DESM, MRCVS
Equine Reproductive Services
Messenger Farm
Ryton
Malton
North Yorkshire YO17 6RY

M. C. Schramme
MedVet, CertEO, PhD, MRCVS, DipECVS
The Equine Unit
Animal Health Trust
Lanwades Park
Kentford
Newmarket
Suffolk CB8 7UU

M. J. Senior
BVSc, CertVA, MRCVS
Division of Equine Studies
Department of Veterinary Clinical Science and Animal Husbandry
University of Liverpool
South Wirral CH64 7TE

J. D. Slater
BVM&S, PhD, MRCVS
Department of Clinical Vet Medicine
University of Cambridge
Madingley Road
Cambridge CB3 0ES

S. J. Stoneham
BVSc, CertESM, MRCVS
Rossdale & Partners
Beaufort Cottage Stables
High Street
Newmarket CB8 8JS

S. L. Taylor
BVetMed, MRCVS
Division of Equine Studies
Department of Veterinary Clinical Science and Animal Husbandry
University of Liverpool
South Wirral CH64 7TE

A. J. Wise
BVSc, MRCVS
Division of Equine Studies
Department of Veterinary Clinical Science and Animal Husbandry
University of Liverpool
South Wirral CH64 7TE

Foreword

The dramatic advances in equine medicine and surgery of the last twenty-five years, have necessitated the development of a group of support staff, which has carried the label of 'equine nurses'. They have performed increasingly sophisticated duties with skill and good humour, but illegally! Schedule Three of the Veterinary Surgeons Act in the UK has specifically precluded the nursing of equidae. Not surprisingly, there has been an increasing clamour for this apparently illogical law to be changed. I am delighted to say that after much hard work behind the scenes by the Royal College of Veterinary Surgeons, the British Equine Veterinary Association and the British Veterinary Nursing Association, the situation is about to be remedied. In fact the year 2000 saw the first batch of qualified Equine Veterinary Nurses (EVN).

Currently these people must already have achieved VN status, before sitting the examination. However it is hoped that the qualification will be available soon to people who do not wish to undergo training in small animal nursing.

How appropriate it is then, to welcome the first book devoted to the subject of equine nursing.

The gestation of the manual was under the care of Karen Coumbe who has had a particular interest in equine nursing and who was one of the first examiners for the EVN Certificate. She has had the most demanding task of obtaining manuscripts from a variety of highly experienced clinicians, scientists and nurses, whilst simultaneously nurturing her own second child; two major achievements!

I would like to congratulate her in particular and all those involved with the production of what I confidently expect to become the definitive work on the subject.

As a surgeon I have always recognised the value of highly trained nursing staff. I have also had the good fortune to have been involved with the challenge of setting up an officially recognised equine nursing qualification. Although there is clearly still much work to do, the future of equine nursing in the UK is secure. Furthermore, there is potential for the evolution of a profession with its own specialties, which will provide satisfying opportunities for people with an equine interest, who want a career in veterinary nursing.

Tim Greet FRCVS
(Immediate Past President of the British
Equine Veterinary Association)

Preface

The purpose of this manual is to provide the definitive textbook for equine veterinary nurses. It will also be useful to all those involved in the care and management of the sick horse. There are a multitude of excellent books available on managing the well horse. For this reason, the basics of equine management such as routine bandaging techniques are not included here, since they are well explained elsewhere. Instead the aim of this book is to provide new information on the care and consideration, as well as the art and science involved in looking after any sick horse or pony.

The Royal College of Veterinary Surgeons has devised an extremely detailed objective equine veterinary nursing syllabus, which this book has followed as comprehensively as possible. This explains the breadth and depth of subject matter. The authors include some of the first veterinary nurses to obtain the qualification in Equine Veterinary Nursing (EVN), following the first examinations held in July 2000. They are to be congratulated on writing their chapters and passing the exam in the same year! Also included amongst the authors, are many of those involved in drafting the original syllabus and all those involved in examining for this qualification. As such it should be a very useful guide for any would be equine nurse. Horses should benefit from those who read it and so improve their knowledge of equine nursing and welfare.

I am extremely grateful to all the contributing authors for all their hard work and for the many people who helped and advised throughout the project. In particular Adam Coumbe, Sue Dyson, Louise Harvey, Tim Mair, Katie Snalune and Sarah Stoneham provided invaluable editorial assistance and advice.

This is the first edition of a textbook on a new syllabus on the evolving subject of equine nursing. Inevitably there will be areas that need improvement, but I hope this is a suitable start. Feel free to comment and constructively criticise.

Karen Coumbe
Kent
Easter 2001

Figures 2.1, 2.3, 2.4, 2.7, 2.8, 2.10, 2.14, 2.19, 2.20, 2.22, 2.23, 2.30–2.44, 2.46–2.48, 2.50–2.53, 3.1, 3.3, 3.4, 4.16, 5.1, 5.2, 8.4, 13.1, 16.7, 17.3, 17.7–17.12, 17.16, 17.18, 17.21, 17.34 17.35, 20.3, 20.4 redrawn courtesy of Vicki Martin.

Abbreviations and Acronyms

ACTH	adrenocorticotrophic hormone		EGT	exuberant granulation tissue
ADH	antidiuretic hormone		EHV	equine herpes virus
AI	artificial insemination		EIPH	exercise-induced pulmonary
ANS	autonomic nervous system			haemorrhage
AP	alkaline phosphatase		EIV	equine influenza virus
ASA	American Society of Anaesthesiology		ELISA	enzyme-linked immunosorbent assay
ASIF	Association for the Study of Internal		EMEA	European Medicines Evaluation
	Fixation			Agency
AST	aspartate aminotransferase		ERS	equine rhabdomyolysis syndrome
BAL	bronchoalveolar lavage		ERV	equine rhinovirus
BAR	Bright Alert Responsive		EVA	equine viral arteritis
BP	blood pressure		EVN	equine veterinary nurse
BUN	blood urea nitrogen		FEI	Federation Equestre Internationale
BW	bodyweight		FFA	free fatty acid
CBC	complete blood count		FFD	film focal distance
CD	controlled drug		FSH	follicle-stimulating hormone
CDE	common digital extensor		GGE	glyceryl guaiacolate ether
CFT	complement fixation test		GGT	gamma-glutamyl transferase
CID	combined immunodeficiency disease		GIT	gastrointestinal tract
CNS	central nervous system		GLDH	glutamate dehydrogenase
COPD	chronic obstructive pulmonary disease		GnRH	gonadotrophin-releasing hormone
COSHH	Control of Substances Hazardous to		GSL	general sales list medicine
	Health		Hb	haemoglobin concentration
CPK	creatinine phosphokinase		hCG	human chorionic gonadotrophin
CPR	cardiopulmonary resuscitation		HSAWA	Health and Safety at Work Act
CRT	capillary refill time		HSE	Health and Safety Executive
CSF	cerebrospinal fluid		HYPP	hyperkalaemic periodic paresis
CT	computed tomography		ICF	intracellular fluid
CVS	cervical vertebral stenosis		ICL	inferior check ligament
DCP	dynamic compression plate		ILRD	infectious lower respiratory tract
DDF	deep digital flexor			disease
DDSP	dorsal displacement of the soft palate		IPPV	intermittent positive pressure
DE	digestible energy			ventilation
DM	dry matter		IURD	infectious upper respiratory tract
DOD	developmental orthopaedic disease			disease
ECF	extracellular fluid		LDH	lactate dehydrogenase
eCG	equine chorionic gonadotrophin		LH	luteinising hormone
ECG	electrocardiogram		LMN	lower motor neurone
EDTA	ethylenediaminetetraacetic acid		MAC	minimum alveolar concentration
EED	early embryonic death		MCH	mean corpuscular haemoglobin

MCHC	mean corpuscular haemoglobin concentration
MCV	mean corpuscular volume
MDP	methylene diphosphonate
MRI	magnetic resonance imaging
MSH	melanophore-stimulating hormone
NE	net energy
NILRD	non-infectious lower respiratory tract disease
NIURD	non-infectious upper respiratory tract disease
NMS	neonatal maladjustment syndrome
NRC	National Research Council
NSAID	non-steroidal anti-inflammatory drug
OCLL	osseous cyst-like lesion
OP	organophosphate
P	pharmacy medicine
PAS	perinatal asphyxia syndrome
PCR	polymerase chain reaction
PCV	packed cell volume
PET	polyethylene tube
PLGE	protein-losing gastroenteropathies
PML	pharmacy and merchant's list medicine
POM	prescription-only medicine
PTH	parathyroid hormone
QAR	Quiet, Alert, Responsive
QAU	Quiet, Alert, Unresponsive
RBC	red blood cell
RCVS	Royal College of Veterinary Surgeons
RIA	radioimmunoassay
RIDDOR	Reporting of Injuries, Diseases and Dangerous Occurrences Regulations
RJB	Robert Jones bandage
RLN	recurrent laryngeal neuropathy
RPA	radiation protection advisor
RPS	radiation protection supervisor
SCBC	subchondral bone cyst (*see* OCLL)
SDF	superficial digital flexor
SDH	sorbitol dehydrogenase
SFT	superficial flexor tendon
SL	suspensory ligament
SOP	standard operating procedure
SRH	single radial haemolysis
STA	Special Treatment Authorisation
STH	somatotrophic hormone
TBW	total body water
TL	tracheal lavage
TPN	total parenteral nutrition
TPR	temperature, pulse and respiration
TRH	thyroid-releasing hormone
TSBA	total serum bile acid estimation
TSH	thyroid-stimulating hormone
TSO	The Stationery Office
UMN	upper motor neurone
USP	US Pharmacopeia
VHS	Video Home System
VMD	Veterinary Medicines Directorate
VMP	veterinary medical product
VN	veterinary nurse
WBC	white blood cell
WSW	written system of work

CHAPTER 1

Basic Management

L. C. Marlborough & D. C. Knottenbelt

Veterinary legislation

The Veterinary Surgeons Act 1966

Accessibility and accountability are expected of every self-regulating profession. The Veterinary Surgeons Act 1966, which governs the veterinary profession, aims to protect the public interest by ensuring a high level of education and training, combined with personal and professional integrity. Section 19 of the Act restricts the practice of veterinary surgery to registered members of the Royal College of Veterinary Surgeons (RCVS) with a number of exceptions. This includes treatment by listed veterinary nurses in accordance with the Schedule 3 (Amendment) Order 1991.

Schedule 3 procedures

Under this Schedule the privilege of giving medical treatment and carrying out minor surgery, not involving entry into a body cavity, is given to listed veterinary nurses (VNs), including equine veterinary nurses (EVNs), under the direction of a veterinary surgeon employer to companion animals under the employer's care. Any VN is not, however, entitled independently to undertake either medical treatment or minor surgery. A student VN learning to perform or performing Schedule 3 procedures must be under the direct and constant supervision of a vet at all times. When a VN is negligent, the liability may rest in part with the directing vet. Equally, nurses must be responsible for their own actions. At the time of writing, Equidae are not included as companion animals under Schedule 3. Legislation may change, possibly as the result of some form of exemption order. The power to delegate acts of veterinary surgery is currently under review.

The RCVS Guide to Professional Conduct

Vets and VNs must follow the RCVS *Guide to Professional Conduct*, in which animal welfare is paramount. Also emphasised are client and colleague relationships and trust, the integrity of veterinary certification and compliance with legal obligations with respect to veterinary medicinal products.

Points that are particularly relevant for equine nurses include:

(1) Responsibility to patients:
  (a) patient welfare,
  (b) provision of a 24-h emergency service (immediate first aid and pain relief are vital),
  (c) maintenance of proper standards in practice premises and equipment in relation to inpatient care.
(2) Responsibility to clients:
  (a) the client is the person who requests professional services for an animal,
  (b) clear information about practice arrange-

ments and out-of-hours services should be provided,

(c) comprehensive case records and accounts should be kept,

(d) the client's informed consent to treatment should be obtained, unless delay would adversely affect the animal's welfare,

(e) the client must be aware if procedures are to be performed by staff who are *not* vets,

(f) the client's concerns and wishes must be considered where these do not conflict with the patient's welfare.

(3) Responsibility to the general public:

(a) reporting to the appropriate authority any suspected occurrence of notifiable disease or adverse reaction to medication,

(b) promoting responsible animal ownership.

(4) Responsibilities in relation to professional colleagues: poor relationships between vets and VNs undermine public confidence in the whole profession.

(5) Legal responsibilities: vets and VNs should be familiar with and comply with relevant legislation, including:

(a) Veterinary Surgeons Act 1966,

(b) Medicines Act 1968,

(c) Health and Safety at Work, Radiation Protection and Control of Substances Hazardous to Health (COSHH) legislation,

(d) Data Protection Acts 1984 and 1999 as they apply to professional and client records,

(e) Protection of Animals Act 1911,

(f) relevant employment legislation, e.g. Employment Rights Act 1996.

(6) Disclosure of records:

(a) client confidentiality—with certain exceptions relating to disclosure of information to insurance companies (undertaken by vets), no information about clients or their animals must be disclosed to any third party,

(b) case records and client details—all notes must be comprehensible and legible.

(7) Maintaining practice standards:

(a) Support staff, including VNs, should not suggest a diagnosis or give any clinical opinion to an owner, but their nursing input and opinion is invaluable in clinical care,

(b) veterinary nurses should discharge animals only on the instructions of a vet,

(c) continuing professional development is vital for both vets and VNs to ensure the continuous progression of capability and competence, it is essential to keep up to date with continual changes and developments in knowledge and nursing skills.

(8) Euthanasia: the Protection of Animals Act 1911 states that failure to destroy an animal to prevent further suffering may amount to cruelty. The duty to destroy falls on the vet, who has the skill and training to make the correct assessment. Firearms are still used for this purpose by many equine vets. Proper storage and management of firearms is essential (see Chapter 9 and contact the police for further information).

Stable management and inspection

Medical reasons for stabling

For nursing horses, stabling is often essential, e.g. for long-term orthopaedic problems requiring continued box rest:

- Monitoring of intensive-care patients usually requires the horse to be stabled.
- It may be necessary to advise owners to keep horses stabled or part-stabled as a preventative measure for certain conditions such as laminitis, *Culicoides* midge bite hypersensitivity (sweet itch) or horses suffering from mud fever or rain scald.
- Stabling is required in situations where isolation is desirable.

Requirements of a stable

Good hygiene is essential. With the large throughput of animals in an equine hospital, there may be an increased risk of infections, e.g. salmonellosis. Stable building requires planning permission and the conversion of existing buildings may be difficult.

Appropriate professional expertise should be sought.

General considerations of a stable

- Stables should be warm and dry and have adequate drainage.
- Stables should be easy to clean and disinfect, particularly in hospital situations.
- All precautions should be taken to minimise the risk of fire.
- Ventilation, lighting and water and food provision should be considered.

Water provision

Adequate clean water always should be available:

(1) Automatic water bowls are efficient but they must be checked regularly to ensure that they are working and a back-up supply of buckets should be available. A major drawback of automatic fillers in an equine hospital is that monitoring the water intake is impossible.

(2) Water buckets should be cleaned and refilled daily. Buckets can be secured in holders, old tyres or on hinged rings off the ground to prevent them from being knocked over.

Food provision—mangers

(1) Mangers should be easy to clean. Ideally, mangers should be large, broad and have a completely smooth surface with all corners well rounded.

(2) Mangers on the floor reproduce the horses' natural way of eating. For some medical conditions, e.g. sinusitis, it may help the horse to eat from floor level to enable good sinus drainage.

Food provision—hay

(1) Hay racks fitted above head level oblige the horse to feed at an unnatural level and there is a risk of getting dust and seeds in the eyes.

(2) Hay nets are commonly used and are useful. However, they should be tied high enough to prevent the horse getting tangled when it rolls.

This is more of a danger in horses shod with long-heeled shoes.

Hay nets should be tied with quick-release knots and attached to twine that will break easily if the horse gets caught and struggles.

(3) Hay also may be fed on the floor, reproducing the natural way a horse eats.

(4) Sometimes it may be desirable to scatter the feed around the bed in order to encourage the horse to forage and take longer over eating a limited quantity of food. This practice can be useful for horses on a restricted diet, e.g. those with laminitis .

Food provision—feed stores

Biosecurity of feed stores is very important. Rodent control programmes should be in place in all equine hospitals.

Stable fittings

Fittings should be minimal and, where possible, flush with the walls with no sharp projections. Firmly fixed rings at shoulder level for tying the horse to, and another ring at eye level for a hay net, should be the minimum requirements.

Ventilation

Good ventilation is particularly important for stabled horses:

(1) There is a tendency among horse owners to see large well-ventilated stables as being too cold. Rugs can provide extra warmth but still permit the horse adequate fresh air.

(2) Often, windows and top doors are the main source of ventilation. Windows should be arranged so that they can be opened with an inward slant while ideally being protected by iron bars.

(3) In barns, louvre boards at the apex of the roof are ideal. These consist of two or more overlapping boards separated from each other by a few inches and set at such an angle that the elements cannot enter. Wind blowing across the top of buildings

will aspirate air. Heat loss from horses also causes air to rise within the building. These factors contribute to the upward and outward flow of air, called *the stack effect*.

In many barns, large doors at one or both ends allow an influx of air. Wind blowing from side to side and end to end is known as *perflation*. Yorkshire boarding assists perflation.

(4) Barns often have better ventilation than individual loose boxes. However, there are disadvantages in that a group of horses share the same air space, which can encourage the spread of respiratory disease. In addition, hay and straw are commonly kept in the same air space and can exacerbate respiratory diseases.

(5) Draughts should be avoided, particularly in foal accommodation.

(6) Mechanical ventilation can be employed in long or wide buildings.

(7) In a stable with a monopitch roof, an open top door will provide an adequate inlet for air. A second inlet in the front wall and an outlet in the back wall are ideal. Boxes with peaked roofs ideally should have a fourth opening in the form of a capped chimney.

Ventilation and respiratory disease

The level of dust and spores in the centre of a box is dependent on the rates of release of the contaminant into the air and on the ventilation rate. Release rates depend on the activity in the stable and on the level of contamination of bedding and hay. Good ventilation combined with the use of bedding and hay with low levels of antigens is important, because improving the ventilation alone may be insufficient.

Heating of stables

(1) Extra heat may be supplied to stables in the form of electric fans, heat lamps or central heating.

(2) Provision of heat is particularly important for sick foals. Rugs, leg bandages and even sweaters worn as rugs (sleeves over fore legs) can be employed as additional sources of heat.

(3) Fire regulations should be observed.

(4) The potential for patient burns from heat sources should not be overlooked.

Lighting of stables and electrical equipment

(1) Take great care with water and electricity!

(2) Be aware that if fires originate from electric heat sources, the first action to take is to turn off the electricity. Know the whereabouts of the mains supply and trip switches, and also of back-up generator supplies if they are available.

(3) Artificial lighting is desirable, particularly in hospital situations. There should be even lighting in stables.

(4) Light switches should be outside stables and have waterproof safety covers. All other wiring should not be exposed. Plugs should be placed well away from water supplies and incoming elements.

(5) Circuit breakers should be employed when using any electrical equipment that potentially could give an electric shock.

Specialised hospital stabling requirements

Provision for cross-tying

Cross-tying may be needed as part of the management of long-bone fractures. This can be achieved by having two rings at eye level placed either side of a corner. It is best to measure the horse's combined neck and head length and calculate how short the ropes need to be to prevent the horse from lying down (even with its head and neck fully stretched out).

Provision for fluid administration (Fig. 1.1)

An overhead system with a hook attached to a rope and pulley is ideal. This allows the hook to be lowered easily so that fluid bags can be changed. The bags then can be raised to a level well above the horse's head and a spiral extension-type giving set can be employed to help the horse to move around.

In non-hospital situations, overhead beams or high structures may be adapted.

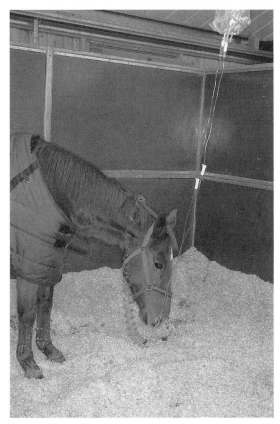

Fig. 1.1 Intensive care facilities: fluid administration.

Yard board for patient details

There should be room to write details for each loose box, such as patient and owner name, treatments and special management requirements.

Stable door details

A removable waterproof hospital card should be in place on each stable door. These also should carry patient details and are particularly useful for individual information such as 'nil by mouth'.

Intensive-care facilities

These are an important part of an equine hospital. They should include:

(1) Facilities for provision of additional heat and good lighting.

Table 1.1 Indications for isolation

- Individual acutely sick animals
- In-contact animals not showing clinical signs. Particular attention should be paid to animals that may be immunocompromised (e.g. old horses, foals and Cushing's disease cases)
- Non-contact unaffected animals in an epidemic
- Animals not showing clinical signs but in the recovery stages of disease (shedders)
- Quarantine procedures preceding entry into the herd

Table 1.2 Some equine infectious diseases in the UK

- Equine influenza
- Equine herpes virus infections
- Other respiratory virus infections
- Equine viral arteritis
- *Streptococcus equi* infections (strangles)
- Other streptococcal infections (e.g. *Streptococcus pneumoniae*)
- Infectious enterocolitis (e.g. salmonellosis, clostridial disease, rotavirus, cryptosporidia)
- Ringworm

(2) Facilities for intravenous fluid administration.

(3) Colic boxes should have ample deep bedding right up to the door. Alternatively they can be constructed with a rubber floor and walls. Such boxes should have minimal fittings so that the horse does not injure itself if it rolls violently.

(4) Specialised bedding for sick foals should be available (see Chapter 15). Intensive-care systems for mares and foals should include a separation box, where the foal can be separated to facilitate treatment while the mare can still have some contact.

Isolation facilities

Forward planning is vital to good isolation and the control of infectious disease outbreaks.

Tables 1.1 and 1.2 list the indications for isolation and some infectious diseases.

Principles of isolation

If a serious infectious disease is suspected, then stop all movement on and off the premises immediately. If it is suspected that an animal has an infectious disease, it must be isolated immediately. *Isolate first and confirm diagnosis later!*

Isolation accommodation

The stable should be used only for isolation purposes and should be cleaned and fully disinfected between patients. The horse should have no contact with others and should be downwind of other stables. Ideally an isolation box should be at least 35 m away from other animals, feeding and bedding stores and regular thoroughfares. A completely separate set of feeding, watering, mucking out, grooming and veterinary equipment should be used. These must be thoroughly disinfected between horses. Disinfection methods should be considered in advance. It may be necessary to adjust these according to the pathogen involved. The efficacy of a disinfectant against the organism involved also can be evaluated.

All hospital boxes, but particularly isolation boxes, should have floors of roughened concrete or rubber mats with sealed edges. Walls should be impervious with central floor drains. There should be minimal fittings in the accommodation and these should be easy to disinfect. Ledges and windowsills also should be minimal because they can promote a build-up of debris.

All waste feed and bedding should be burned or disposed of in sealed containers as clinical waste. Carcasses should be burned or disposed of as clinical waste once the appropriate samples have been taken. The drain from isolation accommodation should be away from other animal accommodation and natural watercourses.

Nursing isolation cases

(1) An isolated horse should have one person ascribed to its nursing and management. There should be minimal contact with the animal and no contact with normal non-isolated animals. In situations where a VN has to deal with isolated horses and others, the isolated animal must be dealt with last.

(2) Overalls, shoe covers and a head cover should be kept outside the box and used whenever the

Table 1.3 Important questions to ask about an infectious disease

Clinical signs and diagnostic tests:
- What samples need to be collected?
- What is the incubation period?

Transmission of pathogens between animals:
- How does the animal contaminate its environment?
- How important are fomites or other animal vectors?
- Over what distance can aerosol transmission occur?

Survival of pathogen outside the animal:
- How long can the pathogen survive?
- What environmental conditions enhance its survival?
- Does the pathogen produce resistant spores?
- What disinfectants is the pathogen susceptible to?

Protection of susceptible animals:
- Will treatment/vaccination help?

During isolation:
- What is the incubation period and for how long can animals shed the pathogen following recovery?
- Can asymptomatic carriers be identified (a recognised problem with strangles)?

horse is dealt with. Latex gloves also should be worn. These protective items should be disposed of in a clinical waste bin outside the horse's box.

(3) There should be full facilities for staff to disinfect at entry/exit to the box. A shoe dip also should be provided outside the horse's box.

(4) Personnel in contact with the isolated horse should thoroughly scrub hands and other exposed skin with a surgical scrub immediately afterwards.

(5) Fomites (i.e. inanimate objects such as feed buckets) can be a cause of disease transmission. Care should be taken to reduce this risk.

Duration of isolation

Duration of isolation is often difficult to assess and implement, and owner compliance is likely to be very much reduced following cessation of clinical signs. The period of isolation will depend on the disease involved (see Table 1.3).

Bedding and cleaning of stables

Table 1.4 summarises the basic bedding materials available.

Table 1.4 Summary of bedding materials

Type of bedding	Comments
Hay	Generally not suitable because it is edible and expensive
Hemp	Low dust and mould free. Good for horses with COPD. Some horses try to eat it
Paper	Excellent for dust-free environment. May be expensive
Peat moss	Inedible. Dust free. Becoming less readily available. Peat extraction is an ecological issue
Straw: barley straw	Often cheapest but can be poor quality and cause skin irritation. Not suitable for horses with COPD. Any straw can cause impactions if eaten
Straw: oat straw	Often cheaper, but edible. Not suitable for horses with COPD
Straw: treated straw	Treated straw to prevent horses eating it is now available. It is more expensive than traditional straw
Straw: wheat straw	Generally considered the best straw bedding. Light, durable and not usually eaten. Not suitable for horses with COPD
Sawdust	May block drains. If damp, can cause foot problems such as thrush
Wood shavings	Less dusty than sawdust, but can also cause foot problems if damp or if hygiene is poor
Other: rubber, peanut hulls, corncobs, etc.	Ensure a fresh clean supply. Easy to muck out

Cleaning and changing of bedding

Deep litter systems
Deep litter stables are maintained by removing just the droppings on a daily basis. This type of management is not suitable for a hospital situation because of the lack of hygiene.

Complete mucking-out systems
Faeces and urine-soaked litter should be removed daily. Ideally bedding should be removed completely between different horses. Personnel involved in the cleaning of stables should be aware of good personal hygiene and the potential problems of handling urine and faeces. Regular washing of hands and wearing clean protective clothing daily is important.

Disposal of bedding waste

A muck heap should be created in a suitable area, not too close to the stables or other hospital buildings because it may attract flies. Rotting mounds of bedding provide another source of potential pathogens and spores. Regular disposal of bedding, at least every third day, should be arranged.

Bedding for special cases

Chronic obstructive pulmonary disease (COPD)
Horses with COPD suffer from an allergy to fungal spores in hay and straw. If this condition is to be controlled it is vital that the horse is not exposed to materials containing spores. The spore content of feed or bedding depends largely on the moisture content. Straw, hay and grains harvested with high moisture contents mould heavily. It should be noted also that other bedding types that have been allowed to mould will exacerbate COPD. Non-biological beddings do not provide a base medium for fungal growth.

Intensive care
Bedding should be chosen for ease of mucking out, cleaning and disinfection. In some situations, e.g. acute laminitis, the horse should be encouraged to lie down as much as possible.

Orthopaedic cases
When such cases lie down they tend to land heavily on the dependent limb. A deep bed is essential.

7

Colic cases

Colic patients may be violent and roll repeatedly. Adequate deep bedding is essential, with deep banks to help prevent the horse from getting cast.

Convalescence

Attention to bedding of horses is often neglected in their convalescence after surgery or illness. Recumbent horses, horses with lung compromise after an anaesthetic or pneumonic foals may inhale millions of spores into an already compromised respiratory system.

Cleaning and disinfection

The design and construction of stables should be such that they can be cleaned and disinfected readily and routinely. To minimise the risk of microorganisms becoming established in the fabric of stables, there should be a regular programme of depopulating the accommodation and subjecting it to a thorough disinfection. It is only possible to do this effectively if all internal surfaces have impervious and easily disinfectable concrete walls and floors. The materials used must withstand pressure cleaners, strong detergents and a full range of disinfectants.

Stable hygiene is of utmost importance in the prevention of infectious and contagious disease (see Chapter 14).

Stable yards

Daily mucking out is important and stables should be kept clean and dry with plenty of fresh bedding. As far as possible, horses should keep the same stables. A routine of removing all the bedding and thorough disinfection should be employed on a regular 3–6 monthly basis.

Equine hospitals

As with any stable yard, hygiene is vital. Hospitals should be organised so that stables are grouped according to the following categories. Notes on cleaning and hygiene are made for each category:

(1) Routine hospital cases: stables should be washed and cleaned between cases, depending on individual hospital policy.

(2) Intensive-care hospital cases: particular care should be taken with the routine cleaning of intensive care boxes. It is important to observe the amount of faeces and urine produced.

(3) Isolation boxes: removal of all bedding (and ideally subsequent burning) should be carried out. Thorough disinfection is essential. Ideally the stable should be left vacant for a period of time before being re-used. This often depends on the microorganism implicated in the contagious disease, because different microorganisms can survive for differing lengths of time in the environment, even after disinfection.

(4) Quarantine: as with isolation boxes, quarantine boxes should be disinfected thoroughly between occupants. It would be advisable when working in such situations to obtain specific information (from the State Veterinary Service) about where the horse has come from and the nature of potential diseases it may carry.

Disinfectants and antiseptics

- *Disinfection* is the removal or destruction of pathogenic microorganisms, although not necessarily of bacterial spores. The number of 'vegetative' microorganisms thereby is reduced to a level that is not harmful to health. Disinfection can be achieved using chemical solutions, by heat treatment or by physical removal.

- A *disinfectant* is an agent usually applied to inanimate objects to destroy microorganisms. Many disinfectants are harmful to living tissue. It is therefore important that anyone using disinfectants be aware of this and take the appropriate precautions as advised by manufacturers. It is essential always to read the labels of disinfectants used and adhere strictly to safety instructions.

- *Antiseptics* destroy microorganisms, but not bacterial spores, on living tissue. They prevent the growth of microorganisms and may be applied safely to living tissue.

- *Sterilisation* is the destruction of microorganisms and spores.

Table 1.5 Disinfectants and their properties

Active ingredients (product name)	Inactivated by organic material (Yes / No)	Effective against rotavirus	Comments
Chlorine compounds (bleaches)	Yes	No	
Quarternary ammonium compounds	Yes	No	
Phenolic compounds	No	Yes	Generally not utilised due to toxic and irritant properties
Iodophors	No	Yes	Usually utilised more for handwashing during outbreaks
Halogenated tertiary amines (e.g. Trigene)	No	Yes	Non-toxic and biodegradable. Commonly utilised
Halogenated peroxides (e.g. Virkon)	Yes	Yes	Commonly utilised. Has fungicidal properties

- *Contamination* is the presence of microorganisms in tissues, which may or may not result in infection.

Principles of disinfection

(1) It is important to establish whether a disinfectant is bactericidal (actually destroys the organisms) or bacteriostatic (stops bacterial growth). Bactericidal chemicals with activity against spores are preferable but such substances are more likely to be harmful to the operator.

(2) Chemicals that are not inactivated in the presence of organic material (such as pus, blood and faeces) should be chosen. Removal of gross contamination is paramount and pressure hoses can be very useful for this.

(3) Selection of a chemical that is effective against the pathogens that are most difficult to destroy is appropriate.

Susceptibility of microorganisms

(1) Gram-positive bacteria are destroyed most easily by disinfectants. Streptococcal organisms are susceptible to drying and heat but *Rhodococcus equi* is resistant to drying and heat under natural conditions.

(2) Gram-negative bacteria, acid-fast bacteria and bacterial spores are increasingly resistant.

(3) Rotavirus and cryptosporidia are most difficult to destroy. Rotavirus commonly causes diarrhoea in foals, from newborns up to 5 months of age. It is a heat-resistant virus that is known to survive in the environment for up to 9 months. Choosing a disinfectant that is effective against rotavirus also will control most other commonly encountered pathogens.

(4) Cryptosporidia are a special case and only a minimum of 18h of fumigation of buildings with formaldehyde or ammonia will disinfect adequately. However, formaldehyde is highly toxic and has noxious fumes, making it impractical to use routinely in stable environments. Fortunately their role in neonatal diarrhoea is questionable because they can be found in both normal and sick foals.

Practical disinfection

Table 1.5 outlines the common disinfectants and their properties. Practically, it is best for a hospital to have one main type of disinfectant to be used for most circumstances. Halogenated peroxides and tertiary amines are highly effective against all bacteria and most viruses, including rotavirus.

Loading and unloading of horses from transporters

Transport by road

Horses may be transported by road in trailers or horse boxes, which come in varying forms and may have side and/or end-unloading facilities.

Many horses are accustomed to travelling and load and unload easily.

However some horses can be very difficult. Common problems include:

- Unfamiliarity with vehicle or trailer
- Ramp too steep or poorly positioned
- Previous bad experience
- Compartment size too narrow (e.g. in end-loader trailers)
- Lack of suitable training
- Reluctance to travel alone

General points for loading and transporting

The trailer should be in a safe loading area with a closed gate between the loading area and a road. Many horses load more readily when the vehicle and trailer have been positioned with one side along a solid high wall. Backing the trailer into a barn could be considered for horses that readily run out of either side of the ramp. Many horses will enter a transporter more readily if a second ramp is open so as to create the impression of a thoroughfare.

Ideally all horses should be loaded in a bridle or with a Chifney bit. Where two or more horses are to be transported, load the easiest and more sensible horses first. Many horses that are nervous and reluctant to load will do so much more readily with a companion already in the transporter.

Trailers and horseboxes should be safe and roadworthy. Regular safety checks and compliance with regulations, as with any vehicle, are important. This includes safety within the transporter, such as ensuring a strong enough floor for any horse travelling.

Trailers

The following points should be considered:

- The vehicle always should be attached to the trailer before loading the animals.
- When loading the first horse it may be easier to move the central partition across to give the impression of a larger compartment.
- It is illegal for persons to travel in the back of trailers.

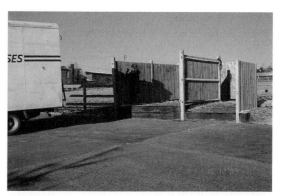

Fig. 1.2 A loading ramp. Difficult horses often will load more readily using a loading ramp.

Loading ramps

Loading ramps (Fig. 1.2) decrease the gradient of the transporter ramp in order to make the entrance to the vehicle seem more inviting for the horse. A purpose-built ramp should have room for boxes with both front and side doors to manoeuvre. There should be solid walls either side of the ramp to 'funnel' the horse in. It is usually necessary to have a lower ramp for trailers and a higher one for lorries.

Unloading

As with loading, all safety precautions should be taken. Horses often exit from vehicles with unexpected speed. A bridle or Chifney bit (see Fig. 1.5, p. 13) should be used, particularly where there is direct access to a road.

Problem horses

There are many tricks to getting problem horses to load. Generally owners should be encouraged to practise loading problem horses so that they learn not to fear transporters, e.g. walking horses through a front- and end-unload vehicle daily, and even feeding in the trailer can be excellent methods of getting animals used to vehicles. Shy loaders should be rewarded with food when they enter the vehicle.

Clothing for transport

Opinion as to how much protective clothing should

be worn by the horse during transport varies greatly. Certainly some form of lower limb protection is advisable. Horses that violently raise their heads or rear may benefit from a poll guard. Tail bandages and tail guards also may be useful.

Transport of sick or injured horses

Dehydration

Transport of even a healthy animal incurs a certain amount of stress, even if the animal looks completely calm and healthy. It is always important to advise owners to provide adequate water, and to offer water during the journey if it is longer than 1 h (particularly in the summer).

Respiratory problems

Horses with respiratory problems may experience sudden flare-ups during transport, particularly on long journeys where conditions are hot and dusty. Normal management factors, such as reduced exposure to hay and straw and adequate ventilation, should be considered. Acute pleuropneumonia can occur when horses travel for very long distances (e.g. across North America). This condition has been linked to the fact that horses are tied in a head-upright position for long periods of time and are thought to be more prone to aspiration of pharyngeal contents.

Horses that have been sedated should be fully recovered before travel. Not only does a sedative make an animal more unstable on its legs, but aspiration of food and choke is also possible. It is always unwise to transport a horse with a hay net after sedation.

Choke

Horses with choke travelling to a clinic should be transported without any food.

Colic

Horses travelling to a clinic for colic investigation may be extremely restless or violent. Such animals should have no food offered to them. Restraint of horses with colic can be very difficult.

Fractured limbs

With any suspected or diagnosed fracture, a vet should apply proper support and splinting before moving the horse, because travel can exacerbate the injury. Great care should be taken when loading, transporting and unloading animals with limb splints.

Equine ambulances

Specialist trailers and lorries are now available for the transport of animals requiring treatment. Such vehicles are fitted with accessories such as winches, belly support straps and drag mats.

Basic training and management

Training

Training a horse so that it learns to live with humans should begin from birth. From a very early stage a foal should be used to people being in its environment and similarly used to human-associated noises. There are no definitive rules for training but continuity and reward are very important. Always remember the nature of the horse and its natural behaviour. Aim to be gentle and not frighten the young horse, so as to produce a horse that is calm and confident to ride and handle. Horses, like people, differ in their natural ability and in their capacity for learning. In addition, different horses are required for different purposes, e.g. the early backing and racing of juvenile thoroughbreds is a particularly highly skilled area.

Early handling

The foal has acute hearing, good eyesight and is sensitive to touch. If properly handled, a foal quickly will become accustomed to people and will learn to trust them. The foal should be touched and spoken to in the first few days of life. As soon as the foal is used to being touched and approached it should be fitted with its first headcollar, which is called a foal slip. Gentle handling of the head and ears in the early stages is important in preventing a headshy horse later in life. Foals often resent being led by a halter. A recently developed device is a figure-of-eight halter, which fits over the whole body of the foal and guides its body rather than just its head.

Leading

Ideally a led animal should walk forward freely. An unwilling foal should never be pulled or it will learn to resist by running back or rearing. Leading the foal while it is following the mare is a good way to teach it, accompanied by the use of quiet but firm verbal aids and a hand around the hind quarters to push and guide steadily.

Traditionally horses are led from the left (i.e. the 'near' side), yet they should be trained to accept approaches from both sides. For example, when leading on the road the handler always should be between the horse and the traffic. The lead rope should be held near the horse's head, with the free end in the other hand. The rope should never be wound around the hand.

Release and catching

If a foal is being properly handled it should not be difficult to catch. Patience and positive rewards should be encouraged when releasing and catching animals.

Lungeing and loose schooling

Lungeing (Fig. 1.3) and loose schooling may be used in the early stages of training, but only by those with experience. This is hard work for a horse and should be used with care and in moderation in young horses with growing joints.

Backing

Before backing a horse it is a good idea to be aware of the animal's natural state and behaviour. A horse has a blind spot behind him and a natural fear of anything landing on its back. In addition, the horse has to get used to an increased weight. Gradual introduction of increasing weights on the saddle should precede the first attempt of a rider in the saddle. Many trainers make use of a dummy jockey.

Aids to training and restraint

For most procedures around the stable yard the horse can be restrained by a halter or headcollar. A foal slip, which will break easily, is preferable for young ani-

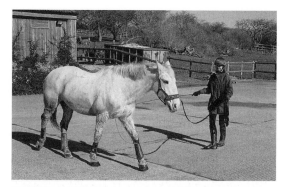

Fig. 1.3 Lungeing with a lunge cavesson and bridle for control. Note the protective brushing boots on the horse and the gloves and hat worn by the handler.

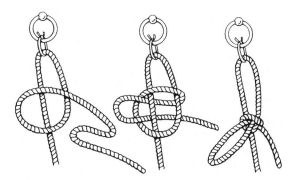

Fig. 1.4 Tying a quick-release knot.

mals. All horses should be trained to stand quietly when tied up. This should be achieved at an early age. A quick-release knot (Fig. 1.4) always should be used, and ideally the animal should be tied to a sturdy ring or post via a piece of string that will break if the horse pulls back violently.

Additional control

For additional control a normal bridle or in-hand bridle may be used. A Chifney or anti-rearing bridle is a very useful device that is fitted with three rings—two for the cheek pieces and one for the lead rein—and has a shallow inverted-port mouthpiece (Fig. 1.5). In animals that are too young to wear a bit, a lunge cavesson with lunge rein may provide better control. The lead rein or lunge line attaches to the front of the noseband on a lunge cavesson. A special halter de-

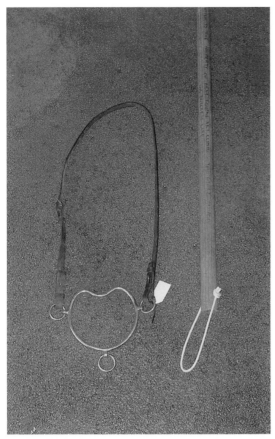

Fig. 1.5 Aids to restraint. The twitch and Chifney bit are two devices commonly used for restraint.

veloped by Monty Roberts can be used to discourage a rearing horse, without using severe forces of bits in the mouth. It puts pressure on the poll and the nose. This device can be very useful for loading difficult horses.

Additional restraints

Twitch
A traditional twitch (Fig. 1.5) is made of a short pole 50–70 cm in length, with a loop of rope 6–7 mm thick at the end. The loop, which should be 40–50 cm long, is twisted around the horse's upper lip. The twitch works partially by causing pain and distracting the horse's attention, so should be used only when *absolutely* necessary. It also causes the release of natural endorphins, which have a narcotic effect. It can be an extremely useful method of restraint, but modern sedatives are often a more humane solution. Other methods of restraint include:

- Skin twitch: taking a firm grip of a fold of neck skin can distract some horses.
- Ear twitch: similar to a skin twitch; holding and gently twisting the ear may control some horses, particularly youngsters.
- Raising a foreleg: this can be useful if you are confident that you can keep the leg up when the horse tries to move.
- Stocks: stocks limit horse movement, but must be designed to maximise horse and human safety.

Approaching an unfamiliar horse

When approaching a horse, particularly a nervous animal, always speak to let it know your presence. Approach from the front and slightly to the side, and walk towards the shoulder. Handle the horse first on the lower neck or shoulder, and then put a lead rope around its neck. At this stage many animals will consider themselves caught. Difficult individuals should wear a headcollar when turned out or even in the stable until they learn to be caught submissively. Headcollars with rubber pieces that break if the headcollar snags on something are ideal.

Using food to tempt horses can be useful, although they should not come to expect it always. Placing the noseband of a headcollar around the inside of a bucket may help when catching a difficult animal. Speed and technique are always important in such situations.

The horse's natural behaviour

Most horses behave better if handled with confidence, firmness and kindness. Only deliberate bad behaviour should incur reprimand, and this should be immediate.

When persuading horses to do something unfamiliar or frightening, their primitive instincts for food and companionship can be utilised. Much work has been carried out recently in new methods of training the horse (e.g. Monty Robert's work) that involve gaining the horse's trust by using common sense and thinking in terms of a horse as a wild pack animal. Kicking, biting, bucking and running away were methods of survival in primitive horses. These instincts remain but can be modified by training.

Signs of certain types of behaviour

When horses flatten their ears, bare their teeth and lunge towards other animals or people, this is very often a sign of aggression rather than fear. If afraid, a horse may flatten its ears, yet turn away.

Remember that fear can manifest as aggression. In certain clinical conditions a horse's behaviour changes, e.g. mares with ovarian granulosa cell tumours may show particularly aggressive behaviour towards people and other horses.

Sexual behaviour

Stallions may demonstrate inter-male aggression, a form of competitive aggression. Inter-female aggression is less commonly encountered.

Some mares may show undesirable behavioural changes when they are in season. It is possible to manage these behavioural changes pharmacologically. Mares can be extremely protective and possessive over their foals. Care must be taken with even the most trustworthy mares. Conversely, some mares show inadequate maternal behaviour and may even reject their foal.

Horses in groups form relationships where there is dominance and a form of 'pecking order'. Many people prefer to keep field-kept mares and geldings separately because traditionally male–female aggression is thought to be a problem, although some geldings and mares can be managed together safely. Horses, particularly young stock, also play together. This may be observed particularly in young entire males.

Each horse is an individual. There are no set rules, and specific types of behaviour should never be taken for granted.

Vices, stereotypies and redirected behaviour

In the past certain types of abnormal behaviour were

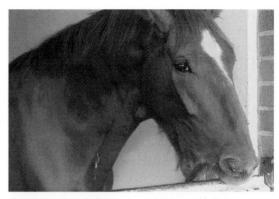

Fig. 1.6 Stereotypical behaviour: horse cribbing on stable door.

known as vices. We now know that many 'vices' are the horses attempt to cope with a stressful environment. Their significance to equine health is widely disputed, e.g. many link crib biting with colic, whereas others refute this.

Stereotypies are invariant and repetitive behaviour patterns that seemingly have no function. Horses are naturally free-ranging social-grazing herbivores. In stables, horses are provided with food, water and shelter, but their choice of food, social interactions and movement are limited. It is under these conditions that undesirable stereotypical behaviours develop. Locomotor stereotypies, such as weaving and box walking, may be related to lack of exercise. Oral stereotypies, such as wind sucking and cribbing (Fig. 1.6), have been associated with feeds of high digestibility but little dietary fibre. Giving the horse greater time in paddocks with *ad libitum* forage and social contact may be a successful means of reducing the frequency of crib biting.

Redirected behaviour occurs when a certain type of motivational behaviour is prevented. The horse will perform another type of behaviour to replace that lost. Weaving bars, for example, may reduce the over-the-door weaving but horses can continue to weave out of sight in the stable. Self-mutilation is a compulsive behaviour that is seen occasionally, particularly in stallions. Castration often resolves this problem and it therefore may represent a redirected behaviour motivated by sexual frustration. Stallions also tend to show a higher rate of cribbing and weaving compared with mares and geldings.

Certain behaviours such as pawing, digging or door kicking may be reinforced by attention. Many horses carry out these 'vices' prior to feeding, and are subsequently 'rewarded' for the abnormal behaviour. Stereotypical and redirected behaviours do not consistently cause direct harm to the horse. They are considered undesirable and may represent a welfare problem. It is important to understand the motivation behind these abnormal behaviours, rather that resorting immediately to drugs or surgical means to prevent them.

Grooming methods and equipment

Grooming equipment

Grooming is carried out in order to promote good health of the coat and skin, as well as for aesthetic reasons. The key items include brushes, curry combs and hoof-care equipment.

Curry combs
Plastic and rubber curry combs are used to remove dried mud, sweat and dead hair. Metal curry combs are used for cleaning the body brush during grooming.

Brushes
Dandy brushes are designed to remove heavy dirt from a horse's coat. Body brushes are softer and are used on the body, mane and tail for the removal of fine dust, scurf and grease from the coat. This is best carried out once removal of the gross debris has been completed.

Whisps, sponges and stable rubbers
Whisps and stable rubbers are traditionally used after a full and thorough groom (known as 'strapping') in order to massage and tone underlying muscles and give a good finish and shine to the coat. Wisps are made from hay or soft straw fashioned into a rope.

Other grooming equipment
Mane and tail combs, scissors and sweat scrapers are just some of the many additional items that may be found in a grooming kit.

Hygiene

All items should be cleaned and disinfected regularly. Grooming kit should be confined to one horse. Cleaning of brushes after each grooming can be a useful diagnostic tool for skin diseases. For example, examining brushings either with the naked eye or under the microscope can reveal mites such as *Trombicula autumnalis* (harvest mites) and lice.

Clipping horses

Horses are clipped for various management and veterinary reasons.

Management reasons for clipping
- To enable horses to work hard without excess sweating.
- To reduce grooming.
- It is traditional not to clip after January, to allow the subsequent summer coat to develop properly. It is also advisable not to clip horses' lower limbs because this removes the waterproofing of the hair. However, many horses are fully clipped and suffer no ills provided that the legs are adequately cleaned and dried as necessary.

Veterinary-related reasons for clipping
- Investigation of trauma sites and wounds.
- When cleaning wounds prior to repair. This may not be possible in some cases, e.g. wounds along the eyelids.
- Preparation of a site for surgery or aseptic techniques, e.g. arthrocentesis.
- Cushing's cases often grow a thick curly coat, which they fail to lose in summer. They may be managed with full body clips during the summer months.
- Skin diseases: rain scald and mud fever develop in damp microclimates, such as that afforded by long hair. One of the steps to control these skin conditions is trimming the thick coat.

Types of clippers
Clippers may be battery or mains operated. Hand-held cordless rechargeable clippers are invaluable in hospital situations. Mains-operated clippers should

have a safety-approved insulating cord. Clipping using such equipment should not be undertaken on wet floors and the horse must be prevented from standing on the electrical flex. Ideally, shod horses should be clipped on rubber mats and a circuit breaker should be used.

General points

The coat must be clean and dry for clipping. Efficient use of clippers is dependent on clean, sharp, cool blades used at the correct tension. Poorly cared for equipment is noisy, pulls the hair and may burn the animal. Clipper rashes or wounds can occur with poor clipping. Periodically clippers need to be lubricated. Clippers can be oiled and left to cool during use if they get very hot. This is particularly relevant where horses are being clipped all over for management reasons. After use, machines should be stripped, cleaned and oiled before storage.

Difficult animals

Some horses can be dangerous and difficult to clip. The horse should be taught that the touch and sound of the clippers are not something to fear. Allowing the horse to see and smell the clippers turned off can be useful. The clippers then can be run over the horse without being activated. Getting a horse used to the sound of the clippers can be more difficult and may take several training sessions. It should be considered that horses are genuinely afraid and punishment may exacerbate this. Terminating clipping due to bad behaviour reinforces this and future attempts can be even worse. Counter-conditioning or behaviour modification uses the principle of associating food and pleasurable activity with the noise of the clippers. This can be achieved using a tape recording of clippers during feeding.

Additional restraint in the form of a bridle or Chifney bit is often advisable for difficult horses during clipping and other veterinary procedures. Some horses are completely intractable to clipping and sedation is required.

Preparation of sites for ultrasound examination

Preparation is particularly important where ultra-sound examination involves the use of a high-frequency probe (such as 7.5 MHz), as used in tendon scanning. Although asepsis is not required, thorough cleaning of the area as for surgical preparation is recommended. This degreases the skin, so facilitating better contact between the probe and the skin. Even better contact is afforded if the gel is allowed to soak in for at least 10 min before scanning.

Bathing horses

Non-medical reasons include bathing for the removal of sweat, dirt and scurf, and for aesthetic reasons. Horse shampoos can wash away the natural oils of the coat and should not be over-used.

When horses suffer from various parasitic infections and skin diseases, bathing with medical preparations may be necessary. Medical reasons for bathing horses include:

- Mud fever and rain scald
- Ringworm
- Lice infestation (pediculosis)

For guidance and information, see Chapters 9 and 14. Other medicated shampoos or washes are sometimes prescribed by the vet for specific skin conditions.

Basic foot care

Daily foot care

Daily care of the feet is vital. This involves picking out the horse's feet and cleaning away debris with a hoof pick and stiff brush. This should be performed at least once daily, plus each time the horse returns from work. Stable hygiene is also a vital part of foot care. Conditions such as thrush and white line disease occur in dirty stabling (see equine lameness, Chapter 16). It should be noted that youngsters and unshod horses turned away to grass still require regular foot care and attention.

How frequently a horse is shod depends on the type of work it is doing, how fast its feet grow and are worn, and the need for special types of remedial shoes.

Hoof oil

This has traditionally been used to form an impermeable barrier to regulate water loss from the hoof. However, in well kept healthy hooves the periople serves naturally to protect the hoof from dehydration. Good stable hygiene is also a vital part of foot care.

Removing a shoe

A shoe is removed by:

(1) Raising the clenches, by placing the blade of a buffer under each clench and giving it a sharp blow with the shoeing hammer.
(2) By using the farriers pinchers (also referred to as pulloffs), the inside heel of the shoe is eased, followed by the outside. This is continued alternately along each branch until the shoe is loose.
(3) At this point the shoe can be grasped at the toe and pulled backwards across the foot and off. Most pinchers have knobs at the ends so that they are less likely to be confused with nippers.

Alternatively a nail puller is an effective tool to remove each nail individually after raising the clenches (Fig. 1.7). It is important that nails are safely disposed of immediately, to reduce the risk of the horse treading on them.

Chaps or a farriers apron are very useful for protection while removing shoes and manipulating feet.

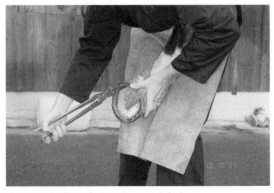

Fig. 1.7 Nail pullers to facilitate the removal of a shoe.

Farriery tools

Hoof testers

Hoof testers are useful in identifying generalised or focal pain in the foot. Generally hoof testers are used prior to hoof knives when an abscess is suspected, because it is important to localise sensitivity within the foot.

Hoof knives

These come in many designs, but the basic style is a curved handle with a blade that is gently curved throughout its body, with a sharp hook at the end. Right- and left-handed versions are available. Hoof knives are used to remove redundant sole from the bottom of the horse's foot and to trim the frog. These knives are used also to search the foot for abscesses.

Rasp

The rasp is a long, thin rectangular piece of metal that has sets of metal teeth on both sides as well as at the edges. On one side the teeth are much longer and angle towards the handle. This side is used for coarse work, such as levelling the foot after trimming. The other side of the rasp usually has a cross-hatched pattern that is used for finishing the foot or smoothing off any rough areas of metal. This side of the rasp can be used to remove nail clenches prior to pulling shoes. This can be carried out with the foot supported on the operator's leg.

Nippers

Nippers are used for removing large portions of outer hoof wall, most commonly when trimming the foot. The handles are opened and closed while perpendicular to the foot in order to maintain a flat weight-bearing surface. They should never be used to remove shoes because this may damage the blades.

Cleaning and preparation of the foot

Extensive cleaning and preparation is often required for radiographic investigation of the foot. For a full examination, the shoes must be removed (see Chapter 17). Similar cleaning of the foot (without the packing) is often required when horses are taken into the operating theatre, in order to reduce contamination.

Care and safety of farriery equipment

Farriery equipment should be cleaned regularly and stored carefully. Knives and nippers should be kept as sharp as possible.

Clothing and rugging of horses

Rugs

Rugs can be important fomites in the transmission of contagious diseases, particularly ringworm. Confining rugs to one individual is a sensible precaution in controlling infection.

General fitting and care of rugs

It is very important to use rugs that fit a horse properly, particularly if they are to be worn for long periods of time. Common areas to develop rubs are over the shoulders, pectorals and withers. Ill-fitting rugs are also more likely to slip if the horse rolls or lies down. This is an important consideration with hospitalisation of colicking horses. Some horses benefit from the use of anti-cast rollers. These utilise a large stiff loop over the withers that prevents the horse from rolling right over. Commonly used rugs include:

- New Zealand rugs: these are made of a waterproof outer layer with a wool, quilt or cotton lining. They are primarily used for horses that are field kept or turned out for part of the day during the autumn and winter months. Clipped horses usually need to wear a New Zealand rug when turned out in the cold or rain. Care should be taken that rugs are checked and refitted daily and are not rubbing.
- Stable rugs: traditionally clipped stabled horses wore a 'jute' rug, made of natural material such as jute or hemp. These are half- or fully lined with wool, and warmth can be augmented with several layers of underblanket. Today there is also a vast array of man-made rugs. Many of these are of excellent quality, being rot-proof, readily washable, durable and warm. Modern rugs also tend to have enough built-in straps to prevent movement of the rug. This precludes the use of rollers and surcingles, which can be poorly fitting and cause rubs.

Traditional natural-fibre rugs and blankets will still suffice if they are properly managed.

- Day rugs: a traditional day rug is made of wool and is used to replace the night rug of a stabled horse after exercise. However, such rugs are increasingly synthetic and of varying thickness and design. Day rugs are now often used for travelling and at shows and events.
- Summer sheets/fly sheets: these replace day rugs in warm weather. They are used to protect the horse from fly irritation and to prevent stable stains. However, horses that really suffer from fly irritation, to the extent that they are allergic to fly bites (fly bite hypersensitivity or sweet itch), require more aggressive anti-fly treatment. Special rugs are now available for sweet itch sufferers. These include extensions up the neck and around the proximal limbs.
- Anti-sweat rugs: the rationale behind anti-sweat rugs is that they create many air pockets and provide an insulating layer in which there is sufficient air movement for evaporation. In cold weather it is wise to use another rug over the top of the sweat rug to prevent over-rapid cooling. Straw or hay can be used underneath the sweat rug to increase the insulative effect. Modern rugs that 'wick' sweat away are available.

Bandages and boots

Bandages

Bandages should be applied with even pressure, so that they do not cross or rub bony prominences. The frequency with which a bandage should be changed depends on the type of bandage and its purpose. A bandaged horse should be checked daily for rubs and sores.

Tail bandages

Any veterinary examination involving the perineal region is greatly facilitated by the horse wearing a tail bandage. This is particularly important during gynaecological work. Such bandages are also useful during hindlimb lameness investigation or evaluation of traumatic wounds. When a site has been aseptically prepared in the caudal region of the body, it is vital that the site is not contaminated as the horse swishes its tail. Full tail bandages for horses with diarrhoea are also very useful in reducing contamination and keeping the perineal area clean. A rectal sleeve over the bandage is also very useful (Fig. 1.8). Full tail bandages should be applied also before a horse enters the operating theatre, in order to reduce contamination.

Stable and travelling bandages

Almost all bandages require some form of conforming material between them and the leg to ensure even pressure distribution. These bandages provide protection against trauma and support to the limb. Traditionally bandaging is used after strenuous exercise to reduce synovial effusions such as windgalls (digital sheath effusions). Stable bandages are frequently made of non-elastic material.

In veterinary situations stable bandages have some specific roles, e.g. a serious limb injury on one leg means that the contralateral (opposite) leg will, effectively, be bearing extra weight, so firm stable bandages for such limbs are extremely important to provide additional support.

Exercise bandages

Exercise bandages are used primarily to protect the digital flexor tendons from injuries such as over-reaches and trauma. They are not as impact resistant as boots, but are conforming, which is important for horses in fast work.

Boots

Brushing boots

Brushing occurs when the supporting limb is struck by its advancing partner. Modern brushing boots are usually made of synthetic materials, and are durable and easy to clean. It is important that boots are cleaned after each use, because dried mud and sweat can create sores and encourage skin disease.

Over-reach boots

An *over-reach* injury is produced by the advancing hindfoot on the back of the forelimb of the same side. Such injuries typically occur at the bulbs of the heel and are caused by the inside toe of the shoe if the

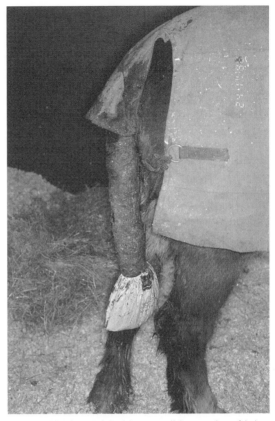

Fig. 1.8 Tail bandages and plastic bags or rectal sleeves can be useful when nursing patients with diarrhoea.

horse is moving at speed. Over-reach boots fit around the pasterns and cover the coronary bands and bulbs of the heel. Over-reach injuries sustained above the fetlock are known as *speedy cut* injuries. Speedy cutting boots are available, and these afford protection to the flexor tendons above the fetlock.

Serving or covering boots

Serving boots are fitted to mares' hindfeet to protect the stallion from the impact of kicks. They are usually made of felt or soft leather.

Other types of boot

A plethora of boots are available for protection of different parts of the horse. These include:

- Heel boots
- Tendon boots

- Fetlock boots
- Fetlock rings
- Coronet boots
- Knee boots
- Hock boots.

Travelling boots are sometimes used in place of stable bandages during transport. Some types of travelling boots have extensions for protection of the knees and hocks. Sausage boots are thick padded rings of leather fitted around the pasterns to prevent the heel of the shoe from traumatising the elbow when the horse is lying down, thus predisposing to a 'capped elbow'.

Tack and harness equipment

A saddle and bridle is the basic tack required for riding. Proper fitting and regular care and inspection is critical. All tack and harness equipment has the potential to cause serious rubs and sores. It is critical that it is fitted properly and maintained carefully. There are many specialist books on this (see the further reading list).

Marking methods

Identifying an individual horse relies on noting their individual natural features (i.e. markings) or using an acquired method of marking, e.g. microchipping. Different markings forms (Fig. 1.9) may vary slightly in their horse outlines and also in the information required. However, in general the following apply:

- Any white marking on the horse must be shown in red and any other marks must be shown in black on the form.
- The use of ballpoint pens is recommended because this ensures good results if the document is to be photocopied.
- The narrative and the completed diagram must agree.

Further information is available in the booklet entitled *Colours and Markings of Horses*, published by the RCVS. Several important parts of the identification should be noted:

(1) Whorls occur where there is a change in direction of flow of the hair, usually radiating from a single point (see Fig. 1.11, p. 23) Whorls must be in dicated by an 'X' in the case of simple or tufted whorls. Linear and feathered whorls are indicated by placing an 'X' where the whorl starts and a line from this to indicate the direction and extent of the whorl.

(2) White markings are outlined in red and hatched in with red diagonal lines. A few white hairs may be indicated by a few short lines in red. White markings from surgery, freeze branding, etc. should be indicated as for other white markings.

(3) Bordered markings should be indicated by using a double line.

(4) Spots: a white spot must be indicated as for a white marking. A spot within a white marking should be outlined in black and left blank. Extensive spots should be noted only in the description.

(5) Flesh marks. These should be outlined and shaded completely in red. Any spots on the mark should be outlined in black and left unshaded.

(6) The prophets thumb mark. This is a natural dimple in the muscle, usually on the neck, which is shown on the diagram by a black triangle.

(7) Permanent scars should be arrowed.

(8) Others: hairs of a different colour on parts of the coat should be described with accuracy and indicated with a few diagonal lines; if the horse is docked or the ears nicked, this should be stated in the description; wall eyes (lack of pigment in the iris, causing the eye to be blue/grey in colour) should be noted; The Jockey Club recently has required that chestnuts (horny deposits on insides of limbs) are marked on the forms for whole coloured or grey animals.

Colours

There are four basic coat colours in horses. These are black, brown, bay and chestnut, but deciding the true colour, particularly of a foal, can be difficult. It is suggested that a decision can be based on the colour of the hairs of the muzzle.

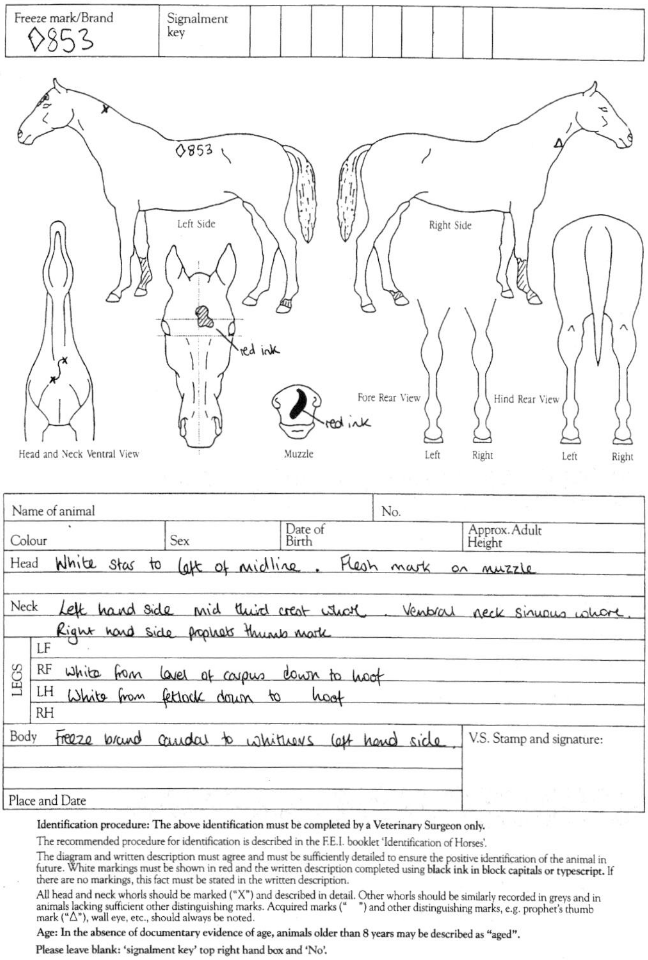
Freeze mark/Brand
◊853
Signalment key
◊853
Left Side
Right Side
red ink
red ink
Fore Rear View
Hind Rear View
Head and Neck Ventral View
Muzzle
Left
Right
Left
Right
Name of animal
No.
Colour
Sex
Date of Birth
Approx. Adult Height
Head White star to left of midline. Flesh mark on muzzle
Neck Left hand side mid third crest whorl. Ventral neck sinuous whorl.
Right hand side prophets thumb mark
LEGS
LF
RF White from level of carpus down to hoof
LH White from fetlock down to hoof
RH
Body Freeze brand caudal to whithers left hand side.
V.S. Stamp and signature:
Place and Date
Identification procedure: The above identification must be completed by a Veterinary Surgeon only.
The recommended procedure for identification is described in the F.E.I. booklet 'Identification of Horses'.
The diagram and written description must agree and must be sufficiently detailed to ensure the positive identification of the animal in future. White markings must be shown in red and the written description completed using **black ink in block capitals or typescript.** If there are no markings, this fact must be stated in the written description.
All head and neck whorls should be marked ("X") and described in detail. Other whorls should be similarly recorded in greys and in animals lacking sufficient other distinguishing marks. Acquired marks ("   ") and other distinguishing marks, e.g. prophet's thumb mark ("Δ"), wall eye, etc., should always be noted.
Age: In the absence of documentary evidence of age, animals older than 8 years may be described as "aged".
Please leave blank: 'signalment key' top right hand box and 'No'.

Fig. 1.9 An example of a markings form. A basic markings form of the left and right sides of the horse, a front view of the head, a ventral view of the muzzle and underside of the neck and rear views of the fore- and hindlimbs.

Black
The skin, mane, tail and body hair are black. No other colour is present except that white markings on the face and limbs are permitted.

Brown
The skin is dark and the coat hairs are a mixture of black and chocolate. The limbs, mane and tail are brown or black.

Bay
The coat is dark red to yellowish brown in colour, whereas the mane, tail and lower limbs are black. Black on the limbs is referred to as black points.

Chestnut
A chestnut horse has yellow hairs in its coat. The proportion of yellow hair varies to give a coat that ranges in colour from reddish brown (liver chestnut) to light yellowish brown.

Palamino
A palamino could be considered a type of chestnut. The body hairs are a bright golden yellow, whereas the mane and tail are flaxen or white.

Dun

Dun colours are the result of dilution of the basic coat colour, whereas the mane and tail remain dark. For example, a yellow dun has a dark skin with a black or chocolate mane and tail. A withers stripe, list (or dorsal stripe) and zebra markings are often present in duns.

Roan

A roan horse has a body colour that consists of a mixture of white and coloured hairs in approximately equal quantities. The solid colour tends to predominate on the head and the limbs, and the colour of the roan is determined from this. A roan differs from a grey horse, which has an uneven mixture of white and coloured hairs and where the percentage of white increases with age.

Grey

The coat of a grey horse is an uneven mixture of white and dark coloured hairs with the skin darkly pigmented. As the animal ages, the coat becomes whiter. Foals are rarely born grey but become grey when they lose their foal coat.

Skewbald

The coat consists of large irregular patches of white and any other colour except black. The line of demarcation between the patches is usually well defined.

Piebald

The coat consists of large irregular patches of white and black. The patches are well defined.

Odd coloured

The coat consists of large irregular patches of white and more than one other colour.

In the USA such coats are termed as Pinto or Paint.

Appaloosa

The Appaloosa is a breed of horse originating in the USA. True Appaloosas have a mottled skin, with white around the eye and hooves that are vertically striped in black and white.

Albino/cream/Cremello

There is no pigmentation of the skin or hair. The eyes are also devoid of pigment and are pink in colour.

Gender

The gender of an animal and whether it is neutered should be noted on identification forms.

Height

The height of an animal at the time of completion of the form should be stated in centimetres.

Acquired identification marks

Tattoos

Tattoos are rare in the UK, but they are sometimes found on the inside of the upper lip.

Hoof burns

These are not strictly permanent markings because they grow out with hoof growth. Some hooves are still burnt, usually by the farrier with post codes or other individual marks (Fig. 1.10).

Freeze brands

This method of marking is common. There is a national scheme such that no two horses have the same number and letter combination. Very cold blocks in the shape of letters or numbers are applied to the skin of the animal. This causes a scar, and subsequent hair

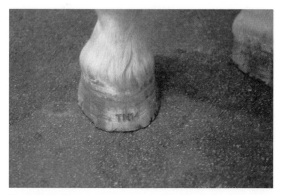

Fig. 1.10 Hoof burns are used as a means of identification but they need to be repeated as the hoof grows.

growth is white. It is common for these markings to be placed on the back just behind the withers, to the left of the midline. Less commonly they are seen on the neck or shoulder. In light coloured horses the freezing effect may be prolonged to prevent any hair growth at that site (Fig. 1.11).

Hot branding

Red-hot irons are applied to the skin to burn and scar it. There is no subsequent hair growth. This method of identification is still used for certain breeds, particularly Warmbloods (Fig. 1.12).

Microchipping (identichip)

This newer form of identification is also organised as a national scheme, so that each microchip code is different. A small chip is implanted on the left side of the

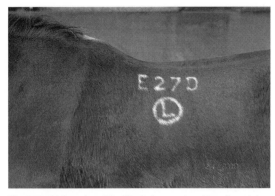

Fig. 1.11 This freeze brand identifies the horse as the subject of a settled permanent incapacity insurance claim.

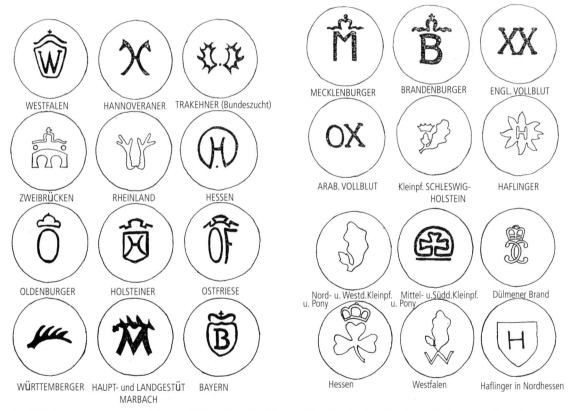

WESTFALEN · HANNOVERANER · TRAKEHNER (Bundeszucht)

ZWEIBRÜCKEN · RHEINLAND · HESSEN

OLDENBURGER · HOLSTEINER · OSTFRIESE

WÜRTTEMBERGER · HAUPT- und LANDGESTÜT MARBACH · BAYERN

MECKLENBURGER · BRANDENBURGER · ENGL. VOLLBLUT

ARAB. VOLLBLUT · Kleinpf. SCHLESWIG-HOLSTEIN · HAFLINGER

Nord- u. Westd.Kleinpf. u. Pony · Mittel- u. Südd.Kleinpf. u. Pony · Dülmener Brand

Hessen · Westfalen · Haflinger in Nordhessen

Fig. 1.12 Some examples of common hot brands. All German Warmbloods have used three breeds as foundation stock, with other breeding then being introduced. These three breeds are the Hanoverian, the Trakehner and the Holstein, as illustrated.

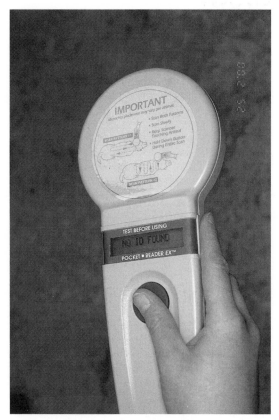

Fig. 1.13 Example of a microchip scanner being used.

middle third of the neck, into the *ligamentum nuchae* 2.5–3.75 cm from the dorsal midline (1.25 cm in foals). The chip is then read using an electronic machine that reads the individual code (Fig. 1.13).

To be eligible for registration in the *General Stud Book* (GSB) or *Weatherbys Non-Thoroughbred Register* (NTR), foals born after 1 January 1999 must be implanted with a Weatherbys microchip by a vet. These are implanted in the same place as other microchips.

Microchips are being used increasingly as a means of permanent identification.

Breeds

It is thought that the horse was first domesticated in around 3000 BC and has evolved into the several hundred breeds of horse in the world today. More information may be found from the further reading list.

Further reading

Bracher, V., McDonnell, S., Stohler, T. & Green, R. (1998) Equine clinical behaviour. *Equine Vet. Educ. Suppl.* **27**.

Brazil, T.J. (1995) Isolation of infectious equine cases. *Equine Vet. Educ.* **7**(4), 220–224.

Cooper, B. & Lane, D.R. (1997) *Veterinary Nursing* (Formerly *Jones' Animal Nursing*, 5th, Edn). Butterworth-Heinemann, Oxford.

Dwyer, R.M. (1992) Practical methods of disinfection and management during outbreaks of infectious disease. *Proc. Am. Assoc. Equine Pract.* **38**, 381–388.

Gogh, M.R. (1997) Clipping horses. *Equine Vet. Educ.* **9**(3), 161–165.

Harris, P.A., Gomersall, G.M., Davidson, H.P.B. & Green, R.E. (1999) *Proc. BEVA Specialist Days on Behaviour and Nutrition.* Equine Veterinary Journal Ltd, Newmarket.

Hickman, J. (1987) *Horse Management*, 2nd Edn. Academic Press, London.

Knottenbelt, D.C. & Pascoe, R.R. (1994) *Diseases and Disorders of the Horse.* Wolfe Publishing, London.

Knottenbelt, D.C. & Pascoe, R.R. (1999) *Manual of Equine Dermatology.* Harcourt Brace and Company, London.

Martinelli, M.J. & Ferrie, J.W. (1997) A basic guide to farriery tools. *Equine Vet. Educ.* **9**, 45–50.

RCVS (1984) *Colours and Markings of Horses* (revised 1984). RCVS, London.

Roberts, M. (1996) *The Man who Listens to Horses.* Hutchinson, London.

Stafford, C. & Oliver, R. (1991) *Horse Care and Management.* J.A. Allen, London.

CHAPTER 2

Anatomy and Physiology

P. D. Clegg, C. L. Blake, R. C. Conwell, E. Hainisch, S. A. Newton, E. M. Post, M. J. Senior, S. L. Taylor & A. J. Wise

This chapter is aimed as a general overview of the subject, concentrating on points specific to Equidae. Readers are recommended to study the further reading list for more detailed information.

Cell structure

The cell is the basic unit of life. Cells of one type are grouped together in *tissues* to perform particular functions, e.g. muscle. The *nucleus* is large and normally in the centre of the cell. It is surrounded by the *nuclear membrane*. The nucleus consists of *DNA* (deoxyribonucleic acid), which contains the genetic code. The nucleus is surrounded by *cytoplasm*. The cytoplasm contains *organelles* with specific roles, such as *ribosomes* for protein synthesis and *mitochondria* for energy production. The whole cell is enclosed by a *cell membrane* that controls what substances enter or leave the cell.

Cell types include:

- *Connective tissue cells*, which bind other cells together.
- *Muscle cells* (see below).
- *Cartilage cells*, found where strength and flexibility are needed.
- *Bone cells*, found within small spaces in the 'ground substance' in bone tissue.
- *Nerve cells* (*neurones*), which send signals (impulses) to other cells.

Basic tissue types

A *tissue* is a collection of cells with a common function, e.g. cardiac muscle. A structure in which one type of tissue predominates and has a specific function is an *organ*, e.g. the heart. A collection of tissues and organs that share some common function is a *system*, e.g. the cardiovascular system.

Types of tissue include:

- *Epithelial tissue* covers the outside of the body and also lines airways, digestive tract and genitourinary tract. Its role is protection and secretion. *Glandular epithelial tissue* is a specialised epithelium that secretes substances. The secretory epithelial cells are often grouped together with a duct connecting to the outside surface (*glands*). Sometimes glands do not communicate with the external epithelium (ductless or *endocrine* glands) and secrete *hormones* that regulate the body's metabolism.
- *Connective tissue* has many supporting functions and contains large amounts of intercellular material (matrix or ground substance). *Cartilage* is connective tissue with the property of being both rigid and flexible, found principally in joints, the larynx, nose and ears. *Bone, cartilage* and *adipose* (or fatty) *tissue* are all forms of connective tissue.
- *Muscle tissue* contains muscle cells that are

arranged as fibres. There are three types: *skeletal* (striated / voluntary) *muscle*, which attaches to the skeleton; *smooth* or *involuntary muscle*, which responds to unconscious impulses, e.g. in the gut wall; *cardiac muscle* in the heart.

- *Nervous tissue* is made up of *neurones* sending signals (i.e. *nerve impulses*) to other cells. The *central nervous system* includes the neurones and specialised support cells found in the brain and spinal cord. The *peripheral nervous system* includes all nervous tissue elsewhere in the body.
- *Vascular tissue* comprises blood (see later) and blood vessels. *Arteries* convey blood away from the heart. They vary in size from small (*arterioles*) to large (e.g. the aorta in the horse is several centimetres wide). *Veins* convey blood back to the heart. They also vary in size from small (*venules*) to large (e.g. the vena cava). *Capillaries* form networks called *capillary beds* within organs. They allow blood to pass into tissues and consist of a single layer of endothelial cells.

Blood

Blood cells are constantly being made (*haematopoiesis*) and destroyed. Blood cells are made by *myeloid tissue*, mainly in the bone marrow and spleen. Blood consists of both fluid (plasma) and cells (see Chapter 12).

Haemostasis and blood clotting

Three mechanisms stop bleeding (*haemostasis*):

(1) Constriction of blood vessels—spasm of smooth muscle within the vessel walls.
(2) Platelets plug the gap, stick to the vessel walls and release factors to stimulate further development of the clot.
(3) Blood coagulation involves enzymes and clotting factors that start a cascade of chemical reactions. This cascade ultimately involves a protein (*thrombin*), forming another protein (*fibrin*) that acts like a mesh to trap platelets and produce a clot.

With an increased blood clotting time the horse is at a greater risk of bleeding following injury. Factors that may increase the clotting time in the horse include:

- Reduced numbers of platelets (thrombocytopenia)
- Liver failure
- Some poisons
- Some infections

A decreased clotting time means that the blood will clot more easily. This can be dangerous because in severe cases the blood can form spontaneous clots inside the body.

The lymphatic system

Some tissue fluid that diffuses from the capillaries will return to the bloodstream, with the rest draining into thin-walled, blind-ended vessels called *lymphatics*. The fluid is then called *lymph* and has a similar composition to plasma but with less protein. The functions of lymph include:

- Transport of nutrients from the villi in the intestine.
- Return of tissue fluid to the blood circulation.
- Transport of lymphocytes from the lymphoid tissue to the blood.

A network of lymphatic vessels is formed within the tissues, starting with lymph capillary vessels that join together to form a network of lymphatic vessels of increasing diameter. Eventually the fluid is discharged into the bloodstream, via the *thoracic duct*, the main collecting channel for the lymph. There are collecting vessels within the small intestine, known as *lacteals*, found within the villi. The drainage into the lacteals is copious and differs from other lymph fluid in that it contains products of digestion, particularly fats.

The movement of the lymph depends on compression of the lymphatic vessels by the muscles, with valves within the vessels to prevent backflow. When the lymph reaches the larger vessels, it is filtered through *lymph nodes* before entering the bloodstream.

The immune system

The immune system protects the body from invading microorganisms. There are two types of immunity:

(1) *Natural immunity* includes defences such as the skin, sweat and mucus.
(2) *Acquired immunity* is the ability of the body to improve the efficiency of the natural mechanisms and to remember and recognise the *antigen* (foreign material) when it is next encountered. There are two types of acquired immune response:
  (a) *Humoral* immunity conveys protection via *B lymphocytes* and the production of antibodies.
  (b) *Cell-mediated* immunity conveys protection via *T lymphocytes* and the direct destruction of foreign cells.

Lymph nodes

Lymph nodes act as filters to remove foreign material, bacteria and viruses from the lymphatic fluid before it reaches the systemic circulation. They are present throughout the lymphatic system and may form chains to drain a specific organ or area of the body. Several *afferent* lymph vessels take lymph into the node. A single *efferent* vessel exits every node. As well as acting as a filter, the node provides a site for the lymphocytes to interact with antigen and therefore plays an important part in the body's defence (Fig. 2.1).

The node can be divided into three main areas

- *Cortex*: contains mainly B cells within primary follicles. These form secondary follicles once stimulated by antigen.
- *Paracortex*: contains T cells and antigen-presenting cells.
- Central *medulla*: contains cords around the sinuses for the lymph drainage from the node into the efferent lymphatic vessel.

Palpation of lymph nodes
There are several groups of superficial lymph nodes but few are easily palpable in the normal horse.

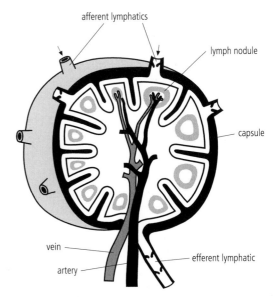

Fig. 2.1 Lymph node anatomy.

- The *submandibular* lymph nodes are arranged in a forward-pointing V shape within the intermandibular space under the jaw. In the normal horse these are the only superficial nodes that are easily palpable.
- The *parotid* lymph nodes are linked to the parotid salivary gland and usually are not palpable unless enlarged.
- The *superficial cervical* lymph nodes lie just in front of the cranial border of the scapula and again are only palpable when enlarged.
- The *intra-abdominal* nodes in the caudal abdomen can be palpated per rectum when enlarged.
- The *superficial inguinal* lymph nodes may be palpable within the groin when enlarged.

The spleen

The spleen is a vascular organ that lies within the left craniodorsal abdomen under the caudal ribs and attaches to the stomach, the intestinal mass, the greater omentum and, via the nephrosplenic ligament, the left kidney. The spleen has several functions:

- Storage of blood
- Removal of particles from the circulation

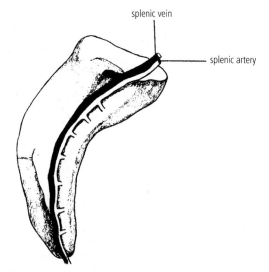

Fig. 2.2 Anatomy of equine spleen.

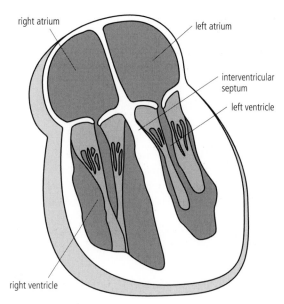

Fig. 2.3 Longitudinal section through equine heart.

- Destruction of aged red blood cells
- Production of lymphocytes

Blood supply to the spleen is via the *splenic artery* and drainage is via the *splenic veins* (Fig. 2.2). It has a thick capsule that contains a large amount of smooth muscle, allowing the spleen to contract to release blood in times of stress. When relaxed, the spleen becomes engorged and may increase in size several fold.

The spleen contains two main types of tissue, the *red pulp* and *white pulp*. The red pulp removes and destroys aged red cells. The white pulp consists of lymphoid tissue.

The heart

The heart acts as a pump, driving blood around the body and to the lungs. It consists of four chambers — two thin-walled *atria* or priming chambers, and two *ventricles* or main pumps. In the adult the left and right sides are completely separate and they are divided by a *septum* (Fig. 2.3). The left ventricle has to pump at high pressure to drive blood around the body and therefore has a thicker muscular wall than the right ventricle.

The heart tissue consists of three layers:

(1) The *endocardium* lines the inside of the heart and also forms the valves, which ensure that blood flows unidirectionally. The atrioventricular valves separate the atria from the ventricles and are attached by thin *chordae tendinae* to extensions of the cardiac muscle, the papillary muscle, which prevent the valve flaps from everting into the atria. Reverse flow of blood is prevented at the aorta and pulmonary vessels by *semi-lunar* valves.

(2) The middle layer is the *myocardium*, which is made up of cardiac muscle.

(3) The *epicardium* is the third layer and this surrounds the myocardium.

The *pericardium* is a fibrous sac around the heart that acts as a barrier to infection, prevents overexpansion of the ventricles and allows free movement of the heart within the thoracic cavity.

The heart contracts in a rhythmical manner. The electrical activity originates in special 'pacemaker' cells in the *sino-atrial node* in the wall of the right atrium. Spontaneous impulses are discharged rhythmically from the sino-atrial node and cause the atria to contract. The impulse then is conducted more slowly at the *atrio-ventricular node*. Conduction spreads very rapidly through the myocardium via the *bundle of His* and *Purkinje* tissue, a system of fast-conducting fibres in the *interventricular septum*, to ensure that the whole ventricular muscle contracts almost simultaneously.

During one heart beat a sequence of mechanical events also occurs in the heart, known as the *cardiac cycle*: *diastole* is the period of relaxation when the heart is filling with blood; *systole* is the period of contraction, during which the blood is ejected from the heart.

The volume of blood ejected by one ventricle in one beat is called the *stroke volume*.

The *cardiac output* is the volume of blood ejected by one ventricle in one minute and can be calculated as:

Cardiac output = Stroke volume × Heart rate

The heart rate is the number of beats per minute. The horse's normal resting heart rate ranges from 25 to 42 beats per minute. The horse has the ability to increase its cardiac output enormously by increasing the heart rate up to 220–240 beats per minute.

The heart is also responsible for maintaining the *blood pressure*, together with the rest of the cardiovascular system. It is greatest when the heart contracts, i.e. the *systolic* blood pressure, and lowest when the heart relaxes, i.e. the *diastolic* blood pressure.

Circulation

Deoxygenated blood from the body enters the right atrium of the heart and passes through the right *atrioventricular (tricuspid)* valve into the right ventricle. Blood then is pumped from the right ventricle through the *pulmonary valve* into the *pulmonary arteries* to the lungs for oxygenation. The *pulmonary veins* carry the oxygenated blood back to the heart to the left atrium. This is the *pulmonary circulation*. From the left atrium blood passes through the left *atrioventricular (mitral)* valve into the left ventricle. The left ventricle is responsible for driving the blood through the aorta via the *aortic valve* and around the body, where oxygen and nutrients can be delivered to the tissues. Blood drains from the tissues into veins and returns to the right atrium of the heart via the

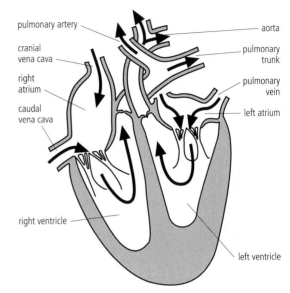

Fig. 2.4 Direction of blood flow through the heart.

vena cava. This is known as the systemic circulation (Fig. 2.4).

Blood vessels

Blood vessels are the system of tubes through which the heart pumps blood. *Arteries* transport blood away from the heart. They have thick walls of smooth muscle and elastic fibres that allow the artery to stretch when the blood flows at high pressure. The arteries divide into smaller tubes called *arterioles*. They influence the peripheral blood pressure by affecting the resistance to blood flow and connect the arteries to the capillaries.

Capillaries are very narrow tubes that are found within almost every tissue and act as the functioning part of the circulation, because at this level the blood is able to give up nutrients and oxygen to the tissues and remove waste products. After applying digital pressure to the mucous membranes, the time taken for the colour to return should be approximately 2 seconds. This is called the *capillary refill time* and is an indicator of peripheral perfusion.

Blood returns to the heart via *venules*—thin-walled vessels that collect the outflow from the capillary bed

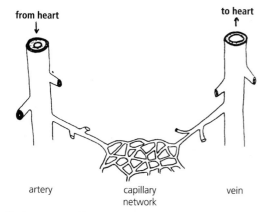

Fig. 2.5 Anatomy of the peripheral circulation.

and act as low-pressure blood reservoirs. Venules have valves to prevent the backflow of blood. From the venules, blood passes into the larger veins and then back to the heart (Fig. 2.5).

Respiratory tract

Nostrils

The nostrils are large and widely spaced in the horse, with flexible margins allowing the nasal opening to be dilated to increase airflow during strenuous exercise. The alar cartilages support the dorsal and lateral margins of the nostrils. The *alar fold* divides the nostril into a dorsal and ventral part. The dorsal part of the nostril leads to a blind-ending pouch known as the *false nostril* or *nasal diverticulum*. The ventral part of the nostril leads into the nasal cavity. Instruments, such as a stomach tube, are therefore guided into the lower part of the nostril to gain access to the nasal cavity or the pharynx. The entrance to the *naso-lacrimal duct* is found ventrally, just inside the nostril, about 5 cm from the entrance, and is easily visible in the horse.

Nasal cavity

The nasal cavities are narrow air-filled spaces that extend caudally from the nostrils to the front of the cranial cavity, divided in the midline by the *nasal septum*.

The septum extends along the whole length of the hard palate so that each nasal cavity communicates with the pharynx via a separate opening (*choana*). The embedded portions of the upper cheek teeth and the extensive paranasal sinus system in the horse reduce the space occupied by the nasal cavities. The *turbinate bones* or *conchae* project into the nasal cavities from the dorsal and lateral walls, further reducing the potential space. In the rostral part of the nasal cavity, the large dorsal and ventral conchae divide the nasal cavity into three spaces called the *dorsal, middle* and *ventral meati*. At the caudal aspect of the nasal cavity, the conchae form the complex *ethmoidal labyrinth*. The ethmoturbinates are covered by *olfactory mucosa*, which is important in the sensation of smell. The function of the turbinates is to warm, moisten and clean inhaled air before it reaches the trachea (Figs 2.6 and 2.7).

Paranasal sinuses

The paranasal sinuses are extensive air-filled cavities within the skull. The sinuses communicate with the nasal cavity via relatively small openings and are lined with respiratory epithelium similar to the nasal cavity. The largest and clinically most important sinuses are the *caudal* and *rostral maxillary sinuses* and the *frontal sinus*. The maxillary sinuses communicate directly with the nasal cavity, where they drain into the middle meatus via the *nasomaxillary opening*. The frontal sinus drains indirectly into the nasal cavity via the *caudal maxillary sinus*. The frontal sinus is triangular in shape and occupies the dorsal part of the skull, medial to the orbit. The maxillary sinuses occupy a large part of the upper jaw (Fig. 2.8). The exact extent of the maxillary sinuses varies depending on the individual horse and the age of the animal. The embedded roots of the four caudal cheek teeth (premolar 4 and molars 1, 2 and 3) extend into and form the floor of these sinuses.

Pharynx

The pharynx is the portion of the upper airway that begins behind the nasal septum and ends rostral to the larynx. The nasal passages open caudally in the throat into an area called the *nasopharynx*. The oral

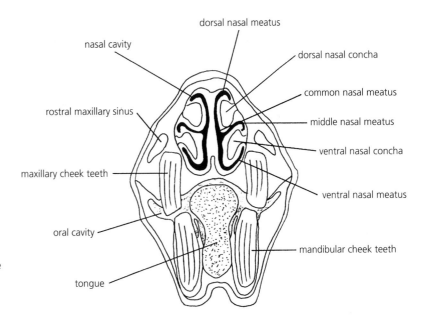

Fig. 2.6 Transverse section of the equine head at the level of the rostral maxillary sinus: illustration of the structure of the nasal cavity.

Labels: dorsal nasal meatus, nasal cavity, dorsal nasal concha, common nasal meatus, middle nasal meatus, ventral nasal concha, ventral nasal meatus, mandibular cheek teeth, rostral maxillary sinus, maxillary cheek teeth, oral cavity, tongue

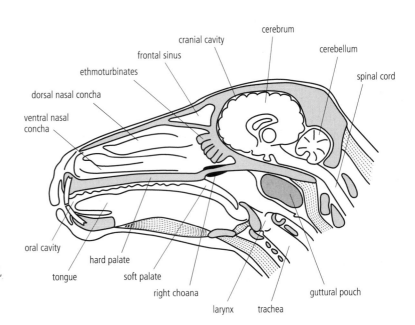

Fig. 2.7 Median section of the equine head, with the nasal septum removed. The figure illustrates the passage of air from the nasal cavity, through the choana, into the trachea.

Labels: cranial cavity, cerebrum, cerebellum, frontal sinus, spinal cord, ethmoturbinates, dorsal nasal concha, ventral nasal concha, oral cavity, hard palate, tongue, soft palate, right choana, larynx, trachea, guttural pouch

cavity opens at the back of the mouth into the *oropharynx*. The nasopharynx and the oropharynx both communicate with the *pharynx* but are separated by the soft palate (Fig. 2.9). The guttural pouches form the dorsal and lateral borders of the pharynx. The openings of the guttural pouches are called the *ostia* and are seen as slit-like openings on either side of the pharyngeal wall. Rostral and dorsal to the pharynx is a distinct concave depression, the *dorsal pharyngeal recess*. The pharyngeal mucosa is lined with a stratified squamous epithelium and the submucosa contains clumps of lymphoid tissue.

31

Guttural pouches

The guttural pouches are paired enlargements or *diverticulae of the eustachian tube* lying on each side of the head, between the base of the skull and atlas dorsally and the pharynx ventrally (Figs 2.7 and 2.8). A thin median septum divides the two guttural pouches in the midline. The caudal border of the mandible, the parotid and mandibular salivary glands overlay the pouches laterally. Each pouch is divided into a large medial and a small lateral compartment by the *stylohyoid* bone. Each pouch has a capacity of 300–500 ml. The function of the guttural pouches is unknown. The guttural pouches are important in many clinical conditions of the horse due to their unique anatomic relationships. Several nerves and blood vessels are contained within the guttural pouches, including the *internal carotid artery*, the *glossopharyngeal nerve* (cranial nerve IX) and the *vagus nerve* (cranial nerve X) within the medial compartment of the pouch and the *external carotid artery* in the lateral compartment.

Larynx

The larynx is a biological valve lying at the most caudal aspect of the mouth and forms the entrance to the trachea. It consists of a complex arrangement of muscles, ligaments and cartilages, and is lined with mucus membrane. The larynx lies in the midline. The *hyoid apparatus* forms a bony sling, which suspends the larynx and the tongue from the base of the cranium (Fig. 2.10).

Laryngeal functions include:

- Protecting the airway during swallowing, so that ingesta do not enter the trachea.
- Controlling the flow of air into the trachea during exercise.
- Producing vocal sounds.

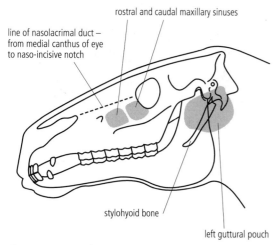

Fig. 2.8 Lateral view of the equine head, showing position of guttural pouch and maxillary sinuses.

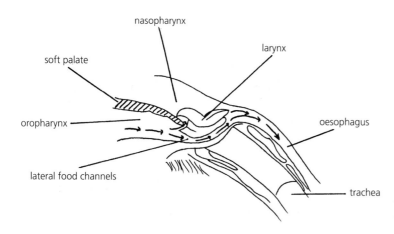

Fig. 2.9 Schematic diagram of the equine pharynx. The arrows illustrate the passage of food material from the oropharynx into the oesophagus via the lateral food channels.

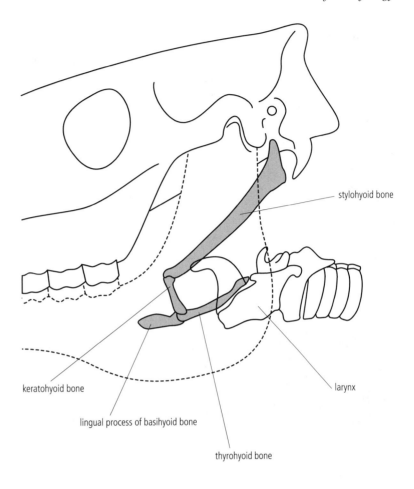

stylohyoid bone

keratohyoid bone

lingual process of basihyoid bone

thyrohyoid bone

larynx

Fig. 2.10 The hyoid apparatus of the horse.

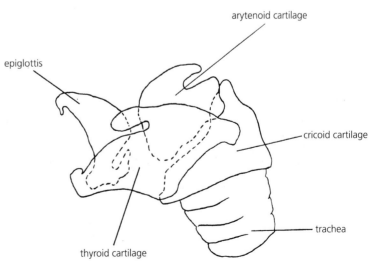

arytenoid cartilage

epiglottis

cricoid cartilage

trachea

thyroid cartilage

Fig. 2.11 The cartilages of the equine larynx.

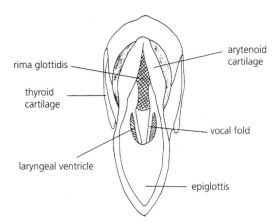

Fig. 2.12 Cranial view of the equine larynx as seen endoscopically.

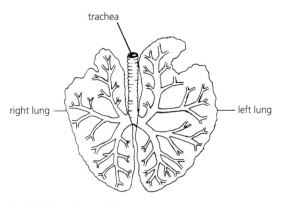

Fig. 2.13 The equine bronchial tree.

There are three single cartilages and one pair of cartilages within the larynx (Figs 2.11 and 2.12):

(1) The *epiglottis*: a valve between the pharynx and trachea.
(2) The paired *arytenoid cartilages* lie caudal and dorsal to the epiglottis on either side of the midline. The *vocal ligaments* are attached to these cartilages dorsally. The vocal ligaments attach ventrally to a midline structure, forming a V shape. The vocal ligaments are covered with mucous membrane, which forms the *vocal folds*. The space bounded by the vocal folds and arytenoid cartilages is known as the *rima glottidis*. The arytenoid cartilages move towards and away from the midline to increase and decrease the size of the rima glottidis and so regulate the flow of air into the trachea.
(3) The *thyroid cartilage* consists of two large lateral plates that meet ventrally and form the majority of the larynx floor.
(4) The *cricoid cartilage* is ring shaped and is the most caudal of the laryngeal cartilages.

The trachea

The trachea is a tube transporting air from the larynx to the lungs. The trachea divides into two smaller *bronchi* within the thorax. The inner layer, the *mucosa*, contains glands that produce a protective covering of mucous to trap dust and bacteria. Other mucosal cells contain *cilia* that constantly beat to move the mucus up to the pharynx, where it is swallowed or exhaled down the nostrils, thus protecting the lungs. The middle layer of the trachea is composed of incomplete rings of cartilage joined together by sheets of elastic connective tissue. They prevent the trachea from collapsing and allow for adjustments in length when the neck is extended.

The bronchial tree

The bronchi further divide into *lobar bronchi* and then into smaller airways called *bronchioles*. The bronchioles subdivide into smaller and smaller branches. Like the trachea, mucous glands line the bronchioles and ciliated cells that function to remove debris from the airways. The smaller bronchi and bronchioles also contain smooth-muscle cells, allowing contraction and relaxation to alter the diameter of the airway (Fig. 2.13).

The terminal bronchi end in *alveolar ducts* that open into the *alveoli*. The alveoli have very thin walls, no cilia and a rich capillary blood supply to allow the interchange of respiratory gases.

The lungs

The left and right lungs have no fixed shape or size and are able to alter during respiration according to the dimensions of the thorax. The lungs contain elastic connective tissue that allows expansion and collapse of the lung. The main bronchus, pulmonary artery and pulmonary vein combine to form the root of the lung and enter at its base. Un-

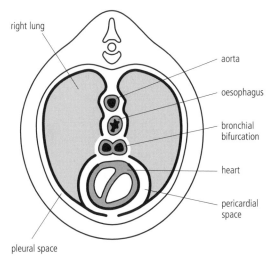

right lung

aorta

oesophagus

bronchial
bifurcation

heart

pericardial
space

pleural space

Fig. 2.14 Transverse section of the thorax at the level of the heart.

like cats and dogs, the lungs of the horse have very poor lobation and lobulation.

The pleural cavity

Two thin layers of serous membrane called the *pleura* line the thorax: the outer layer, the *parietal* pleura, covers the inner wall of the thorax on either side of the chest; the inner layer, the *visceral* pleura, covers the corresponding lung. A thin film of fluid exists between these two layers, allowing them to slide over one another.

The pleura effectively form two closed sacs on each side of the thorax, with the space between them forming the *mediastinum* in which the heart and other thoracic organs are found (Fig. 2.14).

Breathing

During inspiration the external intercostal muscles contract, moving the ribs and sternum upwards and outwards, increasing the width and depth of the chest. The diaphragm contracts and descends, causing the capacity of the thorax to increase. The pressure between the pleural surfaces becomes more negative and stretches the elastic tissue of the lungs, causing them to expand to fill the thoracic cavity. As the air pressure in the alveoli is now lower than

atmospheric pressure, air is sucked into the lungs (Fig. 2.15).

During expiration the external intercostal muscles relax, moving the ribs and sternum inwards and downwards, reducing the width and depth of the chest. The diaphragm relaxes and ascends, decreasing the capacity of the thorax. The elastic tissue of the lungs recoils and, because the air pressure in the alveoli is now greater than atmospheric pressure, air is forced out of the lungs.

Ventilation

The movement of air in and out of the lungs is termed *ventilation*. The volume of air (measured in litres) inspired in each resting breath is the *tidal volume*. At the deepest possible inspiration more air can be inhaled and this is known as the *inspiratory reserve volume*. Likewise, at the deepest possible expiration more air can be exhaled and this is the *expiratory reserve volume*. Both of these reserve volumes are vital during exercise when the resting tidal volume is inadequate for gas exchange. It is not possible to empty the lungs completely, even after maximal expiration, and the air remaining in the lungs is the *residual volume*. Combinations of sums of these volumes are called *capacities* (Fig. 2.16).

Dead space

The *dead space* is the total volume of air channels that conduct air to the alveoli but do not take part in gaseous exchange. The *anatomical dead space* is made up of the nose, pharynx, trachea and bronchi. The *alveolar dead space* is the volume of air that enters the alveoli but does not take part in gaseous exchange, usually due to poor blood supply to the alveoli involved. The *functional dead space* consists of the anatomical dead space plus the alveolar dead space.

Gaseous exchange

Inspired air within the alveoli has a high oxygen pressure whereas venous blood entering the lungs has a low partial pressure of oxygen. Therefore,

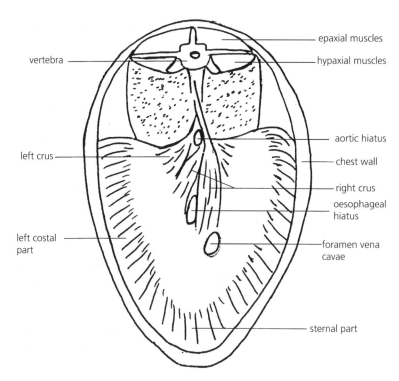

Fig. 2.15 Caudal view of the equine diaphragm.

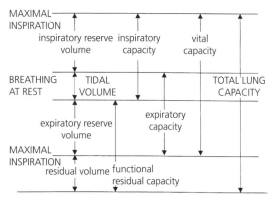

Fig. 2.16 Respiratory terminology.

oxygen moves from the air into the blood where it combines with haemoglobin, the oxygen carrier within the blood. Carbon dioxide is one of the waste products produced by the tissues and is carried via the plasma in venous blood to the lungs. The alveolar air has a lower pressure of carbon dioxide and hence carbon dioxide will move from the blood into the air for expiration.

The tissues of the body require oxygen in order to metabolise food to provide energy — a process called oxidative metabolism. In the absence of sufficient oxygen, e.g. during strenuous energy, the tissue cells must rely upon *anaerobic respiration* to provide the required energy. The cells utilise the glycogen stores, producing lactic acid in the process.

Control of respiration

Normal respiratory movements are involuntary, i.e. carried out without conscious control. The controlling centres are within the medulla and pons of the brain and they discharge rhythmical impulses to the *phrenic* nerves of the diaphragm, the thoracic segments and the intercostal nerves of the intercostal muscles.

During normal breathing the respiratory rate and rhythm are influenced by the *Hering-Breuer reflex*.

This reflex is a negative feedback pathway initiated by the stimulation of stretch receptors in the bronchioles following alveolar distension at the end of inspiration. Respiration is also influenced by chemical factors. The respiratory centres in the brain monitor the levels of carbon dioxide, oxygen and hydrogen ions in the blood and the latter two also are measured by *chemoreceptors* in the heart. Elevations in hydrogen ions and carbon dioxide and lowering of oxygen stimulate respiration.

Digestive system

Oral cavity

The entrance to the mouth or oral cavity is via the lips. This long narrow cavity is divided into a *vestibule* and *central mouth cavity*. The vestibule is the area between the outer surface of the teeth and the inner surfaces of the cheeks and the lips. The central area is bounded by the teeth and gums on either side, the hard and soft palates dorsally and the tongue ventrally. The entire inside of the oral cavity is lined by mucous membrane. In the upper jaw the mucous membrane is tightly attached to the bones forming the hard palate and it is especially thick in this region, with many folds or *rugae*. In the horse there is a large gap (the *diastema*) between the incisor teeth and the cheek teeth. The oral cavity of the horse has several important functions. The sensitive mobile lips and incisor teeth are designed to prehend food, which is then formed into a *bolus* by the tongue and moved caudally in the mouth. Grinding or mastication of food takes place by the side-to-side movement of the cheek teeth. The bolus then is moved caudally into the oropharynx where swallowing or *deglutition* of food takes place.

Teeth

The teeth are embedded within specific bone sockets in the jaw called *alveoli*. The dentition consists of *incisor*, *canine*, *premolar* and *molar teeth*. The premolars and molars are similar in structure and function and are usually referred to as the cheek teeth. The line of teeth in each jaw is called a *dental arcade*. The horse's teeth, as with other mammalian teeth, consist of three calcified, dense and hard tissues: *enamel*, *dentine* and *cement*. The grinding surface of the teeth is known as the *occlusal surface* or *table*.

The incisor and cheek teeth are known as *hypsodont* (high-crowned) teeth, which means that they are tall and continue to grow in length after erupting. The part of the tooth that protrudes from the gum and is visible is called the *clinical crown*. In the horse, a large part of the crown is concealed beneath the gum line and is gradually extruded as the tooth is worn down (*reserve crown*). Thus, teeth are able to withstand the considerable wear that occurs during mastication of fibrous material. The *tooth root* is the deepest part of the tooth that remains embedded within the bone.

Deciduous teeth

In the foal, only the deciduous or temporary teeth are present. These are gradually replaced by permanent teeth in the adult horse.

The horse's *dental formula* is:

Incisors	Canines	Premolars	Molars	
3	0	3	0	upper jaw
3	0	3	0	lower jaw

Or: 2 (Di 3/3 Dc 0/0 Dp 3/3) = 24

The deciduous incisors are smaller and whiter than the permanent teeth. The approximate age of eruption of the deciduous incisors is:

- Central — 6 days
- Lateral — 6 weeks
- Corner — 6 months

The deciduous premolars are erupted at birth or do so within a week or so.

The eruption of both deciduous and permanent teeth can be used to estimate the age of horses up to 5 years with a reasonable degree of accuracy.

Permanent teeth

The mature horse has 40 teeth or 42 if wolf teeth are present.

The dental formula is:

Incisors	Canines	Premolars	Molars	
3	1	3	3	upper jaw
		(or 4 if wolf teeth)		
3	1	3	3	lower jaw

Or: 2 (I 3/3 C1/1 P3 or 4/3M3/3) = 40 (or 42 with wolf teeth)

The age of eruption of the permanent incisors is:

- Central — 2.5 years (fully in wear at 3 years)
- Lateral — 3.5 years (fully in wear at 4 years)
- Corner — 4.5 years (fully in wear at 5 years)

The canine teeth erupt at 4–5 years.

The age of eruption of the permanent premolar teeth is:

- Second premolar (first cheek tooth) — 2.5 years
- Third premolar (second cheek tooth) — 3 years
- Fourth premolar (third cheek tooth) — 4 years

The age of eruption of the permanent molar teeth is:

- First molar (fourth cheek tooth) — 1 year
- Second molar (fifth cheek tooth) — 2 years
- Third molar (sixth cheek tooth) — 3.5 years

Incisors

The incisor teeth are embedded in the incisive bone of the skull, with three pairs of incisors in each jaw (*central*, *lateral* and *corner*) (Fig. 2.17). The occlusal surfaces are worn down by eating, as well as the incisor teeth being extruded from their bone sockets. The appearance of the occlusal surface therefore varies with time and the appearance of this surface on the lower incisors aids in the assessment of age.

Canine teeth

The canine teeth are fully developed in the permanent dentition of the male and are usually erupted by 5 years of age. These teeth are *brachydont* (low-crowned) and so do not grow after eruption. Mares have poorly developed canines, usually in the lower jaws, or none at all.

Wolf teeth

The term *wolf tooth* applies to the *first premolar tooth*.

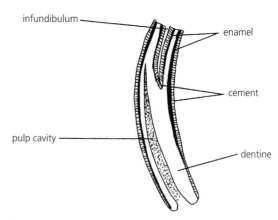

Fig. 2.17 Longitudinal section of an equine incisor tooth.

This often fails to develop or is just a very small peg-like structure with a short root, usually found just in front of the second premolar tooth in the upper jaw.

Premolars and molars (cheek teeth)

The second, third and fourth premolar teeth and the three molar teeth are four-cornered pillars that have three roots in the upper jaw and two in the lower. Once the permanent cheek teeth have erupted, they continue to grow for about 7 years. The cheek teeth are worn down by about 2–3 mm per year and the teeth are concurrently pushed out of the jaw. In these teeth, as with the incisors, the cement and dentine wear down more rapidly, leaving protruding sharp *enamel ridges*. The upper jaw is slightly wider than the lower jaw. Therefore, as the teeth are worn, the outer edges of the upper cheek teeth and the inner edges of the lower cheek teeth tend not to be worn as much.

Tongue

The large tongue lies on the floor of the oral cavity, extending into the oropharynx. The caudal parts of the tongue, i.e. the root and body, are attached to the hyoid bones and mandible, respectively. The tongue is supported by paired (mylohyoideus) muscles that sling it between the lower jaws. The tongue is also a highly muscular organ capable of precise movement and is important in

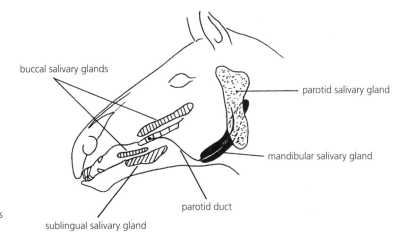

buccal salivary glands

parotid salivary gland

mandibular salivary gland

parotid duct

sublingual salivary gland

Fig. 2.18 Position of the major salivary glands in the horse.

the prehension and manipulation of food within the mouth.

Salivary glands

The salivary glands are several paired glandular structures. Their main function is to produce saliva, which moistens and lubricates food to facilitate chewing and swallowing. Some enzymes in saliva aid sugar breakdown. Saliva also has antibacterial properties. Feeding stimulates an increased flow of saliva.

The major salivary glands of the horse are the paired *parotid, buccal, mandibular* and *sublingual* glands (Fig. 2.18). The parotid glands empty into the mouth via the *parotid salivary ducts*, which are located under the mandible lying near the facial artery and vein.

Palate

The *hard palate* forms the rostral part of the oral cavity roof. It is a bony shelf made from the incisive, maxillary and palatine bones. The hard palate is continued caudally, without visible demarcation, by the *soft palate*. The soft palate is a long muscular membranous structure extending into the oropharynx. The caudal, free border of the soft palate is normally located ventral to the epiglottis. Because of the location of the soft palate, it is impossible for horses to normally breathe through their mouths.

Oropharynx

The caudal part of the oral cavity is known as the oropharynx. This area is bordered dorsally by the soft palate and caudally by the larynx. Food material enters the oropharynx from the oral cavity and then passes around each side of the larynx to enter the oesophagus. The passages around the sides of the larynx are known as the *lateral food channels* (Fig. 2.9).

Oesophagus

The oesophagus is a tube-like structure extending from the oropharynx to the stomach. The oesophagus is located near the trachea in the ventral neck. The cranial oesophagus lies dorsal to the trachea, but moves to lie on the left side of it for the majority of its course. The oesophagus is too soft to palpate in the neck but may be visualised during swallowing. The oesophagus extends through the thorax and diaphragm to enter the stomach at the cardia within the abdominal cavity. The cranial two-thirds of the oesophagus consists of striated muscle, whereas the caudal one-third is smooth muscle. The mucosa of the oesophagus is arranged in many longitudinal folds that allow the oesophagus to distend and contract as food passes down it. Food boluses are passed along the oesophagus by involuntary movement (*peristalsis*).

Stomach

The stomach is the dilated portion of the digestive tract between the oesophagus and small intestine, where the process of digestion begins and where food is stored for a short time. The horse's stomach is comparatively small, with a capacity of 5–15 L. The stomach lies in the cranial abdominal cavity, entirely within the rib cage, mostly to the left of the midline. The cranial part of the stomach is related to the diaphragm and liver, and the caudal surface is in contact with the intestines.

The oesophagus enters the stomach via the *cardia* (Fig. 2.19). The *cardiac sphincter* is thick and well developed in the horse so only very rarely can horses regurgitate food from the stomach. The interior of the stomach is divided into the *fundus*, the *body* and the *pyloric part*. The muscular *pyloric sphincter* controls the entry of food from the stomach into the small intestine.

The mucosal lining of the stomach is divided into:

(1) *Non-glandular* (*squamous*) portion within the fundus and body of the stomach.
(2) *Glandular* (*non-squamous*) portion in the rest of the body and the pyloric part.

The division between these two areas is known as the *margo plicatus*.

There are different types of secretory glands in the glandular area of the stomach that produce *gastric juice*. This consists of mucus, hydrochloric acid and enzymes that start the process of breaking down ingested protein and fats. Bicarbonate is also released in this area to neutralise the strong acid before it enters the small intestine. The average time taken for ingested food material to travel from the stomach to the caecum is about 2 hs.

Small intestine

The equine small intestine connects the pylorus of the stomach to the caecum. The small intestine is a metabolically active complex organ with several important functions:

(1) Transport of ingested food material and secretions by *peristalsis*.
(2) Secretion of fluids and intestinal juice to digest food.
(3) Mixing food and secretions together.
(4) Absorption of food and fluid into the surrounding lymphatic and blood vessels.

There are four main layers that make up the wall of the small intestine (Fig. 2.20):

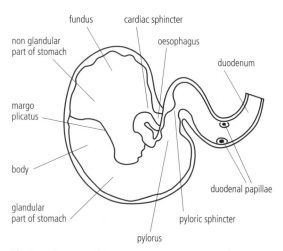

Fig. 2.19 The interior of the equine stomach.

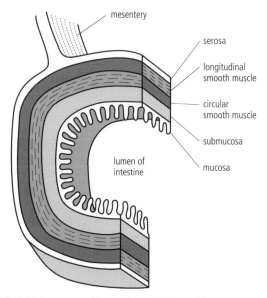

Fig. 2.20 Cross-sectional diagram showing the layers of the small intestine.

(1) *Serosa*—continuous with the peritoneum and is attached to the dorsal abdominal wall by a thin, fibrous connection (*mesentery*) that carries its vascular, nervous and lymphatic supply.
(2) *Longitudinal* and *circular smooth muscle.*
(3) *Submucosa.*
(4) *Mucosa*—this layer has many small finger-shaped projections (*intestinal villi*).

The villi increase the surface area of the small intestine, enormously maximising its ability to absorb digested food material. Epithelial cells line these villi.

Glands in the intestinal mucosa produce *intestinal juice*, which consists of enzymes that enable the breakdown of carbohydrates, proteins and fats into molecules small enough to be absorbed. Bicarbonate is secreted to neutralise the stomach acid, and mucus is produced to protect the intestinal lining. Additionally, enzymes secreted from the pancreas and bile from the bile ducts are involved. Digestion and absorption of all but insoluble fibre is thus completed in the small intestine.

The small intestine is approximately 22 m long in the average horse and is divided grossly and histologically into three distinct areas.

Duodenum

The duodenum is about 1 m long and can be divided further into three sections—the descending, transverse and ascending parts—as it bends around the root of the mesentery. The mesentery of the duodenum is short so the intestine is relatively immobile and closely fixed to the body wall. Both the bile and major pancreatic ducts empty into the descending duodenum.

Jejunum

The jejunum is the longest part of the equine small intestine (approximately 20 m). The mesentery attaching the jejunum to the body wall is also long so that the jejunum can move quite freely within the abdominal cavity.

Ileum

The ileum is the short terminal portion of the equine small intestine (approximately 50–70 cm long). The ileal wall is thicker and more muscular than the wall of the jejunum. The ileum meets the caecum at an area known as the *ileocaecal valve*. At this point, the lumen of the gut is narrowed.

Large intestine

The large intestine of the horse has three main parts.

Caecum

The caecum into which the ileum empties is a large, blind-ending, comma-shaped organ about 1 m long with a capacity of approximately 35 L. The base of the caecum occupies the right flank but also extends forward to lie under the cover of the last few ribs. The apex of the caecum reaches the ventral abdominal wall. There are four fibrous bands that run along the length of the caecum from base to apex; these are called *taeniae*. Blood vessels that supply the caecum run in the two lateral bands. The taeniae gather up the caecal wall into characteristic sacculations or *haustrae*.

Large colon

The colon consists of three main parts—the ascending, transverse and descending parts (Fig. 2.21). The first two together constitute the large colon, whereas the third is the small colon. The large (ascending) colon is about 4 m long and holds on average 80 L. Anatomically, the large colon is folded together to form a double loop consisting of *right* and *left ventral colons* and *left* and *right dorsal colons*, separated by three flexures.

Taenial bands are present on all parts of the large colon, with the number varying according to anatomical location. Except at its origin (the caecum) and its termination (the transverse colon), the bulky ascending colon is free to move within the abdomen. The dorsal and ventral regions are attached together by a short peritoneal sheet, the *mesocolon*.

The two important physiological functions of the large colon are:

(1) The storage and absorption of fluid.
(2) The retention of ingested food material for microbial digestion.

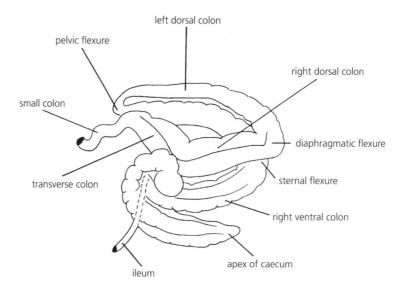

Fig. 2.21 The structure of the equine large colon.

These functions are extremely important in maintaining fluid and electrolyte balance and providing adequate nutrition. Food material is retained in the dorsal and ventral colons where the majority of microbial digestion occurs. The bacteria in these sites break down the ingested fibrous food material into organic acids known as *volatile fatty acids* (VFAs) that are then absorbed into the bloodstream. On average, food is retained in the caecum for 5 h and in the large colon for 50 h.

Small colon and rectum

The *small* (*descending*) *colon* connects the transverse colon to the *rectum*. It is a similar diameter to the small intestine and about 3 m long. Further resorption of fluid from ingesta during passage along the small colon leads to the formation of faecal balls. The rectum is the continuation of the small colon into the pelvic inlet, where it terminates at the *anus*. The rectum is about 30 cm in length. Faecal balls are moved down the small colon to the rectum and are expelled at the anus.

Peritoneum

This is a shiny protective layer of membrane that lines the inside of the abdominal cavity and covers the abdominal contents, i.e. *viscera*. The peritoneum

lining the abdominal cavity and attached to the body wall is called the *parietal peritoneum*. The layer around the viscera is the *visceral peritoneum*. The gaps between the different viscera within the peritoneum are known as the peritoneal cavity. The peritoneal membrane is a *serous endothelium*: serous because it secretes a watery fluid, i.e. *peritoneal fluid*; and endothelium is the term used to describe an epithelium lining a body cavity.

Skeletal system

Components and functions of the skeleton

The skeletal system is made up of bone and cartilage, i.e. it is the hard structures of the body that support and protect the soft tissues and provide leverage for locomotion. Bone also plays a physiological role in the formation of blood cells and mineral homeostasis. *Cortical* bone is the outer shell of dense compact bone. *Cancellous* or spongy bone is made up of linked layers or trabeculae and is found at the extremities of long bones. It also forms the majority of short bones. The cancellous bone absorbs force and provides a surface for the bone marrow.

A *medullary* cavity is present in the centre of long bones. The *endosteum* is a thin fibrous membrane that lines this cavity. Bone marrow fills the interstitial spaces of the spongy bone and the medullary cavity of long bones. Red marrow predominates in the young and is composed of blood-forming connective tissue. As the animal ages this is replaced by fat cells called *yellow marrow*. The *periosteum* is a dense connective tissue membrane that lines the outer surface of the bone, except where it is covered by cartilage.

Bone receives its blood supply from its periosteum at the soft tissue attachments and from the medullary artery that enters at the nutrient foramen. Large veins present in the cancellous bone generally emerge near the articular surfaces. The periosteum has sensory nerve endings, otherwise the nerves generally follow the distribution pattern of the blood vessels.

There are two types of cartilage found in the skeletal system:

(1) *Hyaline* cartilage, making up the gliding articular surface of most joints.
(2) *Fibrocartilage*, found in menisci and ligamentous insertions.

Cartilage is relatively acellular, so repairs poorly.

Skeletal development

Development of the skeleton begins in the fetus and continues in the foal. Although it is necessary to know the time of growth plate closure, it is more important to realise when the exponential or fast growth occurs. It is during this rapid phase that medical or surgical intervention may significantly alter angular limb deformities in the foal (Table 2.1).

Bone tissue consists of bone cells surrounded by a matrix containing collagenous fibres and cement (*calcium hydroxyapatite*). Bone is a living tissue that is constantly remodelling and is formed in one of two ways:

(1) *Intramembranous ossification* occurs when bone is formed from no cartilage precursor. The bone cells are situated between two membranes and directly form bone. This is how the bones of the skull are formed.
(2) *Endochondral ossification*: most bones develop by endochondral ossification. A cartilage precursor of the bone is formed, which calcifies. *Osteoblasts* (i.e. bone-forming cells) gradually produce bone as *osteoclasts* remove the calcified cartilage and produce tunnels through the bone. They are followed by blood vessels that bring further osteoblasts (Fig. 2.22). This is how the majority of longitudinal bone growth occurs.

Long-bone structure and growth

Long bones have a shaft and two ends (Fig. 2.23). They are divided into separate regions with different physical and physiological characteristics:

- *Diaphysis*: the midshaft composed of a dense outer rim—the cortex—and a soft inner core—the medulla.
- *Metaphysis*: the broadening end of the bone with a more uniform density but overall quite soft in the young horse.
- *Physis*: the growth plate where cartilage cells multiply and lay down collagen and ground substance, which subsequently becomes mineralised and organised into metaphyseal bone.
- *Epiphysis*: the end or head of the bone, which is covered in articular cartilage. It is also an active growth area in youngsters, with new bone being laid down as a result of articular cartilage cell activity.

The equine skeleton can be divided into two:

(1) The *axial* skeleton is the skull, vertebral column, ribs and sternum, which run along the long axis of the body.
(2) The *appendicular* skeleton consists of the limb bones.

Table 2.1 The clinically important growth plate closures

Physis	Rapid growth phase (months)	Functional closure (months)	Joint involved
Distal radial	6	12	Carpus
Distal metacarpal / metatarsal	1	3	Fetlock
Distal tibial	4	9	Hock

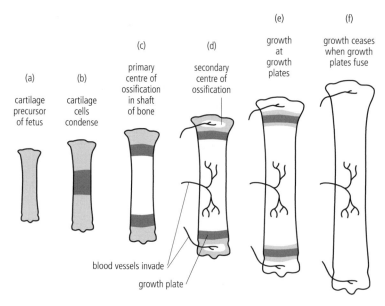

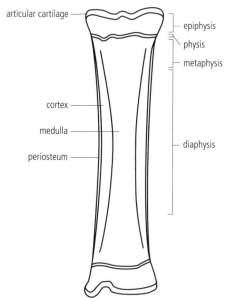

Fig. 2.22 Long-bone growth.

Axial skeleton

Skull

The equine skull consists of a mosaic of bones that together form a rigid structure comprising the cranium and nasal chambers (Fig. 2.24). The mandibles (jaw bones) and the hyoid apparatus are suspended from the cranium, which is the dome of the skull and other bones that surround the brain to make up the cranial cavity. Many blood vessels and nerves enter and leave this cavity via holes known as foraminae, e.g. the *foramen magnum* is in the base of the occipital bone through which the spinal cord connects to the brain.

The *mandible* (or jawbone) has a *horizontal ramus* (containing the mandibular cheek teeth) and a *vertical ramus*. The two mandibles are joined at the *mandibular symphysis* at the level of the chin. The vertical ramus of the mandible has two processes: the *condylar process* (a point of attachment for muscle) and the *coronoid process*. There is a shallow notch on the ventral aspect of the mandible on the caudal horizontal ramus. The facial artery, vein and parotid duct run through this notch, and it is a useful site to palpate the horse's pulse.

Fig. 2.23 Immature equine tibia showing the different regions of a long bone.

Vertebral column

The vertebral column is a linked series of bones along the body midline, extending from the skull cranially to the tail caudally. It is divided into regions according to the part of the body in which it is present:

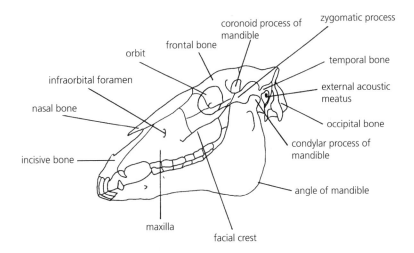

Fig. 2.24 The equine skull.

- Cervical (neck, C1–C7)
- Thoracic (chest, T1–T18)
- Lumbar (loins, L1–L6)
- Sacral (croup, S1–S5)
- Coccygeal or caudal (Cy/Cd–Cy/Cd 1–Cy/Cd 15/21)

The basic vertebra consists of a body (cylindrical) with a flattened dorsal surface that forms the floor of the vertebral foramen. The arch of the vertebra rises up on either side of the body and completes the foramen. The vertebral foramen of a series of connected vertebrae forms the vertebral canal, in which the spinal cord and associated structures are situated. The spinous processes rise dorsally from the middle of the arch. A pair of articular processes is present on the cranial and caudal edges of the arch. These articular processes form synovial joints with those of adjacent vertebrae. Small notches in the cranial and caudal borders of the arch meet in adjacent vertebrae and form intervertebral foramina through which pass the nerves and blood vessels. Transverse processes are paired and project horizontally at the junction of the body and arch. An intervertebral disk is present between each vertebral body that consists of a firm, fibrous outer layer—*annulus fibrosis*—and a softer, amorphous centre—*nucleus pulposis*.

Ribs
Eighteen pairs of ribs form the walls of the bony thorax, one for each thoracic vertebra. Each rib has an articulation at the proximal end with the vertebral column. The distal extremity of the first eight ribs (i.e. sternal ribs) articulates with the *sternum* (a flat bony structure that helps support the thorax). The other ribs do not reach the sternum and are known as floating or asternal ribs. The distal end of each rib is made up of cartilage and is called the costal cartilage. The cartilages of the asternal ribs overlap each other and attach to each other. The line of the last ribs and the cartilages is called the costal arch. The space between each rib, occupied by the intercostal muscles, nerves and blood vessels, is called the intercostal space.

Appendicular skeleton

The basic skeletal anatomy of the limbs is summarised in Figs 2.25 and 2.26.

Foot
The foot of the horse comprises three main bones:

(1) The *distal phalanx* (pedal or coffin bone, otherwise known as P3) is enclosed entirely within the hoof. Paired lateral cartilages arise from the inner and

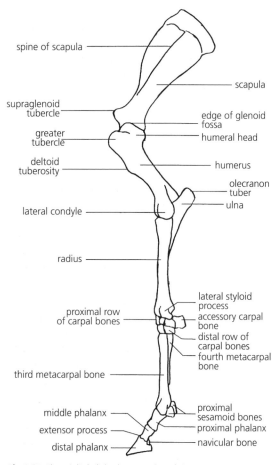

Fig. 2.25 Thoracic limb skeletal structure: lateral view.

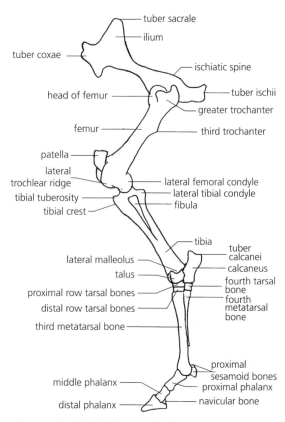

Fig. 2.26 Pelvic limb skeletal structure: lateral view.

outer sides of the pedal bone. They project above the hoof in the heel area, where they can be felt in the living horse just beneath the surface of the skin. When the lateral cartilages ossify, the condition is known as sidebone (Fig. 2.27).

(2) The distal phalanx articulates with the *second phalanx* (short pastern bone or P2) to form the distal interphalangeal joint (coffin joint).

(3) A sesamoid bone, known as the distal sesamoid or navicular bone (Fig. 2.28). The distal sesamoid (navicular bone) is a small, irregular, shuttle-shaped bone situated at the back of and forming part of the distal interphalangeal (coffin) joint. One side articulates with the second and third phalanx, whereas the tendon of the deep digital

flexor passes over it, enabling this tendon to change direction before inserting on P3.

The hoof encloses two tendons:

(1) The common digital extensor inserts on the extensor process of P3.

(2) The deep digital flexor (DDF) tendon runs deep to the navicular bone and inserts on the base of P3.

The navicular bone is suspended from P1 by the paired collateral or suspensory ligaments and is stabilised distally to P3 by the midline impar ligament. The impar ligament further stabilises the coffin joint.

The middle phalanx (short pastern or P2) lies between the proximal and distal phalanx. The proximal phalanx (long pastern or P1) is situated obliquely between the cannon bone to P2. Both P1 and P2 together form the proximal interphalangeal or pastern joint.

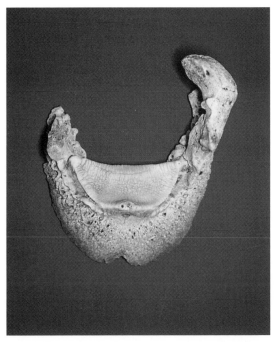

Fig. 2.27 Pedal bone, with ossified lateral cartilage (sidebone) on right.

Hoof

The hoof is the covering of horn that protects the internal structures of the horse's foot. It is non-vascular and insensitive and comprises the wall, sole and foot (Fig. 2.29). The junction of the hoof and skin is called the *coronet*. The *periople* is a thin band of soft greyish flaky horn, which runs above and parallel to the main coronary band. From the periople is produced the thin outer convering of the wall of the hoof, the *stratum tectorium* or *externum*, which gives the healthy hoof its water-resistant properties.

The hoof substance is made up of tubular and intertubular horn that varies in proportion according to site (Fig. 2.30). The horn of the wall of the hoof is predominantly tubular. The softer horn of the sole and frog has a greater intertubular component. Horn tubules are produced by the hair-like dermal papillae of the coronary band and of the sole and frog. The hollows between the dermal papillae produce the softer intertubular horn. The papillae of the coronary band and the papillae of the sole and frog all point in the same direction. This means that all parts of the hoof grow as a single unit. If a horse injures the coronary band, it will result in defective growth of the wall of the hoof below the site of the injury.

The inner surface of the wall of the hoof is attached to the outer covering of the pedal bone by a sliding

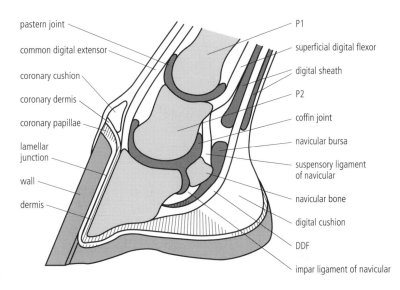

pastern joint
common digital extensor
coronary cushion
coronary dermis
coronary papillae
lamellar junction
wall
dermis

P1
superficial digital flexor
digital sheath
P2
coffin joint
navicular bursa
suspensory ligament of navicular
navicular bone
digital cushion
DDF
impar ligament of navicular

Fig. 2.28 Sagittal section of the equine digit.

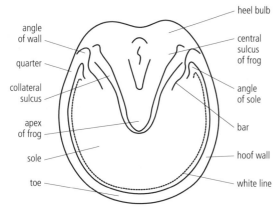

Fig. 2.29 Ground surface of the foot.

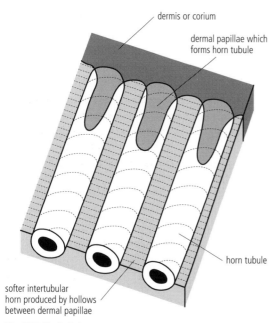

Fig. 2.30 Hoof tubule structure.

joint similar to that found between the human finger-nail and its nail bed. In the hoof the attachment is between the sensitive and insensitive laminae, both of which have a pleated or fluted appearance and dovetail together. As the hoof grows towards the ground, the insensitive laminae slide very slowly over the sensitive laminae. The horn of the insensitive lami-nae is usually unpigmented and can be seen on the bearing surface of a freshly trimmed foot as the *white line*. This joint between sensitive and insensitive lam-inae is important in the transmission of the weight of the animal from the limb, via the pedal bone, to the wall of the hoof. The sole is slightly concave so that the distal walls of the hoof and the frog are the weight-bearing surfaces of the feet.

The digital cushion is a wedge of fibro-elastic tissue at the back of the foot. It is moulded to the sensitive frog below and plays an important part in reducing concussion by expanding when the foot takes weight. The foot has a good blood supply from the medial and lateral palmar/plantar digital arteries, which end in a terminal arch.

Joints

A *joint* is the connection between two or more bones. They are classified by:

(1) The type of tissues involved.
(2) The type of movement permitted.

Synovial or diarthrodial joints

Synovial or diarthrodial joints are formed when a synovial membrane connects two bones and there is a space between the ends of the bones or joint cavity that is filled with synovial fluid. The ends of the bone are always covered in articular (hyaline) cartilage. These joints usually move freely (Fig. 2.31).

Synovial fluid is a viscous substance made from the fluid component of plasma plus hyaluronic acid. It acts as a lubricant between the cartilage of the two bone ends and nutrients diffuse from the synovial fluid into the articular cartilage. *Synovial membrane* lines the joint and produces the synovial fluid. A dense connective-tissue joint capsule surrounds the whole joint. Some joints contain a pad of fibrocarti-lage called a meniscus, e.g. the stifle of the horse contains two menisci that are firmly attached by ligaments to the tibial plateau. Hyaline *articular cartilage* allows low-friction articulation between apposing bones.

Synovial joints are also classified depending on the

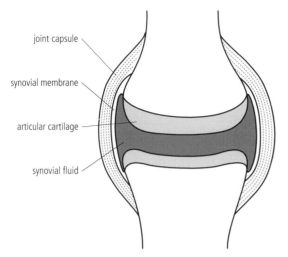

Fig. 2.31 Anatomy of synovial joint.

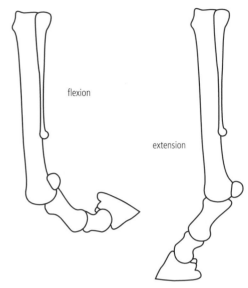

Fig. 2.32 Hinge movement of fetlock.

number of articular surfaces involved and how they move in relation to one another:

(1) *Simple joints* involve only two articulating surfaces.
(2) *Composite joints* have more than two articulating surfaces and movement may occur at more than one level within a single joint capsule.
(3) *Plane joints* involve one surface sliding over another, e.g. articular processes of the vertebrae.
(4) *Hinge joints* involve a convex surface moving upon a concave surface. Movement is only in one plane, e.g. fetlock (Fig. 2.32).
(5) *Pivot joints* allow rotationary movement, e.g. atlanto axial joint.
(6) *Condylar joints* involve two convex structures or condyles articulating with two corresponding concave articular surfaces, e.g. the stifle. Movement is primarily in one plane but some rotation may occur.
(7) *Ellipsoidal joints* have an oval convex surface with a corresponding concavity. There is predominantly movement in two planes and some rotation, e.g. radiocarpal joint.
(8) *Spheroidal* or *ball and socket joints* are composed of part of a sphere that fits into a concave socket, e.g. shoulder and coxofemoral joints.

Fibrous joints/synarthroses

These joints have fibrous tissue connecting the adjacent bones. Little movement occurs between the bones and these joints, e.g. sacro-iliac joint. In older animals the fibrous tissue may become ossified (replaced with bone) and fuse the joint, e.g. sutures in the skull.

Cartilaginous joints/amphi-arthroses

These joints are formed when cartilage connects two or more adjacent bones. When this involves a connection of two corresponding bones on opposite sides of the body, the joint is called a *symphysis*, e.g. pelvic symphysis.

Muscles, tendons and ligaments

A *tendon* is a tough fibrous band of tissue connecting a muscle to bone (Table 2.2 and Figs 2.33 and 2.34). Synovial fluid-filled bursae are often located between the tendon and any site of friction, such as a bony prominence (Figs 2.35 and 2.36; Table 2.3). Alternatively, a portion of tendon may be wrapped in a synovial cushion termed a sheath, particularly overlying joints. The tendon then can glide over

Table 2.2 Tendinous muscles of the forelimb and hindlimb

Muscle/tendon	Origin	Insertion	Function
Forelimb			
Extensor carpi radialis	Humerus	MCIII	Extend carpus, flex elbow
Lateral digital extensor	Radius, ulna, collateral elbow ligament	P1 , common digital extensor tendon	Extend digit, extend carpus
Ulnaris lateralis	Humerus	Accessory carpal bone	Extend elbow, flex carpus
Common digital extensor	Humerus, radius, ulna	Extensor process P3	Flex elbow, extend carpus, extend digit
Flexor carpi radialis	Humerus	MCII	Extend elbow, flex carpus
Flexor carpi ulnaris	Humerus, olecranon	Accessory carpal bone	Extend elbow, flex carpus
Superficial digital flexor	Humerus, radius	P2	Extend elbow, flex carpus, flex digit
Deep digital flexor	Humerus, olecranon, radius	Base of P3	Extend elbow, flex carpus, flex digit
Hindlimb			
Cranial tibial	Tibia	MT3, T1	Flex tarsus
Peroneus tertius	Femur	MT3, T3, T4, calcaneus	Flex tarsus with stifle
Long digital extensor	Femur	P3	Extend stifle, flex tarsus, extend digit
Lateral digital extensor	Stifle collateral ligament, tibia, fibula	Tendon of insertion of digital extensor	Flex tarsus, extend digit
Gastrocnemius	Femur	Point of hock	Flex stifle, extend tarsus
Superficial digital flexor	Femur	Point of hock, P1, P2	Extend tarsus, flex digit
Deep digital flexor	Tibia, fibula	Base of P3	Extend tarsus, flex digit

Table 2.3 Important bursae of the forelimb and hindlimb

Bursa	Located between	Region
Forelimb		
1. Infraspinatus	Infraspinatus tendon and humeral greater tubercle	Shoulder
2. Bicipital	Biceps tendon and humeral greater and lesser tubercles	Shoulder
3. (+/−) Olecranon	Olecranon tuber and skin	Elbow
4. Subtendinous lateral digital extensor	Lateral digital extensor tendon and cannon	Fetlock
5. Subtendinous common digital extensor	Common digital extensor tendon and cannon	Fetlock
6. Navicular	Deep digital flexor and navicular bone	Foot
Hindlimb		
1. Trochanteric	Gluteal and femoral greater trochanter	Hip
2. Proximal infrapatellar	Proximal middle patellar ligament and femur	Stifle
3. Distal infrapatellar	Distal middle patellar ligament and tibia	Stifle
4. Subcutaneous calcaneal	Skin and tuber calcanei	Hock
5. Subtendinous calcaneal	Cap of superficial digital flexor and tuber calcanei	Hock
6. Subgastrocnemius calcaneal	Gastrocnemius tendon and tuber calcanei	Hock
7. Cunean	Medial tibialis cranialis tendon branch and medial collateral ligament	Hock
8. Navicular	Deep digital flexor tendon and navicular bone	Foot

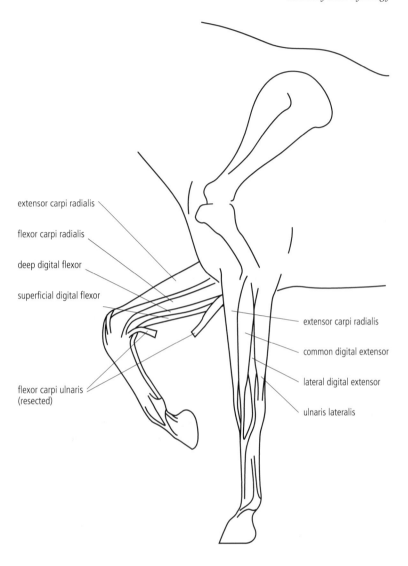

extensor carpi radialis

flexor carpi radialis

deep digital flexor

superficial digital flexor

extensor carpi radialis

common digital extensor

lateral digital extensor

flexor carpi ulnaris
(resected)

ulnaris lateralis

Fig. 2.33 Tendinous muscles of the forelimb.

joints in a lubricated sac. *Ligaments* are tensile bands that run from bone to bone. They function to stabilise or support joints or positions of bones so that they do not move outside of the desired range of motion. *Collateral ligaments* stabilise joints from the medial and lateral sides. There may be multiple collateral ligaments for a given joint. They form relatively short taught bands that attach above and below the joint capsule. They are often extracapsular but can be part of the fibrous joint capsule.

A *muscle* is contractile tissue that controls movement. There are three types:

(1) Skeletal, also called striated or voluntary.
(2) Smooth, also called involuntary.
(3) Cardiac or heart muscle.

Skeletal muscle is found attached to the bones of the body. The origin of a muscle is the more proximal or central attachment of the muscle. Most muscles contract and pull the insertion towards the origin. The *insertion* is usually the more distal attachment of the muscle, which is pulled towards the origin. The muscle *belly* is the fleshy part of the muscle that is made up of cells organised into *fibres*.

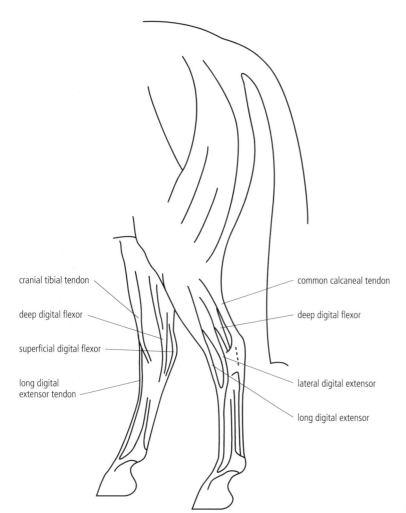

cranial tibial tendon

deep digital flexor

superficial digital flexor

long digital
extensor tendon

common calcaneal tendon

deep digital flexor

lateral digital extensor

long digital extensor

Fig. 2.34 Tendinous muscles of the hindlimb.

Muscle fibres consist of thick and thin fibres: the thick fibres are the protein *myosin* and the thin ones are actin. Muscle contraction is the consequence of stimulation of muscle fibres by nerve impulses from the brain arriving at the neuromuscular junction. This activates a pathway releasing calcium into the cytoplasm of the muscle cell. The calcium enables the production of energy so that the actin and myosin fibres within the cell can attach and slide over each other. The actin and myosin fibres are firmly attached to the cell wall, so this causes cell shortening (Fig. 2.37).

Muscle activity is inefficient, with much heat energy also released. *Isotonic* contraction involves shortening of the muscle during contraction and occurs during movement. *Isometric* contraction is tensing of the muscle without shortening. The motor unit is the complex of a nerve and the muscle fibres that it innervates. The number of fibres supplied by one nerve depends on the level of muscle control required, e.g. there are fewer muscle fibres innervated by one nerve in muscles involved in delicate movement.

Epaxial muscles lie dorsal to the transverse vertebral processes of the spine. They include the dorsal muscles of the neck, back and tail. They are organised in three parallel columns. The lateral, middle and medial columns work together to extend the neck, back and tail, as well as to flex the trunk laterally. The epaxial muscles also include a number of muscles that function to rotate or extend the head. The *hypaxial* muscles are located below the vertebral column and mostly function to flex the head, neck or tail.

The muscles of the proximal limb and abdominal musculature are summarised in Tables 2.4 and 2.5.

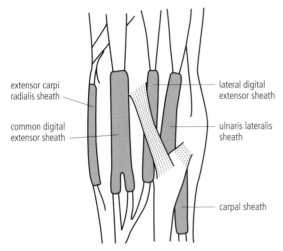

Fig. 2.35 Extensor sheaths of the carpus: lateral view.

Stay apparatus

The passive stay apparatus allows the horse to rest while standing. It consists of several ligaments, tendons and muscles that stabilise the joints and prevent the collapse of the limb. The suspensory apparatus is an important part of the stay apparatus. It consists of:

- The suspensory ligament
- The intersesamoidean ligament
- The proximal sesamoid bones
- The distal sesamoidean ligaments

These together prevent overextension of the fetlock. The suspensory ligament (SL) is a strong, flat, tendinous band. It runs from the palmar carpal ligament and proximal cannon bone and divides at the fetlock to attach to the sesamoid bones and gives off two extensor branches to join the common digital extensor (CDE) tendon of insertion. The cruciate, oblique and straight sesamoidean ligaments run between the proximal sesamoid bones and the proximal and middle phalanges. The suspensory apparatus is reinforced by tension in the distal DDF tendon, including the accessory (or check) ligaments. The inferior check ligament of the DDF tendons attaches to the palmar carpal ligament. The superior check

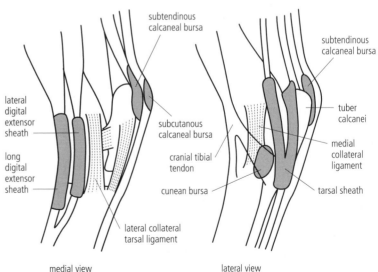

Fig. 2.36 Synovial sheaths and bursae of the tarsus.

53

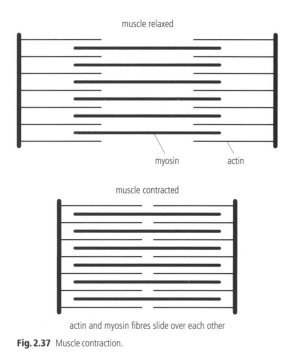

muscle relaxed

myosin   actin

muscle contracted

actin and myosin fibres slide over each other

Fig. 2.37 Muscle contraction.

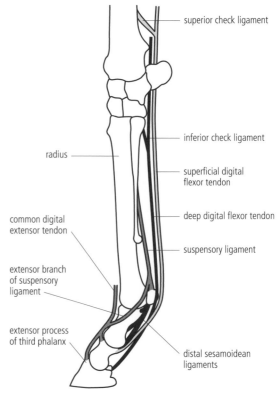

superior check ligament

inferior check ligament

radius

superficial digital flexor tendon

deep digital flexor tendon

common digital extensor tendon

suspensory ligament

extensor branch of suspensory ligament

extensor process of third phalanx

distal sesamoidean ligaments

Fig. 2.38 Suspensory apparatus of the forelimb.

ligament of the superficial digital flexor (SDF) tendon attaches to the distal radius (Fig. 2.38).

The main mechanisms involved in the stay apparatus of the hindlimb are the patella-locking mechanism, the reciprocal apparatus and the suspensory apparatus. Below the tarsus or hock, the suspensory apparatus is similar to that of the forelimb, except that the accessory or check ligament of the DDF tendon is small or sometimes absent. The SDF tendon compensates by firmly attaching to the point of the hock. The fixation of the stifle and the hock depends on locking the stifle in extension and the reciprocal apparatus (Fig. 2.39).

Hooking the parapatellar cartilage and medial patellar ligament over the large medial femoral trochlear ridge (Fig. 2.40) locks the stifle. The quadriceps muscle and the tensor fascia lata pull the patella into a locked position. This locked position is maintained by the pull of the biceps femoris from the lateral side and the gracillus and sartorius from the medial side. Two strap-like tendons link the equine stifle and hock. The peroneus tertius runs along the dorsolateral aspect of the hindlimb and joins the tar-

sus and third metatarsal bone to the stifle and femur. The SDF tendon runs from the femur, distally along the plantar aspect of the limb, to attach to the tuber calcaneus or point of the hock before terminating on the lower digits. These two straps are always tense; thus the stifle and hock normally must extend and flex together.

The anatomical arrangement of the stay apparatus enables the horse to stand while expending minimal energy.

The nervous system

The nervous system can be divided into three parts: the *central*, *peripheral nervous* and *autonomic nervous systems*. The nervous system allows a horse to control its bodily functions and respond to demands in an appropriate and coordinated manner. The nervous system receives external stimuli, which

Table 2.4 Muscles of the proximal limb

Muscle name	Position	Innervation	Action
Supraspinatus	Supraspinous fossa of scapula to the cranial aspect of humeral tubercles	Suprascapular nerve	Extension and stabilising shoulder joint
Infraspinatus	Caudal to scapula spine and tendons insert on the cranial humerus. Synovial bursa protects longer tendon over caudal aspect of tubercle	Suprascapular nerve	Stabilises shoulder joint and tendon acts as a lateral collateral ligament
Triceps	Three heads, one from scapula and two from humerus; all insert on the olecranon with a bursa between the tendon and bone	Radial nerve	Extension of elbow
Biceps bracchi	Supraglenoid tubercle of the scapula over a bursa to the radial tuberosity, has a connection with the carpal extensor	Musculocutaneous nerve	Flexion of elbow and assisting with carpal extension during weightbearing
Brachialis	Caudoproximal humerus to the craniomedial radius	Musculocutaneous	Flexion of elbow
Quadriceps	Four heads combine to insert on the patella	Femoral nerve	Extension and stabilisation of the stifle
Semimembranosus	Two heads: one caudal pelvis to the medial epicondyle of femur and the other medial collateral to the medial tibial condyle	Sciatic nerve	Extension of hip flex stifle when non-weightbearing and extends it when planted
Semitendinosus	Sacrum and adjacent area and pelvis to the medial tibia, crural fascia and joins calcaneal tendon	Caudal gluteal and sciatic nerves	Extension of hip flex stifle when limb raised and extends it when limb planted. Part of stay apparatus
Superficial gluteal	Tuber coxae and gluteal fascia to the third trochanter	Cranial and caudal gluteal nerve	Flexion of the hip and abduction of the limb
Middle gluteal	Caudal back and dorsal pelvis to the caudodistal femur	Cranial gluteal nerve	Extension of the hip and abduction of the limb
Deep gluteal	Dorsal pelvis to cranial aspect of greater trochanter	Cranial gluteal nerve	Abduction of limb
Gastrocnemius	Two heads from supracondylar tuberosities of femur to calcaneal tendon and inserts on calcaneus. Associated bursa	Tibial nerve	Extends hock
Biceps femoris	Sacrum and pelvis to the fascia lata, patella, lateral patellar ligament, tibial crest and joins calcaneal tendon	Caudal gluteal and sciatic nerves	Flexion of the stifle and possibly contributes to extension of the hip
Cranial tibial	Lateral tibia through tendon of peroneus tertius, splits and larger to metatarsal tuberosity and smaller to first tarsal bone	Peroneal nerve	Flexion of hock and counteracts bending action of tibia by other muscles
Peroneus tertius	Almost totally tendinous from distal femur, splits lateral to 4th tarsal and dorsal to 3rd tarsal and metatarsal bones	Peroneal nerve	Part of stay apparatus. Links actions of hock and stifle

Table 2.5 Summary of abdominal musculature

Muscle name	Origin and direction	Additional information
External abdominal oblique	Most extensive, from lateral aspect of thorax 5th rib with digitations into serratus ventralis and caudoventrally to linea alba. Small crus to tuber coxae	The split between the two crura forms the superficial inguinal ring
Internal abdominal oblique	From the tuber coxae and dorsocaudal edge of external abdominal oblique. Runs cranioventrally to costal cartilages and linea alba	A caudal slip provides the cremaster muscle, which passes onto the spermatic cord
Transverse abdominis	Lumbar vertebrae and medial last ribs. Aponeurosis deep to rectus and inserts on linea alba	Least extensive and does not extend more caudally than the level of the tuber coxae
Rectus abdominis	4th–9th costal cartilages and sternum and runs sagitally either side of the linea alba, inserting on the prepubic tendon	Narrow in thorax and widens over abdomen before narrowing again just prior to insertion

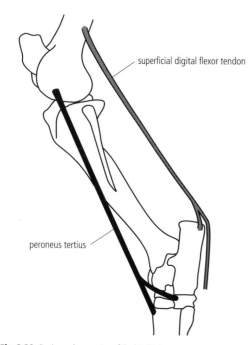

superficial digital flexor tendon

peroneus tertius

Fig. 2.39 Reciprocal apparatus of the hindlimb.

are analysed and integrated and then a response is produced. A *neurone* is the cell that is mainly responsible for transporting information to and from the body and the nervous system. It has long processes that carry information as electrical impulses and a cell body that processes this. Processes trans-porting impulses to the cell body are called *dendrites* (*afferent*) and those carrying them away from the body are called *axons* (*efferent*). Impulses pass from one neurone to another at a *synapse*, which is a gap between the processes where information is transported only one way by the release of chemicals (neurotransmitters).

The receptors are known as *sensory* nerve endings and the processes transmitting the impulses are *sensory* fibres. These carry information on stimuli received. The impulse is carried by the axon (second part of the neurone). If a response is evoked, the impulse has to be transmitted to a muscle or gland. The neurone process carrying this impulse is a *motor* fibre, which will cause muscle movement. The simplest functional unit of the nervous system consists of a sensory fibre synapsing with a motor fibre. An additional neurone is usually carrying the impulse from the sensory to the motor unit. This is called a *connector* or *intercalated neurone*.

Nerve fibres are further classified relating to the structures in which the sensory and motor nerve endings are found. Internal organs, smooth muscle, glands and mucous membrane are principally innervated by *visceral fibres*. Somatic fibres innervate all other structures. Fibres receiving and processing impulses are also called afferent neurones. The fibres sending impulses to structures to initiate an action are motor and called efferent neurones. A *ganglion* is a

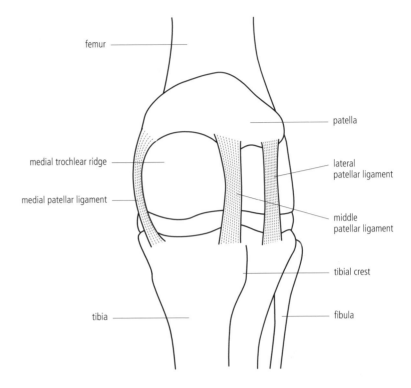

femur

patella

medial trochlear ridge

lateral patellar ligament

medial patellar ligament

middle patellar ligament

tibial crest

tibia

fibula

Fig. 2.40 Patella in locked position.

group of nerve cells where synapses occur, enabling the interchange of signals.

Central nervous system (CNS)

The CNS consists of the *brain* and *spinal cord*, which are protected within the bony cranium and vertebral column and are covered by *meninges* consisting of three layers:

(1) *Dura mater*: a thick outer fibrous layer. The protective dura mater is interwoven with the periosteum on the inner surface of the cranial bones.

(2) *Arachnoid*: a thin middle layer that consists of a network of delicate collagenous fibres. The subarachnoid space between the fibres is occupied by the *cerebrospinal fluid* (CSF).

(3) *Pia mater*: an inner layer that is closely applied to the CNS. It is a delicate and very vascular membrane covering the brain and spinal cord.

The CSF is a clear, colourless fluid that surrounds and permeates the entire CNS, thus protecting, supporting and nourishing it.

The CNS contains collections of neuronal nerve cell bodies, nuclei and columns of grey matter. Tracts, sheets and pathways of dendritic and axonal processes of these cell bodies make up the white matter.

Spinal cord

The spinal cord extends from the foramen magnum of the cranium to the cranial sacral region (S2) in the horse. At the termination of the spinal cord a tail of spinal nerves continues, enabling them to reach the exit foraminae (*cauda equina*). In the spinal cord, the sensory and motor fibres combine to form a mixed *spinal nerve* with a pair (left and right) related to each vertebra. These nerves enter and leave the canal via the intervertebral foraminae. Each spinal nerve is connected to the spinal cord by a dorsal and ventral root. The dorsal root has a localised

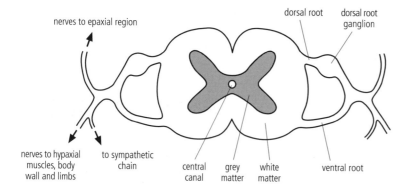

Fig. 2.41 Cross-section of spinal cord.

swelling, the dorsal root ganglion, which lies close to or in the intervertebral foramen. This is where the cell bodies of the sensory nerves are found (Fig. 2.41). All spinal nerves have a communicating or visceral ramus as a ventral branch. The communicating rami have visceral motor fibres running from one to the other to form a continuous nerve on each side of the vertebral column inside the abdominal and thoracic cavities. This is the *sympathetic chain*.

The spinal cord is continued rostrally by the brain, without an abrupt change. It is composed of neurones like the spinal cord but the grey matter is separated into discrete areas by tracts of fibres (white) connecting different regions. The central canal of the spinal cord continues rostrally into the brain tissue. It then expands and has diverticuli to produce a large *ventricular* system. This is filled with CSF. There are four ventricles. The widening of the canal within the medulla oblongata is the fourth ventricle. The ventricular system then narrows again as it travels rostrally into the midbrain as the cerebral aqueduct. Further rostrally, the diameter of the duct widens again and becomes the third ventricle. This is laterally flattened in the midline and has two lateral extensions or diverticuli called lateral ventricles. These each occupy part of the cerebral hemispheres.

Brain

The brain is divided into the *forebrain, midbrain* and *hindbrain*:

(1) The forebrain includes:

(a) Two *cerebral hemispheres*, which are crucial in receiving and processing information. They contain the higher centres, connections with the upper motor neurones and related nuclei, e.g. the visual cortex. It is the largest part of the brain. The surface is arranged in *sulci* (grooves) and *gyrae* (ridges). The most rostral parts of the cerebral hemispheres are the *olfactory bulbs*. These are paired and closely associated with the plate of bone separating the brain from the nasal chambers and convey the sense of smell.

(b) The *thalamus*, which is deep within the brain, relays impulses to and from the cerebral cortex.

(c) The *hypothalamus*, which has important regulatory functions.

(d) The *optic chiasma*, which is a cross-shaped set of nerve fibres associated with the eye.

(2) The midbrain is part of the brainstem that carries nerve tracts between the forebrain and hindbrain. The midbrain is associated with cranial nerves III and IV and their cell bodies.

(3) The hindbrain includes:

(a) The *medulla oblongata*, which contains the respiratory centre and centre for cardiac control. The medulla is associated with cranial nerves VI–XII and their sensory ganglia.

(b) The *pons*, with which cranial nerve V is associated.

(c) The *cerebellum*, which lies on the dorsal part of the hindbrain over the fourth ventricle. Its function is to help maintain balance and equilibrium by coordinating muscular activity.

Reflexes

Reflexes are important physiologically and aid in the diagnosis of a region/nerve affected in neurological disease (see Example 2.1). A neurological examination basically involves testing simple and complex reflex pathways and then interpreting the effected reflex activity and complex responses. A reflex action is a fixed involuntary response, which is always similar for a given stimulus. The reflex arc is the pathway along which the stimuli travel.

Simple reflex arc

A classic example is the *patellar reflex*. This is a simple spinal reflex that is quite difficult to elicit in the adult horse compared with small animals. It is composed of three neurones. Stimulation of a sensory stretch receptor in the tendon of the quadriceps muscle and its sensory neuronal cell body in the dorsal root ganglion stimulates an intercalated neurone. This effects the contraction of the quadriceps muscle via a lower motor neurone (LMN). The LMN has its cell body in the ventral grey matter of the spinal cord. There are no ascending or descending connections with the brain. This reflex can take place even if the spinal cord is cut, as long as the damage does not occur at the segments used by the reflex.

Complex reflex arcs

These involve input from and output to the higher centres in the brain. The various reflex pathways, with their respective LMNs throughout the brainstem and spinal cord, are controlled for voluntary movement by higher motor centres via their upper motor neurones (UMNs). Descending UMNs take specific tracks, e.g. corticospinal synapse, on the LMNs of the reflex pathways. The higher centres help to control the LMNs within the reflex arcs. There are also sensory inputs to the reflex arcs, which are relayed to higher centres to give feedback on proprioception (position sense) and nociception (touch/pain perception). These ascending pathways travel to the thalamus and sensory cerebral cortex.

Example 2.1

'Slap reflex'

The skin behind the shoulder is slapped gently during expiration while the larynx is palpated for movement of the contralateral, dorsolateral laryngeal musculature. Observation of the larynx via endoscopy will allow visual observation of the reflex response. The afferent pathway is through the segmental dorsal thoracic nerves, cranially to the contralateral spinal cord white matter and to the contralateral vagal nucleus in the medulla oblongata. The efferent pathway is through the vagus nerve to the cranial thorax and then back up the neck in the recurrent laryngeal nerve to the larynx.

Cranial nerves

The cranial nerves arise from the brainstem in pairs. They are numbered I–XII, rostral to caudal. The nerves do not attach to the brain with regular dorsal and ventral roots and nor do many have both motor and sensory fibres like the spinal nerves. Special sensory and special motor fibres are found in the cranial nerves. All the nerves innervate only the structures in the head region, except for the vagus (X), which also supplies the thoracic and abdominal organs. Three nerves are concerned only with the special senses and are therefore called 'special sensory' nerves:

- Olfactory (I)
- Optic (II)
- Vestibulocochlear (VIII)

The trigeminal (V) is the largest of the cranial nerves, with both sensory and motor fibres. For a list of the cranial nerves and their functions, see Summary 2.1.

Summary 2.1

Cranial nerves and their major functions

I Olfactory: sense of smell
II Optic: afferent pathway for vision/light
III Oculomotor: pupillary constriction/extra-ocular muscles
IV Trochlear: responsible for eye position muscles
V Trigeminal: sensory to side of face; motor to muscles of chewing
VI Abducens: also responsible for eye position muscles
VII Facial: motor to muscles of facial expression
VIII Vestibulocochlear: vestibular (balance) and cochlear (hearing)
IX Glossopharyngeal: sensory and motor to pharynx and larynx
X Vagus: sensory and motor to pharynx and larynx; also supplies abdominal and thoracic organs
XI Accessory: sensory and motor to pharynx and larynx
XII Hypoglossal: motor to tongue

The peripheral nervous system

This consists of the *spinal* and *cranial* nerves. There are four basic functional types of fibres:

(1) Somatic sensory enter through every dorsal root of the spinal nerves.
(2) Somatic motor leave the spinal cord through the ventral root of every spinal nerve.
(3) Visceral sensory.
(4) Visceral motor.

The swelling on the dorsal root is the dorsal root ganglion containing cell bodies of these fibres. Some of the dorsal roots also may contain visceral sensory fibres. The visceral motor fibres are distributed slightly differently from the rest of the fibre types. These form part of the autonomic nervous system. The ventral roots of the thoracic and lumbar spinal nerves contain visceral motor fibres. In these regions these fibres are called *sympathetic* fibres. The ventral roots of some of the sacral spinal nerves and the corresponding parts of some of the cranial nerves contain visceral motor fibres. These are called *parasympathetic* fibres.

The autonomic nervous system (ANS)

This system directs many of the homeostatic functions necessary for basic life processes and is also involved in response to emergencies. It is a physiological and anatomic system with both central and peripheral components.

It consists of three main components:

(1) The *sympathetic* component is associated with the body's response to emergencies, the 'fight or flight' response. It innervates smooth muscle, cardiac muscle and glandular organs in a rapid response to potential life-threatening situations. It increases the heart rate, opens up airways, and increases the blood supply to skeletal muscle.
(2) The *parasympathetic* part is associated with homeostasis, maintaining the normal processes ongoing in the body. It generally has a more local effect than the sympathetic system and works in the opposite way in that it slows down the heart and breathing rates and increases bowel motility (Table 2.6).
(3) The *enteric nervous system* consists of a diffuse network of neurones that occur in the muscular walls of the hollow viscera. The system receives input from the other two divisions of the ANS but it can act independently of the CNS.

There is also input from higher centres in the CNS. The hypothalamus is the primary integrating centre of the ANS and itself receives input from higher centres in the cerebral cortex. The route of transmission is from the hypothalamus via the midbrain, pons and medulla, and down the spinal cord where the supply leaves as general visceral efferent neurones in the cranial and spinal nerves. These carry information to smooth muscle, cardiac muscle and gland target organs. Some neurones in the parasympathetic arm leave the CNS in the cranial nerves.

The sympathetic system

Axons of the visceral efferent neurones leave via the ventral root and synapse with the post-ganglionic neurone in the sympathetic chain ganglia. The post-ganglionic neurone then runs to the target visceral structures. In addition there is an alternative sympa-

Table 2.6 Summary of sympathetic and parasympathetic systems

Sympathetic nervous system stimulation by noradrenaline	Parasympathetic nervous system stimulation by acetylcholine
Increased heart rate	Decreased heart rate and myocardial responses
Dilation of airway passages	Constriction of air passages in lungs
Lacrimal, parotid and submandibular gland secretion	Increased secretion of lacrimal, parotid and submandibular glands
Sweat gland secretion	
Increased gut motility	Increased peristaltic and segmented motility of gastrointestinal tract
Increased blood glucose	Reduced blood glucose via effects on liver and pancreas
Reduced urine production	
Pupillary dilation	Constriction of pupils and ciliary muscle
Arteriole constriction, general	

thetic pathway supplying vessels of the abdominal viscera. The preganglionic neurone goes to the visceral ramus and the visceral rami combine to form splanchnic nerves, ending in collateral ganglia. These ganglia are located along the dorsal aorta and here the preganglionic neurones synapse with the post-ganglionic neurones.

The parasympathetic system

Similar input from cerebral cortex to hypothalamus and other nuclei. In a similar way to the sympathetic system the nerve fibres emerge from the brain or spinal cord and pass to the organs concerned. The main structural difference is in the position of the ganglia. In the sympathetic system the ganglia lie alongside the vertebrae close to the spinal cord, with the result that the preganglionic fibres are short and the post-ganglionic fibres are long. In the parasympathetic system the fibres synapse close to their target organ, so there are only short post-ganglionic fibres.

The ear

The ear consists of the external ear, the middle ear and the inner ear.

The external ear

The external ear consists of the pinna and the external auditory meatus. The pinna is a cone-shaped structure made of cartilage and covered by skin. The pinna is highly movable so the horse is able to con-

centrate on the source of a sound. The ear position is an important indicator of emotional expression in the horse. Cartilage rings (annular cartilage) surround the external auditory meatus. The meatus then courses into the temporal bone of the skull and ends at the eardrum (Fig. 2.42).

The middle ear

Both middle and inner ear lie in cavities in the temporal bone. The eardrum is the border between the external and the middle ear. The eardrum is vibrated by sound waves. From the eardrum, sound is transferred and amplified mechanically by the three auditory ossicles—the *malleus, incus* and *stapes* (hammer, anvil and stirrup)—in the middle ear (Fig. 2.43). The stapes transfers the vibration onto the oval foramen and from there into the inner ear. The Eustachian tube connects the middle ear to the pharynx. The purpose of the Eustachian tube is to allow the equilibration of pressure between the external and the middle ear. The horse has a large diverticulum of the Eustachian tube (the guttural pouch).

The inner ear

The bony cavity of the inner ear is known as the *bony labyrinth* and is filled with *perilymph*. Within the bony labyrinth is the *membranous labyrinth*. The membranous labyrinth forms the organs of the inner ear. The membranous labyrinth contains *endolymph*. The systems of cavities containing perilymph or endolymph

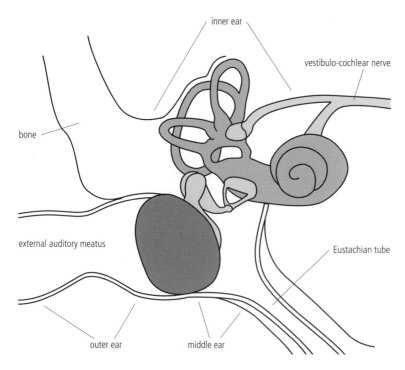

Fig. 2.42 Overview of the ear.

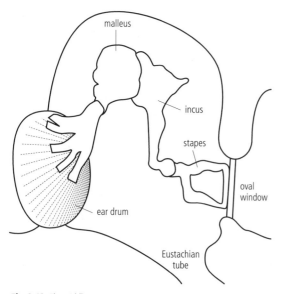

Fig. 2.43 The middle ear.

are not connected. The inner ear contains two organs (Fig. 2.44):

(1) The *vestibular* apparatus is responsible for sending information about balance and acceleration to the brain via the *utricle* and *saccule*. The utricle is the origin of the three *semicircular ducts* that are orientated in the three different perpendicular directions. Endolymph movement due to inertia is measured in these canals, providing the brain with information about acceleration. The saccule is responsible for measuring how the head is orientated relative to gravity. It contains several calcium carbonate crystals (otoliths) that rest on sensory hairs and is the organ responsible for assessing balance. All information from the vestibular apparatus is sent to the brain via the vestibular part of the VIII cranial nerve (vestibulocochlear nerve).

(2) The *cochlea* receives vibration caused by sound through the oval window. The oval window is a membranous interface between the middle and

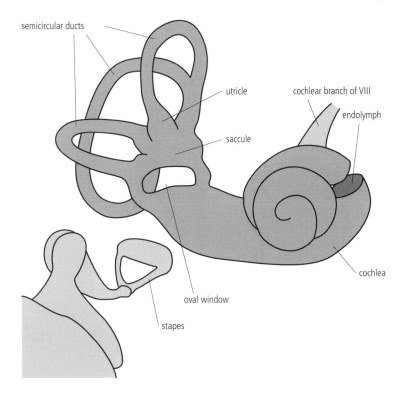

semicircular ducts

utricle

cochlear branch of VIII

endolymph

saccule

cochlea

oval window

stapes

Fig. 2.44 The inner ear.

inner ear. The region of sensory cells bearing fine sensory hairs in the cochlea is called the *organ of Corti*. The endolymph in the cochlea transmits the vibrations onto the sensory hairs. The bases of these hairs, the sensory cells, are connected to nerve endings. The information is transported to the brain by the cochlear part of the VIII cranial nerve (vestibulocochlear nerve). The round window is another interface between the cochlea and middle ear whose purpose is to allow compensation for vibrations reaching the cochlea via the oval foramen.

The eye

The eyeball

The eyeball is made up of three layers of tissue:

(1) The external tunic consists of tough fibrous tissue and forms the *sclera* that surrounds most of the eye-bulb. In the anterior part of the eye the exter-

nal tunic is clear (*cornea*) to allow light into the eye-bulb. The junction between sclera and cornea is called the *limbus*.

(2) The middle layer is the pigmented and vascular *uvea*. Its anterior part forms the *ciliary body* and the *iris*. The part of the uvea surrounding the posterior chamber is called the *choroid*.

(3) The innermost layer is called the *retina*. Only the posterior part of the retina contains light-sensitive nerve cells. The rest of the retina forms a lining for the inside of the posterior chamber and the posterior surface of the iris (Fig. 2.45).

The cornea is a clear tissue that covers the anterior pole of the eye and lets light in. To do this, the exterior surface of the cornea needs to be moistened constantly with tears and lubricated by the secretions of the *tarsal (meibomian) glands*.

The *anterior chamber* stretches from the posterior surface of the cornea to the iris. It is filled with clear fluid (*aqueous humour*), which is produced at the rear of the iris. The flow is anterior through the

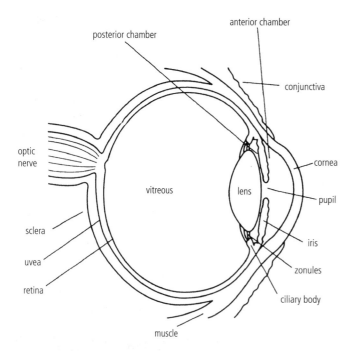

posterior chamber

anterior chamber

conjunctiva

optic nerve

cornea

vitreous

lens

pupil

sclera

uvea

iris

retina

zonules

ciliary body

muscle

Fig. 2.45 Anatomy of the eye.

pupil. The fluid is then absorbed in the angle between the anterior surface of the iris and the cornea.

The *iris* is a circular structure that sits disk-like between the anterior and posterior chamber. The opening in the middle of the iris is the *pupil*, which is oval shaped in the horse. To allow the iris to control the amount of light that enters the eye, pupil size can be changed. When it is dark the pupil is dilated, which is known as *mydriasis*. *Myosis* is the opposite when the pupil is constricted in bright light. The horse has small black granules attached mainly to the superior margin of the pupil, which can grow up to pea size. These are the normal *granula iridica* (*corpora nigra*) in the horse.

The *posterior chamber* stretches from the iris to the back of the eye. The region right at the back of the eye, where the sensory cells are located, is called the *fundus*. Structures filling the posterior chamber are the *lens* and the *vitreous*.

The *lens* is a round, clear structure enclosed in an elastic fibrous capsule. The posterior convexity has a greater curvature than the anterior convexity. The zonular fibres suspend the lens from the ciliary body.

Disruption of these fibres will result in the lens being displaced either anteriorly or posteriorly. Muscles in the ciliary body, which are weak in the horse as compared with other animals, change the shape of the lens and therefore allow the eye to accommodate to view near objects.

The *vitreous* is a clear, gelatinous mass within the posterior chamber behind the lens. It acts to transmit and refract light.

The *retina* is a layer of tissue that is rich in sensory cells in the region of the fundus. Two kinds of sensory cells exist in the retina:

(1) *Rods* are more numerous and are responsible for detecting light and dark difference only.
(2) Cones provide colour vision.

Nerves originating from the rods and cones are bundled into the *optic nerve*. The spot where the optic nerve exits the fundus is not covered by retina and is therefore blind. The *tapetum* (tapetum lucidum) is a reflective non-pigmented part of the retina, which acts as a light amplifier by reflecting light that has already passed once through the retina.

The orbit

The eye is situated in the *orbit*, which is a bony structure surrounding most of the eye and protecting it from trauma. This includes:

- the frontal bone medially
- the temporal bone caudally
- the zygomatic bone laterally
- the lacrimal bone rostrally

These bones form a cavity in the skull that is open rostrolaterally for the anterior structures of the eye.

Structures around the eye

Eye muscles

The eye is attached to the orbit by several muscles. The purpose of these muscles is to hold the eye in place and to enable the eye to be moved actively. A body of fat is situated between the back of the bulb and the bones of the orbit.

Lids

The eyelids protect the front of the eye. The upper and lower eyelids are covered with normal skin externally. The insides of the upper and lower eyelids are covered by *conjunctiva*—a very elastic tissue that allows the eye and the lids to move freely while effectively sealing the eye-bulb into the orbit. The reflection of the conjunctiva covering the insides of the lids and the conjunctiva that attaches to the eye-bulb is called the fornix, i.e. an arch-shaped structure. The free margins of upper and lower lid contain mucoid tarsal (meibomian) glands. Long eyelashes are situated on the free margin of the upper eyelid to protect against sunlight and dust particles.

The third eyelid is drawn over the eye from the medial corner, beneath the upper and lower eyelids. Its base is the third eyelid cartilage, which is covered by conjunctiva on both surfaces. The free margin of the conjunctiva is pigmented in most horses.

Lacrimal apparatus

The purpose of the lacrimal apparatus is to provide the eye with tears to lubricate the anterior surface of the eye and to flush out foreign material. The lacrimal apparatus consists of the lacrimal gland, the two lacrimal puncta and the nasolacrimal duct. The lacrimal gland lies in the lateral orbit between the orbital muscles and the zygomatic bone. It produces tears that are secreted into the conjunctival fornix by several short ducts. The tears are collected at the medial canthus into two small slit-like openings, the lacrimal puncta. From there the tears are conveyed through the nasolacrimal duct to the nostril.

Eyesight

The horse has a field of vision of about 300°. Blind spots exist behind the horse and directly in front of the animal ventrally. Head movement can compensate for these blind spots. The wide, almost circular field of vision makes it easy for the horse to detect movement in its peripheral vision. It can be difficult to detect partial blindness in the horse.

The endocrine system

An *endocrine* gland is a ductless gland that releases its secretory product—a hormone—directly into the bloodstream for general circulation. A *hormone* acts as a 'chemical messenger' that can influence the activity of other organs or tissues, mainly involving the control and coordination of processes such as metabolism, fluid balance, growth, resistance to stress, maintenance of a stable internal environment, sexual development and reproduction.

Pituitary gland

The pituitary gland or *hypophysis* produces many hormones, including some that directly affect the activities of the other endocrine glands. It is suspended beneath the hypothalamus by a stalk and sits within a depression in the floor of the skull on the ventral surface of the midbrain (Fig. 2.46).

The hypophysis is composed of three parts:

(1) The *neurohypophysis* (posterior lobe)
(2) The *adenohypophysis* (anterior lobe)
(3) The *pars intermedia* (intermediate lobe)

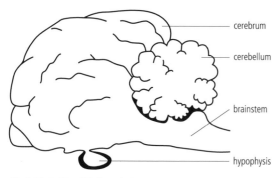

Fig. 2.46 Position of the hypophysis.

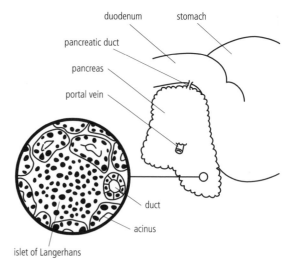

Fig. 2.47 The equine pancreas.

Numerous important hormones are produced by the hypophysis and they are often named using the suffix '*-trophin*' or '*-trophic*' at the end of a word to indicate the target organ.

The adenohypophysis produces the following hormones:

- Growth or *somatotrophic hormone* (STH): no specific target organ but affects many tissues and metabolic processes, in particular the control of skeletal growth.
- *Adrenocorticotrophic hormone* (ACTH) acts on the adrenal cortex to stimulate the release of other hormones, primarily the *glucocorticoids*. The release of ACTH is controlled by cortisol under negative feedback.
- *Thyroid-stimulating hormone* (TSH) acts on the thyroid gland to stimulate the synthesis of thyroid hormones.
- *Gonadotrophic* hormones: *follicle-stimulating hormone* (FSH) stimulates follicular growth in the ovary, whereas *luteinising hormone* (LH) causes maturation of the follicle.
- *Prolactin* acts on the mammary gland to stimulate the production of milk.

The neurohypophysis does not directly produce hormones but acts to store and then release those produced by the hypothalamus. These include:

- *Oxytocin*, a hormone acting on the smooth muscle in the uterus during parturition and on the myo-epithelial cells of the udder, causing uterine contractions and milk release, respectively.

- *Vasopressin*, or *antidiuretic hormone* (ADH), promotes fluid resorption by the kidney.

The pars intermedia produces *melanophore-stimulating hormone* (MSH).

Pancreas

The pancreas is a small, soft, yellowish gland, triangular in shape, lying mainly on the right-hand side of the abdomen. It is attached to the duodenum within the sigmoid flexure and is composed of glandular tissue. The pancreas is a mixed gland with two main functions:

(1) *Exocrine*, involving digestive secretions into the duodenum. Two main ducts carry the digestive secretions collected from many smaller ducts within the pancreatic tissue. The *greater pancreatic* duct opens into the cranial duodenum with the hepatic duct, and the *accessory* duct opens on the opposite side of the gut (Fig. 2.47).
(2) *Endocrine*, which involves the secretion of hormones directly into the bloodstream.

Pancreatic functions

The exocrine, or *acinar*, cells are responsible for the secretion of the digestive enzymes that break down fat, carbohydrate and protein into smaller components to aid absorption.

The endocrine function is located in the *islets of Langerhans*, which are small islands of tissue scattered within the pancreatic acini. They secrete three hormones:

(1) *Insulin*, which is released into the blood in response to a rise in glucose levels. Insulin causes an increase in the conversion of glucose to glycogen for storage within the cells. It also accelerates the uptake of glucose into skeletal tissue. The control of insulin is dependent upon the level of blood glucose.

(2) *Glucagon*, which has the opposite effect to insulin. Low blood glucose levels circulating through the pancreas stimulate the release of glucagon. Glucagon acts to initiate the breakdown of glycogen into glucose, thus raising the blood glucose level. In turn, this elevation in blood glucose to normal levels inhibits the release of glucagon.

(3) *Somatostatin*, which prevents excessive levels of nutrients in the plasma by reducing the rate of food digestion and absorption.

Thyroid gland

The thyroid gland consists of two lobes, palpable as soft ovoid structures dorsolateral to the proximal trachea. The gland contains spherical follicles that synthesise the thyroid hormones *thyroxine* and *triiodothyronine*. There are also parafollicular cells that synthesise *calcitonin*, a hormone responsible for calcium homeostasis.

Parathyroid glands

The parathyroids are four small glands situated behind the thyroid. They secrete *parathyroid hormone* (PTH), a hormone involved in calcium and phosphate metabolism.

Adrenal glands

There are two adrenal glands, irregular in shape and situated along the cranial aspect of the medial border of each kidney. The adrenals are essential for life and play an important role in states of stress (Figs 2.48 and 2.49). Each gland consists of:

(1) The outer *cortex*, which secretes *steroid* hormones. Steroids are all derived from cholesterol and thus have a common basic biochemical structure.
    (a) The *zona glomerulosa* secretes *mineralocorticoids*. The most important of these is *aldosterone*, a hormone acting mainly on the kidney tubules to promote the retention

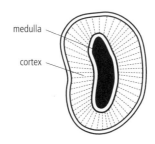

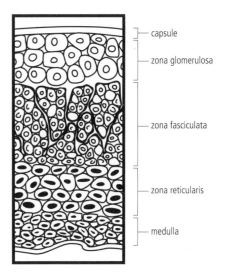

Fig. 2.48 The equine adrenal gland.

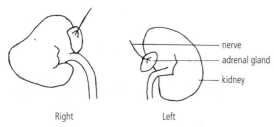

Fig. 2.49 Relationship between the kidneys and adrenal glands.

of sodium and therefore of water, with increased loss of potassium and hydrogen.

(b) The *zona fasciculata* secretes *glucocorticoids*. The main hormones are *cortisol* and *corticosterone* and they have many important effects. One such effect is to cause protein catabolism. The amino acids thus formed are used to make glucose in the liver and therefore cause increased blood sugar. Glucocorticoids also have anti-inflammatory, anti-allergic and anti-insulin actions.

(c) The *zona reticularis* secretes the *anabolic* or sex hormones.

(2) The inner *medulla*, which secretes mainly *adrenaline* but also *noradrenaline*. Secretion is controlled by the sympathetic nervous system and is stimulated in times of stress or fear. Adrenaline is responsible for the 'fight or flight' function.

The liver

The liver is the largest gland in the body and accounts for approximately 1% of the bodyweight in the adult horse. It is made up of four lobes: left, quadrate, right and caudate lobes. The latter two lobes are difficult to differentiate, whereas the former are separated by a fissure containing the round ligament.

The liver is supplied with blood from two main sources. The *portal vein* carries blood that is low in oxygen but very high in nutrients absorbed from the gastrointestinal system. The liver is responsible for the storage, metabolism and transformation of these nutrients. The *hepatic artery* provides a rich source of oxygen to the liver cells (Fig. 2.50).

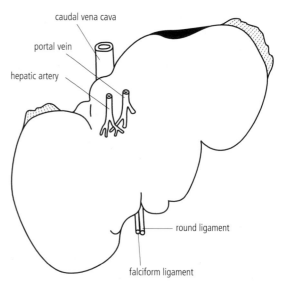

Fig. 2.50 The equine liver.

The liver is positioned asymmetrically in the abdomen, mainly on the right-hand side. It lies entirely under the ribs, up against the diaphragm. In the young foal the liver is more symmetrical and larger, extending beyond the rib cage. Certain diseases also may cause the liver to enlarge in adult horses (*hepatomegaly*).

Bile is secreted by the hepatocytes (i.e. liver cells). The horse does not have a gall bladder, instead the bile drains continuously into ductules and ducts, which converge to form the hepatic duct. The *hepatic duct* opens into the cranial duodenum where it shares a papilla with the major pancreatic duct.

Functions of the liver

• Production and secretion of bile: *bile* acts like a detergent to break down fat in the intestinal lumen, it aids the absorption of lipids and lipid-soluble substances such as vitamins A, D, E and K. Bile consists mainly of bile acids, more than 95% of which are reabsorbed from the intestine and returned to the liver. This recycling is called the *enterohepatic circulation*.

• Lipid metabolism: the liver is involved in converting fat into simpler substances for transport to and use in other tissues. Fatty acids also can be converted for use as an energy source if there is insufficient glucose due to either reduced intake or increased energy demands. Excess carbohydrate is converted to fat by the liver. This is under the control of the hormone insulin.

- Carbohydrate metabolism: the liver is involved in the synthesis, storage and release of carbohydrates, and in this way maintains a normal blood glucose level. Glucose is absorbed from the gut and transported to the liver via the portal blood, where it is converted to glycogen and stored.
- Protein metabolism: the liver is responsible for the production of 90% of the plasma proteins, including proteins such as clotting factors, albumin and fibrinogen. If there are excess amino acids, or if there is insufficient carbohydrate for energy production, the liver is able to convert amino acids to useful precursors for the synthesis of glucose. This leads to the production of ammonia, a substance that is produced also by other tissues and the intestinal microflora and released into the circulation. Ammonia is toxic and so is converted in the liver to urea—a less toxic material—before transport to the kidneys for excretion.
- Detoxification of harmful substances by a process called biotransformation, which alters the toxic compound so that it can be excreted more easily in the bile or urine.

- Formation of red blood cells (haematopoiesis) in embryonic life.
- Storage of minerals and vitamins.

The urinary system

The kidneys

The kidneys of the horse have a flat surface and are a brown-red colour. They are situated either side of the midline ventral to the epaxial musculature in the retroperitoneal space. The left kidney resembles a bean in shape and is 15–20 cm long and 11–15 cm wide. The cranial pole lies approximately at the level of the 17th rib (16–18). It is very slightly mobile. Laterally it borders onto the dorsal part of the spleen with which it is connected via the nephrosplenic ligament. The right kidney of the horse is heart-shaped and is situated more cranially. It is about 13–15 cm long and 15–18 cm wide. The cranial pole lies at the level of the 16th rib (14–17). It reaches the liver where it forms the renal impression into the caudate lobe of the liver. The ventral surface of the kidney is covered by the fibrous attachment of the caecum to the dorsal body wall (Fig. 2.51).

On the medial and ventral aspect of the kidney, the *hilus* is the location of entry for the renal artery and the exit portal for the renal vein and the ureter. On the cut surface of a kidney, the cortex and medulla can be

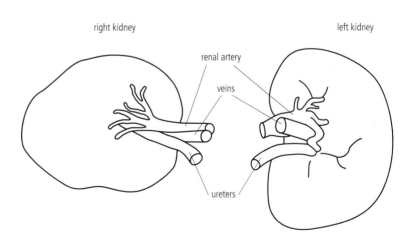

Fig. 2.51 The equine kidneys.

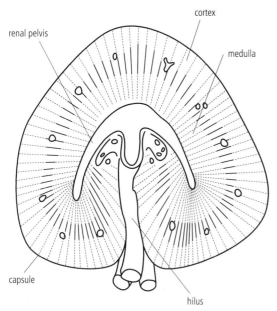

renal pelvis

cortex

medulla

capsule

hilus

Fig. 2.52 Section through equine kidney.

distinguished. The *cortex* is the outer part containing the glomeruli and the *medulla* is the inner part containing mainly the *loops of Henle* and collecting ducts. The innermost part of the kidney is occupied by the *renal pelvis*. The pelvis acts as a collection vessel and transports the urine into the ureters (Fig. 2.52).

The functional unit of the kidney is the *nephron*. The nephron consists of:

(1) The glomerulus.
(2) The proximal convoluted tubule.
(3) The loop of Henle.
(4) The distal convoluted tubule that ends in a collecting duct.

The physiological functions of the kidney are:

• Excretion of metabolic waste products, especially urea.
• Maintaining the homeostasis (biological balance) of water, electrolytes and ions.
• Endocrine (hormonal) functions.

The tubular system and the blood vessels are intimately related so that substances can be passed easily between them. The kidney has an extremely

good blood supply with 20–25% of cardiac output going to the kidneys. Three processes lead to the production of urine.

• Glomerular filtration
• Tubular reabsorption
• Tubular secretion

Water and soluble contents of the blood are pressed into the glomerular capsule by a process called glomerular filtration. A healthy kidney does not allow larger molecules such as proteins or even larger blood cells to escape into the urine. The primary filtrate is produced in large volumes. This process is not selective for any substances. The kidney therefore needs to reabsorb substances that are important to the body.

Selective reabsorption of water and electrolytes takes place in the tubules, primarily in the loop of Henle. The body therefore can retain sufficient water to maintain fluid balance. Electrolytes are also reabsorbed in a way that keeps their plasma concentration constant. Ions like bicarbonate also are selectively reabsorbed to keep the blood pH constant. All of the glucose that is contained in the primary filtrate is reabsorbed. Tubular secretion also is important for the body to dispose of foreign organic substances (Fig. 2.53).

The kidney's endocrine role is:

(1) To produce *renin* when blood pressure is low. Renin triggers the production of angiotensin, which effects vasoconstriction and therefore increases blood pressure. Renin also stimulates the production of *aldosterone*, a hormone that regulates the secretion and reabsorption of sodium and potassium.
(2) To produce *erythropoietin*, which stimulates the production of red blood cells in the bone marrow.

The ureter

The ureters are small tubes about 70 cm long that transport urine to the bladder. The ureters leave the pelvis of the kidney at the hilus and travel caudally in the retroperitoneal space to reach the bladder. The ureter is constructed of three layers:

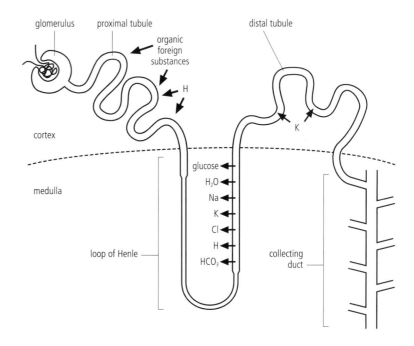

Fig. 2.53 Kidney function.

(1) The innermost, mucosal layer has longitudinal folds and is covered by transitional epithelium. In the proximal part of the horse's ureter, the mucosa also contains mucous glands, which are responsible for the typical mucoid appearance of the horse's urine.

(2) The muscular layer consists of three strata: an inner longitudinal, a middle circular and an outer longitudinal stratum.

(3) The outermost layer is the adventitia.

Urine is transported by rhythmic peristaltic contractions.

The bladder

The bladder is an expansile sack-like organ. Its function is to store urine between episodes of *micturition* (urination). The bladder is roughly cone shaped, with a blunt end (vertex) pointing cranially, a body (corpus) and the pointed end—the neck (cervix)—caudally leading into the urethra. The wall of the bladder has three layers, similar to the ureters.

The ureters join the bladder at the bladder neck. After penetrating the bladder wall they run

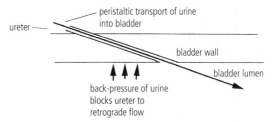

Fig. 2.54 The equine ureter.

obliquely through the whole thickness of the wall and end in small slit-like openings in the bladder lumen. The purpose of this oblique angle of the ureter penetrating the bladder is to form an effective valve to prevent urine flowing back from the bladder into the ureter. The area on the inside of the bladder neck, where the two ureters insert and the urethra takes its origin, is called the *trigone* of the bladder (Fig. 2.54).

The urethra

The female urethra is relatively short. It transports the urine during micturition from the bladder into the vestibule of the vagina. The male urethra is considerably longer, because it passes along the bottom of the pelvis, around the ischium and then ventral and cranial into the penis. The urethra has the same wall structure as described for the ureters.

Skin

The skin is the largest organ of the body. It forms a barrier between the horse and its environment. The skin is composed of:

(1) The *epidermis*, which is the thinner superficial upper layer made up of multiple layers of different cell types.

(2) The *dermis* is the thicker layer below the epidermis. It is composed of fibres, ground substance and cells. It also contains the *erector pili* muscles, blood and lymph vessels and nerves. It accounts for most of the tensile strength and elasticity of the skin and is involved in remodelling, maintenance and repair.

(3) The *subcutaneous layer* is below the dermis. It consists of areolar and adipose tissues. Fibres from the dermis extend into this layer and anchor the skin to it. The subcutis in turn attaches to the underlying tissues and organs. It functions as an energy reserve (due to its high adipose content), as a heat insulator and maintains the surface contours.

At each body orifice the skin is continuous with the mucous membranes. Skin and hair coat varies with species, breed, age, gender and area of body.

Functions of the skin

- Acting as a barrier *and* also creating an internal environment for all other organs by preventing loss of water, electrolytes and macromolecules.
- Protection from physical abrasion, bacterial invasion and UV radiation.
- Regulation of body temperature: using cutaneous blood supply, sweat glands and the support of the hair coat.
- Adnexa production, i.e. producing keratinised structures such as hair and the horny layer of the epidermis.
- Sensation: primary sense organ for touch, pressure, pain, itch, heat and cold.
- Secretion: various glands.
- Excretion: limited function, e.g. urea.
- Immunity: keratinocytes, lymphocytes and other cells form important components of the skin's immune system.

Sweat

Horses have the most numerous and best developed sweat (or sudoriferous) glands of the domestic species. They are found in most areas but are less developed on the skin of the mane, tail, middle of back and limbs. They are absent on the lips close to the mucocutaneous junction and around the margin of the ergot and hoof.

Horses will sweat profusely in response to exercise, pain, excitement or high temperatures.

Hair

Hairs are epidermal growths whose primary function is protection. A hair consists of columns of dead keratinised cells welded together. It is made up of a root (which penetrates the dermis) and a shaft (a superficial portion projecting from the skin surface). Hair growth is cyclical. In horses this happens twice yearly in autumn and spring when the summer coat is shed for winter, and vice versa. The hair cycle is influenced by several factors such as nutrition, hormones, general health and genetics.

In the growth stage (*anagen*) the hair is formed by the differentiation of matrix cells that divide, keratinise and die. As new cells are added at the hair root, the hair gets longer. In the resting stage (*telogen*) the matrix becomes inactive and the follicle partially atrophies. After this period a new growth stage starts and the new hair pushes the old one out of the follicle.

There are four types of hair in horses:

(1) General coat or cover hairs that are shed in response to environmental or hormonal factors.

(2) Coarse, permanent or 'guard' hairs found on the mane, tail, forelock and over the ergot.

(3) Fine hairs on the ears, nares, lips, anal region, teat and ventral tail.

(4) Special hairs (cilia, eyelashes, sinus hairs or vibrissae). The vibrissae project beyond the coat hairs and are stiff and tactile. Eyelashes have specific protective function, particularly with the prominent eyes of the horse.

Further reading

Hickman, J. & Humphrey, M. (1987) The foot and shoeing. In: *Horse Management*, 2nd edn, ed. by J. Hickman, pp. 246–253. Academic Press, London.

Pearson, A.J. (1997) Anatomy and physiology. In: *Veterinary Nursing*, ed. by D.R. Lane & B. Cooper, pp. 255–319. Butterworth-Heinemann, Oxford.

Skerritt, G.C. & McLelland, J. (1984) *An Introduction to Functional Anatomy of the Limbs of Domestic Animals*. Wright, Bristol.

CHAPTER 3

Genetics

G. A. Munroe

Genetics is the study of inheritance and its effect on health and disease.

Chromosomes

Within the nucleus of each cell in the body are structures called *chromosomes*, which hold the 'genetic blueprint' for that particular animal. Each species has a characteristic number of chromosomes:

Horse = 64
Donkey = 62
Wild ass = 56
Man = 46

Two of these chromosomes in each species are called the *sex chromosomes*, designated X and Y, because they determine the sex of the individual. Male animals have an X and Y chromosome, termed XY, whereas females have two X chromosomes, i.e. XX. The remaining chromosomes are called *autosomes*.

Chromosomes are normally present in pairs (i.e. *diploid*). Thus, the horse has 32 pairs, with one of each pair being derived from each parent. When two chromosomes forming a pair are alike, they are said to be *homologous*.

Chromosomes consist of long molecules of deoxyribonucleic acid (*DNA*) and associated proteins. The genetic code is contained within the complex structure of the DNA molecule (Fig. 3.1).

Genes

A gene represents a particular segment of a chromosome, which codes for a particular characteristic in the individual, e.g. coat colour. The gene serves as a code for the exact structure of a specific protein. Its location at a particular point on the chromosome is referred to as the *gene locus*. Genes that are located on the sex chromosomes are termed *sex-linked genes*. Because the X chromosome is larger, this contains more genes than the Y chromosome.

The genetic make-up of an animal is termed the *genotype*, whereas its actual physical appearance is termed the *phenotype*. Without access to sophisticated genetic investigation techniques, the genetic make-up of an individual has to be judged on the phenotype and the results of breeding. Many traits in animals are influenced by a number of genes and environmental factors and therefore the genotype and phenotype are not identical.

Mutation

Damage to a chromosome at a gene locus may disrupt the gene code and alter the original characteristic for which it was responsible. This is called gene *mutation*. Over 99% of mutations that have been studied have been found to be harmful to the animal. Less than 1% of mutations give the individual an advantage, thus forming a basis of evolution and possible progress in breeding.

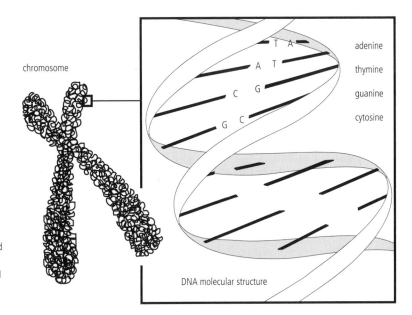

chromosome

adenine
thymine
guanine
cytosine

DNA molecular structure

Fig. 3.1 The molecular structure of DNA and its organisation into a chromosome showing the base pairs adenine, thymine, guanine and cytosine. (Reproduced with permission from Harrison, 2000).

Alleles

Alleles are two or more alternative versions of the same gene, only one of which will be present on one particular chromosome. They arise because of small mutations in genes. One allele at a time occupies the locus, but there are two loci (one on each homologous chromosome) derived from the mother and father, leading to two alleles per cell.

Dominant/recessive genes

If the two alleles in the cell are different but both are expressed, the genes are said to be *co-dominant*. Some genes are expressed only if there are two copies of the same allele in the cell, i.e. *recessive* genes. Other *dominant* genes are expressed when only one copy is present because it suppresses the other allele. In genetic terminology the dominant gene is given a capital letter, e.g. B, whereas the recessive gene is given a lower case letter, e.g. b.

If there are two copies of the same allele then the term *homozygous* is used (BB, bb), whereas *heterozygous* denotes two different alleles (Bb). A simple hypothetical example to illustrate this is shown in Fig. 3.2 using coat colour. This example could be applied to any other pair of genes. In reality, in the horse, most coat colour inheritance involves independent inheritance or complex gene interactions.

Epistasis

Some genes are able to suppress other genes' expression even though they are not the same allele (i.e. at a different gene locus). This is called *epistasis*. An example is the albino gene that blocks the expression of all other coat colour genes.

The cell cycle

Replication of the cell involves a period of synthesis when new genetic material is manufactured, a brief resting stage and then nuclear division that allows separation of new genetic material into the two daughter cells. The process of cell replication in the majority of cells in the body is called *mitosis*. This allows exact replication of the genetic material into each new cell.

Meiosis is the process of gamete formation. This is similar to mitosis but is a longer and more complicated process (Fig. 3.3). The chromosomes are separated to reduce their total number by half

P	BB x BB	Bb x BB	Bb x Bb			
F₁	BB (black)	BB (black)	Bb (black)	BB (black)	Bb (black)	Bb (black)	bb (chestnut)
P	bb x bb	bb x BB	bb x Bb			
F₁	bb (chestnut)	Bb (black)	bB (black)	bb (chestnut)	bB (black)	bb (chestnut)

Fig. 3.2 Hypothetical example to illustrate coat colour inheritance by considering only one pair of alleles without interference in expression by other genes. If B = black and b = chestnut, with the former dominant, three types of horse can be produced; BB (black, homozygous), Bb (black heterozygous) and bb (chestnut, homozygous). There are six possible matings involving these three kinds of individuals. P = parent and F₁ = first filial generation, i.e. offspring.

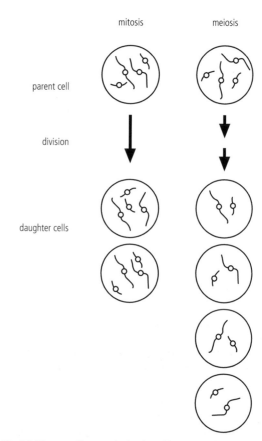

Fig. 3.3 Diagram to illustrate what is achieved by mitosis and meiosis. A standard cell will contain pairs of chromosomes, illustrated as two pairs in this simplified example. Mitotic division maintains this, i.e. the diploid condition. Meiosis results in the daughter cells each containing only one of each type of chromosome, the haploid condition.

(*haploid*) so that each gamete contains one copy of each pair of alleles. Following copulation and gamete fusion, the zygote is formed with the correct number of chromosomes for the species. Thus, any foal has half of its chromosomes and genes from each parent.

During the process of gamete formation, Mendel's First Law of Genetics states that alleles separate to different gametes. The Second Law of Genetics states that each pair of alleles separates independently of every other pair of alleles, which leads to the inheritance of large numbers of genes without being influenced by the presence of other genes. Exceptions do, however, occur due to the phenomenon of *linkage*.

Linkage

The separation of genes independently during meiosis is achieved less easily if they occur on the same chromosome. Such genes are said to be linked. If the genes are on the sex chromosomes they are said to be sex-linked. Animals that inherit a linked gene are highly likely to inherit the other associated gene, which may or may not be an advantage. The phenomenon of *crossing-over*, which occurs during meiosis, does allow some separation of genes, but the closer they are on the chromosome, the more likely they are to be inherited together (Fig. 3.4).

Sex-linked genetic disease in the horse is rare. Haemophilia (a blood-clotting problem) is an example of a sex-linked recessive trait reported in Thoroughbreds, Standardbreds, Arabians and Quarter horses. This disease is also an example of a sex-limited gene disease, i.e. genes expressed only in one sex because only the homozygous male is affected clinically.

Multifactorial inheritance

The characteristics of a particular animal can be determined by a single gene or, more commonly, by

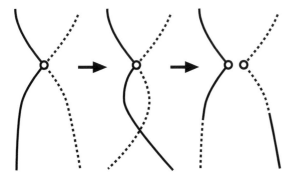

Fig. 3.4 Schematic diagram to illustrate linkage and crossing over of genetic material on a pair of chromosomes during meiosis.

a number of genes in variable combination (i.e. it is *polygenic*). The variable combination can lead to variation in the expressed characteristic.

The degree of gene expression can be influenced also by environmental factors, leading to a multifactorial characteristic. An obvious example in the horse is the ability to run fast. This is influenced not only by the breeding of the animal but also by environmental factors such as nutrition, training, disease, rider ability and many other factors. It is difficult to control and modify polygenic characteristics by selective breeding because of the large number of factors involved.

The development of a horse throughout its life is determined by a complex interaction between genetic and environmental factors. Rarely, some diseases have a simple straightforward genetic cause, such as combined immunodeficiency disease (CID) in Arabian foals. Some genetic abnormalities of the horse are described as lethal, i.e. causing death. True lethal factors that are expressed prior to or shortly after birth include CID and lethal white syndrome (see inherited diseases below).

Breeding strategies

Inbreeding

This is defined as the breeding of two individuals more closely related than the average of the breed or population. Horsebreeders aim for specific traits, which in genetic terms involves obtaining homozy-

gosity for those particular traits, so-called 'breeding true'. This quest is most often achieved by breeding animals that are related to each other to increase the likelihood of the same alleles being present and therefore similar offspring. The closer the inbreeding, i.e. brother/sister, father/daughter, the more rapidly homozygosity is achieved. Unfortunately, both desirable and undesirable gene combinations will be produced in the increasingly homozygous state. Ruthless selection is required to remove the unwanted gene expressions. Masking of desirable genes may occur by some undesirable homozygous recessive genes. Generally a slower rate of inbreeding leads to more effective selection. All inbreeding results show an initial improvement, but once 62.5–75% homozygosity is reached, loss of vigour usually occurs.

Linebreeding

The most common form of inbreeding is *linebreeding*. Linebreeding is an attempt to get as much genetic material of a particular animal (usually a stallion or outstanding mare) into the animals of the herd/breed as possible, while keeping the amount of inbreeding as low as possible. It relies heavily on the correct selection of the particular horse, which should be vigorous and based on the assessment of many traits, preferably including performance. The term linebreeding comes from the common practice of mating within a family or line. Matings are often cousins, grandparents or children, which increases the homozygosity to some extent, but the offspring have more variety, allowing further selection for specific traits and less culling of bad alleles. Linebreeding has been practised for hundreds of years in many breeds of horse, especially Thoroughbreds and Arabians, leading to considerable homozygosity.

Outcrossing or outbreeding

Outcrossing is defined as mating two individuals together that are less closely related, i.e. breeding two unrelated lines. This produces individuals that are less likely to have the same alleles and are more heterozygous. This tends to mask the effects of recessive genes, leading to *hybrid vigour* or *heterosis*. The theory is that bigger and/or better offspring are produced (heterozygous for bad recessive genes) but such horses do not necessarily breed true, i.e. you may produce a great racehorse but they do not necessarily go on to produce great horses.

Outbreeding or crossbreeding increases heterosis even further, e.g. Anglo-Arabs or Thoroughbred crosses with warmbloods or cold breeds, such as draft horses. An extreme example involves the production of an infertile mule, i.e. jack donkey to horse mare, which is actually cross-species breeding.

Progeny testing

Progeny testing is an effective method of determining the genetic make-up of breeding stock and, in particular, the degree of homozygosity. In addition, it is useful in identifying heterozygous breeding animals that are carrying a recessive gene. Progeny testing involves keeping careful breeding records on planned matings, so that genotypes can be determined.

Genetic diseases

Congenital abnormalities

The term 'congenital' is often misinterpreted to mean an inherited or genetic problem. In fact, *congenital* is defined as a malformation of the body present at birth. It may or may not be genetic in origin. Genetic investigation of diseases and defects is difficult. Breeders may be unwilling to participate in surveys to evaluate defects, because it may affect the value of their stock. Many congenital abnormalities are said to be inherited, purely on suspicion or on comparison with other species, but this is frequently unproven.

Inherited defects

These defects or diseases of the horse are caused by genes acquired from either or both of its parents. They may or may not manifest themselves at birth. Some are inherited multifactorially (Tables 3.1 and 3.2).

Table 3.1 Known or strongly suspected inherited defects in the horse

Agammaglobulinaemia

Aniridia

Aplasia cutis (epitheliogenesis imperfecta)

Arabian fading syndrome

Cataracts

Combined immunodeficiency disease

Curly coat

Fell pony syndrome

Gonadal dysgenesis

Haemophilia A

Hereditary multiple exostosis

Hyperkalaemic periodic paralysis

Ileocolonic aganglionosis (lethal white syndrome)

Intersexuality

Junctional mechanobullous disease

Lavender foal syndrome

Linear keratosis

Night blindness

Occipitoatlantoaxial malformation

Selective IgM deficiency

Spotted and reticulated leukotrichia

Von Willebrand's disease

Specific inherited diseases in the horse

Combined immunodeficiency disease

Combined immunodeficiency disease is an inherited, autosomal recessive disease of Arabians and Arabian crossbred horses. This genetic defect prevents maturation of both T and B cells in affected foals, so their immune system malfunctions. The passive transfer of immunoglobulins from the dam allows protection for the first 3–8 weeks but as these are destroyed opportunist infections (bacterial, viral, fungal or protozoal) become established.

Foals are produced only when heterozygous stallions are mated with heterozygous mares and therefore confirmation of the diagnosis in the foal confirms that the mare and stallion are carriers and should not be rebred. Continued use of heterozygous horses in breeding programmes perpetuates the problem by increasing the pool of carrier animals (25% of Arabian horses in the USA in one estimate).

A recent discovery of the actual base pair in the DNA of the encoding gene means that heterozygous animals now can be identified. A genetic test is available to identify carriers.

Table 3.2 Those diseases and disorders thought to be examples of multifactorial inheritance or where there appears to be evidence of a genetic predisposition

Angular limb deformities
Atresia coli
Cardiac defects, e.g. ventricular septal defects
Cerebellar abiotrophy
Cerebellar hypoplasia
Cervical vertebral malformation (wobbler syndrome)
Cleft palate
Contracted foal syndrome
Dermoid cysts
Epididymal aplasia
Hair follicle dystrophy
Hydrocephalus
Idiopathic laryngeal hemiplegia
Lack of libido
Lateral luxation of the patella
Maxillary/mandibular prognathism
Myelodysplasia/vertebral anomalies
Polydactylism
Sterotypies
Sweet itch (Culicoides hypersensitivity)
Umbilical and inguinal hernias

Lethal white syndrome (ileocolonic aganglionosis)

This is a rare disorder in paint foals reported in association with a recessive lethal white gene. Affected newborn paint foals demonstrate albinism coupled with congenital defects of the intestinal tract, which are not compatible with life.

Two types of lethal white syndrome have been reported: a dominant gene that causes early embryonic death in the homozygous condition; a recessive gene that results from breeding of two overo paints (overo is a term used to describe different spotting patterns of the coat in paints and pintos). When the recessive gene is homozygous, the lethal white syndrome occurs. Affected foals are small at birth and rapidly develop functional obstruction of the gastrointestinal tract, leading to euthanasia or death.

Fell pony syndrome

This disease appears to be due to a single recessive,

autosomal gene leading to a bone marrow stem cell problem (aplasia) and poor immunity. A variety of secondary infections occur insidiously after approximately 7 days of age, causing 100% mortality at 3–16 weeks of age despite treatment. Investigation of the condition is ongoing, in the hope that an effective control programme may be introduced.

Hyperkalaemic periodic paresis (HYPP)

This is a disorder affecting Quarterhorses and their crosses, American paint horses and Appaloosas. Affected horses experience episodes of muscle tremors and weakness, which may produce collapse. This inherited trait is transmitted as autosomal dominant, similar to the condition in man. The gene responsible has been identified in descendents of the Quarterhorse sire 'Impressive'. Although the majority of animals survive, they should not be bred. A DNA blood test is available to identify carriers of the HYPP gene.

Ophthalmic diseases

Congenital cataracts are seen occasionally (Fig. 3.5) that may have a variety of causes, including *teratogenicity* (i.e. toxic causes of congenital conditions). They are more common in some breeds but inheritance, although suspected, is not proven. The only definite inherited cataracts have been described in the Morgan horse, although the exact mode of inheritance is not yet known.

Aniridia is a rare condition in which there is partial or complete absence of the iris. It occurs with associated secondary cataracts and other problems as an inherited condition in Belgian draft horses.

Equine night blindness is a congenital, non-progressive disease that produces visual disturbance in conditions of reduced light. Appaloosas are particularly predisposed and a hereditary basis has been proposed. The exact mode of transmission has not been defined but it is thought to be recessive or sex-linked recessive with the defect on the X chromosome.

Immunogenetics

This is a branch of genetics concerned with the inheritance of antigenic and other characters related to the immune response.

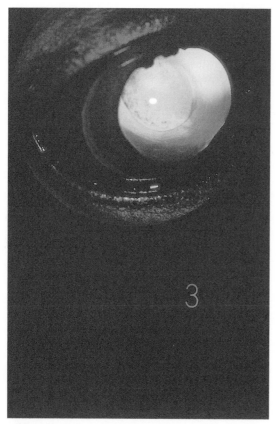

Fig. 3.5 A nuclear cataract in a foal. In the Morgan there is evidence that this may be inherited.

Blood typing

In the horse the genetics of red blood cell antigens is important in breed blood typing. The surfaces of cells are covered with molecules of various types and with various functions, the presence or absence of which is genetically determined. These red blood cell alloantigens form the basis for blood groups and there are seven different genetic systems or loci identified with them (A, C, D, K, P, Q and U). Within the seven systems there are 34 serologically detectable factors that are recognised internationally. The most common factors involved in neonatal isoerythrolysis are Aa and Qa.

Genetic markers in the horse, such as red blood cell and other protein markers, are used for identification and verification of parentage, known as *blood typing*. The effectiveness of blood typing depends on the number of genetic systems tested and the number and distribution of various alleles. Using a battery of 20 loci, blood typing is estimated to be 94–96% effective for recognising incorrect paternity in Thoroughbreds, Standardbreds, Arabians, Quarterhorses and Morgans; DNA fingerprinting (e.g. from hair samples) will increase the efficiency of parentage testing to almost 100%.

Another application of genetic markers is for the study of the inherited basis of disease. Already a number of diseases have been 'associated' with one or more genetic markers, suggesting that some direct cause and effect exists. By mapping the equine genome, it is possible to study the linkage between genetic markers and disease traits, allowing the detection of carriers and the genes and their involvement in disease.

Further reading

Harrison, S. (2000) A brave new world? Thoroughbred genetics in the 21st century. In: *Guardians of the Horse: Past, Present and Future*, ed. by P.D. Rossdale, T.R.C. Greet, P.A. Harris, R.E. Green & S. Hall, pp. 275–285. Romney Publications, Newmarket.

Jones, W.E. (1982) *Genetics and Horse Breeding*. Lea & Febiger, Philadelphia, PA.

Long, S.E. (1998) Genetics and animal breeding. In: *Veterinary Nursing*, 5th Edn, ed. by D.R. Lane & B. Cooper, pp. 399–408. Butterworth-Heinemann, Oxford.

Nicholas, F.W. (1987) *Veterinary Genetics*. Oxford University Press, Oxford.

Trommerhausen-Smith, A. (1980) Aspects of genetics and disease in the horse. *J. Anim. Sci.* **51**, 1087–1095.

CHAPTER 4

Reproduction

J. F. Pycock

Reproductive anatomy of the mare

The mare's reproductive organs are situated within the pelvic and abdominal cavities (Fig. 4.1):

(1) The *vulva* forms the external opening of the reproductive tract. This is directly ventral to the anus. The two vulval lips should be full and firm and meet evenly in the midline (Fig. 4.2). Mares with an abnormal vulval shape can suck air and foreign material into the vagina and uterus. Consequently, infections develop and conception will be prevented.

(2) The *clitoris* is contained within a depression (the clitoral fossa) at the lower end of the vulva. It is important because particular bacteria can live there and these cause potentially serious venereal infections. Infected mares show no outward signs of these venereal bacteria, which are detected only when the vet takes a swab from the clitoris (see Chapter 12). When a mare is in oestrus (i.e. heat), the clitoris is repeatedly exposed; this is termed 'winking'.

(3) The *vagina* is a potentially hollow tubular structure that extends from the vestibulovaginal constriction to the external opening of the cervix. At the junction between the vagina and the vestibule there is a fold of skin overlying the external urethral opening. In maiden mares (mares that have not been mated by a stallion) this fold may continue on either side of the vagina forming the hymen. If the hymen is complete it may have to be broken gently to allow breeding. The vagina is mostly retroperitoneal (i.e. it lies outside the peritoneal cavity.) This means that penetrating injuries to the vagina do not usually enter the peritoneal space.

(4) The *cervix* is a thick-walled tubular structure that can be identified by palpation transrectally. The cervix forms an important protective physical barrier for the uterus, providing the last line of defence between the uterine lumen and the external environment.

(5) The *uterus* is a Y- or T-shaped muscular organ that is made up of a cranial body and two more caudal uterine horns. At times the uterus is intermingled with the intestines and bladder. Its position may be changed depending on the degree of filling of the bladder or intestines. The uterus is lined by a secretory epithelium and has a thick muscle layer. Changes in the latter are responsible for the differences in uterine tone at oestrus, dioestrus and early pregnancy. Prominent glands open into the uterine lumen and extend into the depth of the *endometrium*, which is the uterine lining. These glands have an important function in early pregnancy because they secrete the uterine 'milk' that is responsible for the nutrition of the early embryo.

(6) The *uterine tubes* (fallopian tubes or oviducts) lie at the end of each uterine horn and are long

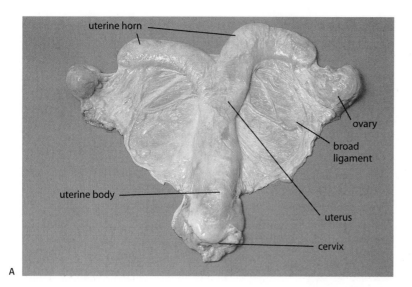

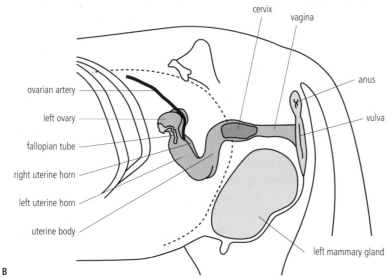

Fig. 4.1 The reproductive tract: (a) gross specimen; (b) schematic diagram.

B

(20–30 cm), extending from the horns of the uterus to the ovaries. They are the site of fertilisation and where the early embryo resides for 5.5 days before entering the uterus. The mare has a unique ability to retain unfertilised ova within the uterine tubes.

(7) The *ovaries* are broad bean-shaped and vary in size. The mature *oocyte* (i.e. egg cell) is shed from the follicle and captured by the uterine tube. During spring and summer the ovary often has several follicles of different sizes developing before ovulation. The ovaries are smaller during the autumn and winter, when they are hard with no large follicles. The actual location of the ovaries in the abdomen is variable but they are usually below the 3rd / 4th lumbar vertebrae.

(8) *Suspensory apparatus, vessels* and *nerves*: the uterus is suspended within the pelvic cavity and abdomen by two large ligamentous sheets called the *broad ligaments*. These not only provide attachment to the body wall but also provide an avenue for blood vessels, lymphatic vessels and

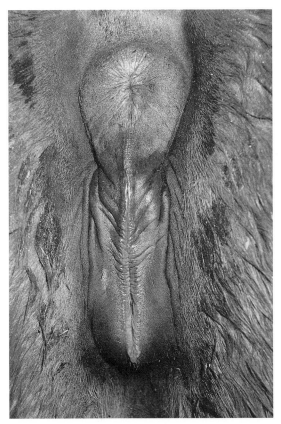

Fig. 4.2 The normal vulva.

old and above. However, many mares are bred successfully as 2-year-olds. The best approach is to consider each mare as an individual and to decide if she is cycling normally and is mature enough to conceive and carry a foal successfully to term.

The normal oestrous cycle

- The mare is seasonally polyoestrous with cyclical ovarian activity occurring during the spring, summer and autumn. Non-domesticated, feral mares do not normally undergo cyclical ovarian activity (anoestrus) during the winter and early spring months. However, some domesticated mares will cycle regularly throughout the year.
- The mare does not suddenly start to cycle regularly, but enters what is known as a 'transitional phase'. This is the period between winter anoestrus and the onset of normal cyclical activity.
- The horse is a long day breeder, daylight being the most important influence. This seasonality means that foals are born in the spring and early summer, which is the time when the environmental conditions should be optimal for foal survival. Therefore, the natural breeding season of the horse is from May until July. This is the time when highest pregnancy rates are likely to occur.

Man has superimposed his requirements of when mares should foal on this natural pattern. Since the early 19th century, when 1st January was declared the official birth-date for thoroughbred foals in the UK, irrespective of their actual birthdates within that year, horse breeders have had difficulty in breeding mares early in the year. For some types of horse, notably thoroughbreds, an operational breeding season exists, which is the 15th February until the first week of July. This artificial 'man-made' breeding season means that mares are in the transitional period between winter anoestrus and the regular cycles of summer when they are bred.

During the transitional period there is prolonged oestrus, and thus the time of ovulation, which is the optimum time to breed mares, is difficult to determine. Before the first ovulation of the year there is poor correlation between sexual behav-

nerves. The main blood supply to the uterus is from the uterine artery. Occasionally at foaling, rupture of the uterine arteries can occur with very serious consequences.

Puberty

Puberty precedes the development of physical maturity and occurs in the mare by 2 years of age, (average 18 months). Some mares may ovulate as yearlings in late summer if they were born in late winter, therefore a mare can conceive at an early age. Puberty can be delayed by poor nutrition, being in heavy work (e.g. racehorses in training) and/or the administration of drugs such as anabolic steroids.

It is not recommended to breed from immature mares. Although 2-year-old mares often cycle, the heat periods may not be as regular as in horses 3 years iour and ovarian activity. However, once ovulation has occurred, regular cycles usually follow.

The oestrous cycle can be divided into two phases:

- The *follicular phase* (also known as *oestrus*) is when the mare will allow the stallion to mate her. Typically oestrus lasts an average of 6 days.
- The *luteal phase* (also known as *dioestrus*) is when the mare is not receptive to the stallion.

Dioestrus lasts 14–15 days on average and is usually more constant in duration than oestrus. The oestrous cycles last on average 22 days. Cycle length is very variable and the cycle tends to be longer in the spring and shortest from June to September.

At the end of oestrus, the follicle has enlarged and ovulation releases the oocyte. Ovulation occurs up to 48 h before the mare stops showing signs of oestrus. After ovulation, the cavity occupied by the previously mature follicle becomes filled with a blood clot to form the corpus luteum.

Normally a single oocyte is released at ovulation, but twin ovulation (associated with the maturation of two follicles) is common, particularly in thoroughbred mares where double ovulations can occur with an incidence of 30%.

The oocyte enters the uterine tube and if a stallion has mated the mare in the last 2 or 3 days there should be sperm there. The sperm then will penetrate the oocyte and fertilisation occurs.

Reproductive endocrinology in the mare

The hormones of the hypothalamic–pituitary–gonadal axis control the regular pattern of the oestrous cycle.

Central nervous system involvement

Pineal gland

Light is the major modulator of seasonal reproductive rhythms in the horse. Light perceived by the retina of the eye results in a signal being transmitted to the pineal gland. During light stimulation, the function of the pineal gland to produce the hormone melatonin is inhibited, which influences hypothalamic–pituitary function.

Hypothalamus

The decline in melatonin secretion stimulates the hypothalamus to produce increased amounts of gonadotrophin-releasing hormone (GnRH), which stimulates the release of the gonadotrophins: follicle-stimulating hormone (FSH) and luteinising hormone (LH).

The pituitary

The gonadotrophin hormones FSH and LH are released by the anterior pituitary gland in response to GnRH release. Follicle-stimulating hormone stimulates the growth and development of follicles in the ovary.

The study of the growth and development of follicles has advanced with ultrasonography. It is apparent that follicles develop in groups, know as follicle waves, and initially grow in synchrony (approximately the same diameter and growth rate) but eventually dissociate.

Luteinizing hormone is also secreted by the anterior pituitary and is involved in the final maturation of the follicles, maturation of the oocytes within the follicles and ovulation. Plasma LH levels begin to rise steadily at the end of dioestrus as the suppressive effects of progesterone are removed during luteolysis. A pre-ovulatory surge of LH brings about ovulation of the mature follicle to release the oocyte and form the corpus luteum. Unusually LH peaks 1 or 2 days after ovulation in the mare before levels fall rapidly due to the suppressive effects of progesterone secreted by the new corpus luteum.

Gonadal involvement

The ovaries

Both FSH and LH stimulate the ovaries to produce oestrogens, which cause the mare to be receptive to the stallion. Concentrations are low during most of the oestrous cycle but rise in early oestrus to peak 12–36 h before ovulation and before the LH surge.

Peripheral plasma progesterone concentrations rise rapidly after ovulation, peak at about day 6 after ovulation and then plateau. The corpus luteum produces progesterone for about 15 days, before prostaglandin F2α produced from the endometrium causes regression (luteolysis) of the corpus luteum and the mare returns to oestrus. If the mare is pregnant, the primary corpus luteum continues to produce progesterone until about day 160 of gestation. Progesterone does not suppress FSH release in the mare and so follicular development occurs during pregnancy.

Progesterone prepares the uterus for entry of the embryo and maintains pregnancy by increasing the activity of the secretory glands in the endometrium while inhibiting the motility of the myometrium. A mare will rarely show behavioural signs of oestrus when plasma progesterone concentrations exceed 2 ng/ml, even when large follicles are present on the ovaries. This is why it is important to remember that a large follicle in itself does not mean that the mare will be in oestrus.

The uterus

The uterus produces two reproductive hormones:

(1) Equine chorionic gonadotrophin (eCG, which used to be called pregnant mares' serum gonadotrophin).
(2) Prostaglandin F2α.

Cyclical changes in the reproductive tract

During winter anoestrus, the ovaries are small and the mare is usually indifferent to the attentions of a stallion. This period of sexual quietness centres on the shortest day of the year (21st December). Signs shown by the mare may include:

- A closed vulva
- A pale (blanched) and dry cervix and vagina
- A partially closed cervix, but it may gape open in some mares
- Little glandular activity in the endometrium
- A flaccid uterus
- Low oestrogen and progesterone levels

As follicles begin to grow during the spring transitional period, mares typically show intermittent oestrous behaviour towards the stallion. The transitional period is roughly centred on the spring equinox (21st March). The cervix does not close tightly until the mare has had her first ovulation of the year. Once a follicle has ovulated and the corpus luteum is formed, the mare has regular oestrous cycles.

During oestrus:

- The ovaries are large and the mare shows the signs of oestrus (raised tail, urinating frequently and everting the clitoris, i.e. 'winking').
- The vulva is relaxed and long; the cervix is pink, moist and open.
- The uterus is relaxed on palpation.
- Concentrations of oestrogen are high, whereas levels of progesterone are low.

Once the mare has ovulated:

- The ovaries become smaller because the smaller corpus luteum has replaced the big follicle.
- The oedema in the endometrium subsides.
- The mare is no longer receptive to the stallion and is often aggressive to him.
- The vulva becomes closed and the cervix is pale, dry and closed.

The middle of the mare's natural breeding season is around 21st June. As autumn approaches, cyclical activity normally wanes.

Controlling oestrus

Artificial lighting

Artificial lighting can be used to advance the onset of the breeding season. Experience has shown that 16 h of light stimulus (artificial + natural) is adequate. This means providing light from 7 a.m. until 11 p.m. The extra light is best added at the end of the natural daylight period. The artificial light works by suppressing the release of melatonin.

A 200-W clear bulb in the middle of a box will provide sufficient artificial lighting for 4 m × 4 m. If a strip light is used (40 W) this should be 1.3 m long. Care should be taken to eliminate shadows because they can prevent a good response. A practical method of checking that there is sufficient light is to see if it is easy to read a newspaper wherever you stand in the box. Often breeders term this procedure as 'putting the mare under lights'.

There are two important points to note when using artificial lighting regimens:

- Generally it must be started a minimum of 8–10 weeks before the mare is required to be covered. Thus, mares should be exposed to the lighting system by 1st December so that they will begin to cycle normally by 15th February. A shorter time period of artificial lighting will be ineffective.
- Mares should be in good body condition at the start of the artificial lighting regimen. It may be necessary to increase the mare's body condition by extra feeding beforehand.

Some breeders also like to expose pregnant mares to artificial lighting to ensure that the mares return to cyclical activity after foaling.

Hormones

Hormones are also used to manipulate the cycle:

- Mares coming to the end of a 2-month artificial light programme may be treated for 10–15 days with a synthetic *progestagen* to assist in the stimulation of the onset of cyclical ovarian activity. It is a liquid designed for in-feed medication. It is administered daily for 10–15 days and then stopped. The mare should come into oestrus and ovulate about 10 days later.
- To ensure that mares ovulate at a predictable time, *human chorionic gonadotrophin* (hCG) is sometimes used. Once a mare has a follicle of 35 mm and is showing good signs of oestrus, most mares will ovulate within 48 h after hCG administration. This hormone is sometimes called a '*holding injection*'. This is misleading because it implies that the mare will remain in foal following breeding. This is not true; the hormone only hastens ovulation.
- Prostaglandins (prostaglandin F2α or an analogue) can be used to shorten the normal luteal phase (or dioestrus), with oestrus occurring 3–6 days later. This will not work for the first 4–5 days after ovulation when the corpus luteum is refractory to the action of prostaglandins. In addition, prostaglandin F2α can have unpleasant side effects such as sweating, transient colic, diarrhoea and respiratory distress. Owners should be warned that these might occur but usually need no treatment. The synthetic analogues, such as cloprostenol, usually have fewer side effects.

Reproductive anatomy of the stallion

(1) The *penis* of the stallion is of the musculo-cavernous type and consists of three regions (Fig. 4.3):

the *base* (site of attachment to the skeletal system);

the *body* or shaft (main portion);

the *glans penis* (enlarged free end of the penis). The distal part of the penis is usually contained within the sheath. Two independent compartments of erectile tissues form the functional components:

(a) the *corpus spongiosum penis*, which surrounds the urethra in its entire length and is responsible for the marked enlargement (known as 'belling') of the glans at the time of erection and ejaculation;

(b) the larger *corpus cavernosum penis*, which is the main cause of erection of the penis.

An *erection* occurs during sexual excitement due to the filling of the corpus cavernosum penis with arterial blood. This, together with restricted venous drainage, leads to the drop and swelling of the penis. This blood normally cannot escape until after ejaculation. During ejaculation, further swelling of the tip occurs. This swelling dilates the mare's cervix and helps to ensure that most of the ejaculate enters the uterus. The extra swelling can be seen if the stallion dismounts from the mare before ejaculation is complete.

(2) The *prepuce* or sheath is the skin that covers and protects the retracted penis.

(3) The *urethra* is a membranous tube common to the urinary and genital system that extends from the neck of the bladder to the urethral process on the glans penis. The urethra serves as the joint excretory duct for urine and semen. The urethral fossa at the tip of the penis is where smegma often accumulates, and is one of the sites required to be swabbed for the control of venereal diseases.

(4) The *scrotum* consists of two sacs and is located in the inguinal region. It should contain two testicles in a pendulous location. However, during manual palpation or extreme cold ambient temperatures the scrotum might appear smaller and

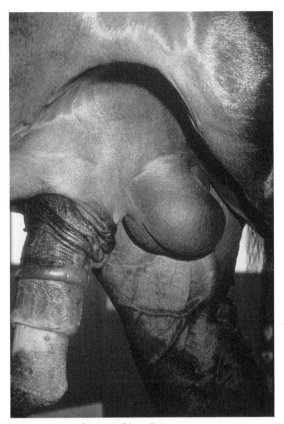

Fig. 4.3 Anatomy of the penis of the stallion.

testes will be pulled towards the abdomen. The scrotum is an important structure in regulating testicular temperature.

(5) The *testes* are two ovoid, similar-sized, freely movable organs within the scrotum. It is common to find a small percentage of stallions with rotation of one testis. Rotations of 90–180° do not appear to have an adverse effect on fertility, although total sperm output and volume can be lower in such stallions. Testicular size correlates well with daily sperm production and therefore testicular volume is an important parameter to record.

The endocrine role of the testes is the production of testosterone and oestrone sulphate, whereas the exocrine role is limited to the production of spermatozoa. Spermatogenesis (i.e. sperm production) occurs in small tubules called seminiferous tubules, which make up 70% of the testis.

These tubules are supported by interstitial or *Leydig cells*, which produce testosterone. The seminiferous tubules drain into the epididymis, where spermatozoa mature. Located within the seminiferous tubules are *Sertoli cells*, from which developing spermatozoa obtain nourishment.

(6) The *epididymis* is a single lengthy convoluted duct into which the seminiferous tubules drain. The epididymal duct enlarges as it enters the spermatic cord, forming the *deferent* duct or *vas deferens*. Spermatozoa mature in the epididymis.

(7) The *spermatic cord* contains:
   (a) the testicular artery;
   (b) veins (pampiniform plexus);
   (c) nerves;
   (d) lymphatics;
   (e) the cremaster muscle;
   (f) the vas deferens.

The testicular vein fans out and surrounds the testicular artery, thus cooling blood going to the testis. The cremaster muscle either retracts or relaxes, depending on ambient temperatures. This ability to move the testes away from the body wall affects their temperature. It is important that the testes are not at the same temperature as the rest of the body. If the temperature within the testis is elevated to body temperature for a long time or to 40°C for as little as a few hours, cells in the testis can die and sperm production is impaired.

(8) The *internal genitalia* of the stallion (Fig. 4.4) include:
   (a) three accessory sex glands (bulbo-urethral glands, prostate gland and the seminal vesicles);
   (b) the inguinal canal;
   (c) the vas deferens.

There are two *bulbo-urethral glands*, which are ovoid structures surrounded by heavy musculature located on the dorsal surface of the pelvic urethra. The secretion of the bulbo-urethral glands is a clear fluid. Its purpose probably is to clean and neutralise the pH of the urethra prior to ejaculation. The *prostate gland* is situated on both sides of the pelvic urethra. Besides providing a portion of the fluid suspension for sperm, it is believed that the prostatic fluid provides some energy to the sperm cells. The *seminal vesicles* or vesicular glands are two elongated glands located dorsally to the bladder, just cranial and slightly lateral to the prostate gland. The function of these glands is not well documented but appears to be the source of the gel or last fraction of the ejaculate. Despite their name, they do *not* contain spermatozoa.

Testicular development

The *inguinal canal* is a channel formed by a gap in the abdominal muscles, immediately anterior to the scrotum. Inguinal passage of the testis usually occurs during the last month of pregnancy or the first 2 weeks after birth. After this time, the foal's testicles should have descended through this canal and entered the scrotum. Occasionally the vaginal rings contract to prevent descent of an abdominal testis and the condition known as *cryptorchidism* results. If only one testis is undescended, the foal is termed a unilateral *cryptorchid*; if both are undescended, it is bilateral. Stallions with one or both testicles in a location other than the scrotum are referred to as *cryptorchids* or *rigs*. The cause is unknown but it may have a genetic (inheritable) component.

If the inguinal canal is too large, intestine may pass through it and cause an inguinal hernia. This occurs very rarely as a complication of castration. When the intestine extends into the scrotum, this herniation is sometimes referred to as scrotal rather than inguinal.

Puberty

Puberty can be defined as the age at which a colt is able to mount, copulate and successfully impregnate a mare. This normally occurs during the second spring after the year of birth. Season, age, breed and nutritional status affect the onset of puberty. Puberty should not be confused with sexual maturity, which occurs after the age of 5 years when the stallion attains maximum reproductive capacity. Daily sperm production is usually stable from 5 to 20 years of age. After 20 years, it may decline.

Reproductive endocrinology in the stallion

Like mares, the functioning of the stallion's reproductive system occurs in response to changes in hormone production. Although there is an apparent reduction in testicular size, testicular volume and daily sperm production in winter, the seasonal effect it is not as marked as its effect on ovarian function in the mare. Most stallions will breed all year round, but reproductive capacity is maximal

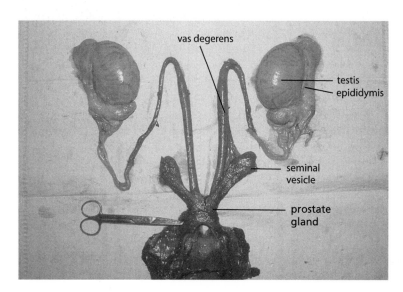

Fig. 4.4 A dissected specimen of the internal genitalia of the stallion. The scissors mark the opening of the urinary bladder into the urethra.

during the spring and summer months. Stallions usually are not exposed to artificial lighting patterns like mares.

Hypothalamic–pituitary–gonadal axis

Daylight acts via the pineal gland on the hypothalamus to release GnRH, which stimulates the pituitary gland to produce FSH and LH. The FSH acts on the Sertoli cells, whereas LH targets the interstitial or Leydig cells. These cells are the main sites of testosterone production. Through this production of testosterone, Leydig cells control the process of:

- spermatogenesis (the production of sperm cells);
- secondary sex characteristics of a stallion, which include the development of a large, thick neck and aggression towards other males;
- libido.

Spermatogenesis (sperm production)

Spermatogenesis involves growth and division of cells to produce the millions of spermatozoa (sperm) voided in each ejaculate. The development of each individual sperm takes 55–57 days and is not affected by frequency of ejaculation or season. There is a prolific production of sperm, with billions being produced daily in the mature stallion.

Spermatozoa morphology

The spermatozoon is the male gamete. It is a highly specialised cell that comprises three parts (Fig. 4.5):

(1) a sperm head formed by the nucleus and acrosome;
(2) a mid-piece;
(3) a tail.

It contains half the chromosomes (genes) of a horse, such that when fertilisation with the female gamete occurs a cell containing the full complement of genes is formed.

Libido and copulatory behaviour

Horses in the wild are long-day seasonal breeders that breed in a relatively stable social group (harem). Free running stallions also will interact with a female for hours or even days before copulation. Normally the sociosexual activity of the domesticated stallion is severely restricted. Usually, breeding stallions are confined to a paddock or a stable, and frequently do not have any interaction with mares or other horses. This type of management can result in overly aggressive and dangerous stallions. Mating and / or ejaculation normally is permitted only under one of three conditions:

(1) *Pasture breeding*, where the stallion runs with the mare (s) continuously.
(2) *Hand mating*, where the stallion is presented with a mare in oestrus; after he has covered her, they are separated.
(3) *Mount of a phantom or dummy mare* (for semen collection).

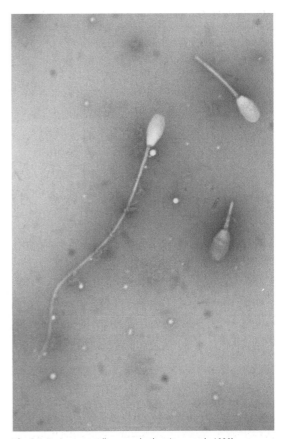

Fig. 4.5 Equine sperm cells seen under the microscope (× 1000).

Mating behaviour

There are several behavioural responses that stallions display either during teasing and / or breeding. The sexual response, also known as *libido*, is highly dependent on breeding experience, management and, in some cases, season. Libido is influenced also by olfactory, visual and auditory stimuli. Typically a normal stallion that has never bred a mare will take a longer time to mount; however, he will display good libido. On the other hand, a stallion that has had a negative previous experience might show no interest in the mare or in mounting.

A normal stallion should show interest in the mare, drop the penis within 1–2 min of exposure to a quiet mare in standing oestrus and will try to mount within the first 3 min. Once they are allowed to mount they will have several (5–8) intravaginal thrusts, followed by 3–5 short thrusts synchronous with ejaculation, urethral pulsation and flagging of the tail. A single stallion tends to be consistent in his breeding behaviour, provided that the conditions under which he is used are the same. There are three basic processes involved in the release of semen:

(1) *Erection*: the lengthening and stiffening of the penis.
(2) *Emission*: the movement and deposition of sperm and fluid from the vas deferens into the urethra.
(3) *Ejaculation*: the culmination of the process of copulation, which involves the expulsion of semen.

Normal semen characteristics

Semen (or the ejaculate) is a fluid or gelatinous suspension consisting of:

- spermatozoa
- fluid secretions (seminal plasma)

Besides these two components, semen contains a low number of epithelial cells and some bacteria originating from the lower urinary tract.

Characteristics such as volume, sperm concentration and pH of the stallion's ejaculate are highly variable and dependent on factors such as breed, frequency of collection, season and intensity of sexual stimulation before ejaculation. The total volume of the ejaculate is, on average, 30–100 ml, whereas normal sperm concentrations average 100–400 million/ml. The stallion ejaculates in three distinct fractions:

(1) A *pre-ejaculatory* fraction, observed as a translucid fluid dripping from the urethra. This fraction with little or no sperm can be observed consistently once the stallion is aroused during preparation for mating.
(2) The *sperm-rich* fraction, which is the portion of the ejaculate containing the great majority of sperm. This fraction is forcefully delivered due to 5–10 rhythmic contractions of the urethral musculature, which generates successive jets of semen. The first three jets contain three-quarters of the total sperm in the ejaculate. This is the critical part to be collected for use in artificial insemination.
(3) *The gel* or *sperm-poor* fraction, which comprises mainly secretions from the vesicular glands.

Sperm transport

The equine ejaculate is deposited directly into the uterus. Transport to the uterine tube probably occurs within a few minutes for some sperm and it has been confirmed that sperm are present in the uterine tube within 2 h after insemination.

Fertilisation

The uterine tube has the ability to transport sperm towards the ovary while transporting the ovum in the opposite direction. Fertilisation of the ovum occurs in the oviduct in mares. The fertilised egg or conceptus then takes 5–6 days to reach the uterus.

Embryonic and fetal development

The conceptus is highly mobile throughout the entire uterus until day 16 after ovulation. The early movement of the conceptus is thought to play a key role in the 'maternal recognition of pregnancy'. The mobility phase ends 16 days after ovulation, when the conceptus becomes stationary and 'fixation' occurs. The conceptus becomes fixed at the base of the right or left horn. Fixation in postpartum mares tends to occur in the previously non-gravid horn. Implantation occurs gradually and relatively late in the mare, beginning around day 40. It is not complete until around day 140. By convention, the term *embryo* is used up to day 40 and the term *fetus* thereafter.

Placentation

The placenta consists of fetal and maternal tissues that are in apposition for purposes of physiological exchange. The placenta of the mare is:

- diffuse, non-deciduate;
- epitheliochorial, because the uterine epithelium is in contact with the outer layer of the chorion;
- microcotyledonary, with the microcotyledons representing the units of placental exchange.

This non-invasive type of placentation ensures that there is no loss of maternal tissue at parturition.

The placental membranes in the mare are:

(1) The *allantochorion*: the red tougher outer fetal membrane.
(2) The *amnion*: the innermost white fetal membrane.

The umbilical cord crosses the allantoic cavity and consists of two portions (amniotic and allantoic) that can be distinguished readily.

In each placenta there is a vestigial *yolk sac remnant* within the allantoic part of the cord, which may be mistaken for a deformed remnant of a twin pregnancy. *Hippomanes* are soft putty-like aggregates of urinary calculus that form throughout pregnancy. They vary in colour and size and have a layered appearance when cut.

Endometrial cups are a unique feature of the equine placenta. On or about day 28 of gestation the chorionic girdle begins to form at the junction of the yolk sac and allantoic membranes. Specialised cells from the chorionic girdle invade the underlying uterine epithelium between days 36 and 38. Once in the endometrium, they enlarge and become clumped together to form the endometrial cups. The cups are arranged in a circle at the base of the gravid uterine horn. Endometrial cups produce eCG, which stimulates the primary corpus luteum and causes induced secondary follicles to ovulate and/or luteinise. Because progesterone production remains high, mares do not show signs of oestrus at the time of these secondary ovulations. This is independent of the presence of a fetus and so once the endometrial cups are formed, eCG production will proceed even in cases where embryonic/fetal loss occurs.

Pregnancy diagnosis

Diagnosis of early pregnancy

This is possible using ultrasound by rectal examination and, as such, is an act of veterinary surgery:

- The equine embryonic vesicle can be detected at day 11, but mares are not usually scanned that early.
- The 14-day conceptus is 13–18 mm in size and lies centrally in the uterine body. In the event of twin pregnancies, both vesicles usually can be seen at 14 days, even if the second co-twin arose from a later ovulation. This fact, together with the mobility and relatively small size of the concepti, makes 14–15 days the optimal stage of pregnancy to diagnose twins and crush one co-twin.
- By day 26 of pregnancy the embryo is highly echogenic and is clearly visible ultrasonographically, with the beating heart apparent on the scan.

Pregnancy also can be diagnosed in the mare by:

- Rectal palpation by about 28 days, but best at about 42 days.
- Blood tests: these can be used but eCG is unreliable due to the variable length of production by the endometrial cups, and oestrone sulphate cannot be measured in high concentrations until approximately day 90.
- Transabdominal ultrasound from day 80.

Suggested protocol for pregnancy diagnosis

Assuming that the day of ovulation is day 0, ultrasound is used as follows:

- First exam, day 14–15
- Second exam, day 24–27
- ±Third exam, day 33–35
- Autumn exam (rectal), October.

Following an initial examination at day 15, the aim of the examination at day 24–27 should be to assess whether the embryo is developing normally (increase in size, normal echogenicity of the yolk sac, etc.) and to identify the heartbeat. In addition, it can be confirmed that there is only a single conceptus. If twins were inadvertently missed at the earlier examination, it still may be possible to manage them correctly.

Ideally a third examination should be performed around day 33–35. The aim of this examination is to confirm that a single conceptus is developing normally. If there is failure of normal development or if twins are detected, it is usually possible to terminate the pregnancy and re-breed the mare before endometrial cups develop.

A twin pregnancy usually produces abortion at 7–8 months or undersized live or dead foals at term. The reason for the low survival rate of twins is due to competition for placental space.

The duration of pregnancy is 330–345 days, but enormous variation is possible and anywhere from 315 to 360 days is frequently reported. A useful guide to remember is 11 months and 4 days.

Preparation for foaling

Mares should be well cared for during pregnancy to ensure the birth of a normal, healthy foal. This includes:

(1) Adequate but not excessive feeding (see Chapter 5).
(2) Proper parasite control.
(3) Vaccinating the mare 1 month before foaling to ensure that her colostrum has the necessary antibodies. Vaccination of the pregnant mare has the dual purpose of protecting the dam and also the foal.
(4) Moving the mare into the environment where she is going to foal 6 weeks before she is due, so that the mare can get used to her new environment and the handling procedures. It will also ensure that her colostrum will contain the protective antibodies against infections there. Ideally mares should foal in special housing called a foaling box. The foaling box should be at least 4 × 4 m for an average 500-kg mare and be well-ventilated but free from draughts. Bedding should be dust-free, preferably comprising plenty of high-quality straw.

Monitoring the mare for foaling

A mare should be observed closely late in pregnancy. Physical changes indicating impending delivery include:

- Development of the udder or mammary gland. There is an increase in the size of the mammary gland in the last month of pregnancy and this is particularly noticeable in the 2 weeks before birth. Once this increase is noted, the mare should be moved to a foaling box where she can be watched easily during the night.
- Relaxation of the pelvic ligaments.
- Lengthening of the vulva.
- Just before foaling the udder typically becomes very swollen and there is a waxy secretion noticeable on the teat ends. This is know as 'waxing' and is usually a sign that foaling will be within 1–4 days. Sometimes milk can run from the udder ahead of foaling and lose the colostrum. Such foals can be at risk from not getting enough colostrum and must be given extra care in the first few days after foaling.

The best approach to managing a foaling mare is to watch her very closely but without disturbing her. Having an experienced attendant watching the mare and assisting if necessary is the best way of reducing the risk of problems at foaling. However, mares vary tremendously in the signs of impending foaling that they actually show, hence it is possible to waste much time waiting for a mare to foal. To avoid this, options include:

(1) Measuring the electrolyte concentrations in prefoaling udder secretions using kits that are available commercially. These kits measure electrolyte levels in a sample of udder secretion. When the amount of calcium in the milk increases above a certain level, over 95% of mares will foal within 72 h.

(2) Foaling alarm systems, such as a small transmitter lightly stitched to the mare's vulva. When she pushes the fetal membranes through the vulva at the beginning of foaling, a pin in the transmitter is pushed out. This then sets an alarm off, which activates the attendant's pager. The disadvantage is that the alarm only alerts you once the mare starts to deliver, so you need to be nearby.

(3) Foaling alarm systems that strap around the whole mare and sound an alarm if or when she sweats during delivery. The disadvantage of this is that if the mare does not sweat it does not go off.

Closed-circuit TV is also commonly used. Because parturition is very rapid in mares, it is important to monitor them very closely.

Nursing/management checks before foaling

It is important to check if the vulva has been stitched (Caslick's operation). If she has been 'stitched' it is important to 'open' the vulva before foaling. It is not enough just to remove the stitches that were put in when the mare was 'Caslicked', and in any case these should have been removed 2 weeks after the procedure. The stitched area must be cut open before the foal emerges. If this is not done, at best the tissue of that area will tear and bruise severely, making future repair difficult; at worst, the foal will suffocate.

It is also an important hygiene measure to wash and dry the mare's udder.

Parturition

Parturition is the term used to describe the expulsion of the fetus (and its membranes) from the uterus through the maternal passages by natural forces. The most important initiating factor for parturition is the maturation of the fetal hypothalamic–pituitary–adrenal axis. The production of cortisol from the fetal adrenal gland may be the ultimate trigger of the process of parturition. This increase in cortisol indicates the foal's 'readiness for birth'.

Oxytocin is the hormone produced by the dam and plays a key role in all stages of labour. In the mare oxytocin release can be blocked by external stimuli,

which allows the mare, at least temporarily, to resist the fetal signals for birth, e.g. if she is disturbed.

The act of parturition is a continuous process but it is customary to divide it into three stages, as in other species.

First stage

This lasts for 1–4 h and begins with the onset of uterine contractions. The changes are not visible externally but they prepare the birth canal and fetus for expulsion. During this stage the muscles of the uterus begin to contract and push the fetus against the cervix. This helps the cervix to dilate. The foal begins to move of its own accord, rotating itself and extending the front legs and head. The increasing myometrial activity, together with spontaneous fetal movements, will result in rotation of the cranial part of the fetal body into a dorsosacral position. The front legs and head are extended. These processes usually result in discomfort in the mare and the following signs:

- Becoming restless and exhibiting colic-like signs (looking at flanks, tail switching, frequently getting up and down).
- Exhibiting patchy sweating (flanks, neck, behind elbows).
- Yawning.
- When the cervix is fully dilated the allantoic membrane ruptures and several litres of allantoic fluid escape from the genital tract. This is popularly called 'the waters breaking' and indicates the end of the first stage.

As the mare approaches the end of the first stage of labour her tail should be bandaged and her vulval area cleaned and dried. Mares do *not* normally strain during the first stage of parturition.

Second stage

The onset of the second stage occurs abruptly and commences with the onset of forcible abdominal straining and/or the appearance of the amnion. These two features usually occur almost simultaneously. During stage two, actual delivery of the foal takes place. The mare usually lies down and goes into lateral recumbency until the foal is born. The outer red membrane ruptures and the amnion (transparent bluish-white membrane) is quickly visible at the vulva and fluid and a fetal foot should be visible. Straining occurs regularly and both front feet should soon appear. As the amnion emerges at the vulva, one foreleg is in front of the other by some 10 cm. Shortly the nose should appear also. The greatest effort is associated with delivering the head, with the passage of the chest and hips usually occurring relatively easily. As the head and shoulders pass through the pelvis, the amnion should rupture. If necessary, the mare can be assisted by gentle pulling on the foal's front legs.

The foal has a relatively long umbilical cord, which is still intact after delivery. When possible, the cord should be left intact for a few minutes to help the circulation of the newborn foal. Care should be taken not to disturb the mare at this stage or she may rise and rupture the cord. The cord usually ruptures at a predetermined place due to movements of the mare and/or foal several minutes (up to 15 min) after birth. Once the umbilical cord has ruptured, the stump should be checked for haemorrhage and disinfected with dilute chlorhexidine. This disinfection of the navel needs to be repeated several times during the first few days of life. If the mare is still lying down, the foal can be moved towards the mare's head to try to reduce the chance of the foal being stood on when the mare attempts to get up. All disturbances should be kept to a minimum during this stage.

The second stage of labour usually occurs at night; the average duration is about 15 min and normally it should not exceed 1 h.

Third stage

This involves passage of the fetal membranes, often termed 'delivery of the afterbirth', and usually occurs within 1 h on average and should not take more than 2 h. Continuing myometrial activity plays an important role during this process. There is controversy with respect to the time interval for placental expulsion. Recognition of the precise time at which the process has become pathological if the membranes have not been passed is difficult.

The placenta initially should be tied up so that it hangs just above the hocks. This should avoid it being stepped on before it is passed. If the placenta is not passed within 3 h, the vet should be contacted.

The uterus contracts very quickly after foaling and this process carries on for several days until the uterus is almost as small as it was before the mare became pregnant. This process of becoming smaller is known as 'involution'.

Complications

Premature induction of foaling

This is rarely indicated in the mare. Mares for induction have to be selected very carefully because it is difficult to ensure the maturity of the foal when inducing parturition.

Dystocia

Dystocia means difficult birth and is possible if either the first or second stage of parturition does not progress or is prolonged. Speedy recognition of dystocia is necessary to save the life of the mare and foal and prevent injury to the mare's reproductive tract.

Dystocia is usually caused by the foal not being delivered in the right direction or one of its legs being bent backwards. This is more likely in the foal compared with other domestic animals because of its long limbs and neck. Sometimes the foal may be presented 'back to front', i.e. the rump is presented first, which is known as a breech birth. Dystocia can be caused also by problems with the dam, such as not straining properly. Rarely the bony pelvis of the dam, through which the foal must be delivered, may be small.

Studies in thoroughbreds have suggested an incidence of 4%, i.e. 4 in 100 births do not proceed normally. Dystocia is not a common problem and the more severe forms of dystocia are the rarest. There are three main reasons why equine dystocia is so serious:

(1) The mare will continue to push and strain even if the foal is stuck. The mare may strain so hard that her uterus ruptures, leading to peritonitis or fatal bleeding.

(2) During delivery the placenta separates quickly and so the foal loses its oxygen supply and must breathe itself.

(3) The placenta is often retained following dystocia, with serious consequences if not treated.

For an equine nurse, it is important to recognise if the foaling is abnormal. There are six main clues:

(1) Failure of the glistening white amnion, with front legs and nose to appear shortly after the waters have broken.

(2) Appearance of the bright-red allantochorion at the vulval lips at the start of the second stage, with no fluid loss noticed.

(3) Repeated forceful straining with nothing happening.

(4) No straining for lengthy periods once the amnion has appeared.

(5) The mare continually gets up and down and rolls from side to side.

(6) The foal is stuck at the hips once the head, legs and chest are out.

In all potential dystocia cases the vet should be contacted as soon as you realise that things are not right. There is no time to spare with a foaling and it is better to call for help too soon rather than too late (see Example 4.1).

Example 4.1 Foaling difficulties

A nursing emergency

An owner rings your equine hospital to say that a vet is referring a mare to you as an emergency because she has been in non-productive labour for over 30 min. They are currently waiting for transport and the mare is very distressed and straining hard.

Your initial response is to reassure the owner and recommend that the mare is kept walking TO REDUCE STRAINING until the vet is able to either place a nasogastric tube in the trachea or administer an epidural to stop the abdominal efforts or administer other medication to help. You establish how long it will take for the mare to arrive and arrange for the duty vet to talk to the referring vet. Meanwhile, you organise a team and equipment, with a plan of action ready to deal with the mare as soon as she arrives. This is an emergency requiring effective nursing teamwork.

The vet informs you that the problem is thought to be one of fetal oversize, i.e. the foal is simply too large to deliver normally and assisted vaginal delivery (attempts to deliver the foal in the awake mare with sedation and epidural) have failed. Together you plan to:

- Perform controlled vaginal delivery under general anaesthesia if possible to do so.
- If the foal cannot be delivered within 15 min or it becomes obvious that it will not be possible to do so within 15 min, then a Caesarean section will be performed.

- If the foal is obviously dead on arrival, consider a fetotomy (cutting up the dead fetus to extract it from the mare).

As nurse in charge you rapidly set up equipment and organise personnel for:

- General anaesthesia.
- Foaling equipment, including sterile ropes, lots of obstetric lubrication, stomach pump and tubes.
- Equipment for midline laparotomy for Caesarean section.
- Fetotomy equipment, including fetotome, wire saw and handgrips.
- Equipment to revive the newborn anaesthetised foal, including separate oxygen supply, towels and staff to receive and revive it.

When the mare arrives soon thereafter you take her straight to the anaesthetic knockdown box, where the vets perform a rapid clinical examination and general anaesthesia is induced. When the mare is recumbent, hobbles are attached to the hindpasterns and a hoist used to elevate the hindquarters. This effect of gravity sometimes helps the clinician to repel and reposition the fetus. While controlled vaginal delivery is attempted, you concentrate on clipping the abdomen and preparing the mare for surgery.

Because the foal is alive but too big for delivery through the mare's small pelvis, the clinician elects to perform a Caesarean section. The mare is moved into the operating theatre and surgery is performed rapidly under light general anaesthesia to avoid fetal respiratory depression. The most

(Continued on p. 96.).

important factor in foal survival is rapid delivery and immediate neonatal care. When the surgeon lifts the foal up and out of the uterus by its hindlimbs, it is transferred to you and a second nurse to hold adjacent to the mare until the umbilical cord has finished pulsing. You clamp the cord, while the other nurse concentrates on getting the foal breathing. It is then moved away from the dam to administer oxygen and be dried while being held in a sternal position.

After surgery, colostrum is milked off the mare in recovery and given to the foal by stomach tube. The foal is introduced to the dam, once she is fully awake and on her feet under careful supervision. It is important to supervise the foal's nursing efforts because they may distress the mare by traumatising the surgical site; for this reason, a belly bandage is used on the mare. The mare is watched carefully until the placenta and normal droppings are passed, because retained fetal membranes and ileus are common complications of the procedure (see Chapter 18).

After foaling

After a Caesarean section, mare fertility is adversely affected. This may in part be due to trauma by attempts at vaginal delivery as much as the surgical procedure itself. Dramatic swelling and bruising of the vagina and vulva can occur with normal deliveries. This usually resolves within a few days of foaling. Sometimes vulval tears may have to be stitched, known as Caslick's procedure. There are a range of other conditions that are more serious, usually requiring immediate veterinary assistance. In rare cases the damage to the vulva and/or vagina may be much more serious. The foal's foot may tear completely through the vagina and may even rip completely between the anus and vulva.

First postpartum oestrus

First postpartum oestrus or foal heat is characterised by normal follicular development and ovulation by day 20 postpartum in almost 100% of mares. By day 10 postpartum around half of all foaled mares have ovulated.

As the uterus decreases in size (involutes), so *postpartum luminal fluid* (lochia) is discharged from the uterine lumen. This uterine discharge is normal and often noticeable as a vaginal exudate (bloody, brown or mucopurulent) about 3 or 4 days after parturition. The colour generally becomes paler by day 5. Delayed uterine involution invariably follows dystocia, abortion, placentitis and placental retention.

In the early postpartum stages (first 2–3 days) the mare may exhibit systemic signs such as dullness,

inappetence and mild colic. In severe cases, usually subsequent to placental retention or dystocia, there may be evidence of septicaemia and laminitis.

Most commercial stud farms aim to produce as many healthy foals, as early as possible, from mares mated the previous year, hence they will breed at foal heat. Against the obvious time-saving advantage of this, there are two negative issues to consider:

(1) Pregnancy rate at foal heat: there is a lower pregnancy rate for mares mated at the first postpartum oestrus.
(2) Subsequent foaling rate of mares diagnosed pregnant from a foal heat mating: there may be an increased incidence of early embryonic mortality.

Infertility (subfertility) in the mare

Very few mares are permanently and completely infertile, but subfertility of varying degrees is a major problem. There are many causes of subfertility, which can act either alone or in combination with each other. Broadly, they can be categorised into infectious or non-infectious factors, with the latter being further divided into anatomical abnormalities and functional aberrations (Table 4.1). To calculate the reproductive efficiency of a mare, several parameters are used (see Key points 4.1).

Pregnancy failure

Pregnancy failure is a source of major economic loss to the horse industry. *Embryonic death* occurs before

Table 4.1 Summary of the causes of mare subfertility

I Anatomical	II Functional	III Infectious
Defective vulva	Anoestrus	Endometritis: bacterial/fungal
Defective vestibulovaginal constriction	• Seasonal (winter/early spring)	Metritis
Vesicovaginal reflux (urine pooling)	• Poor body condition	Pyometra
	• Disease	Pregnancy failure:
Vaginal bleeding	• Chromosome abnormality	viral/bacterial/fungal
Persistent hymen	• Lactation related	
Abnormal cervix	• Prolonged luteal function	
Uterine tumour	• Pregnancy/pseudopregnancy	
Uterine haematoma	• Silent heat	
Uterine adhesions	Irregular or prolonged oestrus	
Uterine cysts	• Transitional ('spring') oestrus	
Partial dilatation of the uterus	Ovulatory dysfunction	
Abnormal oviduct	Pregnancy failure	
Ovarian tumour	• Early embryonic death	
Pituitary abnormality	• Abortion	

Key points 4.1

Mare reproductive efficiency

Below are some of the parameters used. The percentages in parentheses give likely figures on a well-managed stud farm.

- *Fertilisation rate*: number of ova fertilised/number of ovulations (85–90%).
- *Pregnancy rate*: number of mares pregnant on a specified day (often day 15) per breeding cycle (50–70%) or per breeding season (80–95%).
- *Live foal rate* (most reliable indicator of overall reproductive efficiency): number of mares foaling/number of mares bred (65–90%); this figure is likely to be below owner expectations.
- *Pregnancy loss rate*: number not foaling/number pregnant on a specified day (day 15) (15–20%).
- *Early embryonic death*: conceptus loss before organogenesis is complete (day 15–40) (5–15%).

---

40 days of gestation when organogenesis is complete, with *early embryonic death* (EED) occurring before the maternal recognition of pregnancy. *Early fetal death* occurs before 150 days of gestation; thus, *late fetal death* occurs afterwards. *Abortion* is defined as expulsion of the fetus and its membranes before 300 days, whereas a *stillbirth* is expulsion of the fetus and its membranes from day 300 onwards.

Fetal death/abortion

An overall abortion rate of 10% after 60 days of gestation is usually cited for the horse. In practice, it is important to distinguish infectious from non-infectious causes. Signs of an impending or recent abortion include:

- vaginal discharge
- running milk
- colic

When abortion occurs, the mare should be isolated, a history obtained and the fetus and fetal membranes sent to an approved laboratory for autopsy. The causes of equine abortion can be broadly divided into non-infectious (70%), infectious (15%) and unknown (15%).

Non-infectious causes of abortion and stillbirth: twinning

Historically, twins have been the single most important cause of abortion. However, it is now much less common due to the widespread use of ultrasonography.

Umbilical cord abnormalities

In mares, the umbilical cord is twisted, usually in a clockwise spiral. The normal length is 36–83 cm (mean 55 cm). Increased cord length has been associated with excessive cord torsion, which can cause vascular obstruction of the urachus. This can result in abortion of an autolysed fetus. Decreased cord length can cause premature tearing of fetal membranes, leading to fetal asphyxia.

Premature placental separation

When placental separation occurs shortly before parturition, the thickened placenta often does not rupture through the cervical star, and the allantochorion bulges out of the vulva ('red-bag' delivery). The foal can become hypoxic, resulting in neonatal maladjustment syndrome (NMS).

Infectious causes of abortion

The main causal agents of infectious abortion are:

- Viruses, including equine herpes virus (EHV) and equine viral arteritis (EVA), and equine infectious anaemia.
- Bacteria that gain access to the placenta, which can cause abortion in the mare. They are often opportunist pathogens that can be isolated from normal mares, i.e. *Streptococcus* spp. and *Escherichia coli*. Others are considered to be venereal pathogens, i.e. *Pseudomonas* spp. and *Klebsiella* spp. Recently, leptospirosis has been diagnosed in association with abortion.
- *Aspergillus* spp. are the most common cause of mycotic placentitis and mycotic abortion in the mare.

Endometritis

Reduced fertility associated with endometritis has been recognised for many years in broodmares. The term 'endometritis' refers to the acute or chronic inflammatory process involving the endometrium. These changes frequently occur as a result of microbial infection, but they can be due also to non-infectious causes. One of the main obstacles to producing the maximum number of live, healthy foals from mares bred during the previous season is susceptibility to persistent acute endometritis following breeding.

Artificial insemination (AI)

This involves the collection, evaluation and dilution of semen from the stallion and then the timely infusion of an adequate number of viable sperm into the mare's uterus.

A successful AI programme depends upon various factors in the stallion and the mare:

(1) Stallion:
  (a) A thorough examination for breeding soundness on the stallion being used.
  (b) Confirmation that the stallion has semen of sufficient quality.
  (c) Appropriate cooling and storage of the semen sample after collection.
(2) Mare:
  (a) A satisfactory breeding soundness examination.
  (b) Induction of an ovulatory oestrus.
  (c) Accurate prediction of ovulation.
  (d) Correct timing of insemination relative to ovulation.
  (e) Appropriate storage, thawing and handling of semen.
  (f) Correct insemination technique.
  (g) Post-insemination examination and treatments as required.
  (h) Correct pregnancy diagnosis 14–16 days after insemination.

Artificial insemination in the horse requires a high degree of veterinary input and is not a cheap alternative to natural breeding.

Advantages and disadvantages of AI

Although AI has many advantages there are also drawbacks that must be considered.

Advantages of using AI:

(1) Maximises the efficiency of stallion usage because more mares can be inseminated from one ejaculate, which means that a stallion can breed more mares per year.

(2) Transport of semen across or even between countries is possible.

(3) Can evaluate the semen on a regular basis.

(4) Use of semen extenders with proper antibiotics to preserve the longevity of sperm and minimise bacterial contamination.

(5) Implementation of minimal contamination breeding techniques for mares that are susceptible to uterine infections.

(6) Enhances the safety of animals and animal handlers.

(7) The mare (and foal) can be kept at home and the risks of infection and injury from transport are reduced.

(8) Reduces the risk of venereal diseases spreading throughout a breeding population.

Disadvantages of using AI:

(1) Higher costs due to labour and paperwork.

(2) Requirement of adequate infrastructure and capable skilled vets.

(3) Risk of genetic, viral or bacterial disease transmission.

(4) Semen from some stallions will not tolerate the cooling and/or the freezing and thawing process, therefore stallion variability is an added problem.

(5) Some breed societies, notably the thoroughbred registration authorities, will not allow the registration of foals born by AI.

For an AI programme to be successful, strict attention should be paid to health precautions and hygiene. Guidelines and Codes of Conduct to reduce the risk of disease transmission should be strictly followed.

Storage of semen: fresh, chilled and frozen semen

The temperature at which semen should be stored depends on the period of time for which it needs to remain viable. In general:

- Semen that is going to be used within 12 h after collection can be stored at room temperature in a dark environment.

- If semen is intended to last longer than 12 h, either because of stallion unavailability or need for semen transport, it should be chilled down to 5–8°C over a 2–3 h period.

- If life expectancy of the semen is longer than 72 h, cryopreservation (freezing) should be considered.

Semen that is collected should be diluted with an appropriate extender regardless of its intended use. Extenders used for the storage of stallion semen are typically based on egg-yolk, skim milk or a combination of both. The extenders contain sugars, other nutrients and antibiotics to optimise the survival time of the sperm.

Frozen semen is the most difficult and conception rates may be very poor if strict stallion selection and careful insemination routines are not practised. Technically, frozen semen requires a lot of veterinary input to determine the optimal time and frequency to inseminate mares. There are many other problems associated with the use of frozen semen. One of these is that mare owners are often charged large amounts of money for semen of unknown potential. Unfortunately it is not easy to do controlled fertility testing of frozen–thawed equine semen and at present, therefore, standardisation is almost completely absent in this industry.

Nurse's role

A nurse's role in AI may include:

- Checking the mare's identity from a passport or similar document.

- If semen has been imported, the accompanying documentation should be checked and confirmed that the stallion is seronegative for EVA.

- Ensuring that semen storage is adequate, e.g. by regularly filling liquid nitrogen flasks and maintaining clear records.

- Preparing the mare for insemination, preferably by using stocks for restraint. The tail should be bandaged and tied out of the perineal region (Fig. 4.6). The vulva and perineal area should be cleansed thoroughly with dilute povidone iodine solution or mild soap. This is then rinsed off thoroughly with fresh warm water and the perineal

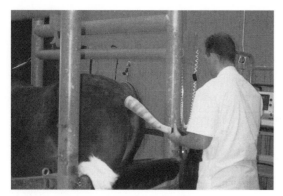

Fig. 4.6 Preparing a mare for AI.

area dried with clean, soft, disposable (paper) towels. Because there may be a small delay between cleaning the mare and insemination, the vet may empty the mare's rectum of faeces to prevent contamination of the area after cleansing.

• Observing the mare for oestrus behaviour, because correct timing of the AI is critical. The clinician may use hormonal treatments, e.g. hCG, to facilitate this.

Further reading

Davies-Morel, M.C.G. (2000) *Equine Reproductive Physiology, Breeding and Stud Management.* CABI Publishing, Wallingford, Oxon.

England, G.C.W. (1996) *Allen's Fertility and Obstetrics in the Horse.* Blackwell Science, Oxford.

Knottenbelt, D.C., LeBlanc, M.M. & Pascoe R.R. (with contribution from Asbury, A.C.) (2001) *Handbook of Equine Stud Medicine.* WB Saunders, London.

Pycock, J.F. (1997) *Self Assessment Colour Review of Equine Reproduction and Stud Medicine.* Manson Publishing, London.

Samper, J. (2000) *Equine Breeding Management and Artificial Insemination.* WB Saunders, Philadelphia, PA.

Nutrition

P. A. Harris

Horses are fundamentally non-ruminant herbivores, which means that they are suited to eating high-fibre diets owing to continual microbial fermentation within the caecum and colon. The horse evolved to eat mainly grass with some other herbage and, when available, 'wild' cereals and other starch-containing feedstuffs. The horse naturally is a social animal, living in groups and spending the majority of its time foraging in a diverse and seasonally variable environment.

Domestication has meant that horses now tend to be kept in stables and/or on managed pastures and we are responsible for their feeding. This, together with the increasing demand for horses to perform at levels that require energy intakes above those able to be provided by their more 'natural' diet, has resulted in the addition of cereal grains and their by-products, as well as supplemental fat, in modern equine diets. This has benefits but also potential disadvantages, including:

- The close confinement of horses
- Restriction of access to buddies
- Restriction of feeding to 'meal times'

Optimal feeding of horses uses both art and science: the science provides the information about the digestive and metabolic processes, the nutrient requirements and the principles behind feeding practices; the art is the ability to convert this theory into practice for the individual horse, its needs and its likes and dislikes. Although good nutrition cannot improve the basic ability of a horse, poor nutrition may limit performance.

Overview of the digestive system of a horse

The horse's digestive system can be considered in two sections. The first section has similarities to the precaecal digestive system of a monogastric (i.e. single-stomached) animal; the second is more like the rumen of a cow (Fig. 5.1).

First section: precaecal (mouth, oesophagus, stomach, small intestine) monogastric-like

- Chewing involves complex jaw movements incorporating lateral and vertical components.
- The jaw sweeps approximately 60 000 times a day when grazing.
- The type of feed influences the movements of the jaw during chewing and the speed of ingestion. The average 500-kg horse takes about 40 min or 3400 chews to eat a kilogram of hay or about 10 min and just 850 chews for a kilogram of oats, leaving more time to get 'bored'.
- Chewing movements are relatively long and wide in horses eating grass but are reduced when hay, cereals or pelleted feeds are fed, increasing the chances of lateral and medial hooks (enamel points) developing.
- Saliva in horses is produced in response to chewing food rather than in anticipation of eating. Feeds that are chewed less result in swallowed boluses with higher dry matter (DM) content, e.g. with a hay bolus the DM content is around 20%

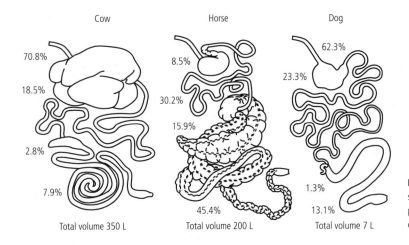

Fig. 5.1 Comparative guide to the digestive system of the cow, horse and dog. By permission of Pedigree Masterfoods (a Division of Mars UK Ltd.).

whereas that of a cereal-based feed bolus is more like 30–40%.

- The equine stomach is relatively small in size and inelastic. Horses have evolved to eat high-fibre diets almost continuously, i.e. they are 'trickle feeders'. In general the rate of gastric emptying is proportional to the square root of the volume, i.e. the larger the meal, the more rapid the gastric emptying. In addition, the larger the meal, the more quickly it passes through the small intestine with less digestion time.

- A limited amount of bacterial fermentation occurs in the stomach of horses in the initial stages, especially of easily available sugars and starches, which is stopped on mixing with the gastric juices. With large cereal-based meals there is slower and/or reduced mixing of the feed with the gastric juices and therefore an increased risk of abnormal fermentation (see Fig. 5.2).

- The basic digestive processes (enzymatic degradation of proteins, fats, starches and sugars) are similar to those of other monogastric animals but the activity of several of the enzymes is lower in horses.

- Amylase activity is limited in horses, so they have a finite capacity to digest starch—a major component of cereal grains—in the small intestine (recommended intake of starch is $\leqslant 2\,g/100\,kg$ bodyweight (BW) per meal). Adult horses also appear to have a limited ability to digest lactose (it is suggested not to feed >75 g/100 kg BW of milk

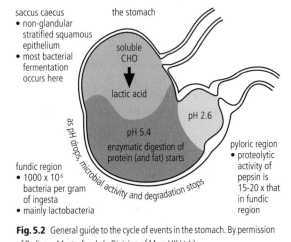

Fig. 5.2 General guide to the cycle of events in the stomach. By permission of Pedigree Masterfoods (a Division of Mars UK Ltd.).

powder otherwise there is an increased risk of diarrhoea).

- When large meals of either pellets or cereal grains are fed infrequently, a transient state of hypovolaemia results because of upper gastrointestinal secretions, including saliva. In quick or greedy feeders there can be a large loss in plasma volume. Horses should be prevented from bolting their feed, e.g. by adding large stones to the feed bucket or spreading the feed over a large trough area. Adding chaff can be beneficial. If a lot of grain is fed, it should be spread over several meals.

- The majority of minerals and trace elements given to horses are absorbed in the small intestine, as are most of the dietary vitamins. Phosphorus, however, is mainly absorbed in the hindgut; high phosphorus intakes, especially plant phytates, may interfere with calcium absorption but this does not work the other way around.

Second section: caecum/colon–rumen-like

- A high proportion of the available starch ingested is degraded to glucose before absorption in the small intestine, unless its digestive capacity is overwhelmed.
- The rest is subjected to microbial fermentation, mostly in the large intestine along with dietary fibre. (NB: Some fermentation will occur in the small intestine but to a varying extent according to the individual, the feedstuff concerned, and the feeding practices followed). Mammals cannot break down the linkages between the glucose molecules of cellulose. Horses rely on bacterial fermentation to accomplish this initial step in fibre digestion. The breakdown products are predominantly short-chain or volatile fatty acids. These can be used directly as an energy fuel by the gut cells themselves, but the majority are absorbed and converted to either glucose or fat. This is ultimately less efficient than obtaining energy from carbohydrate sources directly, via glucose (see Fig. 5.3).

- Unlike the ruminant, this microbial fermentation obviously occurs after the 'monogastric'-like section rather than before.
- Microbial protein, which is synthesised in the large intestine, cannot be utilised to any great extent by the horse. This means that animals with a high demand for protein (foals, lactating mares and probably intensively exercising horses) must be fed high-quality protein, which can be broken down and absorbed primarily in the precaecal section of the gut.
- The colonic fermentation cycle of fluid-shifts and changes in bacterial populations is a meal-induced event and basically is not seen in horses fed continuously.
- The extent to which cereal starch provides glucose or volatile fatty acids as the end result of digestion depends on its precaecal and even pre-ileal digestibility. This in turn varies according to the feedstuff under consideration and the process-ing to which the feedstuff has been subjected (see Fig. 5.4).
- Large grain meals (or pastures with high sugar contents) may overwhelm the digestive capacity of the small intestine, leading to rapid fermentation of the carbohydrate in the hindgut, a decrease in the pH and excessive growth of those bacteria that can live under such conditions. Consequently there may be a degree of lysis of those bacteria that cannot live at such low pH, allowing the release of endotoxins and damage to the mucosa of the caecum and colon. This may allow the

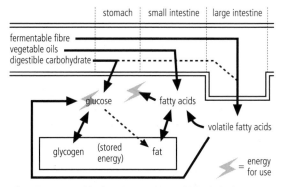

Fig. 5.3 Overview of the digestive processes involved with the three main energy sources in the horse. Copyright of Pedigree Masterfoods (a Division of Mars UK Ltd.).

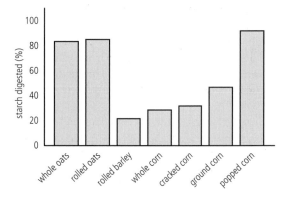

Fig. 5.4 Effect of feedstuff and processing on pre-ileal starch digestibility. Meyer *et al.* (1995).

absorption of endotoxins and other toxic substances with potential clinical consequences, including colic, diarrhoea and laminitis. Hay- or roughage-based diets do not result in such decreases in caecal pH but they may not provide sufficient usable or net energy for some horse's needs.

General comments about feeding horses

Water

The amount of water required by a horse will vary according to the individual, its diet, work schedule and its sweating rate, as well as the environmental temperature. Although non-lactating horses on lush pastures, with shade, undertaking no work can thrive in theory without additional water, this is not advisable.

The recommendations are:

- Provide a constant supply of fresh clean water, including for foals from 10 days old.
- Ensure that water containers are regularly cleaned and checked; any ice must be broken to enable access.
- The environmental temperature will have a large effect on the amount of water consumed; increase supply in hot conditions or if the horse sweats considerably.
- Do not give a horse large amounts of water (especially very cold water) immediately after hard exercise. Let them have repeated small amounts (5–6 swallows).

Feed plenty of suitable roughage

Horses have evolved as hindgut fermenters who naturally live on a predominantly forage-based diet, the fibrous components of which act as a source of energy. Suitable roughage occupies a horse's time chewing and reduces the risk of developing vices.

Thus, roughage should be the foundation of any horse's diet, even those in hard work. Some horses and ponies may not require anything else. Hays with higher energy levels and greater digestibilities

should be considered, especially for those animals in competitive work. Horses in general should be fed as much roughage as possible; grain should be fed only when the horses' energy requirements cannot be met by forage alone (sometimes small amounts of grain or other concentrates may be needed to carry supplemental protein or minerals to balance the ration).

- For the majority of horses, at least 50% of their diet on a DM basis should be suitable forage (around 1 kg/100 kg BW). Even fit, very intensively working horses should be fed at least 35% and preferably 40% of their DM intake as forage. The exact amounts needed will vary according to the forage type and nature.
- One of the major factors affecting the energy content of preserved forage is the stage of maturity at which the plant is cut. Older plants have increased fibre content, a lower percentage of leaves and reduced digestibility. Legume hays tend to have higher energy values than grass hays such as Timothy.
- All forage should be as dust free as possible and free from mould (see Chapter 1).
- Consider mixing additional good-quality, short-chopped fibre (e.g. chaff of >2 cm in length) with concentrate feeds, especially for horses that bolt their food.
- Many pastures and forages will not provide all the nutrients that a horse needs. An appropriate vitamin and mineral mix may be satisfactory for many horses at rest and, depending on the pasture, for those in light/moderate work. Additional feed is likely to be required for the young growing animal, the pregnant and lactating mare and for those in hard work.

Feed little and often

Feed smaller and more frequent concentrate/ cereal-based meals. Ideally feed <500 g/100 kg BW per meal in general and <400 g/100 kg per meal of oats, i.e. ideally ≤2 kg per meal for a 500-kg horse. Increase the number of meals per day rather than the amount per meal. It is important to remember that horses have evolved to bite, chew thoroughly and then swallow small amounts of highly fibrous diets almost continuously for up to 18 h/day. Divide the daily concentrate feed into three to four meals a day rather than having two large feeds.

If a horse appears to require ever-increasing amounts of feed in each of its meals in order to maintain condition and type of ride desired, consider:

• Increasing the number of meals
• Changing to a feed with a higher energy content
• Adding additional oil (see below)
• Seeking veterinary advice if a horse loses weight significantly or rapidly

Add supplementary oil

Most forage-based diets and those based on grains, fat-extracted oilseed meals and hays contain 2–5% oil and typically ~3%. Recently there has been increasing use of supplemental vegetable oil in horse diets:

(1) Feeding oil-supplemented diets, with appropriate training, has been suggested to result in a range of effects on a variety of physiological and metabolic parameters as well as on performance. In order to obtain metabolic benefits from the feeding of oil or oil-supplemented diets, in addition to those associated with its high energy density and lack of starch content, the oil needs to be fed for several months. The suggested benefits include:

    (a) increased mobilisation of free fatty acids (FFAs) and increased speed of mobilisation;

    (b) increased speed of uptake of FFAs into muscle, often considered to be rate limiting;

    (c) a glycogen-sparing effect so that fatigue is delayed and performance improved; this is especially important in endurance activities;

    (d) increased high-intensity exercise capacity.

(2) The increase in the energy density of the feed (vegetable oils have about 2.5 times as much digestible energy as maize/corn and 3 times as much as oats) effectively means that the horse may take in more energy even if its appetite decreases. Many horses when in hard work and regularly competed have a reduced appetite.

(3) More fibre can be fed and less cereal or hydrolysable starch need to be fed while still maintaining the desired energy intake.

(4) An oil-supplemented diet may have behavioural advantages over high cereal starch diets.

(5) Because oil in the diet is converted more efficiently to usable energy than feeds such as hay and cereals, this may help to reduce the heat load on the horse, which may be particularly useful when competing under hot and humid conditions. It also reduces the water requirement.

(6) A low-starch, high-fibre diet that is supplemented, if necessary, with oil is recommended for the feeding of many horses that are prone to suffering from tying up, i.e. equine rhabdomyolysis syndrome.

(7) Additional oil may benefit skin and hoof appearance, but exact requirements of the various FFAs are unknown.

Supplemental fat or oil diets can be supplied in four main ways:

(1) As an oil-supplemented, manufactured diet: such diets should be balanced with respect to the protein, vitamin and mineral intake that they provide when fed with forage (and salt as required); a simple, practical and convenient way to feed high-oil diets.

(2) High-oil supplemental feedstuffs (such as rice bran: ~20–30%) that are also high in fibre and usually low in starch. However, many of the rice brans available have the same disadvantages as wheat bran in that they have a very imbalanced calcium to phosphorus content. Alternatives include whole oilseeds (15–26% oil).

(3) Supplemental animal fat: often unpalatable and generally not recommended.

(4) Supplemental vegetable oils (such as corn oil or soya oil): should be of feed grade and non-rancid.

Any supplemental oil or oil-supplemented feed should be introduced slowly. Dietary oils are usually hydrolysed in the small intestine and the capacity of lipid hydrolysis in herbivores seems to adapt over a week or two. Horses have been shown to be able to digest and utilise up to 20% of the diet as fat, although

~10% of the daily intake has been suggested in the literature to provide the maximal beneficial metabolic effects when incorporated in a complete and balanced feed. Adding oil to existing feed has the potential to create multiple imbalances and therefore it is recommended to add less than the 10% suggested above. Levels of 5–8% in the total diet are more common in some high-performing horses. Many performance horses can be fed up to 400 ml daily in divided doses without any problems, provided that it has been introduced gradually, the extra energy is required and the oil is not rancid.

It is important to note that supplemental oil *per se* does not provide any additional protein, vitamins or minerals (unless fortified by the manufacturer). If the horse is not receiving sufficient of these for its workload from its basal diet, then an appropriate additional mix may be needed or one should consider a manufactured, balanced, high-oil feed. It is also important to ensure a sufficient calcium intake.

It is recommended that additional vitamin E be fed in combination with any supplemental vegetable oil. Exact recommendations are not known but an additional (above requirements) 100 IU of vitamin E for every 100 ml of added supplemental oil is a current recommendation.

When to feed

- There has been considerable debate over when and what to feed horses before exercise. Recently it has been recommended that grain should be withheld from eventers for at least 3 h before exercise, but repeated small quantities of hay should be fed to ensure proper gastrointestinal tract function.

- Glucose peaks at ~1–3 h after a meal, which is associated with a rise in insulin. This may slow the release of FFAs into the circulation (so the horse has to rely even more on stored glycogen). If exercised at this stage, there may be a drop in blood glucose during the first stages of exercise, which may not be desirable because the brain can only use glucose as a fuel.

- A large amount of fluid, which comes effectively from the circulating blood, is secreted into the gut during digestion. Exercising under these conditions would, in effect, be similar to working a dehydrated horse.

- A distended gastrointestinal tract may restrict the space available for lung expansion.

- Following a meal, blood flow is diverted to the gut to enable the products of digestion to be utilised efficiently. This may reduce the blood flow to working muscles and other organs where it may be better employed.

Feed according to the individual and its workload

The amount and type of feed that a horse requires will depend upon many factors including:

- Age, health and temperament
- The amount and type of work carried out
- Environmental conditions
- The body condition required
- The type of ride preferred

It will vary depending on the individual horse and rider.

- Young growing horses, aged horses and pregnant and lactating mares usually will require supplemental feed in addition to forage or pasture. In some cases just adding legume hay such as alfalfa may be sufficient.

- Horses have a finite appetite, which influences what they can be fed in order to meet their energy requirements. This ranges from ~1.5 to 3.0% of BW on an 'as fed' basis for most adult horses, although foals may eat significantly more. On average, most horses eat ~2–2.5% BW/day on an 'as fed' basis and ~2% on a DM basis (i.e. 10 kg DM for a 500 kg horse).

- Compound manufactured feeds are formulated to be fed at certain levels. If a horse eats less than the manufacturer's recommendations for that work load, then an appropriate vitamin and mineral supplement may be needed. Alternatively a different diet that is less energy dense should be fed with the appropriate vitamin and mineral fortification.

- Feed according to workload and individual needs; feed intake should never be increased in anticipation of an increase in workload.

- Reduce the amount of cereal and other concentrates fed from the evening meal on the night before rest days to around one-third until the evening meal on the day they are returned to work. The volume, if required, can be made up with short-chopped fibre/chaff. If rest is likely to be prolonged, consider changing to a feed of lower energy content or rely on roughage alone (with or without a general vitamin/mineral mix, as appropriate).
- Monitor body condition and weight regularly. Obese or underweight horses are unlikely to perform optimally. Certain clinical conditions may result in a loss of weight. Judgement by eye can be inaccurate. Calibrated weighbridges are the most accurate. Weigh tapes provide an approximation but can be out by a significant margin, especially in fit, lean horses or pregnant mares.

Feed by weight not volume

It is important to feed by weight rather than by volume (scoop, bucket, etc.). For example, oats weigh far less for a given volume than corn, so if cereal intakes were changed on a volume basis the horse effectively would be fed less oats (weight for weight) and far less actual energy (see Table 5.1).

Make any change in feed gradually

- The microbial population of the hindgut becomes adapted to the type of feed provided. Rapid changes in diet may cause marked fluctuations in this microbial population, which can result in digestive disturbances. Sudden changes in the amount or type of concentrates fed are particularly likely to produce problems. Try to vary the amount gradually rather than the type of feed.

- Minor changes should be made in a stepwise manner over 3–5 days. More major changes may take up to 2 weeks. Even in a fully grain-adapted horse, the grain (concentrate) ideally should not be increased by more than ~0.5 kg/day (for a 500-kg horse).
- Ponies, especially if pregnant, have an increased risk of developing hyperlipaemia if abruptly starved. It is much safer to reduce the diet to a half-maintenance level than to completely starve a pony for weight loss purposes. Wherever appropriate, the diet can be made up to near appetite levels by substituting low-energy forages. Poorly digested, highly silicated forages such as straw increase the risk of impaction.

Keep to a routine, whenever possible

It is beneficial to maintain a standard routine within the yard. One aim is to adhere to regular feeding times that fit within a workable timetable. For the majority of horses, roughage should be available continually. If the amount of roughage needs to be limited, then switch to a lower energy-dense variety, e.g. from alfalfa to grass hay. Try to maximise the time taken by the horse to eat the amount offered by hanging the hay in a difficult to reach location or using double or treble hay nets to reduce the amount pulled out with each mouthful.

Store all feeds appropriately

Correct storage of feedstuffs is essential to preserve their nutrient value, to ensure that palatability is retained and to prevent pest, fungal or bacterial contamination:

Table 5.1 Guide to the relative feeding value of cereals by weight and volume (absolute values will vary with source)

Feed	Volume (kg/l)	Digestible energy (MJ/kg)	Relative feeding value to corn by weight	Relative feeding value to corn by volume
Corn	0.8	14	100	100
Oats, regular	0.4	12	86	43
Oats, hull-less	0.7	15.5	111	97
Barley	0.7	13.5	97	84

- Store all feeds in cool, dry, well-aired but fairly dark conditions.
- Preferably store coarse mixes in pest-proof bins. Beware of increased moisture levels within certain bins, which might increase the risk of mould growth.
- Remember to empty and clean out galvanised bins between feed loads.
- Do not feed poor-quality hay: haylages where there has been damage to the packaging; spoiled leftover feed; dusty, mouldy or contaminated ingredients.

Feeding supplements

- The use of supplements is widespread and is often based on a myth that some essential nutrient is lacking in the ration or that if X amount is good then 2X must be better. In many cases, although such supplements may not have any positive benefits, there are usually no negatives. Occasionally problems with excessive supplementation can occur (see Table 5.2).
- Only supplement if there is a specific shortfall or likely to be a deficiency in the diet.
- Check whether it would be possible to avoid or reduce the need for additional supplementation by changing the core ration if appropriate (e.g. to one of a lower energy density if feeding far less than recommended for type and intensity of work).
- Mix any vitamins and minerals in with the feed, especially when dampened, just before feeding in order to minimise any interactions. This is especially important for vitamins E and C if elements such as iron and copper are present because they speed up the loss in activity.
- Palatability sometimes can be a problem, so add any supplements gradually and mix well.
- Monitor and be prepared to alter as the requirements change or as responses dictate.
- Beware of oversupplementation, especially if multiple preparations are being fed.

Requirements

Maintenance requirements can be defined as 'the daily intake that maintains constant bodyweight and body composition, as well as the health of a healthy adult horse with zero energy retention, at a defined level of low activity in comfortable surroundings'. For some, but not all, nutrients additional amounts will be needed with exercise to cover, for example, the nutrient losses in sweat and to aid in the repair processes. Growth and reproductive status also impose their own additional demands.

A horse's nutritional needs can be influenced by a number of factors, including:

- Bodyweight
- Weight of the rider and weight of the tack (need to be considered when evaluating energy needs, especially for endurance)
- Body composition and breed
- Age/growth (young horses will require more energy, protein and minerals for growth and an older horse may need more calcium, phosphorus and protein due to decreased utilisation)
- Reproductive demands
- Exercise intensity or workload (intensity and duration)
- Condition and training of the animal
- Environmental conditions

Individual horses vary in their metabolic efficiency (e.g. some horses are 'good doers'), temperament, health status (including level of parasitic burden), appetite, likes and dislikes and other variables. There is a difference between what a horse *can eat* and what it *might need* for maintenance, so that many mature horses will gain weight if fed a free choice of hay and are not exercised.

Feeding plenty of hay can often satisfy maintenance. If legumes such as alfalfa form part of the forage, then the diet may meet maintenance energy, protein, calcium and phosphorus requirements. Light to moderate work can be satisfied by feeding more forage and switching to more digestible forages. If forage alone is insufficient, then additional feeds should be added to meet energy needs. Protein, vitamin and mineral supplements may be needed

Table 5.2 Guide to some of the main functions and sources of the components and nutrients required by the horse (figures given for nutrient content are on an 'as fed' basis if not stated otherwise and are an approximate guide only)

Nutrients	Main functions	Some of the suggested signs of deficiency	Some of the suggested signs of excess	High source	Moderate source	Low source
Energy (not a nutrient per se) in MJ or Mcal (1 Mcal = 4.184 MJ)	Essential to all cellular functions	Weight loss; hypothermia, weakness and depression in terminal stages	Obesity and secondary problems, e.g. laminitis; digestive disturbances if suddenly increased	Vegetable oils ~35 MJ/kg as fed	Oats ~10–12 MJ/kg Barley ~13 MJ/kg Corn ~14 MJ/kg Mature grass hays ~6–12 MJ/kg	Wheat straw ~6 MJ/kg Rice hulls ~2 MJ/kg
Protein, expressed as crude protein (CP) or digestible protein (DP) (DP ~40–80% CP)	Maintaining, building and repairing body tissues; essential amino acids have to be provided by the diet because they cannot be manufactured by the horse	Negative nitrogen balance; loss of protein from the tissues; restricted milk production; growth failure	Increased blood urea, heat production and water requirement; acid–base disturbances on exercise; increased ammonia in stable, possibly leading to increased respiratory problems	Oilseed meals: ~22% sunflower seeds ~45% soyabean meal	Alfalfa hay ~15–20%	Grass hays ~8% Grains variable and influenced by growing conditions ~6–12%
Amino acids (lysine is believed to be the first limiting amino acid in typical horse rations and if the lysine requirement is met, unless synthetic amino acids are used to supplement the diet, then it is believed that the requirement for other amino acids will most likely also be met)	Threonine at 80% of the lysine level is believed to be adequate; methionine is a sulphur-containing amino acid that is essential for optimal growth, provides methyl groups for choline synthesis and can be replaced partially by cystine but not vice versa			Soyabean meal: ~28 g/kg lysine ~20 g/kg threonine ~6 g/kg methionine	Linseed: ~12 g/kg lysine ~11 g/kg threonine ~4 g/kg methionine	Cereals: ~2–3 g/kg lysine Grass/cereal hay: <2 g/kg lysine
Fat, a source of energy (there may be a need for certain fatty acids such as linoleic acid)	Concentrated source of energy and essential fatty acids for metabolism, skin condition and nerve/muscle membranes; fat-soluble vitamins associated with uptake and storage	Possibly poor coat quality	Obesity; digestive disturbances and diarrhoea; always use non-rancid oils	Vegetable oils ~99%	Whole oilseeds ~20% Rice brans ~25%	Grains ~1–3% Hays ~2% Beans ~1%

(Continued on p. 110.)

Table 5.2 Continued

Nutrients	Main functions	Some of the suggested signs of deficiency	Some of the suggested signs of excess	High source	Moderate source	Low source
Sodium (mineral, electrolyte)	Major extracellular cation; nerve and muscle function; water balance	Salt craving; dehydration; decreased feed intake and production; disturbances in acid–base and water balance	Rare except where a dehydrated horse is given access to salt water ad libitum or salt-deprived animals given access to salt	Salt ~11 g/28 g (or oz)	Sugarbeet molasses ~4 g/kg	Cereals usually <0.5 g/kg
Potassium (mineral, electrolyte)	Major intracellular cation; normal cellular function, including heart and muscle	Reduced appetite; growth problems; weakness; muscular problems; rare in horses unless fed a low-forage/fibre diet and sweating considerably	Unlikely when given parenterally in excess—cardiac arrest; note also the condition of hyperkalaemic periodic paralysis where normal intake is too much	Sugarbeet molasses ~30 g/kg	Forages ~15–25 g/kg in hay	Grains <5 g/kg
Chloride (mineral, electrolyte)	Closely inter-related to sodium; osmotic pressure	Appetite loss; weight loss; poor performance	Not really known without any association with sodium	Salt ~17 g Cl/28 g (or oz)	Sugarbeet pulp molasses ~5 g Cl/kg DM	Cereals <1 g/kg DM Salt ~0.6 g Cl/kg
Calcium (mineral, electrolyte)	Bone formation, nerve and muscle function and blood clotting; availability from feeds 45–70%	Disturbances in bone quality and growth, i.e. weak poor quality bones and reduced growth; some grasses contain high oxalate concentrations which may prevent calcium uptake	May interfere with absorption of other minerals such as Zn, Mg and Mn; possibly excessive bone deposition	Limestone flour ~40% Ca, 400 g/kg	Legumes: Alfalfa ~1.2% Sugarbeet pulp ~0.6%	Cereals ~0.15%; some very low, <1 g/kg
Phosphorus (mineral, electrolyte)	Bone formation; energy metabolism; essential component of cell membranes; acid–base buffer in blood and the gastrointestinal tract (GIT)	Skeletal abnormalities; abnormal appetite; ? reproductive problems	Reduced calcium absorption; potentially secondary nutritional hyperparathyroidism (big head), especially if the diet is also low in calcium	Dicalcium phosphate ~23% Ca and 18% P	High content in most cereal brans (~11 g/kg) but due to high phytate level limited bioavailability estimated ~2 g/kg Legume hays ~2 g/kg	Cereals ~0.3–0.6% P (NB still high relative to Ca content)
Magnesium (mineral, electrolyte)	Bone; muscle contraction; metabolism	Ataxia, weakness and muscular tremors unlikely in the horse; low serum levels sometimes seen in horses with severe GIT disturbances	No evidence; claims for behaviour modification not scientifically proven	Rice brans ~0.9% Wheat bran ~0.55% Canola seeds ~0.55%	Sugarbeet molasses ~0.23% Oilseeds ~0.3%	Timothy mature hay ~0.08% Oats ~0.8%

110

Mineral	Function	Deficiency signs	Toxicity signs	Sources	Levels in legume hays/supplements	Levels in cereals/hays
Copper (micromineral)	Cofactor of many enzymes associated with energy metabolism, collagen and elastin synthesis	Potentially implicated in developmental orthopaedic disease (DOD) and lameness in growing horses ?anaemia; ?change in hair colour	Not known	Synthetic sources Molasses can be ~50 mg/kg	Legume hays ~10–16 mg/kg Some cereals may have ~10 mg/kg	Many cereals and hays <4 mg/kg
Zinc (micromineral)	Component of many metalloenzymes involved in protein and carbohydrate metabolism	Inappetence; reduced growth rate and skin problems; potentially implicated in DOD	Potentially linked to bone problems, enlarged joints, lameness in growing animals and DOD	Synthetic sources Inorganic sources	Synthetic sources Chelates and bioplexes Full-fat soya ~50 mg/kg	Legume hays and cereals ~20–25 mg/kg
Manganese (micromineral)	Cartilage (formation of chondroitin sulphate); metabolism	Possibly associated with DOD and bone developmental abnormalities	? Anaemia and infertility; ?neurotoxic; ??aggressive behaviour	Synthetic sources	Legume hays ~30–60 mg/kg Oats can be high, 35 mg/kg, or low	Grass hays Corn ~5 mg/kg Barley intermediate
Iron (micromineral)	Incorporated into haemoglobin, myoglobin and certain enzymes; oxygen transfer; metabolism	Rare to occur, except in chronic blood loss, especially in foals; rare that anaemia in the horse is due to iron deficiency; diets normally more than sufficient for needs	Nutritional siderosis; more likely in young foals, especially if inject iron and provide highly supplemented feed	Inorganic supplements Oaten chaff ~350 mg/kg	Legume hays ~140–210 mg/kg Cereals <100 mg/kg	
Cobalt (micromineral)	Vitamin B12 contains ~4% cobalt and is involved with haemoglobin formation and metabolism	If occurs, will result in vitamin B12 deficiency and anaemia, rough coat and poor appetite	Unknown	Synthetic sources	Legume hays up to ~0.4 mg/kg	Cereals <0.15 mg/kg Oats tend to be low, ~0.05 mg/kg
Selenium (micromineral)	Part of the cellular antioxidant defences	Nutritionally associated myopathy (white muscle disease in foals); some claim an association with poor performance in racing horses and lower fertility rates in stud animals	Hair loss of the mane and tail and sloughing of the hooves; cumulative; lameness	Synthetic sources Certain selenium-accumulating plants	Selenium yeast	Cereals and hays; variable, some plant species can have very high levels Cereals <0.2 mg/kg
Iodine (micromineral)	Essential component of thyroid hormones	Goitre; weak dead foals; poor performance	Goitre; weakness; infertility and abortion	Seaweed meal Iodised salt Potassium iodate	Legume hay ~0.15 mg/kg	Cereals usually <0.1 mg/kg

(Continued on p. 112.)

Table 5.2 Continued

Nutrients	Main functions	Some of the suggested signs of deficiency	Some of the suggested signs of excess	High source	Moderate source	Low source
Vitamin A (fat soluble)	Normal growth; production of visual pigment in the eye; maintenance of skin and epithelial tissue; aids in resistance to infection; bone	Night blindness, poor growth, excessive lacrimation, reduction in disease resistance, reduced appetite; liver has ~2 months of reserves; beta-carotene of feed destroyed by heat, light and oxidation in stored feed	?Teratogenic effects; unthriftyness, poor muscle tone, ataxia and loss of hair; unlikely to result from provision of beta-carotene-rich sources because the horse is believed to be able to reduce the conversion of beta-carotene to vitamin A	Leafy green plants Vitamin A equivalents ~200 000 IU/kg, but will vary with plant maturity, season, etc. Cod liver oil ~200 000 IU/20 ml Different synthetic sources may have different availabilities	Yellow maize ~2000 IU/kg Legume hays, early stage 50 000 IU/kg	'Aged' preserved forages (rapid loss in cured hays) Oats <500 IU/kg Barley<1000 IU/kg
Vitamin D (fat soluble)	Normal bone growth; calcium and phosphorus regulation; synthesised in skin by sunlight; believed involvement in Ca metabolism not as great as in other species	Skeletal abnormalities; associated with reduced calcium uptake; vitamin D may be destroyed by heavy metals and alkaline components of feeds	Hypercalcaemia; hyperphosphataemia; bone resorption; anorexia; soft tissue calcification; poor performance	Action of sunlight on the skin Synthetic sources Cod liver oil ~2000 IU/ 20 ml	Sun-cured forages Alfalfa hay ~1500 IU/kg	Little or none in cereals and preserved aged forages
Vitamin E (fat soluble)	Maintenance of normal growth; maintenance of normal muscle metabolism; antioxidant; promotes immune function; supplementation is believed to be most beneficial if given orally daily	Myodegeneration (white muscle disease); effect on immune system; suggested to have a negative effect on performance; equine degenerative myeloencephalopathy and equine motor neurone disease thought to involve a vitamin E deficiency	Not reported, although has been suggested in very high doses may interfere with absorption of other fat-soluble vitamins, such as vitamin A	Synthetic or natural concentrated tocopherols	Oils of some grain seeds; wheatgerm ~2.1 mg/20 ml Green forage ~ 100–450 IU/kg	Cereals <30 IU/kg Alfalfa hay ~10–30 IU/kg
Vitamin K (fat soluble)	Involved in blood clotting	If hindgut fermentation is suppressed, signs may be seen?; converted to active form in liver so if liver function is compromised signs may be seen; ? some plants may also interfere with action, resulting in haemorrhage	Plant form not well absorbed; injectable can be toxic and said to result in depression, kidney failure, loss of appetite and laminitis	Not thought required in the diet as synthesised in the hind gut Most forages and hays are adequate substrates		

Vitamin	Function	Comments	Toxicity	Synthesis / source	Source	Source
Thiamine (vitamin B1, water soluble)	Growth; energy production; nerve function; intake at 3 mg/kg feed has been suggested to increase growth rate	Reduced growth rate; reduced appetite; muscle tremors; bracken fern poisoning (contains thiaminase) causes nervousness	Claims for tranquillising or behaviour-modifying effect have not been substantiated in controlled experiments	Synthesised by bacteria in the GIT; Brewer's and Baker's yeast contain 150–160 mg/kg yeast as a good source of thiamine as well as other B vitamins	Cereal by-products ~10–15 mg/kg if contain the scutellum and germ, which is rich in thiamine	Legume hays ~3 mg/kg; Cereals ~5 mg/kg
Biotin	Involved with maintenance of hoof, skin, hair and other tissues; metabolism	Some horses with crumbly hooves seem to respond to amounts ten or more times the maintenance for prolonged periods, e.g. ~3–5 mg/100 kg BW for up to 12 months; biotin in wheat, barley, sorghum and bran said not to be available due to phytate binding	Not known	Synthesised by bacteria in the GIT; Brewer's yeast ~1 mg/kg dried yeast	Reasonably good; Sugarcane molasses ~0.7 mg/kg; Wheat bran ~0.4 mg/kg	Oats ~0.3 mg/kg; Peas ~0.2 mg/kg
Folic acid	Associated with vitamin B12 and blood cell production; synthesised by microbial fermentation and higher levels found in plasma of pastured horses	Possible advantage in supplementing horses in training that are stabled; no signs reported; best to add supplements to feed if wish to supplement because intramuscular injections do not raise plasma levels for long	Not known	Brewer's yeast ~10–15 mg/kg	Wheat bran ~0.8–1.8 mg/kg; Alfalfa meal, dehydrated ~1.6 mg/kg; Rice bran ~1.6 mg/kg	Cereal grains, variable, ~0.1–0.6 mg/kg
Vitamin C (ascorbic acid, water soluble)	Formation of cartilage and bone; biological antioxidant; normal growth; immune system and wound healing	Horses do not in theory need vitamin C levels in their diets; ? advantage of supplementation in older horses, horses in intense work or under stress	Not reported	Manufactured within body; absorption from synthetic sources not always good and individuals variable	Pasture contains variable amounts	

to supply the essential nutrients not contained in the forage or the forage/concentrate combination. The nutritional content of forages is often not known but guidelines are available. Analysis of batches of preserved hay is possible, so that supplementation can be based on improved knowledge.

Guidelines to requirements can be provided, which then need to be tailored to individual circumstances. One of the main reference materials used and referred to is the National Research Council (NRC) requirements (NRC, 1989). This provides *minimal* rather than *optimal* requirements.

'Dry matter' versus 'as fed'

'Dry matter' basis refers to the feed or forage after the moisture has been taken out, whereas the term *'as fed'* refers to a feed as it would be fed to a horse. Most concentrate feeds such as cereals, cubes, pellets, etc. contain ~10% moisture, with a DM content of 88–92%. Fresh forage contains 20–60% moisture. Because only the DM contains nutrients, more feed will need to be fed to match requirements if the feed contains more water.

Requirements can be given in a variety of ways. Two of the most common are:

- Per kg DM feed intake
- Amounts per day on an 'as fed' basis

It is important to check which units are being used. Either can be suitable, but obviously the DM intake guidelines rely on horses being fed appropriate amounts of feed for their age, reproductive status, workload, etc. Guidelines on expected intakes are given later in this chapter (see Table 5.10).

To convert from an 'as fed' to a 'dry matter' basis, divide the 'as fed' value by the DM percentage, e.g. pasture protein content on an 'as fed' basis is 4% and the DM content is 40%, so the protein content on a DM basis would be $4/40 \times 100 = 10\%$.

To convert from 'dry matter' to an 'as fed' basis, multiply the 'as fed' value by the DM percentage, e.g. cereal protein content on a DM basis is 12% and the DM content is 90%, so the protein content on an 'as fed' basis would be $12 \times 90/100 = 10.8\%$.

What nutrients are needed

Like all animals, horses need to be provided sufficient of the following in a balanced diet:

- Energy
- Protein
- Vitamins
- Minerals
- Water

A guideline to the various functions and sources of the most important nutrients for the horse is outlined in Table 5.2.

Energy

Critical to feeding any horse for health and vitality is the appropriate and adequate supply of energy. If a horse is fed too little energy for its needs it will tend to become dull and lethargic, it can lose weight and/or become ill. If fed too much energy or inapppropriate energy sources, it may become excessively lively, can gain weight and/or become ill.

Adult horses in particular tend to be fed primarily for energy and then the diet is balanced for protein, vitamins and minerals. Presently there are two main ways used to describe the energy potential of a horse feed: digestible energy (DE) and net energy (NE). Each of these has been determined in a number of ways over the years. The DE is the most commonly used in the UK and USA, with the NE system gaining popularity in France and Scandinavia. Two units of energy are in common use in the horse industry: the joule (J), predominantly in Europe; and the calorie, in the USA (4.184 J = 1 calorie). Some recommendations are given for estimated metabolic bodyweight and others are given for actual bodyweight.

Sources

Certain nutrients in a horse's diet provide the energy intake for that individual, following conversion of their chemical energy to other forms of chemical energy, mechanical energy and heat. Dietary energy is provided to the horse by four principal dietary energy sources:

(1) Hydrolysable carbohydrates, e.g. starch.
(2) Fermentable carbohydrates (e.g. cellulose, pectins and hemicelluloses, which cannot be broken down by mammalian enzymes).
(3) Fats: naturally ~ <3% of total feed intake.
(4) Proteins (not a nutritionally preferred option as an energy source).

With the exception of feeds high in fats or ash, the gross energy content of most feeds is similar. Differences arise mainly from differences in digestibility. Hay is less digestible than cereals and produces much more spare 'lost' heat, so is much more 'internally heating' and is therefore especially useful in winter. The efficiency of conversion of digestible to usable or net energy also differs widely: cereals have higher net energy than hay, which in turn contains more than twice the net energy of straw; vegetable oils contain proportionally more net energy than the cereals and 2.25–3 times the amount of digestible energy. Replacing forage with cereals and/or fat decreases the amount of feed the animal has to eat in order to obtain the required amount of energy (this is important because horses have a finite appetite).

Maintenance requirement

An adult horse at rest requires very approximately 13–15 MJ/100 kg BW (for details, see further reading list) and so typically will need to eat ~1.5–2.0% of its BW in DM (depending on energy content) to meet demands.

If the energy content of the feed is high or the animal is a good 'doer', it may be able to manage on less than this amount of feed to satisfy its energy needs but not its psychological needs. Then, either the diet should be changed to one with a lower energy intake or perhaps be bulked out with a lower energy feed such as more mature hay or chaff.

Pregnant and lactating mares

In late pregnancy some allowance for the energy needs of the fetus is needed. It has been recommended that thoroughbred mares in the 9th, 10th and 11th month of pregnancy should receive 1.11, 1.13 and 1.2 times the maintenance requirements, respectively.

In lactation, mares need maintenance requirements plus an allowance for the energy content of the milk produced. Milk production will vary from around 2 to 4% BW daily, according to body size, how good a milker the mare is and the stage of lactation.

Growth and exercise

Need to allow for growth and exercise if appropriate (see NRC, 1989).

Protein (Table 5.3)

- Essential amino acids have to be provided by the diet because they cannot be manufactured.
- Proteins are not an efficient energy source; nitrogen must be removed because excess protein is not stored, resulting in an increased water requirement and potentially higher ammonia levels in the stable.
- Higher amounts of protein are needed for young growing animals, those in hard work, as well as pregnant and lactating mares.
- The NRC lysine requirements are based on a ratio of lysine to digestible energy. This may underestimate the lysine requirements in rapidly growing horses and overestimate them in older slow-growing horses.

Minerals

Sodium, potassium, chloride (macrominerals and electrolytes)

Traditional forage-based horse diets are rich in potassium and require no further supplementation. A possible exception is for horses working hard on low-fibre diets for prolonged periods of time, especially in hot climates. In contrast, traditional diets contain little sodium, so salt supplementation is common.

Maintenance

A guide to maintenance requirements is given in Table 5.4. Low mineral intakes may reduce the endogenous losses of sodium and potassium and therefore reduce the daily requirements, but this is not believed to be so with chloride.

Table 5.3 Guide to the protein and lysine requirements of horses based on NRC guidelines (NRC, 1989)

Nutrient	Maintenance	Exercise	Growth	Pregnancy /lactation
Protein expressed as: (a) % in total diet on a 90% DM basis (b) g/MJ digestible energy/day (c) g/100 kg BW	(a) 7–8% (b) 9.6 (c) 130–150 g	(a) 8.5–12% (b) 9.6 (c) 170–270 g	Weanling (a) ~13% (b) 11.95 Yearling (a) 11.3% (b) 10.75	9 months, 8.9% 10 months, 9.0% 11 months, 9.5% Lactation <4 months, 12.0% >4 months, 10.0%
Lysine (g/day)	0.035 × g crude protein	0.035 × g crude protein	Weanling 0.5 g/MJ digestible energy/day Yearling 0.45 g/MJ digestible energy/day Two-year-old 0.41 g/MJ digestible energy/day	0.035 × g crude protein

	Assumed availability (%)	Estimated amount in sweat (g/l)	Maintenance (mg/kg BW/day)
Sodium	80–90	3.2	20
Potassium	80	1.6	50
Chloride	100	5.5	80

Table 5.4 Guide to the sodium, potassium and chloride requirements of the horse at rest and the information needed to estimate the requirements for exercise (which varies according to the literature source)

Exercise

- The requirements for exercise should take into consideration the content of sweat and the amount of sweat produced, i.e. for light, moderate, hard and very heavy exercise the values are around 0.5–1, 1–2, 2–5 and 7–8 l of sweat/ 100 kg BW, respectively.
- Salt should be provided for many horses in work. For those horses in little or no work the provision of a salt block may be adequate; ensure that it is sited so that its use by an individual horse can be monitored. In particular, where complementary feed or a vitamin/mineral supplement is being fed, any block should be of pure salt rather than mineralised. It is not recommended to use blocks formulated for other species.
- For those horses in heavy work or who sweat noticeably, the recommendation is that additional salt should be added to the feed or given as a supplement during the period of heavy exertion,

e.g. at the rest stops in a trail ride on a hot day. Advice on how much salt should be needed for a particular horse and diet may be calculated, but as a rough guide: for a 500-kg horse the regular daily amount fed should start at ~14 g (½ oz)/day and build up to ~56 g (2 oz)/day, depending on the core diet, time of year, workload and sweating rate. If, with the addition of salt, the horse either will not eat the feed or obviously urinates more than normal, it may be helpful to reduce the amount by ~14 g (½ oz), leave it at this level for a few days, monitor and reassess. Estimates of sweat loss can be made by weighing a horse accurately before and after exercise and calculating from that: ~0.9 l of fluid is lost for every 1 kg of BW.
- Some horses that are fed low levels of forage, especially if hay is replaced on a weight to weight basis with haylage, may become deficient in potassium.

Table 5.5 Guide to the calcium, phosphorus and magnesium requirements of the horse at rest and the information needed to estimate the requirements for exercise and lactation (see text)

	Estimated availability (%)	Approximate amount deposited in milk, early and late lactation (g/l)		Estimated amount in sweat (g/l)	Maintenance (mg/kg BW/day)
		Early	Late		
Calcium	50	1.2	0.8	0.12	50
Phosphorus	35–47	0.75	0.5	<0.01	22–30
Magnesium	40	0.09	0.045	0.05	15

Pregnancy/lactation/growth

Pregnant, lactating and growing horses probably need ~0.1–0.3% of the total diet as salt (on an 'as fed' basis). Pregnant mares need ~0.35% potassium in the total diet, early lactating mares need slightly more at ~0.4% and growing horses not in work need ~0.3%.

Calcium, magnesium and phosphorus (macrominerals and electrolytes)

The greatest requirements for all three minerals are in young growing animals and mares at peak lactation:

- Losses in sweat are small.
- During prolonged inactivity, the intakes of calcium and phosphorus should be increased to ~20% above recommended levels to compensate for the losses from the skeleton.
- Diets need to be formulated to take into account the calcium content of the hay. Grass hays are likely to be deficient in calcium, particularly for growing and lactating horses. Legume hays contain more calcium and are often sufficient for these animals. Grain is rich in phosphorus but is a very poor source of calcium. Calcium supplementation will be needed with a high grain diet, depending on the legume intake.
- The calcium to phosphorus ratio of the total diet ideally should be between 1.5 : 1 and 2 : 1.

Maintenance

Minimum requirements have been based on estimated endogenous losses and assumed availabilities, as illustrated in Table 5.5.

The NRC gives the minimum requirements on a diet basis as being 0.21, 0.15 and 0.08% of the total diet on an 'as fed' basis for calcium, phosphorus and magnesium, respectively. The author suggests that levels of 0.4, 0.25 and 0.15% of the diet may be more like the target minimal values.

Exercise

As for sodium, potassium and chloride, calculations can be made based on the maintenance requirements with an allowance for the amount of sweat produced and the amounts found in sweat. Because the concentrations in sweat are comparatively low, often little increase is recommended for horses in work. The NRC, for example, suggests minimal requirements for exercise: calcium, ~3 g/kg feed 'as fed'; phosphorus, 1.9–2.3 g/kg; magnesium, 1.0–1.2 g/kg. The author would recommend around twice these levels for calcium, between 150 and 200% of the phosphorus (to keep the Ca/P ratio between 1.5 : 1 and 2 : 1) in order to allow for bone developments and change during exercise and training and 1.5–2 g/kg feed 'as fed' for magnesium. An extra allowance is needed for young growing horses in work.

Growth

For calcium in particular, an allowance is needed for young growing horses that are in work.

Pregnancy and lactation

In pregnancy the minimum requirements based on the NRC would be:

- Ca g/day = 0.45 × MJ/day (~0.4% of total diet 'as fed')
- P g/day = 0.345 × MJ/day (~0.3% of total diet 'as fed')
- Mg g/day = 0.115 × MJ/day (~0.1% of total diet 'as fed')

Vitamin	Maintenance	Pregnancy/ lactation	Growth	Exercise	Maximum upper limit recommended
A	4000	6000–7000	4000–5000	5000–6000	16 000
D	500	900	1000	500	2 200
E	100	160	160	160–250	1 000

Table 5.6 Suggested intakes of the main fat-soluble vitamins in IU/kg DM of feed (will need to be modified with individual circumstances)

In lactation the requirements depend on the amount of milk produced and the amount deposited in the milk. For calcium the requirements for a moderately milking mare in early lactation would be, as a minimum, ~0.5% of the diet on an 'as fed' basis or 5 g/kg feed.

Vitamins

Fat-soluble vitamins A, D, E and K

The author and others tend to recommend that the daily intakes of vitamins A, D and E are 1.5–3 times those recommended by the NRC (see Table 5.6). No requirement has been set for vitamin K, which is involved in blood coagulation. It has been linked anecdotally with exercise-induced pulmonary haemorrhage (EIPH) but there has been no scientific evidence.

Vitamin B (water soluble)

Precise dietary requirements have not been established for the horse. Suggested levels are:

- Thiamine at 3 mg/kg DM feed intake per day for all animals apart from working horses, for which the level is 5 mg/kg DM.
- Riboflavin at 2 mg/kg DM for all horses (levels around twice this have been recommended by some).
- Folic acid suggested levels are 0.55 mg/kg DM feed for adult horses at rest and in light to moderate work, but levels are ~1.1 mg/kg DM in pregnant and lactating mares and ~1.7 mg/kg DM for those in intensive work and for young growing horses with the greatest demands.
- Vitamin B12: 5 μg/kg feed 'as fed' for performance horses and 15 μg/kg feed for young growing horses have been suggested.

Vitamin C

The vitamin C needs in the healthy horse are met by tissue synthesis, but horses that have been subjected to trauma or major surgery may require supplementation using suggested levels of 30–40 mg/kg BW/day. Although the efficiency of absorption from all oral ascorbic acid sources is thought to be relatively poor, it has been suggested that ascorbyl palmitate may have better availability than many others.

Trace elements or microminerals

A guide is given in Table 5.7.

Feedstuffs commonly fed to horses

Exactly which cereal types and forages are most likely to be fed will vary from country to country and area to area. A short overview of some of the more common non-forage-based feedstuffs used for horses is given in Table 5.8. A short overview of the various categories of feedstuffs is given below.

Cereal straights

These are the basic components of home-mixed feeds purchased from a feed mill or feed wholesaler. The most common cereals are oats, barley and maize (corn). Various processes can be applied before sale/use, e.g. bruising, rolling, flaking and micronising, with the aim of improving digestibility/ palatability (and appearance).

Additional separate feedstuffs

These can add to the energy/protein composition of the ration. Commonly fed examples are:

Table 5.7 Guide to the recommended concentrations of trace elements (mg/kg DM) in the diet (modified from NRC, 1989)

Trace element	Maintenance	Pregnancy/ lactation	Growth	Exercise	Maximum upper limit
Copper	15	20	20	15–20	800 (less in growing horses if zinc not elevated)
Zinc	45	60–80	60–80	60–80	500 (Zn : Cu ratio of diet should be 3 : 1–4 : 1 ideally)
Manganese	45	60	60	60	750
Iron	40	50	50	50–70	750
Selenium	0.2	0.2–0.3	0.2	0.2–0.3	2
Cobalt	0.1	0.15	0.15	0.15	10
Iodine	0.2	0.2	0.2	0.2–0.3	5

Meyer (1987) has recommended that the iron requirement of the 500-kg horses is 500, 600 and 1200 mg/day for light, moderate and heavy exercise.

- Sugarbeet, usually soaked before feeding
- Molasses
- Wheat bran
- Rice bran/pollard
- Linseed
- Soybean meal

Compound feedstuffs or complementary complete feedstuffs

These are a mixture of the cereal straights or their products with additional feeding stuffs and vitamins/minerals plus other supplements, produced by a commercial manufacturer. They are designed so that, when fed as directed with appropriate roughage (and usually salt), they provide an adequate and balanced ration for that type of animal. There are three main formats:

(1) **Nuts/pellets/cubes**: very popular, especially for maintenance or light work.
(2) **Extruded feeds**: vary in popularity, depending predominantly on country/area.
(3) **Coarse mixes (sweet feed)**: contain a number of processed cereals together with molasses or glucose syrup and other ingredients such as grass nuts/pellets, locust beans, sugarbeet pellets and protein/mineral/vitamin-balancing pellets.

Compound complete feeds

These are similar to the above but contain sufficient fibre sources to be fed without the need for additional roughage. Not currently popular in the UK but used in areas where roughage is in limited supply or very expensive.

Supplementary complementary feeds

These are designed to complement the basic straights component of the ration and therefore to help correct any likely deficiencies/imbalances and/or to improve the ration. They are produced by a commercial manufacturer and are not designed to be fed in large amounts or on their own. The main examples would be the various cereal (especially oat) balancers.

Supplements

These are fed in rather small quantities, usually obtained from a commercial manufacturer or commercial feedmill; most (apart from fat/oil, which is commonly described as a supplement) are not designed to add substantially to the basic energy/protein content of the diet. They are usually in the form of powders, liquids or small pellets, e.g. vitamin/vitamin sources, minerals/electrolytes,

Table 5.8 Guide to some of the more commonly fed non-forage feeds and typical contents (g/kg DM) in the UK

Feedstuff content	How commonly fed	Good points	Points to consider
Cereals	Whole or more commonly processed; fibre content increases from maize, through wheat, triticale, naked oats, barley and oats; protein content tends to be highest for triticale and decreases progressively for wheat, barley, naked oats, oats and maize	Most are palatable to horses and well digested; included primarily as a source of energy, which is present mainly as starch. The starch grains of different cereals vary slightly in chemical structure and size so that their patterns of digestion differ slightly	Generally low in lysine and methionine; calcium generally low — unbalanced Ca: P ratio as P relatively high; salt and sodium levels generally low (~0.2 g Na/kg DM); contain up to 1% phytates, which make the phosphorus less available and bind calcium — even though the phytates may be broken down in the hindgut, the released minerals cannot be absorbed from there; rancidity and spoilage rate increase with processing
Oats DM 88% CF 100 Oil 40 CP 110 Starch 470 Ca 0.8 P 3.5	Whole most common; bruised, rolled and crushed; 'naked' — without husks — lower fibre, better protein content and quality; clipped or racehorse oats remove part of the fibrous hull and therefore increase the relative starch to fibre ratio	Higher fibre than many cereals in relation to its starch content — oat starch well digested in small intestine, making it a more 'safe' cereal; lowish energy content; sugar ~1.5%	No proven advantage of processing unless horse has poor dentition; not more than 0.4 kg/100 kg BW per meal; lowest energy content of most commonly fed grains — increases the bulk needed for intensively exercising horses to meet energy; high variability in nutrient content
Corn/maize DM ~87% CF 20 Oil 35 CP 90 Starch 700 Ca 0.2 P 3.0	Flaking, steaming, and micronising improves small intestinal starch digestion	Energy-dense cereal more than twice the energy per unit volume of oats, although the difference is only 20% on a DM basis; less waste heat of fermentation so more helpful in hot conditions; fair source of vitamin A unless aged; sugar ~1% on DM basis	Lowest crude protein of common cereals (~8–10% DM); cracked corn commonly fed in the USA but unprocessed corn is not well digested in the small intestine, with an increased risk of excess starch reaching the hindgut; advise not more than 0.25 kg/100 kg BW per meal; corn is prone to mould infestation and production of mycotoxins; adding molasses may substantially increase intake rate
Barley DM ~86% CF 50 Oil 20 CP 120 Starch 530 Ca <1 P 4.0	Generally fed rolled, crimped or soaked to improve palatability (by opening up the closely attached hull) or cooked/micronised to increase digestibility and allegedly improve behaviour in some horses	Higher level of energy than oats but lower than corn; lower oil content so less risk of rancidity after processing; like oats has a hull; sugar ~3.5%	Whole barley is harder and less palatable than oats and starch less well digested in the small intestine than oats; contains hordenine, which can have relevance when testing under Jockey Club or FEI rules; more likely to suffer weevil infestation
Wheat DM ~85% CF 25 Oil 18 CP 120 Starch 660 Ca 0.5 P 3.5	Cracked or coarsely ground — often dusty and must be introduced gradually; can be steam flaked	Small grain — higher energy content on a weight basis than corn and nearly twice as much as oats on a volume basis; naked grain has ~66% starch and 5.5% sugar on a DM basis; low fibre (~2.5% DM)	Often more expensive; hard grain needs to be chewed thoroughly or else increased risk of undigested starch reaching hindgut; if feed is >20% as finely ground wheat, may form a glutinous mass with increased risk of gastric colic; less palatable than corn and oats

Table 5.8 *Continued*

Feedstuff content	How commonly fed	Good points	Points to consider
Wheat bran DM ~88% CF 120 Oil 42 CP 175 Starch 180 Ca 1 P 12	By-product of wheat flour milling—bran consists predominantly of the husk and the thin papery layer from around the starch—very little starch is found in bran; low-density flaky ingredient; various forms are available; nutritional content is very variable	Usually very palatable—warm bran mashes can be used as a feed stimulant in some horses, especially if mixed with molasses; can contain relatively high levels of B vitamins; CF varies 10–13% DM	Very unbalanced Ca: P content—very high phosphorus; high level of phytate, which can bind a variety of minerals; avoid high bran diets because they can lead to digestive disturbances and mineral imbalances; do not suddenly feed a high bran diet as can cause disturbances in the hindgut flora similar to any abrupt change in diet
Soyabean hulls DM ~87.5% CF 400 Oil 34 CP 135 Ca 5 P 2		Soya bean hulls have a high content of fermentable fibre and are well digested in the horse, giving a higher actual energy supply than predicted; palatable and useful as a low-starch, relatively high-energy, high-fibre feed	
Peas DM ~87% CF 60 Oil 18 CP 240 Starch 400–500 Ca 1 P 5	Micronised or flaked or split	Good protein source with a reasonable amino acid profile (lysine ~15–18 g/kg DM, threonine 8–10 g/kg DM); sugars ~55 g/kg DM	Certain varieties including those fed in the UK contain trypsin inhibitors and other anti-nutritive factors and therefore must be cooked before feeding; other varieties from other countries contain far lower amounts and can be fed whole or more commonly rolled or flaked
Beans—winter DM ~85–90% CF 83 Oil 14 CP 280 Starch 400 Ca 1 P 9	Often cracked, crushed or coarsely ground or rolled following micronisation, but can be fed whole; cooked or micronised for certain varieties such as winter horse beans and field beans, where potentially toxic factors are present; field bean is the main variety grown in the UK; not normally fed in large quantities	High in energy (15 MJ DE/kg DM) and protein with a reasonable lysine content, especially the field beans (~15 g/kg), and are suited to horses in hard work or breeding/growing animals, but soyabean has a better amino acid profile; rich in phosphorus but poor in calcium and manganese (~8 mg/kg DM)	Bean protein is not believed to be as well digested in the small intestine, especially if uncooked; most varieties of beans are best cooked before feeding because they contain low levels of a trypsin (the enzyme that breaks peptides into amino acids) inhibitor and other anti-nutritive factors; they are normally micronised or cooked and split open; field beans, for example, also contain tannins, which can have adverse effects—again, appropriate cooking processes are needed to destroy such anti-nutritive factors
Soyabean meal (dehulled) DM ~90% CF 34 Oil 15 CP 470 Starch 34 Ca 3 P 8	Soya is commonly fed to horses with the oil removed (soya meal ~1% oil) or as full fat soya, which contains 18–19% oil and can be used as a meal or more commonly micronised as a flake	Good source of protein—full fat soya ~40% protein as fed, with high levels of essential amino acids (dehulled meal ~36 g lysine/kg DM; full fat soya ~24 g/kg DM); low starch around 1–3% DM and 8–10% DM sugar	Needs to be appropriately cooked or micronised before feeding to destroy the protease inhibitors, anticoagulant factors, allergenic and goitrogenic factors; meal is not always very palatable and may need to be added gradually to the diet; antinutritive factors are destroyed in meal production; micronised or

(Continued on p, 122.)

Table 5.8 *Continued*

Feedstuff content	How commonly fed	Good points	Points to consider
			extruded full fat soyabean flakes have enhanced palatability and digestion and improved stability
Linseed meal DM ~89% CF 100 Oil 80 CP 350 Starch 50 Ca 4.5 P 8.5	Small, oval, flat, shiny, dark brown seeds; linseed meal or cake, where the seeds are cooked and most of the oil extracted and then compressed together into small rectangles, or linseed oil (bought ready prepared) can be used; newer forms of processed linseed now on the market are designed to be safe to feed without cooking	Linseed contains good protein levels (26%) and a very high oil level (39%); mechanically expelled meal has higher protein level of ~35% with a much lower oil content (~4–8%) and a high linolenic acid level and is still thought to have beneficial effects on coat condition; linseed meal contains a mucilage (30–200 g/kg) that may help to maintain softer droppings without any irritation (cf. bran); ?feed at ~10% of a grain mix to help with mild impaction	Contains an enzyme that is thought to release hydrocyanide from the glycoside compounds contained within the seed, especially after soaking unless cooked —therefore seeds tend to be boiled until they spilt open, making a gruel, tea or jelly (dependent on the amount of water added); the cake- or meal-making process will inactivate the enzyme but may not destroy all the antinutritive factors, so amount fed should still be limited; solvent-extracted meal contains low levels of oil (<2%) so has less effect on coat condition; lower lysine content than soyabean meal or other high protein sources such as canola and only ~50–60% of the amount of other essential amino acids
Sugarbeet pulp (molassed) DM ~90% CF 130 Oil 5 CP 110 Ca 6 P 0.8	Can be molassed or non-molassed; no known antinutritive factors	Rich in fermentable fibre and well digested predominantly in the hindgut; some digestion of residual sugars in the small intestine; better calcium content than most cereals but a similar protein content; better salt (~7.5%) and therefore sodium content; molassed has a sugar content of ~250 g/kg DM	Sugarbeet is usually molassed in the UK and sold as dehydrated shreds or pellets that increase considerably in volume when rehydrated, so the tendency is to soak in at least twice their dehydrated volume in water for 12–24 hrs before feeding; extruded sugarbeet has already been expanded; poor source of vitamins
Molasses DM ~74% CP 40 Ca 10 P 5	By-product of sugar cane industry; may be mixed with corn oil, for example, to improve flow	Same energy as barley on a weight basis; often used to improve palatability and reduce dust when added to other feedstuffs; salt ~5 g/kg DM; contains ~50% (up to 64% sugar, depending on what they have been diluted with) of water soluble carbohydrates on a DM basis	Lower protein than barley; sugar content of feeds or forages mixed with up to 10% or 40% molasses, respectively, still have lower sugar content than fresh early grass
Carrots DM ~12% CF 100 Oil 15 CP 90 Starch 110 Ca 5 P 3	Whole or sliced length-wise	No known antinutritive factors; DM content of ~11% and an energy value similar to oats on a DM basis; orange-coloured varieties are rich in carotene	Horses that are not used to eating carrots may bolt them—risk of choke, especially if fed chopped; will go mouldy

Ca, Calcium g/kg DM; CF, crude fibre g/kg DM; CP, crude protein g/kg DM; DM, dry matter; DE, digestible energy; FEI, Federation Equestre Internationale; Oil, total crude fat g/kg DM; P, phosphorus g/kg DM; Starch, strach g/kg DM; WSC, water soluble carbohydrates.

calming agents, fat/oil, ergogenic aids/buffers, haematonics/products with medicinal claims, herbs and salt licks/mineral blocks.

Roughage

Chaff and straw

These are the fibrous protective outer layer of grains and their stems. Straw is more commonly used for bedding and its use as an accepted portion of the roughage intake depends on the type, the country and the age and type of horse being fed. There are various forms of chaff (basically short-chopped hay or other roughage source) available. Typically, apart from alfalfa, they tend to be low in digestible energy, protein and mineral content and are useful in bulking out diets. They can be home produced or purchased, they may be molassed or have other additions, including ground limestone, herbs and vitamins/minerals, and can be processed into cubes/briquettes, etc.

Pasture and hay

There are various types of pasture: legume (e.g. alfalfa), grass (e.g. meadow, seed, tropical, mixed) or a combination. There are different ways of conserving or preserving pasture, including hay, silage and haylage products.

The nutrient content of fresh or preserved forage will depend on the species, the stage of maturity and the season. More mature grasses have higher fibre content and lower energy and protein levels. The mineral content of pastures varies with time quite considerably and so regular analysis of the grass content may be helpful, e.g. on large stud farms. One needs to consider not only the nutritive quality of the hay but also the amount of dust and fungal spores and therefore the potential adverse effects on the respiratory system.

Preserved forage intake can be estimated by weighing the amount offered and allowing for any wastage. Pasture intake is more complicated because it is unclear whether pasture intake is purely limited by the amount of time available for grazing, by the energy requirements of the horse or by the amount of supplemental feed.

UK meadow hays from permanent pastures will tend to provide higher protein (8–12% crude protein/kg DM) and digestible energy (9–11 MJ/kg DM) values compared with seed hays, which usually contain one or two grass species, e.g. rye grass or Timothy. Seed hays are more uniform and tend to be fairly mature at harvesting in the UK, with lower energy (8–10 MJ/kg DM) and protein (4–8% DM) levels. Legume-rich hays (alfalfa/clover, etc.) have high protein and calcium contents.

Haylages (Table 5.9)

Grass and other forage plants such as alfalfa are wilted to ~50–60% DM (12–24 h) and packaged so that a mild lactic fermentation occurs due to reduced oxygen levels. This plateaus out at around pH 4.5, depending on the amount of oxygen and substrate available, and inhibits the proliferation of fungal spores. Damage to packaging allows the influx of oxygen, permitting further microbial action. Haylages contain more water and less fibre, weight for weight, than hay. Big-bale haylage tends to have a higher DM content. Botulism is a low but potential risk with all haylages.

Silage

Fresh grass and legumes are stored immediately in airtight mounds or bales. A rapid pH drop, greater water activity and a decrease in available oxygen and soluble carbohydrate as fermentation progresses all inhibit the development of fungal spores. Dry matter levels of >35% and preferably >50% are recommended, with pH < 6 in order to minimise microbial action. If the pH is 5–6 the DM should exceed 40% to help prevent clostridial activity. Low-pH silage may be unpalatable for horses and may cause problems in donkeys. Specialist advice should be obtained

Table 5.9 Guide to the typical DM content of small- and big-bale haylages and grass and the hay equivalents

Type	Typical DM (%)	Hay equivalent to 5 kg of forage type on a DM basis
Small-bale haylage	50–55	3 kg
Big-bale haylage	60–75	4 kg
Grass	10	0.5

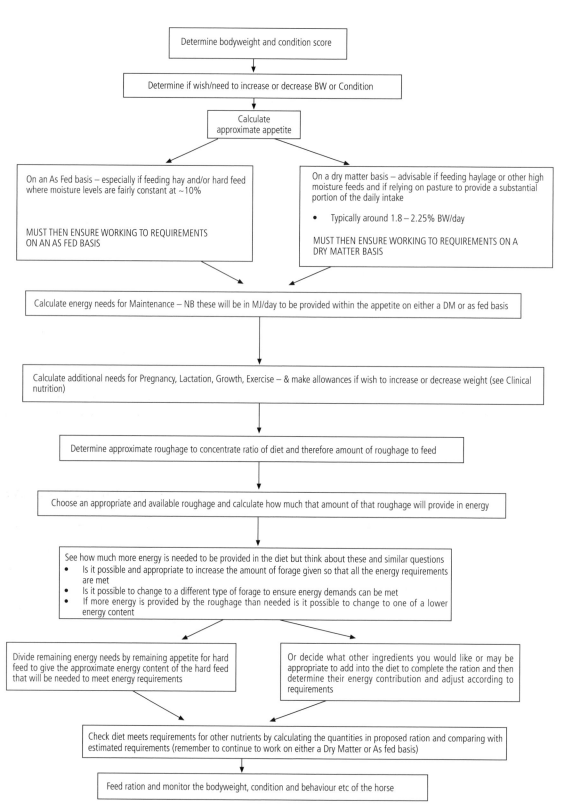

Fig. 5.5 Guide to how to formulate a ration for a horse.

Table 5.10 Guide to the likely food consumption and relative proportions of forage and concentrate based on the NRC guidelines for horses (NRC, 1989) at various lifestages and lifestyles which will vary according to individuals and feedstuffs concerned etc.

Status	Guide to approximate appetite (% BW on as fed basis, 90% DM)	Forage (approximate % of total diet)	Concentrate (approximate % of total diet)
Maintenance	1.5–2.0	100	0
Light work	1.5–2.5	75	25
Moderate work	1.75–2.5	60	40
Intense work	2.0–3.0	40	60
Last third of pregnancy	1.5–2.0	70	30
Early lactation	2.5–3.0	50	50
Weanling	2.0–3.5	30–40	60–70
Yearling	2.0–3.0	40	60
Two-year-old	1.75–2.5	50	50

on suitability before feeding home-made silage to horses, especially that produced for cattle.

One of the main advantages of silage is its decreased challenge to the respiratory system.

How much forage to feed

The amount of forage to feed will depend on the individual, how it is being kept and its energy needs, as well as what forages are available. In general, with increasing workload a decreasing amount of forage will be fed, from ~100% to 40% of the total daily intake, with the high-energy feeds increasing from 0–60%. The exact ratio will vary with the individual. Approximate guidelines for forage and concentrate intakes are given in many of the textbooks but a very approximate guide based on the NRC guidelines (NRC, 1989) is given in Table 5.10. These will need to be modified according to circumstances and individuals.

How to formulate a ration

There are many ways of formulating a ration but one method is illustrated in Fig. 5.5. The tips and sugges-

tions given above should be taken into consideration whenever designing a ration.

This chapter was intended to provide a general guide to the various aspects that should be considered when feeding horses for health and activity. Additional factors need to be taken into consideration when a horse is ill or debilitated and these will be covered in the next chapter, which concentrates on clinical nutrition.

Further reading

Harris, P.A. (2001) *Nutrition and Clinical Nutrition*. Internet site: www.waltham.com.

Meyer, H. (1987) Nutrition of the equine athlete. In: *Equine Exercise Physiology*, vol. 2, ed. by J.R. Gillespie & N.E. Robinson, pp. 645–673. KEEP Publications, Davis, CA.

Meyer, H., Radicke, S., Kienzlo, *E., et al.* (1995) Investigations on pre-ileal digestion of starch from grain, potato and manioc in horses. *J. Vet. Med. Services* **A42**, 371–81.

NRC (1989) *Nutrient Requirements of Horses*, 5th Edn. National Academy Press, Washington, DC.

Clinical Nutrition

P. A. Harris & J. M. Naylor

Assisted feeding

Assisted feeding may be needed for:

(1) Sick horses, because they often have reduced feed consumption.

(2) Horses that have recently undergone certain types of surgery.

(3) Horses that have head or neck injuries.

The horse's immune system and general defences, even in normal horses, are known to be severely compromised by 5 days of total anorexia. If food intake is decreased for long periods of time, death can occur from cardiac or respiratory failure when bodyweight falls to ~60–70% of ideal. Adult horses, provided that water intake is maintained, can tolerate at least 2 days of complete starvation. Foals have lower energy reserves and greater energy demands per unit body mass than adult horses and cannot survive long periods without food. If neonates are deprived of milk for several hours it may have irreversible effects. Premature foals, and other weak, malnourished or small horses, may have even lower energy reserves and yet greater heat loss due to poor body insulation. Many sick adult animals have higher energy needs than a normal horse, especially those in a state of hypermetabolism (catabolic), which is more common in horses suffering from trauma, sepsis and stress.

Correcting malnutrition may help survival rates after illness or surgery. Pre-existing protein malnutrition has been shown to have a more adverse affect on survival from a salmonella infection than energy malnutrition. Most sick, aphagic (unable to swallow) horses should be given vitamins, including the B vitamins, because the gastrointestinal tract (GIT) flora may be disturbed adversely, affecting normal production from the hindgut. A variety of dosages and cocktails have been suggested, but experimentally it takes a long time to produce clinical signs of a deficiency and a multi-B vitamin preparation is probably most useful. Importantly, there is often no advantage in providing additional support to well-nourished animals that soon will be able to feed normally. In such cases, forced feeding may in fact be counterproductive.

Assistance can be given to improve appetite or to provide part or all of the horse's nutrient needs, either

enterally (given by mouth or oesophagus into the gut) or

parenterally (via routes bypassing the alimentary canal, usually intravenously).

When feeding sick horses, knowledge of normal nutritional requirements is necessary. Foals can be particularly vulnerable with respect to weight loss, and an appreciation of the expected weight gain of a foal at a particular age can be useful. Rapid changes in weight, with large growth spurts, are undesirable in foals.

Improving appetite

There are various options:

- Providing fresh, highly palatable feeds such as freshly picked green grass ('Dr Green') can be beneficial, but avoid lawn clippings or very small pieces of fine grasses.
- Molassed feeds and oats often have a high palatability in healthy horses but this can change in sick animals.
- Providing a mixture of feeds, including some poorer quality (in a nutritional sense) forages and feeds, as well as the better ones, because some sick horses will prefer them.
- All feed should be positioned appropriately so that the horse can easily smell and sample the various feeds on offer.
- It can be useful to include feeds that the horse is known to like, as well as new tastes.
- Provide different forms of roughage, not just their normal type.

Treat the reason for the decreased appetite by managing the primary condition and in particular alleviate any pain, toxaemia or fever. In some individuals it may be worth considering directly stimulating the feeding centre with a benzodiazepine. Diazepam and its derivatives have been shown to stimulate appetite in healthy animals but are inconsistent in sick horses. Ataxia and sedation are potential side effects, especially in the more depressed animals (additional caution is needed when there is hepatic dysfunction).

Enteral or tube feeding

Indications

- Horses with an intact functional gut.
- Those willing to eat but oral, pharyngeal or oesophageal problems make eating difficult or undesirable, e.g. post-oesophageal surgery, botulism and cases of dysphagia (difficulty swallowing).
- To provide colostrum and therefore passive transfer of immunity in foals that do not suckle in the critical post-natal period or whose dams have

low immunoglobulin concentrations in their colostrum.
- To administer large volumes of substances that the horse would not eat willingly, e.g. liquid paraffin.

Methods

Nasogastric tube

Nasogastric tube (Fig. 6.1) can be used once for a particular purpose, repeatedly introduced or sutured in place. There are two different types:

(1) Smooth flexible tube, which is less likely to cause irritation.
(2) Large-bore tubes that help with feeding but cause more irritation than the smaller tubes.

Neonatal foals require special narrow-bore soft indwelling feeding tubes. Normal nasogastric tubes are not suitable for indwelling use in foals.

Points to consider

- It is recommended that the feed is introduced slowly via gravity through the tubes (see Example 6.1).

Example 6.1   Types of diet

Examples of types of diet that can be given through a nasogastric tube are given in Table 6.1. The amount of food that is needed to maintain condition will depend to a certain extent on whether the horse is in a hypometabolic state (requires ~50–70% of maintenance energy requirements), at maintenance or in a hypermetabolic state (catabolic and can require up to twice maintenance energy needs), plus whether concurrent conditions such as protein-losing enteropathies are present (increased protein requirements). Careful monitoring of bodyweight and condition should be undertaken.

An example of how gradually to introduce complete feeding through a nasogastric tube is given in Tables 6.2 and 6.3. It is important to ensure that water needs are met. As a minimum 3 l/100 kg bodyweight (BW)/day is needed, but unless contraindicated ~4.5–5 l/100 kg BW should be the target. Casein is a high-quality protein feed with a high digestibility. If dehydrated cottage cheese is used it should be low in lactose for an adult horse, otherwise diarrhoea may occur.

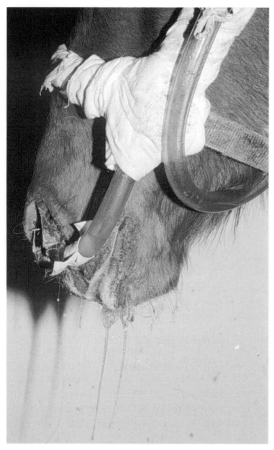

Fig. 6.1 Drooling in a horse with pharyngitis secondary to long-term maintenance of an indwelling nasogastric tube.

- Check that there is no gastric reflux before feeding, especially in foals (see Chapter 15).
- Check the position of the tube carefully (see Chapter 8).
- If the tube is left *in situ* it should be plugged with a syringe case or equivalent between use.
- Check for inflammation, irritation and ulceration around the tube, particularly in the pharynx, if left *in situ*. It can be very irritating and may make a sick horse feel worse. Tube feeding is not practical in a horse in lateral recumbency.

Indwelling oesophagostomy tube

These are occasionally used if tube feeding is likely to be continued for several days, e.g. for a ruptured oesophagus. A fistula tract will form around the tube from the oesophagus to the skin. This will allow food spilling out of the oesophagus to drain to the outside when the tube is removed (during the initial period before the oesophagus heals).

Oesophagostomy tubes are placed either through a trauma-induced fistula or preferably via elective surgery. In the latter, the incision for the tube should be sited to drain in a ventral midline position and the oesophageal incision should be as small as possible. Room should be left for drainage around the skin incision at the tube exit point. The tip of the tube should be placed in the stomach and not the distal oesophagus, because this is less likely to result in displacement or cause reflux oesophagitis. The tube should be sutured in place immediately where it exits the neck, with at least two sutures—each capable of holding the tube in place. It is dangerous to reintroduce a tube once it has come out, because there is a great risk of passing the tube down tissue planes into the thoracic cavity. If replacement is attempted, correct positioning of the replaced tube should be confirmed by endoscopy or radiography before any food is given. Special soft tubes are now manufactured for the purpose. It is best to choose as small a tube as is practical without it blocking.

Complications

Complications include tube dislodgement and severe cellulitis secondary to contamination from the opened oesophagus. Infection can spread to the thorax. Antibiotic cover and appropriate surgical positioning of the tube help to minimise such problems.

Daily maintenance

- Check sutures at each feeding. These should be replaced as necessary.
- Petroleum jelly may be smeared around the surgical site to reduce skin damage from the discharges.
- Blocked tubes are common at feeding times; clearance of a blockage can be aided by extra water or, if refractory, pass a polyethylene tube inside the blocked tube and vigorously flush with water. Fizzy drinks (e.g. carbonated cola beverages) have been used successfully to help unblock the tube!

Table 6.1 Types of diets that may be considered for enteral feeding (nasogastric tube) in horses

Type of diet	Positive aspects	Points to consider
Colostrum for foals	Colostrum contains necessary immunoglobulins and the foal relies on such a passive transfer of immunity from the dam for the first few weeks of life. The gut is permeable to these large proteins for the first 12–18 h (critical period)	If the immunoglobulin levels are <4 g/l and the foal is <12 h of age then equine colostrum should be given by stomach tube; if older, intravenous administration of plasma should be given (see Chapters 14 and 15)
Milk replacer for foals	Milk composition does vary between species, but milk from other species can be used as an alternative to mare's milk if this is not available. Commercial products are available that are more convenient—use those designed for horses rather than cows (different composition, and those for cattle may contain growth promoters or antibiotics)	See Chapter 15. May need to dilute the mare milk replacers more than recommended by the manufacturers to help improve digestibility (10–15% dilution), especially in sick foals with gastrointestinal disorders, but need to increase volume in such cases. Consider multivitamin preparations in addition (low stores of vitamin A in particular). Can add 1–4 ml of mineral oil to each feed if necessary to assist with constipation
Human enteral diets for foals	Low residue and therefore easily digested; high-energy feeds that may help sick foals with a poor appetite but higher energy requirements. They contain more energy, protein and fat than mare's milk and some contain non-lactose carbohydrate (which may help with any lactose intolerance but it is best to confirm this is present)	Use in foals over 7 days of age, either via a nasogastric tube or via the bucket. Digestive disorders often occur (bloat, colic) and the non-lactose products may not be advisable, except if lactose intolerance has been established, because the maltose and sucrose they contain may not be well digested in neonatal foals due to low intestinal maltase and sucrase. The major disadvantage is that, unlike equine foal milk replacers, these products are not designed for foals. If they must be fed, slow infusion of each meal through a feeding tube over a period of 30–60 min is recommended
Soaked pellet slurries made from grass- or alfalfa-based *complete* feed pellets (do not use pellets designed to be fed with long-stem hay)	Relatively inexpensive. Provide fibre to help maintain hindgut function and minimise risk of digestive disturbances. Usually need to be soaked in water for at least 2 h. Depending on the feed, ~5 g complete feed/kg bodyweight soaked in 6 l of water should be considered for a 500-kg horse and up to a further 6 l added to the mash at feeding times to help dilute further and flush the tube. Such a diet would be fed around three times a day. May need to start with lower volumes and increase. Take time to deliver.	Initially no more than 5–7 l of fluid slurry should be given for a 500-kg horse to minimise the risk of colic; less if starved. The amounts can be increased in successive feedings. Do not use a pump for introducing the slurry; use gravity. Different recipes are available. Can add oil as an additional energy source if the ileum is intact and functioning (up to 50 ml/meal and ~1–200 ml/day, building up to 400 ml/day/500-kg horse has been recommended—the higher amounts can be fed more rapidly if horse has already been adapted to an oil-supplemented diet, but caution if there is a risk of liver disease). Practically tubes block: need flushing with water, passing down narrow tubes or fizzy drinks, e.g. 'cola'

(Continued on p. 130.)

Table 6.1 *Continued*

Type of diet	Positive aspects	Points to consider
Liquid diets in general	Compared with soaked pelleted diets they flow more easily, less water is needed and a smaller, less-abrasive tube can be used	These must be introduced gradually to reduce the risk of laminitis and digestive upsets. At present all liquid diets that are fed without a fibre source carry a risk of inducing diarrhoea, especially if the meals are not gradually infused over a period 1 h or more. Risk of diarrhoea can be reduced by feeding at least 2 kg of dehydrated alfalfa per day to maintain large-colon function, if appropriate.
Liquid and soaked ground alfalfa pellet mix Mixture of human enteral diet and soaked alfalfa pellet slurry	Home made can be relatively inexpensive (see Tables 6.2 and 6.3)	Base on the requirements of a horse as described in Chapter 5 Ideally a 450-kg horse at rest needs a minimum of 60 MJ of energy, which would be equivalent to 14 L of full-strength enteral diets, which would be too expensive and still would not support hindgut function. Reported problems with feeding at maintenance levels include diarrhoea and laminitis. Aim for ~50–75% of the energy coming from the enteral diet and the remainder from dehydrated alfalfa meal. Start the human enteral diet at ~25% of maintenance and slowly increase in 25% increments. Problems may be decreased by slowly infusing the human enteral component over a period of 30–60 min through a feeding tube and initially diluting the solution

Table 6.2 Tube feeding regimen for a 450-kg horse (Naylor, 1999): the total daily amounts should be divided between at least three feeds

Regimen	Day 1	Day 2	Day 3	Day 4	Day 5	Day 6	Day 7
Dextrose[a] (g)	300	400	500	600	700	800	900
Casein (g)	300	450	600	750	900	900	900
Oil (canola or corn) (ml)	50	75	100	125	150	175	200
Dehydrated alfalfa meal (g)	2000	2000	2000	2000	2000	2000	2000
Electrolyte mixture (g) (see Table 6.3)	230	230	230	230	230	230	230
Water (L)	21	21	21	21	21	21	21
Digestible energy intake (MJ/day)	28	35	38	43	47	50	52

[a] Sucrose (table sugar) has been substituted successfully in at least one horse but do not abruptly switch sugar types.

- Laminitis is a potential complication (especially of low-fibre, high-carbohydrate diets), so check the digital pulses and feet daily. The incidence of this problem can be reduced by always making sure that increases in the amount of diet are gradual and by including fibre in the diet whenever possible. If more needs to be fed to maintain body-weight, then consider adding an extra feed rather than simply increasing the amount per feed.

Parenteral feeding

Total parenteral nutrition (TPN) involves the provision of a balanced diet and suitable amounts of fluid,

Table 6.3 Maintenance electrolyte mixture: 1-day requirement for a 450-kg horse (modified from Naylor, J. M. (1977) Nutrition of the sick horse. *J. Equine Med. Surg.* **1**, 67–70)

Electrolyte	Amount (g)
Sodium chloride, NaCl	10.0
Sodium bicarbonate, NaHCO$_3$	15.0
Potassium chloride, KCl	75.0
Potassium phosphate, dibasic anhydrous, K$_2$HPO$_4$	60.0
Calcium chloride, CaCl$_2$·2H$_2$O	45.0
Magnesium oxide, MgO	25.0

most commonly by intravenous administration. It can provide part or all of the nutrients that the animal needs. Even though it is an expensive way of feeding horses it can be very valuable and in foals, for example, even if only used for relatively short periods it can significantly improve the clinical outcome.

Requirements can be based on the needs of the normal horse of that size although some allowances may be required, e.g. additional energy/protein demands in response to illness and for any thermoregulatory needs must be made. However, many sick horses have reserves of energy and other nutrients so it may not be necessary to meet 100% of requirements from the start. Intravenous feeding bypasses some of the normal regulatory mechanisms in the gut, so it can be difficult for foals to adapt to this method of feeding. Blood glucose, in particular, can reach very high concentrations or fluctuate rapidly if delivery is not even. For these reasons it may not be desirable to feed more than maintenance levels intravenously.

It usually takes 3 or more days to achieve adequate energy intakes and therefore it is preferable to initiate TPN earlier rather than later if it is likely to be needed.

Indications

- Foals without a sucking reflex; foals with immature/compromised GIT, e.g. premature foals and those with severe diarrhoea or ileus or after surgery, particularly colics; also cases of sepsis.
- Animals with GIT disorders that preclude enteral feeds.

- Those animals that require more energy than can be provided by enteral feeds alone.

Administration

- A dedicated catheter is placed in a central vein, usually the jugular.
- Non-thrombogenic polyurethane (long, 6–8, 16-gauge) catheters are suitable for TPN in foals.
- Place using aseptic techniques and use catheter extension tubing so that the catheter itself is not handled. The catheter should be bandaged/protected and all intravenous tubing changed every 24 h.
- Bags should be hung and maintained at a comfortable temperature and, if necessary, use heated wrappers to keep warm.
- Use coiled intravenous lines if possible.
- Non-TPN fluids should be run through a separate intravenous line to assist in maintaining sterility.
- Replacement of a TPN-dedicated catheter in a foal is considered an emergency procedure, because the sudden cessation will result in marked hypoglycaemia.
- A fluid pump is very helpful in ensuring an even supply of nutrients and is essential in neonates.

How to finish

- Once enteral feed is re-introduced, TPN should be withdrawn over 2–3 days in an adult, starting with the lipids and then decreasing the concentration of glucose and amino acids.
- Foals should be weaned off the solutions slowly over 2 days to prevent possible hypoglycaemia and seizures. On day 1 remove lipids and on day 2 halve the quantities of amino acid and glucose solutions given.

Monitoring

- Check the site for signs of heat or swelling.
- Check the intravenous line for kinks.
- Check actual TPN delivery against intended delivery.
- Daily monitoring of haematology, especially the packed cell volume (PCV), total protein, urea, glucose, electrolyte levels (including Na, K, Ca and P),

triglyceride levels and blood acid–base status. Check plasma for signs of lipaemia if lipid levels cannot be determined. Foals need blood glucose checking 6 hourly and liver enzymes should be monitored.

- Monitor the temperature, pulse and respiration (TPR) at least 4–6 times daily.
- Test the urine for glucosuria (at least four times a day) as well as output and specific gravity.
- If long term, check bodyweight and condition score every few days. In foals, check bodyweight daily.

Potential complications

- Risk of thrombophlebitis and sepsis at the catheter site and septicaemia, especially in the neonate.
- Intolerance to glucose or lipids or other components of the diets used (excess glycine reported to increase glomerular filtration rate, which could further stress a foal with renal damage; excess glutamate has been linked with retinal and hypothalamic degeneration).
- Gastrointestinal atrophy—animal studies have shown that if nutrition is provided exclusively by the parenteral route the GIT begins to atrophy after just 3 days. This is a concern in neonatal foals and is avoided by giving 5–10 ml of milk/h via the GIT to ensure its development.
- Decrease in gastric pH has been shown in the absence of enteral feeds, possibly increasing the risk of gastric ulcers. Anti-ulcer medication via the intravenous route (ranitidine) is essential in young foals.

Types of fluids

Short term

Short term (no more than 12–24 h) dextrose saline is used in foals; this is best by continuous infusion rather than boluses (see Chapter 15).

More long term

For longer periods (>24 h), or when a balanced solution is needed, a more complete combination of carbohydrates, protein, electrolytes and lipids will be needed. Mixing the various components of the TPN

solution must be undertaken under sterile conditions. Many of the bags provided for parenteral use have several inlet tubes that allow for sterile mixing. Alternatively there are now double- or triple-chamber bags that contain the individual solutions in the separate chambers and these solutions can be mixed together when required for immediate use. Although the resultant solution is predetermined, such bags are worth considering because they make it easier to avoid the problems with bacterial contamination of solutions that can occur with other methods of mixing. Care should be taken in the use of lipid solutions in neonates, especially those that have suffered an anoxic insult, because these may develop a fatty liver. It is worth considering using amino acid and glucose solutions; although they do not meet the energy requirements, they do not carry the risk of problems associated with lipid solutions and are available in dual-compartment premixed solutions. Foals can be weaned on and off these solutions over 24–36 h (Table 6.4).

In adult horses similar solutions can be used, but at lower volumes of intakes because energy and fluid requirements are not directly proportional to bodyweight. It is frequently prohibitively expensive. One of the few indications for the emergency use of TPN in adults is hyperlipaemia in ponies (see Chapter 14).

What to feed before and after surgery

In most cases their standard home diet or a variant thereof should be fed before and after surgery because this minimises the problems that can be associated with dietary changes, such as laminitis, colic and diarrhoea. However, high-grain-based feed should be reduced considerably or preferably stopped altogether, unless the time off work will be very short.

- Wherever possible, maximise fibre intake so that time spent chewing and eating is optimised.
- Avoid sudden changes in *bedding* and diet.
- Do not be tempted to overfeed a horse in poor condition; always make changes gradually, find out the type of roughage being fed at home and either gradually increase the amount or switch to a better quality product over a 10-day period. Only intro-

Table 6.4 Type of fluid composition for total parenteral nutrition (TPN) in a foal

Fluid composition	Procedure	Observations
Glucose: 50% dextrose solution (500 mg dextrose/ml, ~7 kJ energy/ml)	Start ~10 g/kg BW/day (20 ml/kg/day) and can increase by 2–3 g/kg BW/day if required. Care and monitor diligently if go over 15 g/kg BW/day; often a sensible ceiling level	Signs of intolerance include diarrhoea, hyperglycaemia and glucosuria. If persistent signs are seen, then reduce the amount of glucose given and the energy lost replaced by lipid until the hyperglycaemia resolves May cause additional demand on the respiratory system (excrete excess CO_2) and therefore use sparingly in foals with respiratory distress
Lipids: 20% solution (200 mg lipid/ml, ~8 kJ/ml)	Start ~1 g/kg BW/day (5 ml/kg/day) and can be increased to 3 g/kg/day if it is well tolerated and done gradually	Signs of intolerance include hyperlipaemia and diarrhoea. Hyperlipaemia is said to be more common if lipid is given at >3.6 g/kg/day Should provide 60% or less of the energy in TPN Advised to be avoided in foals with liver failure or with anoxic liver damage
Protein: 10% amino acid solution (100 mg protein/ml, ~3 kJ/ml)	Start at rate of 2 g protein/kg BW/day (20 ml/kg/day) and can be increased gradually to 3 g/kg BW/day if needed	Ill horses/foals often have an increased protein requirement. To avoid the horse using amino acids for energy, the ration of non-protein calories provided to grams of nitrogen should be kept at 100–200 (take 6.2 g amino acid to contain 1 g nitrogen) or ~400–800 kJ non-protein energy/g nitrogen Branched chain amino acids may have clinical advantages over aromatic amino acids but has not been proven in horses. Has been recommended that for foals with renal failure should reduce amount of glycine in particular that is given Excess protein is not recommended, even in cases of protein-losing nephropathy

duce concentrates if improving the roughage is insufficient (see later).

- Wait to diet obese horses until after the horse has recovered from its surgical procedure. It is usually best to feed at least a half-maintenance hay ration. Starvation can cause complications.
- Following surgery the nutritional regimen will depend on: the surgery that has been undertaken, the feeds available, the individual horse and the potential lay-off time.

In many cases the recommendation is usually a gradual return to normal ration, with hay being introduced first and then grain introduced if necessary. Further comments on particular diets following certain surgical procedures are given in Table 6.5.

How to feed horses with particular clinical conditions

Obviously, before such advice should be given an accurate diagnosis needs to be made. In addition, an accurate assessment of the nutritional status of the horse, as well as its bodyweight and condition, is needed (see Table 6.6).

Thin horse

One of the most common problems in which nutrition can play a large role is the thin horse. This condition is multifactorial and can occur for many reasons—from inadequate energy provision to poor absorption, excessive loss or metabolism of

Table 6.5 Guide to particular diets that may be advantageous before and after certain surgical procedures[a]

Condition	Diet
Hospitalised horses	Be aware of behaviour issues associated with the change in environment. Will need to occupy as much time as possible with eating if appropriate
	Alfalfa grass or high-quality grass-hay diets with *ad libitum* access to water and trace mineralised salt or preferably a vitamin/mineral mix may be best for long-term support of those patients that are not suffering from gastrointestinal tract (GIT) problems. For short-stay patients their regular 'at home' diet may be best, particularly their normal roughage, but it may be advisable to reduce concentrates
	If concentrated energy feeds are to be fed then not more than 0.4 kg/100 kg BW. Supplemental oil may be worth considering for those horses who need a bit more energy but for whom cereal-rich concentrates are not the answer
Pre-surgery	Food deprivation has been recommended to reduce gut fill and abdominal volume, potentially facilitating anaesthesia, particularly respiratory function, and exploration of the abdominal cavity (see Chapter 20). Within a couple of days of food deprivation there may be depression of the immune system and severe changes will be seen by 5 days. Wound healing may be depressed and the risk of diarrhoea increased, as well as potentially increased prevalence of gastric ulceration
Pre-abdominal surgery	Fast for ~12–24 h because 80% of the manure produced by a fasting horse will be passed in the first 24 h and faecal production is minimal by 48 h. This may facilitate surgery when time allows, e.g. for cryptorchids
	Many colics are emergency cases and fasting is not an option. Prolonged fasting makes residual faeces hard, which may make passage past a surgical site more difficult
	Mineral oils (10 ml/kg) or magnesium sulphate (1 g/kg) given 12 h before surgery may help to soften the faeces and empty the distal colon and rectum. Enemas can be used but the resultant stress on the horse and the microflora of such techniques need to be considered. Gastrointestinal ulcers are a risk to consider too
Oesophageal problems, especially those with sutured oesophageal incisions or pericircumferential ulceration	Wound healing can be an issue and feeding a traditional hay grain diet soon after surgery can be fatal in horses that have been sutured to close an oesophageal laceration or incision
	Liquid diets fed through a tube give the best healing rate. An oesophagostomy tube placed distal to the injury or incision gives the best wound healing but nasogastric tubes have a lower overall incidence of complications (see text). Paying special attention to the nutritional management for ~1–2 months following the injury can be very beneficial:
	• Soft mashes (slowest healing rate) for a minimum of 30–45 days
	• Slurries or liquid diets through nasogastric tube (intermediate healing rate)—can use initially and then switch to the soft mashes
	• Liquid diets through a tube placed either at or distal to the site of injury
	• If large amounts of saliva are being lost—increased risk of hyonatraemia and hypochloraemia—advise to increase the amount of salt fed to the horse and ensure an adequate water intake
Choke: occasionally re-impact following successful treatment due to spasm associated with the ulceration or fibrosis and stricture	Feeding a soft mash diet for 30–45 days following choke can help to prevent re-obstruction, reduce trauma to the mucosa and allow strictures, due to fibrous connective tissue or spasm, time to dilate
	Always feed a diet composed solely of soft mashes made from soaked complete feed, alfalfa pellets or alfalfa meal for at least a month if a post-choke oesophagoscopy reveals oesophageal ulceration or the horse rechokes
Removal of caecum	No long-term dietary modifications needed
Extensive large-colon resection: GIT passage time, fibre, protein and	Often recommended after 2–4 days, an alfalfa or alfalfa/grass-hay diet can be gradually introduced
	Add 0.5 kg of bran daily for the required additional phosphorus or add a phosphorus supplement. Grain should not be introduced until 2 weeks after surgery. Only feed in small meals—perhaps a maximum of

Table 6.5 *Continued*

Condition	Diet
phosphorus digestion are reduced, leading to long-term problems with malnutrition	1 kg per feed for a 500-kg horse—to reduce the risks of nutrients escaping small intestinal digestion and overloading the colon Alfalfa pellets may not be tolerated; straight grass hays are likely to be nutritionally inadequate and would need to be supplemented. Avoid straw, mature stemmy hays, coastal Bermuda grass or other forages with high indigestible fibre content at all times post-surgery
Small intestinal surgery:	Usually recommend no feed or water by mouth in the first 24 h following small intestinal anastamosis. Water at 12–24 h once gastric reflux ceases (1 L, ~6–7 swallows per hour) until not thirsty or for at least 12 h and then feed introduced at 36–48 h post-surgery if no reflux for 12–24 h. The best initial diet is probably hand-grazing fresh grass every few hours. After 12 h if no problems, one can start increasing the amount offered over the next 24–48 h until eating *ad lib*. This will vary according to the operation performed. Must provide fluids intravenously during the initial period. Ideally feed some dextrose, amino acids and protein intravenously if the total period of deprivation has been >48 h (rarely done). Based on studies of oesophageal healing it has been recommended to avoid feeding hay diets in the first few weeks postoperatively. Fibrous, stemmy hays, chaff and straw should be avoided. Base diets on soft mashes or gruels made from ground feeds such as ground, dried grass, alfalfa or complete feeds. Palatability can be improved by adding some molasses and salt. Initially meals should be small and separated by 3–4 h. Aim to start at ~25% of maintenance (0.4% BW) on day 2 or 3 after surgery and increase to maintenance by 5 days. Can use liquid diets in some cases if required. If intake does not match this, try additional supplementation by allowing to graze fresh grass
More than 60% small intestinal resection	Long-term problems include malabsorption, weight loss, lethargy and diarrhoea. Long-term diet should be low grain. Diet based on alfalfa, recommended supplemented with corn or canola oil (100–200 ml b.i.d. or t.i.d.) and with a small amount of grain to make it palatable. Oil should be fed only if sufficient ileum is left to ensure absorption. Or pelleted (1–2 cm) alfalfa in many small meals. Soya hulls, unmollassed sugarbeet pulp and other highly digestible fibre sources may be of value
Rectal surgery	Laxative diet to reduce pressure on suture lines. Fresh grass and certain pelleted or cubed complete diets (based on finely ground, not coarsely chopped, alfalfa because the grinding decreases passage time and increases faecal water content). Some complete feeds based on alfalfa can give soft manure

All these regimens vary according to the preferences of the individual vets and their clinic's routine practices. This table is a general guide only (see Mair *et al.*, 2001).

nutrients, and specific diseases such as malabsorption or malignancy. A number of factors may be present in a single individual, e.g. marginal diet made worse by poor dentition. The status of the teeth and the worming programme should be assessed in all cases. An evaluation of the diet and managemental regimen also will be needed. Regular recording of bodyweight and body condition can be very valuable. Hydration must be considered as well.

Rehabilitating thin horses without disease

In the absence of intercurrent disease the simple method to rehabilitate a thin horse is to increase the intake of digestible nutrients. It is very impor-tant that changes are made gradually. The overzealous re-introduction of feed can be rapidly fatal. Successful rehabilitation programmes incorporate gradual ac-climatisation to more or better quality feeds in grad-ual steps over a period of several weeks.

Table 6.6 Body condition scoring for horses (modified from: Henneke, D. R., Potter, G. D., Kreider J. L. & Yeates, B. F. (1983) Relationship between condition score, physical measurements and body fat percentage in mares. *Equine Vet. J.* **15**, 371–372; Ralston, S. L. (1991) Performance horse nutrition. In: *Large Animal Clinical Nutrition*, ed. by J. M. Naylor & S. L. Ralston, pp. 417–422. Mosby Year Book, St. Louis, MI)

Score	Description	Tail–head	Rump	Loin (back)	Withers	Ribs	Neck
1	Emaciated (skin and bones)	Boney	T. coxae and T. ischii very prominent	Spinous processes prominent	Bones visible	Bones protruding	Bones visible
2	Very thin	Boney	T. coxae and T. ischii prominent	Spinous processes, slight fat covering at base, transverse processes feel rounded	Bones faintly visible	Bones prominent	Bones faintly visible
3	Thin	Boney, cannot see individual vertebra	T. coxae rounded, T. ischii not visible	Spinous processes visible, fat covering halfway up; transverse processes cannot be felt	Outline visible	Bones visible	Thin, flat musculature
4	Moderately thin	Fat palpable	T. coxae not visible	Concave	Smooth	Faintly visible	Some fat
5	Moderate	Spongy fat		Flat	Smooth	Easily palpable	Blends smoothly with body
6	Moderately fleshy	Soft fat	Rounded	Rounded	Some fat	Some fat	Some fat
7	Fleshy	Rounded, soft fat		Slight crease	Some fat	Fat between ribs	Some fat
8	Fat	Flabby fat	Crease	Crease	Rounded	Hard to feel	Thickened
9	Obese	Bulging fat	Obvious crease	Obvious crease	Bulging fat	Patchy fat pads	Bulging fat /fat pads

If the horse is not at its maximum dry matter (DM) intake it can be fed more. Problems with competition from other horses may require separate management of the nutritionally challenged animal. Providing a waterproof rug can help to reduce energy expenditure in a cold, wet or windy environment, and general good nursing, e.g. grooming, can improve the feeling of well-being.

If the feed is low in digestible nutrients, or the nutritional demands on the horse are high, e.g. for growth, then the diet will have to be changed to increase the nutrient density. Poor-quality roughage can be improved by replacing it with a legume or roughage harvested earlier in its growth phase, which has a higher digestible energy and protein content. Poorly preserved roughages can be replaced with better preserved forages. It is often easier to get good-quality haylage than hay in the UK. If the roughage is marginal rather than totally unsuitable,

a simple method of improving overall quality is to add some well-preserved alfalfa to the diet; this has a higher digestibility and will increase the concentration of protein and minerals. Alfalfa is a rich source of calcium, which is particularly important for growing or lactating horses. The amount of alfalfa that should be fed depends on the situation. Weanlings can be fed diets in which all the roughage is alfalfa. This would be wasteful for horses that are no longer growing or lactating and there is no point in feeding more than half of the roughage as alfalfa for mature, non-lactating horses. Simply switching to a high-quality grass hay or haylage would be another method of giving suitable roughage to a thin horse in these circumstances. Certain dietary supplements containing live yeast may help to improve digestibility, improve the growth of foals sucking supplemented mares and may improve performance on marginal diets. Brewer's yeast (30–60 g daily for a 500-kg horse) can be incorporated into the diet as a source of B vitamins (feed with a little grain and possibly some molasses) and also may have digestive benefits. Nutrient density also can be improved by feeding concentrates. Those thin horses that are still in their rapid growth phase may require a mixture of grain and a protein supplement to meet both their energy and protein needs.

It is possible to meet all of a horse's needs with a few simple feeds. However, deficiencies of calcium and some of the trace nutrients, particularly copper, selenium, vitamin E and biotin, can occur with simple rations. For this reason a vitamin/mineral supplement may be required. Mineral supplements can be incorporated into the concentrate or top-dressed on the feed. Vitamin E is of particular concern in horses kept in stables for very long periods (months to years) without access to fresh forage. It is thought to be associated with equine motor neurone disease.

The initial therapeutic objective for a horse that is cachectic (extreme weight loss with muscle loss and weakness) as a result of severe feed deficiency is simply to re-acclimatise it to a normal maintenance diet based on roughage alone. Only after this should any consideration be given to feeding a more nutritious 'booster' diet. A period of at least 10 days is thought to be required for this initial digestive and metabolic re-adaptation. Successful rehabilitation of severely thin horses has been described using a roughage-based diet fed in a controlled fashion. On the first day, intake was limited to an amount that would provide only 50% of the maintenance requirements for a horse of similar size but at ideal bodyweight. The amount offered was increased day by day until the horses were eating a 100% maintenance ration on day 10. All horses gained weight on this regimen, mortality was low and there was some suggestion that diets based on poorer quality roughage (oat hay) might give better results than starting with straight alfalfa hay. The most consistent serum chemistry abnormality detected during refeeding was hypophosphataemia, so additional inorganic phosphate or possibly bran starting at ~0.1 kg and gradually increasing to 0.5 kg daily might be appropriate (for a 500-kg horse).

Once the horse has been re-introduced success-fully to a maintenance ration it can be fed a more nutritious diet. Grain is a good source of energy and contains sufficient protein for most situations, but always limit increases to no more than 0.5 kg/day (for a 500-kg horse). The protein and calcium content of the ration can be increased by adding alfalfa to the roughage component or by feeding a protein supplement. Again, changes should be gradual.

With time, even severe loss of condition can be reversed. Young, growing animals also can recover from periods of severe nutritional deprivation. Closure of growth plates is delayed if nutritional deprivation occurs while the horse is growing, and there are only small effects on final mature size or onset of oestrous.

Feeding for specific clinical conditions

Liver failure and hyperlipaemia

See Chapter 14 for horses and Chapter 15 for foals.

Protein-losing conditions

- For nephropathies use high-quality protein sources but do not provide excessive protein because it may exacerbate any azotaemia.
- For protein-losing gastroenteropathies (PLGE) in the acute stage, a plasma transfusion is often needed. If TPN is needed then the maximum percentage of protein energy that should be used in solution should be ~12% (of total energy in kJ).
- In chronic PLGE cases, diets of a high quality (i.e. digestibility, amino acid spectrum and balance) and quantity of protein should be fed (e.g. additional soyabean meal, canola meal or alfalfa hay as roughage) unless the horse is concurrently azotaemic.

Diarrhoea

- Requirements vary with the disease.
- In general, many require additional protein.
- If the diarrhoea is due primarily to small intestinal dysfunction then little or no grain should be fed. Highly digestible fibre is essential in all cases because the volatile fatty acids produced, together

with glutamine and aspartate, are primary energy sources for the enterocytes. Avoid overly mature, poorly digestible hays.

- If the condition is mainly a large-bowel dysfunction, grain could be beneficial. However, the exact site and extent of pathology are often difficult to ascertain in the live horse, making precise recommendations difficult. Start slowly and build the grain component up to 50% of the ration if this does not exacerbate the diarrhoea. A mineral supplement (particularly if not feeding a legume hay) with added oil (up to 20% if introduced gradually and if small intestinal function is adequate) and water-soluble vitamins also may be indicated.
- Frequent small meals are preferable.
- Often diarrhoea occurs in a state of energy, mineral and vitamin malnutrition. If small intestinal fat digestion is impaired for more than 1–2 weeks then fat-soluble vitamins A, D, E and possibly K should be given parenterally. Vitamin B supplementation may be advisable.
- Monitor the electrolyte status, especially in cases of colitis and salmonellosis.
- Probiotics may be worth considering.

Renal failure

- Supply adequate nutrition without excessive protein but it is better to maintain energy intake than to over-restrict the protein (dietary crude protein should be <10% of the DM). Good-quality grass hay, possibly with 1–2 kg of oats or maize, is one suggestion. Avoid oversupplementing with calcium, which can happen if alfalfa hay is used as the roughage or with overzealous mineral supplementation.
- If weight cannot be maintained, consider adding corn oil in grain twice a day, but watch for lipaemia.
- Try to maintain the blood urea nitrogen (BUN) to creatinine ratios (mg/dl) between 10:1 and 15:1 (<10:1 suggests inadequate dietary protein; >15:1 suggests that dietary protein may be excessive and possibly will aggravate the degree of uraemia).
- Avoid alfalfa, but if this is the only thing that the

horse will eat it is preferable to the horse starving. It is important to maintain appetite.

Old horse

- Unless kidney or liver problems are present it may be worth considering a more palatable and digestible diet than traditional maintenance feeds.
- Ideally, provide a diet with 12–14% protein, 0.3–0.4% phosphorus and 0.6–0.8% calcium.
- Roughage should be a good-quality hay, ideally a grass/alfalfa mix.
- If dentition is poor, consider a slurry of cubes or pellets made from grass or alfalfa. Soaked sugarbeet and soya hulls also can be of value.
- If this is insufficient, add a highly digestible concentrate whose digestibility has been enhanced by processing.
- Additional soyabean meal (for lysine), 50–100 g of Brewers' yeast and up to 500 ml of vegetable oil per day (500-kg horse, if thin) may be helpful, but be careful if there is concurrent liver disease.

Equine rhabdomyolysis syndrome (ERS)

- Most, if not all, of the daily intake of feed should be forage, either fresh (pasture) or preserved (nonlegume hay). An appropriate general vitamin and mineral supplement normally will be required to ensure adequate overall nutrition.
- Do not turn the horse out onto lush fast-growing pastures.
- If the horse is kept indoors, prolonged daily periods outside in a sparse paddock is often beneficial.
- If the horse's energy needs cannot be met by forage alone, then provide a fibre-based complementary manufactured feed, i.e. a high-fibre, low-cereal (low-oat) feed. These feeds tend to be 'low-energy' feeds. If the horse requires more energy then consider adding additional supplementary oil, remembering to balance the protein, vitamin, mineral and trace element intake.
- It is advisable to try to ensure that the diet provides a sufficient intake of electrolytes. Ensure that sufficient salt is given. Feed an appropriate electrolyte supplement following or during prolonged exer-

cise, especially in hot weather, to compensate for sweat losses.

- Although vitamin E and selenium supplementation is often advised, these nutrients are actually not deficient in the majority of cases. However, it is advisable to ensure that all horses, *especially* those in hard work, are fed adequate amounts of vitamin E and selenium.
- Avoid the addition of wheat bran to the horse's diet whenever possible, and always avoid large amounts (unbalanced calcium to phosphorus ratio).
- Small amounts of soaked sugarbeet may be fed, but the non-molassed variety is recommended.
- Do not feed in anticipation of an increase in workload; wait until additional energy is needed.

Laminitis

- Prevention is best (see Chapter 16). Feed in a similar way to that described for ERS, based on forage with minimal cereals and, utilising oil as an energy source if required and appropriate.
- Restrict access to grass, especially lush or frosted pastures. Muzzling may be of value in certain cases.
- Obese ponies with a history of laminitis should be restricted to 50–80% of their maintenance requirements using grass hay (plus a vitamin and mineral mix as required) until a normal weight is regained.
- In horses with endotoxic shock or other severe disease, particular attention should be paid to electrolyte status, especially potassium.

Hyperkalaemic periodic paralysis

- The aim is to control the potassium intake. Ideally keep at <1% potassium in the total diet.
- The biggest source of potassium is forage, but this varies tremendously according to type, region, irrigation and stage of cutting, so analysis may be needed. In general, grass-type forages have around half (0.8–1.7% on a DM basis) the potassium content of the legumes (1.5–3%). More mature forage has a lower potassium content than young, rapidly growing forage.
- Satisfactory diets can be made by mixing unmolassed sugarbeet pulp (which is low in potassium) with appropriate hay and a low-potassium vitamin/mineral supplement. Specific diets are now available in the USA.
- It is best to avoid lush grass, early harvest hay, legumes, alfalfa and soyabean meal and sugarbeet molasses.

Further reading

Harris, P.A. (2001) *Nutrition and Clinical Nutrition*. Internet site: www.waltham.com.

Mair, T., Divers, T. & Ducharme, N. (2001) *Manual of Equine Gastroenterology*. Saunders, London.

Naylor, J.M. (1999) How and what to feed a thin horse with and without disease; what to feed pre- and post surgery; feeding the sick horse. In: *Proce. BEVA Specialist Days on Behaviour and Nutrition*, ed. by P.A. Harris, G.M. Gomarsall, H.P.B. Davidson & R.E. Green, pp. 81–86. Equine Veterinary Journal Ltd., Newmarket.

NRC (1989) *Nutrient Requirements of Horses*, 5th Edn. National Academy Press, Washington, DC.

CHAPTER 7

Basic First Aid

N. E. Haizelden & H. J. Hangartner

Basic principles

A client asking for emergency assistance may be stressed. It is essential to respond in a prompt and caring manner, offering them reassurance and helpful professional advice. This is an important nursing role.

Definition of first aid

First aid is the initial help that is given following injury or illness. It may need to be followed up by 'second aid', which could involve more sophisticated treatment or investigations, depending on the severity of the initial problem.

The objectives of first aid are to:

- Preserve life
- Prevent suffering
- Stabilise the patient's condition
- Relieve acute conditions
- Promote recovery

Basic Rules of first aid

Safety

A distressed horse can behave in an unpredictable manner. A vital role of the first aider is to take charge of the situation and ensure the safety of everyone present.

Triage

Triage is the prioritisation of emergencies occurring at the same time. There are a number of rating systems to divide cases into categories to allow their prioritisation, e.g.:

- Life-threatening
- Urgent
- Semi-urgent
- Non-urgent
- Delay acceptable

This categorisation can vary; if a patient's condition alters, a change of category to which it has been allocated may be required. Prioritising emergency cases is difficult. It may need careful explanation to the waiting client: e.g. a horse with choke can be very alarming to a client who has not seen one before but this would rank below a road traffic accident, a wound with severe bleeding (see Example 7.1) or a colic, but above the call to attend the horse that has been lame for 2 weeks.

Immediate treatment—A,B,C

In a life-threatening situation, the immediate points to assess are:

- A: AIRWAY—*is the airway clear?* Straighten head and neck carefully and remove any obstructions (e.g. bedding). Where and when it is feasible to do so, it may be possible to pass a nasopharyngeal tube. Some cases, e.g. a horse with bilateral laryngeal paralysis, may require emergency insertion of a tracheostomy tube.
- B: BREATHING—*is the patient breathing normally?* Look, Listen and Feel. If apnoea is present (i.e. the

Example 7.1   Bleeding

Control of haemorrhage

A horse is presented to the clinic with deep wounds to its hind-limbs, having been caught in fencing. Blood is spurting repeatedly from the inside of the left fetlock and darker blood pours continuously from a wound above the right hock. The horse is shaking, has a weak pulse and a heart rate of 80 beats per minute (bpm). Mucous membrane colour is normal but capillary refill time is >3 s.

Triage

Which wound to treat first? The fetlock wound is probably arterial bleeding due to the pulsatile nature and brighter colouration of the blood lost. The venous bleeding is from a much larger vessel, possibly the saphenous vein, and blood loss such as this could result in hypovolaemic shock and death. Hypovolaemic shock is characterised by depression, fast weak pulse (reduced blood pressure), increased capillary refill time, cold extremities, reduced pulse pressure and hyperventilation.

Attempts are made to apply pressure over the tibial wound with a pad of gamgee. Meanwhile, a blood sample is taken that can be tested later. Swabs, poultice or, in an emergency, any clean material can be used to apply pressure on or near the tibial wound. Pressure should be applied for a minimum of 5 min, timed with a clock (early peeping usually results in renewed bleeding).

The horse will not stand still, so a small dose of an intravenous sedative is given. An alginate dressing is applied to the wound, followed by a pad of swabs tightly bandaged in place with a few tight turns of a conforming bandage. On close inspection the fetlock wound has a piece of wood protruding from it, making direct pressure inappropriate. An examination with a sterile gloved finger following cleaning of the wound indicates a synovial penetration.

A tight bandage with minimal padding is applied above the wound to stem bleeding. This can be left in place for up to 2 h if it is necessary to transport the horse and will be tolerated better than an old-fashioned tourniquet. The blood sample is centrifuged and a packed cell volume of 28% is recorded.

Having stemmed the flow of blood, a thorough examination is carried out with particular attention to the cardiovascular system. Temperature, pulse, respiration, colour and capillary refill are monitored carefully and an estimate of blood pressure and blood loss is made. The horse is prepared for surgery while 10–15 l of warm polyionic fluids are administered. The horse is kept quiet and warm and its clinical parameters are continually reassessed as first aid responsibility is passed over to ongoing hospital treatment.

---

horse is not breathing) then intubate and start positive pressure ventilation at 4–6 breaths per minute, using oxygen if available. If specific airway tubes are unavailable, intranasal oxygen can be given using any wide-bore tubing and the nostrils occluded to expand the chest. Flow rate should be adjusted so that the chest can be expanded in 2–3 s.

- C: CIRCULATION—*does the patient have a pulse*? If not, compress left chest wall over heart (above costochondral junctions just behind the elbow) at 20–30 compressions per minute using hands or knee, while monitoring pupil size. Remember that an airway should be established first. This is difficult to do in the adult horse and is unlikely to be effective in any horse much larger than 300 kg

(see Chapter 20). Successful cardiopulmonary resuscitation (CPR) depends on prompt diagnosis of the arrest and full facilities being available for treatment.

General approach to an emergency

When attending any emergency, the most obvious rule is *don't panic*!

Assessment

The first aider in charge must quickly gather the necessary information required and act on it, as below:

- S: *scan* to evaluate rapidly the patient, client and environment

- I: *identify* the relevant problems and predict the most likely results
- P: *prioritise* and decide where the immediate needs lie
- P: *plan* what action is to be taken and by whom
- E: *execute* the plan
- R: *reassess* and repeat and continue until the patient (and the owner) is stabilised.

Data collection

The more urgent the situation, the less evaluation and more action that is required immediately. Each time the S.I.P.P.E.R. cycle is completed, more detailed information is gathered (see Fig. 7.1).

The general appearance and vital signs (temperature, pulse, respiratory rate and consciousness) of the patient are best used for initial assessment. History taking should be directed to save time, but care should be taken to listen to the client. The priority is to determine the patient's status and not to make a definitive diagnosis initially. Often a clinical examination is carried out at the same time. Economic considerations, including whether the horse is insured and what sort of cover is in force, may also need to be addressed early on. Findings should be recorded as soon as is practical.

Pain

Even if the horse requires euthanasia, some basic first aid, particularly pain control, may be required while decisions are made. *A horse in pain will often react in an unpredictable fashion, making evaluation and treatment more hazardous.*

Restraint

In order to facilitate the safe evaluation and treatment of the patient, it should be securely restrained at all times by a competent handler. Additional restraint, e.g. the use of a skin twitch or sedation, may be needed (see Chapter 1).

Nursing

The patient's environment should be checked to see if it is safe or if improvisations need to be made. This may entail rigging up an electricity supply or extra lighting near the patient, providing shelter for a horse recumbent in a field using a tarpaulin or bales or moving it away from danger such as a road or river. The patient should be kept warm, quiet and calm. This is often a role that the owner can assist with, as long as it is safe for them to do so. Communication of your first aid objectives to owners and handlers will not only allow them to assist your efforts but will also help to relieve their anxieties.

Emergency planning

Forward planning can make dealing with emergencies considerably more efficient. Clients should be encouraged to do this by having a first aid kit and vital telephone numbers to hand. Similarly, nursing staff at an equine practice can be prepared by having a list of emergency contact numbers, e.g. for horse transporters, slaughterers and insurance companies, readily available. A number of basic kits also should be maintained that can be collected instantly with all the necessary components to do a specific task. Such kits may be required for intravenous catheter placement, limb immobilisation, euthanasia, large-volume fluid administration and tracheostomy tube insertion, for example.

Bandaging and immobilisation

Bandages, particularly of the limbs, are an important part of first aid in the horse. An injured horse may

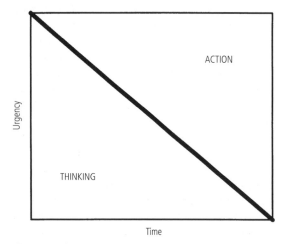

Fig. 7.1 Time for evaluation as urgency increases.

well be excited, anxious and dangerous to bandage without sedation.

Functions of any bandage

- Cover wounds to control bleeding
- Controls swelling
- Protect the injury from further trauma
- Provide a clean environment for wound healing
- Keep a dressing in place
- Restrict movement and reduce pain

In an emergency the aesthetic appearance of a bandage does not matter, but an overtight bandage may cause damage, particularly if left on for >2h. The horse may not make you aware of the discomfort of an excessively tight bandage, so ensure:

- The injured area is adequately protected.
- The bandage fits snugly and is well padded.
- Pressure over the tendons is even.
- Pressure is avoided over bony prominences, e.g. the accessory carpal bone of the knee. They should be adequately padded or the bandage split to avoid pressure sores.
- Soft tissues in the contralateral limb are supported. This is extremely important when a horse is severely lame, especially in heavy individuals.

Bandages

Any bandage is basically made up of three parts:

(1) *The primary layer*: usually this is a non-stick dressing pad, e.g. Melonin® or Rondopad®, which may be held in place by bandage padding such as Soffban®.
(2) *The secondary layer*: this is the padding that protects the injury and controls swelling. With inadequate padding and overtight bandaging there is a risk of causing a so-called bandage bow (i.e. damage to tendons), or a pressure sore. A variety of padding materials can be used. Cottonwool is ideal, because it will conform well to the shape of the leg and is inexpensive. This is compressed evenly with a conforming bandage (KBand®, or Crepeknit®).

(3) *The tertiary layer*: this is the sealing layer that holds the dressing in place and protects the layers underneath. Commonly some sort of stretch bandage is used that sticks to itself, such as Vetrap®, or a sticky bandage such as Elastoplast®. This sealing layer should not extend beyond the edge of the underlying padding in case it causes sores by rubbing. This is particularly true with foot bandages, where the heels and the back of the pastern are easily traumatised by a stiff bandage. On some other sites, e.g. the hock or knee, using a sticky bandage extending onto the skin may be the only way of keeping a bandage in place.

Robert Jones bandage (RJB)

This is a heavily padded limb bandage that is made up of several compressed layers of cottonwool. It aims to provide strength, rigidity and even pressure for:

- Limb support
- Control of limb oedema
- Stabilisation of fractures
- Protection of soft tissues

Half-limb RJB

This should extend from the floor to the proximal metatarsus or metacarpus and will require up to four or five rolls of cotton wool with 8–10 cm conforming bandages. Any wound is covered with a suitable primary layer (e.g. a sterile non-adherent dressing such as Melonin®) held in place with conforming padding (e.g. Soffban®). The first layer of cottonwool is applied adding extra distally, if necessary, to even out the thickness to ~2–3 cm throughout. Conforming bandages (minimum 10 cm width) are used to compress the cottonwool firmly and evenly. At least two further layers are constructed similarly. The cottonwool frequently will be thicker in the middle, so extra padding may need to be added at either end of the bandage to provide even support without any weak points. Splints, if applicable, are incorporated after the final layer and the entire structure is covered in 7.5-cm elastic adhesive bandage (e.g. Elastoplast®) applied with constant even pressure. The finished bandage should be an even tubular cylinder, sounding like a ripe melon when tapped.

Full-limb RJB

This requires 8–10 rolls of cotton wool and 15–20 conforming bandages. In the forelimb it should extend from the floor to the point of the elbow. In the hindlimb it should extend from the floor to the proximal one-third of the tibia. Occasionally splints are incorporated within such a bandage.

Many horses resent immobilisation, especially with hindlimb joints, and will panic and kick out violently when they first try to move, which may be part-way through application of the bandage. An RJB will provide support, but if a fracture is suspected, then a splint also may be incorporated to increase the rigidity of the bandage.

Splints

Objectives of a bandage splint
- To prevent further injury to bone and soft tissues
- To support a limb fracture
- To enable a horse to travel for further treatment

Ideally a splint should immobilise the joints above and below the area of damage. For first aid purposes it must be quick and easy to apply in the field. Proper limb immobilisation requires knowledge of limb anatomy and the types of fractures involved. The forelimb and hindlimb are divided into four areas. Each region requires different splinting techniques and an inappropriate splint may do more harm than good. Figure 7.2 gives a summary of splint placement for fractures and Figs 7.3–7.8 give examples of different types of bandage splints on the forelimb and hindlimb.

Splinting materials

Many materials can be improvised in an emergency, e.g. broom handles, wood (45 × 20 mm), Farriers' rasps, plastic piping or guttering (112-mm diameter cut in half). The material should be sawn to a suitable length and the ends padded. The ideal splint will be light but rigid. It also should be strong enough for the job and if in doubt a double thickness should be used.

Board splint

A board splint is used for suspensory apparatus breakdowns, severe tendon lacerations or distal joint luxations, to support the limb in flexion and prevent further overextension injury to soft tissues. A board of ~40 × 12 × 2 cm is secured to the toe by drilling through the hoof and board and fixing with 18-gauge wire. The limb is bandaged and padded and the board is secured to the caudal aspect of the bandage with elastic adhesive tape so that the limb is fixed in flexion and the weight of the horse bears on the point of the toe (Fig. 7.9).

Commercially available splints
- Farley compression boot
- Kimzey leg-saver splint
- The monkey splint

These are easy to apply and provide excellent support. The drawback is that these splints, to be effective, are made to fit a narrow range of sizes and so the correct size is not always available.

Applied first aid

This section covers examples of common first aid situations encountered in practice, considering conditions related to each body system in turn. Further information is available in Chapter 4 and Chapters 13–16.

Integument

Always consider the anatomy of the skin itself and determine the depth and location of the injury in order to decide on management.

Types of wounds
- *Puncture* or penetrating wound: often has a small entry point, which may be visible only after clipping away the hair. Deeper structures are likely to be involved or contaminated.
- *Laceration*: a tearing or cutting of the skin, variable in depth and tissues involved.
- *Contusion*: bruising, without skin penetration.
- *Abrasion*: usually as a result of friction; removal of superficial layers of skin. Less likely to involve deeper structures, but may be intensely painful.

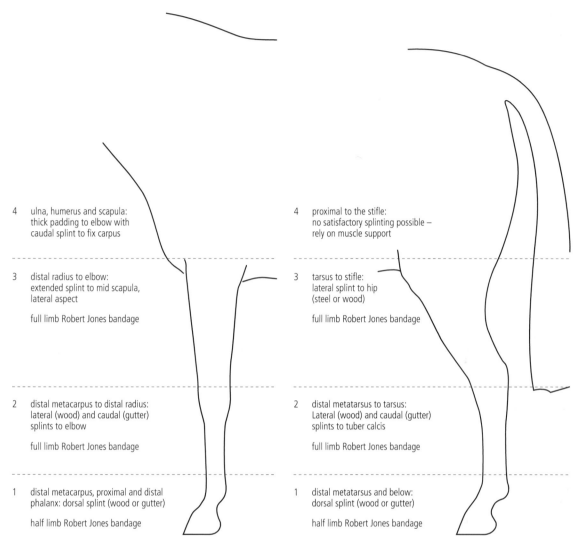

4   ulna, humerus and scapula:
    thick padding to elbow with
    caudal splint to fix carpus

3   distal radius to elbow:
    extended splint to mid scapula,
    lateral aspect

    full limb Robert Jones bandage

2   distal metacarpus to distal radius:
    lateral (wood) and caudal (gutter)
    splints to elbow

    full limb Robert Jones bandage

1   distal metacarpus, proximal and distal
    phalanx: dorsal splint (wood or gutter)

    half limb Robert Jones bandage

4   proximal to the stifle:
    no satisfactory splinting possible –
    rely on muscle support

3   tarsus to stifle:
    lateral splint to hip
    (steel or wood)

    full limb Robert Jones bandage

2   distal metatarsus to tarsus:
    Lateral (wood) and caudal (gutter)
    splints to tuber calcis

    full limb Robert Jones bandage

1   distal metatarsus and below:
    dorsal splint (wood or gutter)

    half limb Robert Jones bandage

Fig. 7.2 Summary of splint placement for fractures of the forelimb and hindlimb.

• *Burn or scald*: determine the area affected and if deeper structures are involved.

The wound's position

A small innocuous-looking wound and, in particular, puncture wounds may have very serious complications due to the involvement or contamination of deeper structures, such as tendon sheaths, joints, blood vessels, body cavities, tendons and ligaments or bones. Such wounds should be investigated further to rule out the involvement of vital structures.

It helps to understand how an injury happened: e.g. the horse that fell on the road and has a large skin deficit over the dorsal carpus will have landed with the limb in a flexed position, exposing a completely different area than that seen when the horse is standing normally. There will usually be a hidden pocket of highly contaminated tissue distal to the wound in these cases.

Key anatomical structures that may be involved in equine wounds causing severe complications include: digital tendon sheath; navicular bursa;

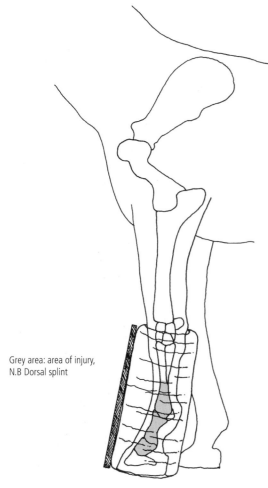

Grey area: area of injury,
N.B Dorsal splint

Fig. 7.3 Splint placement for Group 1 fractures of the forelimb. (Kindly supplied by Lucy Begg.)

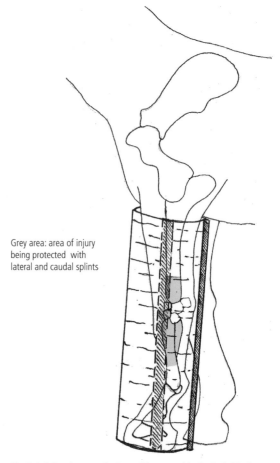

Grey area: area of injury being protected with lateral and caudal splints

Fig. 7.4 Splint placement for Group 2 fractures of the forelimb. (Kindly supplied by Lucy Begg.)

calcaneal bursa; bicipital bursa; extensor tendon sheaths; any limb joint, particularly elbow, fetlock, hock and pastern joints; splint bone.

Assessment of a wound

The key questions to ask are:

- How did the accident happen?
- How long ago did it happen? (Even wounds with minimal contamination repair best within 6–8 h)
- Is the patient bleeding?
- Are there any injured persons?
- What is the clinical state of the patient?
- Where is the damage located?
- Where is the patient located?
- How has the injury been managed up to now?
- Is the injury contaminated?
- Are there any other injuries?
- Tetanus status?

Detailed assessment of a wound may need to wait until is has been cleaned up, at least to some degree, to avoid further contamination of deeper structures. This should be carried out using gloves, and a sterile metal probe and sterile saline may be required by the clinician to explore the wound.

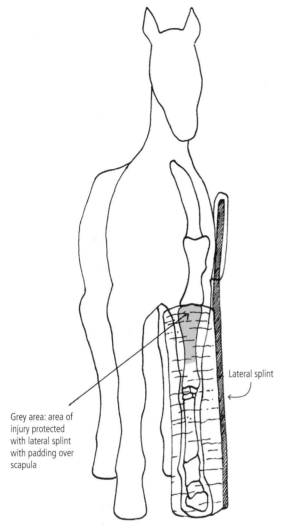

Grey area: area of injury protected with lateral splint with padding over scapula

Lateral splint

Fig. 7.5 Splint placement for Group 3 fractures of the forelimb. (Kindly supplied by Lucy Begg.)

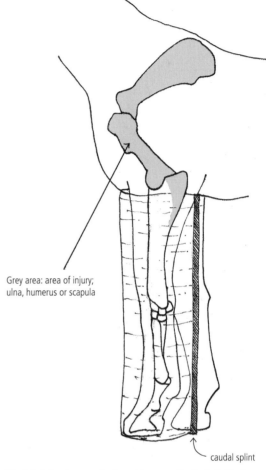

Grey area: area of injury; ulna, humerus or scapula

caudal splint

Fig. 7.6 Splint placement for Group 4 fractures of the forelimb. (Kindly supplied by Lucy Begg.)

Action and procedures

Wounds

After initial assessment of the wound, anatomy and general condition of the patient, the general first aid rule for wounds is Clot, Clean and Cover:

(1) *Clot*: excessive haemorrhage should be dealt with first. Once this is under control, the wound should be cleaned thoroughly.

(2) *Clean*: high levels of bacterial contamination prevent wound healing. This occurs due to initial contamination of the wound, application of unsuitable material or by bacteria multiplying within the wound. Obvious blood, soil and other debris should be removed from around the wound using swabs, cotton wool or paper towel. Ideally the hair then should be removed from a wide area around the wound with scissors or preferably fine clippers, protecting the exposed tissues by packing with damp swabs or a water-soluble carboxymethylcellulose gel (e.g. Intrasite®, Smith & Nephew®). The surrounding skin should be cleaned with damp swabs before removing the packing to remove small particles of hair and debris. The wound then should be

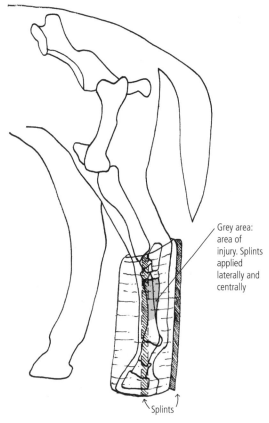

Grey area: area of injury. Splints applied laterally and centrally

Splints

Fig. 7.7 Splint placement for Group 2 fractures of the hindlimb. (Kindly supplied by Lucy Begg.)

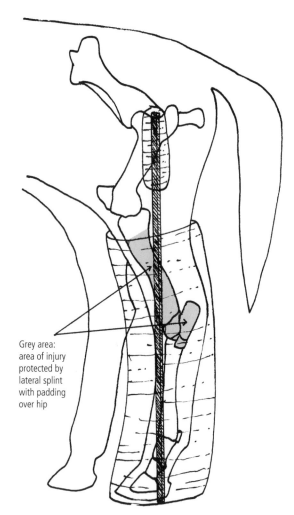

Grey area: area of injury protected by lateral splint with padding over hip

Fig. 7.8 Splint placement for Group 3 fractures of the hindlimb. (Kindly supplied by Lucy Begg.)

lavaged thoroughly using sterile saline, water, dilute povidone iodine (0.1–0.2%) or dilute chlorhexidine (0.05%). Large volumes should be used, ideally at 10–15 psi of pressure. Higher pressure will force bacteria and debris deeper into the tissues. A pump-up garden sprayer (Fig. 7.10), if available, works well or a (clean) hosepipe can be used. If not available, a 50-ml syringe and an 18-g needle will give a pressure of up to 7 psi. Lavage should be continued until the wound appears clean but not so that the tissues become pale and waterlogged. A vet occasionally may prescribe a final lavage of antibiotics, e.g. sodium benzylpenicillin, or, if soil contamination is present, metronidazole.

(3) *Cover:* carboxymethylcellulose gel (e.g. Intrasite®) provides a moist environment for the tis-

sues, protects from further contamination and may encourage migration of bacteria out of the tissues into the gel. The wound should be packed with one of these products and covered with a sterile non-adhesive dressing. In an emergency, a disposable nappy or plastic food wrap can be used to protect the wound. A conventional pressure bandage should be applied in the normal way and the patient transported or prepared for further treatment. Any flaps of skin should be replaced in their normal position. Wounds penetrating the chest should be covered and pressure

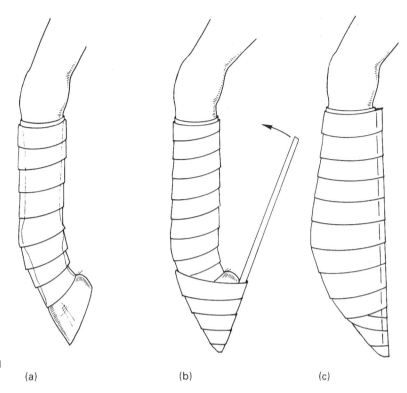

Fig. 7.9 Board splint for suspensory apparatus or flexor breakdown. (From Wyn-Jones, G. (1988). *Equine Lameness*. Blackwell Scientific Publications, Oxford.)

(a)   (b)   (c)

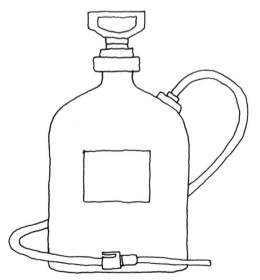

Fig. 7.10 Pump-up garden sprayer used for wound lavage. (Kindly supplied by Lucy Begg.)

applied to seal the hole, to prevent the development of a pneumothorax. Wounds to eyelids, tongue or lips may appear simple but usually will require careful surgical reconstruction.

Burns and scalds
These are fortunately rare, usually superficial and normally heal quickly. Serious burns may result in rapid development of shock and hypovolaemia. Other complications such as corneal injury and smoke inhalation should be considered, so the patient should be examined for other problems and not just skin damage (see Example 7.2).

Chemical burns
Treatment involves copious lavage with water, avoiding contamination of the persons handling the patient. Dry chemicals should be brushed off gently using protective clothing and gloves.

149

Example 7.2 Burns

Treatment of burns

A horse is rescued from a burning stable block and has partial thickness burns over its hindquarters.

The burns are cooled rapidly by lavage with large volumes of water (or normal saline or application of ice in a plastic bag) to reduce further thermal damage. Burnt tissues continue to cook long after the heat source is removed. Pain may be extreme and the vet may prescribe analgesics and tranquillisers. Once cooling has been achieved, the burns are covered with carboxymethylcellulose gel (or dilute povidone iodine, 0.1–0.2%) and protected with a plastic disposable drape or non-adherent sterile dressing to prevent further contamination.

Secondary infection is a serious complication of deep burns. When the eyes are examined for damage, they are swollen and painful. The vet administers antibiotic ointment and atropine eye drops. Lungs are auscultated for signs of smoke inhalation. Intranasal oxygen (10–15 L/min), bronchodilators (such as Clenbuterol) and broad-spectrum antibiotics may be required to combat smoke damage, carbon monoxide poisoning, pulmonary oedema and pneumonia. Polyionic fluids are administered to combat shock.

Example 7.3 Urticaria

Treating nettle rash

A yearling thoroughbred is reported to be staggering around the field in a distressed state, falling over and sometimes rolling. Multiple small raised swellings have appeared on the skin.

The patient may well have rolled in some stinging nettles. Examination is carried out to exclude other causes of ataxia (e.g. neck trauma), keeping the patient quiet and reassured. Hosing or washing with cool water can soothe the skin, or sometimes calomine lotion is used. The vet may prescribe tranquillisers and analgesics.

Nettle rash

If a horse rolls in nettles a variety of dramatic clinical signs may be seen, particularly in thin-skinned breeds. A horse may appear very lame and even stagger as if ataxic. They can mimic colic in their distress and discomfort (see Example 7.3).

Bites and stings

These may cause swelling of the affected part, usually the muzzle or limb. Cold should be applied to help reduce this, and anti-inflammatory and analgesic medication may be administered as required.

Poisoning

A poison is any substance that causes injury or death if ingested, inhaled, absorbed or injected in sufficient quantity.

Examples of the more commonly encountered toxic agents include:

- Bacterial: botulism, endotoxin, tetanus
- Chemical: ionophores, organophosphates, lead, smoke
- Plants: oak, ragwort, yew

Assessment

Suspicion of poisoning is a much more common event than actual occurrence. First aid often will be requested for suspected poisoning when a horse becomes ill for no obvious reason. Until a diagnosis is made the owners may blame poisoning, when in fact a more straightforward cause exists. A diagnosis of poisoning should be made only if a horse was clearly seen to have digested something. Poisoning can cause a variety of clinical signs, including: anorexia, ataxia, collapse, colic, constriction or dilation of the pupils, convulsions, depression, diarrhoea, dysphagia, dyspnoea, excitement, muscle tremors, muscle weakness, sweating, sudden death.

The amount of material that the horse has been exposed to and over what time period is important. Samples of suspect feedstuffs or other materials should be collected as soon as possible and placed into appropriate containers so that further laboratory investigations can be used to confirm the diagnosis. In the case of chemicals, the owner should be warned to take great care to avoid self-contamination. It should be established whether other animals are affected or at risk.

Action and procedures

General first aid for the suspected poison case means providing supportive care and treating severe symptoms, e.g. bleeding. Specific antidotes may be given in the few cases where they are available and the cause is identified with certainty, e.g. bleeding due to ingestion of warfarin is treated with vitamin K1. The condition of the patient should be monitored repeatedly. Drug treatment may be prescribed according to the signs shown (see Example 7.4). In some cases activated charcoal may be given by stomach tube to reduce toxin absorption. Alternatively, liquid paraffin may be given to speed passage of the toxin through the gut.

Useful contacts

- Manufacturer of a particular product.
- National Poisons Information Service Units. (see Appendix, p. 438)

Ocular

Conditions requiring first aid that involve the eye include:

- Lacerations of the eyelid, sclera, or cornea
- Uveitis
- Fracture of the orbit
- Corneal penetrating wound or foreign body
- Corneal ulceration
- Glaucoma

Assessment

Successful treatment of eye injuries depends on prompt and aggressive treatment. It is important to ascertain how and when the injury occurred and whether the horse has had previous occurrences of eye pain, as tends to happen with recurrent uveitis.

The injured eye often is too painful to allow complete examination without sedation and topical or regional anaesthesia (see Example 7.5). *Attempting to force open a painful eye may result in rupture of the globe and should be avoided.*

Action

It is important to protect the eye from further trauma, including self-trauma. This can be done by holding

---

Example 7.4   Suspected poisoning

A farmer rings to say that his horse is showing signs of colic. On presentation the horse is in moderate pain with muscle tremors, sweating and dyspnoea, and has started drooling saliva and passing diarrhoea.

A thorough clinical examination is required to differentiate between a number of causes, including colic, choke, botulism and grass sickness. Examination of the eyes reveals marked miosis. The horse becomes more excitable and the muscle tremors worsen. The vet sedates the horse, an intravenous catheter is inserted and blood samples are taken. Polyionic fluids are administered and the vital signs monitored.

Further questioning reveals that the horse may have been exposed to hay contaminated with sheep dip, and organophosphate (OP) poisoning is suspected. The exact make and concentration of the product is established and checks made with the manufacturer to confirm the active ingredients. Atropine is administered (despite risk of gut side effects) and the effects of the OP (salivation, sweating and miosis) begin to improve. A stomach tube is passed and activated charcoal is given. If available, oximes are a specific antidote to OPs but are not indicated for carbamate poisoning, so it is important to know the precise toxic agent.

Example 7.5   Eye injury

A horse is found in the field with a painful, swollen, tightly closed (blepharospasm) eye with excessive tear loss (epiphora) and a constricted pupil (miosis) and is attempting to rub it against a wall.

Most of the possible eye conditions may present with such signs. After sedation, a hayseed is observed in the medial canthus. This is lavaged from the eye by gentle flushing using sterile water.

the horse or using sedation. Eye protection guards, such as racing blinkers, may be used if available; they may help to avoid bright light.

Gentle palpation of the globe through the eyelids will help to establish if it has ruptured and therefore lost pressure. Cold compresses may help to reduce pain and swelling but care should be taken to avoid pressing on the globe. The vet may administer sedation or regional analgesia to enable a full examination.

Eyelid lacerations

The horseowner always should be advised to have these surgically repaired if the eyelid margin is disrupted. *Flaps of eyelid skin should never be cut off!*

Corneal ulcers

Melting ulcers can progress rapidly to rupture. Fluoroscein dye should be used to determine the depth and extent of the ulceration when the horse will tolerate examination.

Gastrointestinal

Conditions requiring first aid that involve the gastrointestinal tract (GIT) include:

- Anterior enteritis
- Choke
- Colic
- Diarrhoea
- Eventration (see Example 7.6)
- Gastric ulceration
- Herniation
- Peritonitis
- Bowel or rectal prolapse
- Rectal tear

Horses are prone to colic due to the unnatural feeding practices that we impose upon them, together with their low pain threshold. Also, certain anatomical features create potential problems, including:

(1) The horse is unable to open the cardia of the stomach and vomit. This may result in rupture of the stomach before fluid or gas reflux can occur.

Example 7.6 Castration complication

Eventration

A horse that had undergone an open castration earlier in the day has a large pink tubular structure hanging from one of the wounds and is showing signs of pain.

First it is important to establish whether it is bowel or omentum that has prolapsed. Examination confirms that it is prolapsed small bowel. The priority then is to prevent further damage, contamination or loss of bowel that has herniated through the castration wound. The same approach applies for rectal prolapses. The patient should be kept calm using sedation if necessary and the bowel supported and protected by tying a large plastic disposable drape underneath the body. A sheet (damped with clean water) or similar material can be used to improvise some protection. The patient should be prepared for immediate surgery to repair the prolapse.

---

(2) Fluid secretions and gas are produced continuously and will cause rapid distension if a bowel obstruction occurs. Large-colon torsions will cause the horse to bloat quickly, can compromise breathing and rapidly produce severe shock.

(3) The large intestine has a number of tight bends and variations in diameter, which make obstructions more likely.

Colic

Some types of colic can become life threatening very rapidly. Only by quickly recognising the severity of the colic can the chance of recovery be maximised in the more serious cases. *The goal in assessment of the colic case is to determine if the problem is treatable medically or if surgical intervention is needed.* It is important also to differentiate abdominal pain from other conditions such as azoturia, foaling and laminitis. It is a common first aid condition.

Signs of colic

- Absence of, or reduced, gut sounds
- Cool extremities
- Depression
- Elevated pulse rate
- Kicking or biting at the abdomen

- Lack of appetite (anorexia)
- Lack of bowel movements
- Lip curling (Flehmen response)
- Pawing the ground
- Playing with water without drinking
- Rapid respiration and/or flared nostrils
- Repeatedly lying down and getting up
- Rolling, especially violently
- Sitting in a dog-like position or lying on its back
- Stretching out as if to urinate without doing so
- Sweating
- Turning the head towards the flank

Abdominal pain may make the horse violent and dangerous to handlers. In extreme cases the horse must be confined alone to a well-bedded box or left in a sand school until help arrives. Gentle walking (but on a suitable surface in case the horse goes down) may ease the pain, but the horse should not be walked for protracted periods causing exhaustion. Feed should be withdrawn from the patient.

Horses in severe pain may need to be sedated to allow safe and complete examination. Pulse rate (a good prognostic indicator, with >80 bpm being considered very serious) and blood for packed cell volume (PCV) and total protein determination should be taken prior to sedation if possible.

In addition to the parameters described below for diarrhoea, the intensity and duration of pain and whether continuous or intermittent, gut sounds, amount of abdominal distension, passage and nature of droppings, previous colic history, worming status and any treatment given are all important data to collect and record.

Many episodes of colic are related to a recent change in management, feeding or exercise and so these should be checked. The colic patient should be prepared for other diagnostics, including peritoneal tap, rectal examination, passage of a stomach tube or ultrasonography as required by the vet. If a colic case is very shocked and dehydrated, administration of intravenous fluids will be required.

An important role for the equine nurse is to assist the vet in deciding whether the colic case is surgical and then to aid in the rapid preparation of the case for surgery when appropriate, e.g. clip, catheterise, remove shoes.

Choke

Acute obstruction of the oesophagus by impacted feed is commonly known as *choke*. It is a frequent equine first aid problem, which can be alarming when first seen but is rarely life threatening. Horses often arch their necks and cough, with saliva and feed material appearing at the mouth and nostrils.

It is important to establish the duration of choking and what and how much has been eaten.

Action for choke

Remove all feedstuffs immediately and keep the patient calm. Sedation may be prescribed by the vet. It is said that massaging the left side of the neck along the line of the oesophagus may help to shift an obstruction. Prolonged cases may require intravenous fluids. If the obstruction does not clear with conservative treatment, then lavage or even surgery may be required.

Acute diarrhoea

This can be a first aid emergency because severe fluid loss may lead to hypovolaemic shock. History taking is important to determine possible source and any other horses affected or in contact. Salmonella infection should be considered.

With severe diarrhoea cases, it is important to monitor hydration status, including parameters such as pulse, capillary refill time (CRT), skin tenting, total protein measurement and PCV. Severely infected or red mucous membranes are indicative of endotoxaemia. Bounding digital pulses may indicate impending laminitis as a complication. Pyrexia may occur with abdominal pain prior to diarrhoea developing. Faecal samples may be required for laboratory culture and electrolyte disturbances should be identified.

Nursing action for diarrhoea cases

Fluids can be life-saving; the route of administration and the type selected will depend on the clinician's assessment of the individual case. Intravenous hypertonic saline is required if hypovolaemia is severe, followed up with polyionic fluids. Electrolyte disturbances should be corrected. Patients with low plasma protein levels (<45 g/l) may require intravenous plasma slowly to support plasma oncotic pressure.

Urinogenital

Conditions requiring first aid that involve the urogenital tract include:

- Acute renal failure
- Cystic calculi (see Example 7.7)
- Dystocia
- Penile prolapse or trauma
- Post-castration complications (see Example 7.8)
- Prolapsed bladder
- Prolapsed uterus
- Ruptured bladder
- Testicular torsion
- Urethral obstruction

Example 7.8   Castration complication

Post-castration bleeding

A horse gelded earlier in the day has a continuous stream of blood from an open castration wound, having been turned out and cantered round the field.

If the bleeding is continuous, the need for intervention is very likely. If blood is only dripping, the patient should be kept calm and quiet in a loose box to see if clotting will occur. For severe blood loss, see Example 7.1. The castration wound can be packed temporarily with sterile swabs or bandage to attempt to stem bleeding, but further surgery may be required to find and ligate the bleeding vessel(s).

Example 7.7   Urinary problem

Calculi

A gelding is presented with abdominal pain, making frequent attempts to urinate but only passing small amounts of blood-stained urine.

Sedation may be administered at the clinician's discretion before a well-lubricated urinary catheter is passed to relieve the obstruction and prevent possible bladder rupture. The distal penis is grasped in one gloved hand, exposing the glans, and the catheter is slowly introduced. Usually a urethral obstruction can be moved back to the bladder to relieve pressure prior to further investigation. A mid- and end-stream urine sample may be collected for urinalysis.

Assessment

With any urinary condition it is important to assess the stance of the horse during urination, the colour and amount of urine passed and whether urination is painful. Observe if urine is passed in a continuous or intermittent stream and be aware of water intake. Hydration status also can be important in urinary tract disease. Take note of the time of occurrence and amount of any bleeding in relation to urination and, with traumatic injuries or post-castration bleeding, assess cardiovascular status and blood loss.

Nursing action

Penile trauma

Bleeding may be profuse to the extent that surgery may be required. Cold hosing or cooling with ice packs will help to control swelling. Apply pressure or a bandage to control bleeding and swelling. Support the penis using a disposable drape (or similar) to prevent further vascular damage.

Paraphymosis

Paraphymosis is the inability of a horse to retract its penis in the prepuce. It can occur for several reasons, including general debilitation or occasionally following sedation with phenothiazine derivative tranquillisers, e.g. acepromazine.

Nursing first aid action may include:

- Establishing and removing the inciting cause where possible
- Cleaning the penis and prepuce with mild cleansers and antiseptic cream or petroleum jelly
- Reducing swelling and supporting the prolapsed penis with some form of truss

Dystocia

Dystocia is defined as difficulty in giving birth. Emergency veterinary attention should be sought as soon as there is any indication of problems. (See Chapter 4.)

Neurological

Neurological conditions requiring first aid include:

- Brachial plexus injury
- Convulsions
- Equine herpes virus 1 (EHV1) myeloencephalitis
- Electrocution
- Head and spinal trauma
- Hepatic encephalopathy
- Peripheral nerve injuries: facial, supraspinous, femoral, radial
- Tetanus
- Wobbler syndrome

Assessment

Neurological emergencies are usually acute in onset, serious and may deteriorate rapidly. Signs can vary from mild subtle deficits of gait or mental state to terminal convulsions. Convulsing or ataxic horses present a danger to those handling them. They should be handled with extreme caution.

Parameters to assess

- Coordination
- Cranial nerve function
- Head carriage
- Level of consciousness: mental state and behaviour
- Muscle tone
- Pattern of respiration (and changes with therapy)
- Pupil size, symmetry and response to light
- Reflexes, e.g. flexor, patellar and panniculus
- Tail and anal tone
- Urinary retention or incontinence

Note that after exercise or severe stress, adrenaline will abolish many reflexes for 1–2 h. Hence, the horse that is recumbent, e.g. following a fall, can be difficult to assess immediately following the accident (see Example 7.9).

Example 7.9   Recumbency

Nursing first aid for the recumbent horse

A young thoroughbred is discovered down in its box at evening stables, having suffered a fall earlier in the day during exercise. It is bright and alert and showing no other clinical signs.

The first consideration must be the safety of the people with the horse. Recumbent horses can make unexpected attempts to get to their feet and may be suffering neurological deficits resulting in ataxia or even convulsions. The admission of people to a confined area with a recumbent patient should be strictly controlled. No single person should attend to the horse without someone else being present. Any physical objects that may cause the horse further injury should be removed or, if this is not possible, shielded with bales of hay or straw. If struggling or convulsing, sedation may be required to avoid injury to the patient, for safety reasons, and to facilitate a full clinical examination. A blanket spread under the horse's head will limit trauma and contamination to the eyes. If a horse is down in an open area, bedding should be placed under and around the horse. Bales can provide shelter and prop the horse in sternal recumbency. If the horse has collapsed with tack on, this should be removed with care, cutting the girth straps if necessary. A full and careful examination should be carried out to assess the patient's status. Feed and water can be offered at regular intervals, if appropriate. Care should be taken regarding the risk of infection spreading to other horses. The vet may require assistance to roll the horse to check for possible fractures on the horse's 'down' side.

Nursing action

General

Safety of handlers and prevention of further trauma is essential. In some cases, sedation or anaesthesia may be required. Monitor the horse repeatedly for signs of deterioration. Good nursing management of the recumbent horse (see example) is important with neurological cases.

Convulsions or seizures

These are rare in the horse and may be generalised or localised. If generalised there will be muscle spasms, involuntary recumbency and loss of consciousness.

Severe depression and blindness may follow this. Partial seizures may produce localised signs, such as facial or limb twitching, compulsive circling or self-mutilation of a particular area. Poor prognostic signs include increasing frequency or intensity of seizures and poor response to treatment.

Causes of seizures can be classified into:

(1) *Structural brain disease*: neoplasia, abscesses, other masses such as cholesterol granuloma, meningitis, damage following intracarotid injection, etc.
(2) *Metabolic brain disease*: hypocalcaemia, hypoglycaemia, neonatal maladjustment syndrome (see Chapter 15), hyperthermia, etc.
(3) *Idiopathic (i.e. of unknown cause) brain disease*: such as idiopathic epilepsy in Arab foals.

Convulsions sometimes can be difficult to differentiate from the horse that is struggling to free itself or get up. Other differential diagnoses for seizures include:

- A normal foal that may twitch in its sleep
- Colic
- Exertional rhabdomyolisis
- Narcolepsy or cataplexy
- Syncope or fainting arising from various causes
- Tetanus

Treatment to stop a seizure will involve sedation or anaesthesia, and drugs may be required to combat central nervous system (CNS) swelling. Non-steroidal anti-inflammatory drugs, e.g. flunixin, also can be useful. Antibiotics may help if a bacterial cause is suspected or secondary infection is a risk.

Fluids should be given with caution (can cause more CNS swelling). Administration rates should be slow and not changed rapidly. Specific treatments may be needed for certain conditions, e.g. tetanus antitoxin for tetanus.

Metabolic and environmental

Metabolic and environmental conditions that may require first aid nursing include:

- Exertional rhabdomyolysis (tying up, azoturia) (see Example 7.10)

Example 7.10   Rhabdomyolysis

A competition horse comes in from fast exercise and becomes progressively stiff, distressed and unwilling to move, with a raised heart rate. Colic-like symptoms and profuse sweating, accompanied by hard painful muscles over the hindquarters and back. Urine is dark red in colour.

These signs are typical of equine rhabdomyolysis syndrome (ERS). Management should include the following:

(1) Avoid exercise wherever possible. Treat *in situ* or bring transport to the patient, but *avoid prolonged transportation* in order to limit further muscle damage.
(2) Keep the patient calm and warm and away from draughts.
(3) Blood samples should be taken to determine muscle enzyme levels and evaluate the degree of damage.
(4) It is essential to maintain renal function and fluid balance, especially if myoglobinuria is present, i.e. dark red urine.
(5) If the horse has become recumbent, give intravenous fluids rapidly and through multiple large-bore (10–12-gauge) catheters. Commercially available 5-L bags (Hartmanns) are ideal for use in the field.
(6) Monitor urine output.
(7) Drug treatment: analgesia for the reduction of both pain and anxiety is important for the horse's welfare, as well as making it easier to handle; a single dose of steroids is often used in the early stages to combat shock and improve tissue perfusion.
(8) General nursing support: if the horse remains recumbent but can be made to sit sternally it should do so by being propped up, e.g. with bales of straw; the distal limbs should be bandaged; an antimicrobial lubricant should be applied to the eyes to minimise the risk of corneal abrasion; urinary catheterisation may need to be considered.

- heat stroke, heat exhaustion, hyperthermia (see Example 7.11)
- Hypocalcaemia ('thumps', synchronous diaphragmatic flutter and hypocalcaemic tetany)

Assessment of any problem should include the horse's history: particularly recent exercise, diet, lactation and stress. It is always important to monitor

Example 7.11 Heat stroke and exhaustion

A horse completes a long-distance ride on a hot humid day, after which it is depressed, unwilling to move and ataxic, with slow deep respiration. Heart rate is 80 bpm with a weak pulse, and mucous membranes are conjested. The horse is no longer sweating but body temperature is 42°C.

This is typical of heat stroke and it is essential to *start cooling as rapidly as possible*, with as many helpers as possible. To do this, use water (4–10°C) applied all over to effect. Use sponges both sides, in addition to a hose or buckets. Do not use wet towels because they reduce evaporation and convection. This rapid cooling should be done in any horse with a temperature above 40°C (104°F). Move into shade as soon as possible. Alternate 30 s of slow walking (to increase airflow over the patient) with 30 s of cooling. Use fans if available. Offer half-buckets of oral electrolyte solution frequently. If refused, try plain water. Monitor temperature: a cooling rate of 1°C in 10 min can be achieved; continue until a temperature of 38–39°C is reached.

The horse is still distressed and refusing to eat or drink despite a rectal temperature of 39°C. Mild colic and muscle cramps develop. Heart and respiratory rates are high with synchronous diaphragmatic flutter, and pulse is weak and irregular.

Treat for exhaustion: if no colic, 5–10 L of isotonic oral rehydration fluid should be given by stomach tube. It may be difficult to pass a stomach tube and intravenous fluids may be simpler. The response to treatment should be monitored by assessment of pulse rate and quality, mucous membrane colour and, most importantly, the animal's demeanour. Good nursing will include encouraging the horse to eat and drink.

vital signs. Taking blood tests for biochemistry can be helpful.

Tetanic hypocalcaemia

This condition is also called eclampsia or transit tetany. Causes include:

- Blister beetle toxicity in the USA
- Diarrhoea and colic
- Excessive bicarbonate administration
- Exhaustion in endurance horses
- Heavy lactation, particularly in draught mares

- Idiopathic
- Transport and stress

Clinical signs

The most obvious sign is a twitch in the flank area in synchrony with each heartbeat. This may be obvious enough to produce an audible thump, hence the traditional name of 'thumps'. Other signs include sweating, generalised stiffness, muscle twitches, raised heart rate and a raised temperature.

Laboratory findings

A blood sample that shows a low serum calcium level (4–6 mg/dl) confirms the diagnosis.

Action

The horse is kept calm and quiet. Calcium borogluconate (500 ml, 20% diluted 1:4 in saline) is given slowly intravenously, monitoring the heart and pulse. An electrocardiograph (ECG) monitor is useful if available. If extrasystole or an increase in heart sounds occurs, infusion should be stopped immediately. Complete recovery may take several hours and repeat treatments may be required.

Respiratory

Respiratory conditions that may require first aid nursing include:

- Acute respiratory infection
- Acute respiratory obstruction
- Acute small-airway disease
- Anaphylaxis
- Exercise-induced pulmonary haemorrhage
- Pneumothorax
- Pulmonary oedema
- Shipping fever and pleuritis

Anatomical considerations

It should be remembered that the horse is an obligate nasal breather.

Assessment

Firstly determine whether the upper or lower respiratory tract is involved. Upper respiratory emergencies are frequently obstructions and may rapidly become life threatening, so speed is vital. These can be distinguished by the 'snoring' noise that the individual is making when breathing, particularly on inspiration. Lower respiratory disease producing respiratory distress can usually be determined by auscultation of the thorax. Inspiratory difficulty often is more pronounced than difficulty in breathing out with an upper airway obstruction; the opposite is true with lower airway obstructions, such as chronic obstructive pulmonary disease (COPD).

Points to observe are:

- Respiratory rate and effort
- Passage of air through both nostrils
- Nasal discharge
- Temperature
- Stridor (snoring noise associated with difficulty in breathing coming from upper airway)
- Stance (elbows abducted and neck extended)
- Swelling around nose or throat
- Lung sounds on auscultation.

Establishing a patent airway

This can be vital if the horse is seriously compromised.

Nasotracheal tube

Inserting a nasotracheal tube may be difficult to perform on a distressed, conscious horse. It may not be possible unless the patient collapses or is sedated. The tube should be lubricated well and passed through the ventral meatus. A 450-kg horse will take a 22-mm tube, but try a smaller size first and replace with a larger one when possible. Extend neck and rotate the tube as it is passed into the pharynx. If the oesophagus is entered there will be resistance and the tube can be palpated below the larynx. Once in place, the tube should be secured with insulating tape to ensure that it is not lost in the airway!

Tracheotomy

This is the formation of an opening into the trachea for the insertion of a tube, thereby allowing the patient an open airway through which to breathe. This is only justifiable in an absolute emergency to maintain an airway. Usually there is little time for preparation. Ideally the area should be clipped and prepared with a sterile scrub. The site is the junction of the upper and middle one-third of the ventral neck, where the trachea is easily palpable. Under sedation if required, local anaesthesia is infiltrated and a 7-cm midline incision is made down to the trachea. Incise horizontally between two rings no more than 50% of circumference and insert appropriately sized tube. Hold rings apart or improvise a tube if a tracheostomy tube is not available. In a life-threatening emergency, the sterile technique may need to be abandoned and any available tube, e.g. piece of stomach tube, inserted into the airway as rapidly as possible.

To care for the in-dwelling tracheotomy tube, the following steps should be followed:

- A tracheotomy requires maintaining an open wound. Although strict asepsis is not possible, every effort must be made to keep contamination to a minimum.
- The incision and clipped area surrounding the wound must be surgically prepped twice daily to keep clean of exudate and prevent wound infection.
- The tube must be replaced daily with a sterile one.
- Suctioning the secretions from the tube and trachea may be necessary if there is a significant amount present, which can cause decreased airflow. All suction apparatus must be sterile.
- Check that the straps securing the tube (if present) are keeping the tube in place.
- Bandaging the tube in place may be beneficial in keeping the wound clean and free from contamination from bedding.
- Bandaging materials must give and not cause constriction if the horse moves its head up and down.
- Horses with tracheotomy tubes should be fed off the ground so as not to introduce hay and dust into the trachea.

Care must be taken to prevent bedding from entering the tube and airway. A dust-free management protocol must be followed closely.

Orotracheal intubation

This is usually a last resort when the horse is collapsed or needs general anaesthesia. A section of

5-cm diameter pipe is inserted as a gag between the incisors to prevent the tube itself from being chewed. Extend the neck and rotate the tube as it is passed through the pharynx.

Supplementary oxygen

Oxygen may need to be administered to a horse in respiratory distress once a clear airway has been provided by any of the above methods. Sometimes it is possible to pass oxygen tubing into the trachea, or nasal insufflation is performed by passing tubing into ventral nares and occluding the nostrils to expand the chest and then releasing for exhalation. Minimum flow rates of 10–15 L/min are required. Oxygen is best humidified by passing through sterile water, if possible, especially for longer term administration.

Treating anaphylaxis

Occasionally a horse may present with acute difficulty in breathing (*dyspnoea*) and an elevated breathing rate (*tachypnoea*), which may be due to an acute allergic reaction. Treatment is by intravenous administration of steroids (usually dexamethasone). Rarely, adrenaline diluted in water or saline may be required for true anaphylaxis.

Improving alveolar ventilation

For penetrating chest wounds, close and cover as soon as possible to minimise air aspiration and *pneumothorax* (the presence of free air within the chest cavity).

Treating pneumothorax

This is an uncommon emergency, the severity reflecting the amount of free air that has got into the chest cavity. As with other thoracic conditions such as pneumonia or COPD, there will be dyspnoea without dramatic respiratory noise. On auscultation there will be the absence of lung sounds dorsally.

Treatment involves:

(1) Treating the underlying cause, e.g. cleaning and sealing the wound.
(2) Administering oxygen if needed.
(3) Removing the free air from the chest after the wounds are closed. A chest drain should be intro-duced following aseptic preparation. The chest drain should have a one-way valve (e.g. a Heimlich valve) or a valve can be improvised using a glove or condom taped around a catheter with a drainage hole at the far end. This will collapse with negative pressure and prevent the aspiration of air.

Treating nasal obstruction

To cause nasal obstruction, both nostrils must be involved. Causes include bee stings, snake or dog bite, nettle stings, burns, trauma and anaphylaxis.

With nasal obstruction it helps to keep the head up to reduce further swelling, so sedation is contraindicated. Apply cold to decrease swelling. The clinician may prescribe anti-inflammatory medication. In severe cases, pass a tube into the nasal passages and tape in place. Administer supplementary oxygen if required.

Cardiovascular

Cardiovascular conditions that may require nursing first aid include:

- Arrhythmias
- Haemorrhage
- Shock (hypovolaemic, septic, endotoxic, cardiogenic, traumatic, anaphylactic)

Shock

Shock is a profound physiological change in the body with circulatory collapse and consequently inadequate tissue oxygenation, often caused by poor perfusion. It can be assessed by:

- Pulse rate, quality and blood pressure
- Capillary refill time (CRT)
- Mucous membrane colour
- Hydration (PCV/TP)
- Demeanour
- Urine production
- Response to treatment.

Shock can be present in a wide variety of emergency situations and always should be considered, whatever else is going wrong.

Nursing action and procedures

A successful outcome is more likely when shock is treated in the early (hyperdynamic) phase. The aim of treatment is to raise tissue perfusion to higher than normal rates. Aggressive fluid and drug therapy frequently is required.

Haemorrhage

Haemorrhage can cause shock. *Remember that with severe haemorrhage death can occur with little or no change in PCV.* Mucous membrane colour also is a poor indicator of severity of blood loss until levels have fallen very low. Aggressive early treatment, including intravenous fluids and whole blood, may be required.

Cardiac arrhythmias

Cardiac arrhythmias (loss of the normal heart rhythm) occur commonly in the horse and rarely require treatment. Certain cardiac arrhythmias may be rapidly life threatening. An ECG examination is required to determine whether treatment is feasible.

Musculoskeletal

Musculoskeletal conditions that may require nursing first aid include:

- Foot problems (e.g. foot abscess), foreign body penetration and laminitis
- Joint, bursa and tendon sheath infection or trauma
- Sudden non-weight-bearing lameness, e.g. fractures, luxation, and ligament and tendon injury

Nursing assessment (see Summary 7.1)

Catch the lame horse if loose and prevent movement. However, avoid chasing an injured horse that will not be caught until sufficient help is available. Weight bearing on an unstable limb will increase soft-tissue damage, resulting in a poorer prognosis.

Keep the horse calm and warm and monitor for signs of shock. Consider whether the injury is unilateral or bilateral: a horse with bilateral injuries is often reluctant to move. Assess the degree of weight bear-

---

Summary 7.1

Assessing the musculoskeletal system

JEDI	CUTS	PADS
Joint pain	Crepitus	PAin
Effusion	Unnatural movement	Deformity
Digital pulses	Tenderness	Swelling
Immobility	Shock	

---

ing. Carefully palpate and inspect all structures. The order is unimportant but a routine should be established so that the examination is complete and methodical, e.g. work from the foot up.

It may be difficult to make a definitive diagnosis despite the horse being very lame. It should be remembered that as well as fractures there are other causes of severe lameness, such as septic joints, catastrophic tendon injuries and most commonly pus in the foot (subsolar abscessation).

The vet will decide whether the injury warrants immediate humane destruction or whether further investigations are required, particularly radiography and ultrasonography. If the horse is to be moved for further treatment, applying proper support bandages is an important nursing role.

Orthopaedic injuries requiring immediate euthanasia include:

- Multiple fractures
- Complete tibial or femoral fractures
- Complete humeral fractures
- Complete radial fractures in patients >300 kg
- Compound comminuted fractures, especially with severe soft-tissue damage
- Severe long-standing septic joint or synovial sheath or bursa
- Severe loss of or damage to soft tissues

Road traffic accidents and other major accidents

In such public circumstances it is particularly important to consider human safety. Ask for all persons not required to be removed from the scene immediately.

The key points are:

- Triage is important
- Shock is likely
- Arrest any haemorrhage
- Assess for fractures and other major injuries

The clinician may need to sedate an injured horse to prevent further injury to the emergency team, patient and onlookers. In some cases, anaesthesia may be necessary to move the horse or to enable complete assessment if the horse is distressed, particularly if euthanasia looks necessary.

These situations can be difficult but if routine first aid principles are followed the problems can be solved successfully and safely. If in doubt, seek advice from a vet as soon as possible (see Summary 7.2).

Summary 7.2

Major emergencies that require you to contact a vet immediately

- Choke
- Colic
- Collapse
- Eye trauma
- Foaling and related concerns, e.g. retained placenta
- Major wounds
- Profuse haemorrhage
- Respiratory distress
- Road traffic accidents
- Severe lameness

Further reading

Bertone, J.J. (1994) Emergency treatment in the adult horse. *Vet. Clin. N. Am.: Equine Pract.* **10**, 489–728.

Bramlage, L. (1983) Current concepts of emergency first aid treatment and transportation of equine fracture patients. *Comp. Cont. Educ. Pract. Vet.* **5**, 564–574.

Coumbe, K. (2000) *First Aid for Horses.* J.A. Allen, London.

Dyson, S. (1996) *A Guide to the Management of Emergencies at Equine Competitions.* Equine Veterinary Journal Ltd, Newmarket.

Orsini, J. & Divers, T. (1998) *Manual of Equine Emergencies, Treatment & Procedures.* WB Saunders, Philadelphia, PA.

Smith, R. K. W. (1993) Bandages and casts. *Equine Vet. Educ.* **5(2)**, 108–112.

Stashak, T. (1991) *Equine Wound Management.* Lea & Febiger, Philadelphia, PA.

General Nursing

R. J. Baxter

The ability to assess the abnormalities in a horse's appearance or behaviour requires a knowledge of normality and vigilant observation.

As a veterinary nurse it is important not only to be able to recognise signs of disease but also to record and report them accurately. Following a routine helps to avoid omissions. Most clinicians use a system known as SOAP, which refers to:

- Subjective
- Objective
- Assessment
- Plan.

The equine nurse should be able to record both *subjective* and *objective* findings clearly and report them to the vet in charge, whose responsibility it is to *assess* these findings and formulate a *plan* for the future.

Records

Recording of clinical progress should be carried out at least once daily and every equine hospital ought to have record sheets available for this purpose (Fig. 8.1). Animals in intensive care may benefit from the use of separate assessment sheets, which should be completed several times a day (Fig. 8.2). Although details of medication given to the patient should be recorded on these sheets and in the plan section of the horse's clinical records, it is easy to lose sight of the details, so it is best to have a separate chart for recording the administration of medication (Fig. 8.3). Separate sheets should be available for monitoring during general anaesthesia (see Chapter 20).

Subjective assessment

Initially horses should be observed from outside the stable. Note should be made of their demeanour, attitude and responsiveness to stimuli, as well as whether or not they are up, moving around and interested in food. Notes are generally abbreviated, e.g. BAR (bright, alert, responsive), QAR (quiet, alert, responsive), QAU (quiet, alert, unresponsive), etc.

Signs such as a bright eye and a glossy coat are also reasonable indicators of health and well-being, whereas a dull coat can indicate disease. The horse's physique should be noted: underweight with very visible ribs; overweight; any asymmetries due to muscle wastage.

Objective assessment

This involves assessment of measurable characteristics such as the vital signs and hydration status, as well as signs of pain or lameness. First the temperature, pulse and respiration (TPR) values are recorded (Table 8.1) and then a more detailed investigation can be carried out. Also, notes should be made of the quantity and type of food ingested, the water intake and whether urine and faeces have been passed.

The normal horse's water requirement is approximately 40 ml/kg bodyweight/day. *Polydipsia* (increased water intake) can occur due to a variety of conditions, including kidney disease and fever. Reduced food or water intake also should be noted.

CASE NO: ————————
PATIENT'S NAME: ——————
CLINICIAN: ——————

Equine Centre
CLINICAL PROGRESS NOTES

Date	Temp	HR	RR	Notes

Fig. 8.1 Clinical progress records.

Table 8.1 Normal values for temperature, pulse and respiration in the adult horse[a]

Temperature	98.5–100.5°F (37.0–38.0°C)
Pulse	25–42 beats per minute
Respiration	10–20 breaths per minute

[a] The pulse and respiration rates of ponies tend to be slightly higher than those of horses.

Difficulty *prehending* (taking in) or *masticating* (chewing) food or *dysphagia* (difficulty swallowing) may cause an apparent reduction in appetite or abnormal eating.

Respiration

Count the horse's respiration rate by careful observation of rib movements; this is best done from outside the stable before disturbing the animal. The rate of ei-

ther inspirations or expirations should be counted over 1 min to avoid inaccuracies. An alternative method for counting the respiration rate is to feel the expiratory breaths at the nose, but some horses will react to the proximity of a stranger with fear, which can elevate the respiratory rate. In cold weather the exhaled breaths may be seen and counted.

Dyspnoea (difficulty breathing) can result from problems during inspiration, expiration or both. The horse is an obligate nasal breather (cannot breathe through its mouth). Damage or blockage of the nasal passages can therefore obstruct breathing and cause inspiratory dyspnoea even if the mouth is clear. Expiratory dyspnoea can follow lung diseases that reduce the elastic recoil of the lungs, such as bronchitis or pleural adhesions. Mixed dyspnoea occurs if there is impedance of both inspiration and expiration. This can be a consequence of pneumonia or space-occupying diseases of the pleural cavity, such as *pneumothorax* or *pyothorax* (respectively air or pus in the pleural cavity), or it may be secondary to other problems that cause respiratory pain, such as broken ribs. Severe dyspnoea can result in thoraco-abdominal breathing (where the abdominal muscles become involved in helping to force out breath). This is a common consequence of severe expiratory dyspnoea caused by *chronic obstructive pulmonary disease* (COPD). A characteristic 'double' breath (heaves) is seen with the development of a 'heave line' in the caudal abdomen.

Disorders of breathing rate include *apnoea* (stopping breathing), which may occur intermittently during unconsciousness or light planes of anaesthesia. *Tachypnoea* (increased breathing rate) can occur due to pain, fever and heat, acidosis and during/after exercise. *Bradypnoea* (abnormally slow breathing) is rather less common, but can occur as a consequence of metabolic alkalosis as well as during unconsciousness. Alternating periods of deep, rapid breaths followed by shallow breathing and apnoea (*Cheyne-Stokes breathing*) is an indicator of *hypoxia* (reduced oxygen in the blood) or disease of the central nervous system (CNS). Breathing that is rapid and deep may occur:

- Pathologically due to *pyrexia* (a raised temperature), acidosis or *anaemia* (reduction in red blood

INTENSIVE CARE SHEET

HORSE/CASE NO: .... DATE: ....

TIME				
TEMP				
H.R.				
PULSE				
R.R.				
M.M.				
CRT				
PCV				
TP				
ATTITUDE/DEGREE OF PAIN				
GUT MOTILITY				
FAECES/URINE				
DIG. PULSE				
MEDICATION				
FLUIDS ADMINISTERED				
APPETITE				
WATER CONSUMPTION				
RECTAL				
COMMENTS				

Fig. 8.2 Intensive care records.

cells and hence oxygen-carrying capacity of the blood).

• Physiologically due to exercise or anxiety.

Conversely, fast and shallow breathing may be a consequence of restrictive lung disease such as pleuritis (inflamed pleurae), pneumothorax or pyothorax, or may occur due to respiratory pain. Breathing that is slow and deep is usually a consequence of partial airway obstructions, whereas slow and shallow breathing may follow CNS depression or alkalosis (see Chapter 13).

Pulse

The horse should be approached calmly and quietly to avoid false elevation of the pulse rate due to fear. The pulse rate can be counted by palpation of any artery situated near the body surface. The most commonly used arteries are the transverse facial, submandibular, coccygeal and digital arteries, and while the horse is anaesthetised the lingual pulse can be assessed (Fig. 8.4).

To count the pulse rate, an artery is located and partially occluded by finger pressure. This allows the

CASE NO: _____

OWNERS NAME: _____

PATIENT'S NAME: _____

CLINICIAN: _____

HOSPITALISATION SHEET
Drug Record

Drug Idiosyncracy and Previous Relevant Therapy

| TOTAL COST |
| CC525 |

ONCE ONLY DRUGS	Dose	Route	Signature	Date	Time	

REGULAR PRESCRIPTIONS	TIME	DAY:1	2	3	4	5	6	7	
Drug (Approved) Name									
Dose / Frequency / Route									
Signature & Date									
	TIME								
Drug (Approved) Name									
Dose / Frequency / Route									
Signature & Date									
	TIME								
Drug (Approved) Name									
Dose / Frequency / Route									
Signature & Date									
	TIME								
Drug (Approved) Name									
Dose / Frequency / Route									
Signature & Date									
	TIME								
Drug (Approved) Name									
Dose / Frequency / Route									
Signature & Date									

£ _____

Fig. 8.3 Record of administration of medication.

pulsation of the artery to be felt. Finger pressure that is too weak or too strong may prevent the pulse from being palpable. Having located the pulse with the fingertips, the rate is counted over a period of 1 min to avoid inaccuracies. Increased pulse rates can indicate anxiety, pain or heart failure.

Each arterial pulsation should correspond to a contraction of the ventricles of the heart. Placing the hand or a stethoscope over the heart base in the left axilla while palpating the arterial pulse allows concurrent assessment of the heart and pulse rates. Abnormal heartbeats can result in a pulse deficit (a pulse rate that is reduced compared with the heart rate).

The pulse rhythm is normally regular, although it may increase during inspiration and decrease during expiration (*sinus arrhythmia*). In addition, some horses miss occasional heart beats (*dropped beats*) at

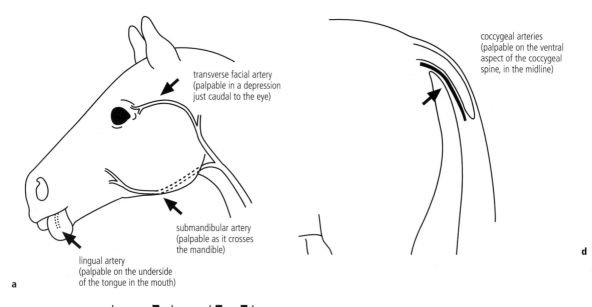

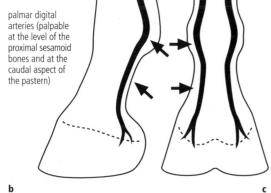

palmar digital arteries (palpable at the level of the proximal sesamoid bones and at the caudal aspect of the pastern)

transverse facial artery (palpable in a depression just caudal to the eye)

submandibular artery (palpable as it crosses the mandible)

lingual artery (palpable on the underside of the tongue in the mouth)

coccygeal arteries (palpable on the ventral aspect of the coccygeal spine, in the midline)

a

b

c

d

Fig. 8.4 Locations of the arterial pulses. (a) Diagram of the head showing the positions where pulses are palpable: the transverse facial artery is palpable in a depression just caudal to the eye; the submandibular artery is palpable as it crosses the mandible; the lingual artery is palpable on the underside of the tongue in the midline. Diagram of the lateral (b) and palmar/plantar (c) aspects of the pastern, showing the location of the palmar/plantar digital arteries and the sites where they are palpable: at the level of the proximal sesamoid bones and at the palmar/plantar aspect of the pastern. (d) Diagram showing the site at which the coccygeal artery is palpable: on the ventral aspect of the coccygeal vertebrae in the midline. (i.e. on the underside of the tail).

rest. However, irregular pulse rhythms can indicate an abnormality.

The normal pulse feels strong and firm. A weak pulse feels fainter or more 'fluttery' than a normal pulse, and may indicate reduced cardiac output due to debilitation, disease or shock as well as anaesthesia, unconsciousness or sleep. A *hyperkinetic* pulse (one with increased pressure), on the other hand, can feel as though it has rather more depth than a normal pulse, and can be associated with increased heart rate due to fever, exercise, hypoxia, pain or fear. A particularly strong and jerky pulse is often referred to as a 'water hammer pulse' and may be associated with anaemia and some forms of cardiac disease, such as valvular insufficiency.

Temperature

The temperature is taken rectally. It is advisable to familiarise yourself with the horse before taking its temperature and then approach the hindquarters carefully, standing close to the side to avoid being kicked. The lubricated bulb of the thermometer should be inserted about 2 inches into the rectum and angled towards the rectal wall to avoid faecal material, otherwise the rectal temperature recorded may be inaccurate. After 1 min the thermometer may be removed and wiped clean prior to reading it. It should then be reset/turned off, wiped clean with antiseptic and stored safely to avoid contamination and breakage. The thermometer should not be left unattended in the rectum.

A digital thermometer, when switched on, takes a few seconds before it is ready for use. After 1 min a bleep sounds to indicate that the temperature can be read. It should be turned off to reset it. A traditional clinical mercury thermometer contains a kink in the mercury tube to prevent backflow, so that the maximum temperature reached is recorded. To reset the thermometer, the mercury within it must be shaken down (avoiding hard surfaces).

Abnormalities in temperature include:

- *Pyrexia/hyperthermia* (increased temperature), which can result from infection, pain, excitement or, occasionally, heat stroke
- *Hypothermia* (reduced temperature), which follows shock, collapse and blood loss.

Although temperature is usually recorded in degrees centigrade (°C), some clinicians are more familiar with the use of Fahrenheit (°F) values. Most thermometers show temperature on both scales but some do not. For conversion, the following equations should be employed:

$$°C = (°F - 32) \times 5/9 \qquad °F = (9/5 \times °C) + 32$$

Clinical examination

Having checked and recorded the TPR values and any abnormalities in character of these vital signs, a full clinical examination should be carried out and the findings recorded.

Mucous membranes

Healthy mucous membranes should be a pale pink colour and the capillary refill time (CRT), assessed by blanching a gum with finger pressure and then recording the time for the normal colour to return, should be within 2 s.

Pallor of the mucous membranes can relate to reduced cardiac output, blood loss and anaemia.

Congestion (filling of the blood vessels, resulting in them becoming visible as fine red lines) can be caused by *toxaemia* (release of bacterial toxins into the blood) and *septicaemia* (release of bacteria into the blood). The mucous membranes may become *cyanotic* (bluish) if blood oxygenation is reduced due to illness or lung disease. With severe colics, the mucous membranes often take on a dull muddy appearance due to a combination of dehydration and toxaemia. In severe cases of toxaemia they become purplish, and petechiation and *echymosis* (haemorrhage from the blood vessels, causing a mottled or bruised appearance) may be seen. Liver disease can cause *icterus* or *jaundice* (a yellowish appearance due to an increase in blood levels of bile pigments). However, a horse that has not eaten recently also may show signs of jaundice (i.e. appear icteric) despite being perfectly well.

Hydration status

Clinical examination is important to assess fluid deficits (see Chapter 13).

Cardiac examination

Cardiac auscultation may be carried out by applying the stethoscope to both sides of the chest in the axillary region. It may be necessary to move the right forelimb forwards in order to listen far enough forward on the right side to hear the heart properly. The heart should be listened to over several minutes so that any abnormal sounds or rhythm irregularities may be identified.

What do you hear when you listen to the heart?

The normal heart beat sounds something like b-lub–dup-d, although often it is only the first and second heart sounds (the lub-dup) that are identified. The first or S1 sound (lub) relates to the start of *systole* (the emptying of the heart) and the second or S2 (dup) occurs as the semi-lunar valves in the arteries close at the end of systole. The S3 (d) sound is that made by the fast phase of blood flow into the ventricles during *diastole* (the filling of the heart). A pause follows and then the S4 (b) sound is heard just before the S1 sound. This is composed of the noise made by the atria contracting just before systole begins and the closing of the mitral and tricuspid valves (the two atrioventricular valves). The S1–S2 period therefore encompasses systole, whereas diastole occurs during the period from S2, through S3 and S4, to S1. Other cardiac noises are referred to as murmurs.

Respiratory system examination

Assessment of breathing should have been carried out initially, but other signs also may indicate respiratory disease, including:

- Swellings of the glands at the angle of the jaw and between the mandibles
- Nasal discharges
- Coughing
- Abnormal respiratory noises

Nasal discharges may be watery, mucoid, purulent or haemorrhagic. In some cases food material may be seen coming from the nostrils, most commonly due to an oesophageal obstruction (choke). Unilateral nasal discharges are likely to come from the nasal passages or paranasal sinuses (which contain molar tooth roots and so may become infected if a tooth root infection occurs). The presence of bilateral nasal discharge often indicates that the cause lies deeper within the respiratory system, such as from the lungs.

Abnormal respiratory noises may be heard; specific noises can relate to specific problems. Sounds caused by pain on breathing, such as grunts and groans, may be heard without using a stethoscope. Most commonly heard at exercise, *stridor* (a loud inspiratory snore) indicates partial obstruction of the upper respiratory tract. However, most adventitious sounds (abnormal noises superimposed on normal respiratory noises) can be heard only with a stethoscope, and some can be heard only when forced hyperventilation (e.g. by making the horse breathe into a plastic bag) is used to maximise respiratory noise.

Abdominal examination

The abdomen is divided into four quarters or quadrants: left upper and lower; and right upper and

lower. Movement of food and liquid through the guts causes gurgling sounds (i.e. *borborygmi*) to be audible, particularly in the left quadrants and the right lower quadrant. The right upper quadrant is dominated by sounds from the caecum, which makes gentle mixing sounds interspersed about every 2 min by a sound not unlike the flushing of a toilet.

Increased borborygmi can relate to recent feeding or may indicate gut hypermotility, which can be associated with colic, particularly after the ingestion of highly digestible and fermentable material. Reduced gut sounds also can indicate problems; impactions can result in gut hypomotility, as can *ileus* (gut stasis), which can result from a range of intestinal conditions or may follow anaesthesia (particularly for colic surgery). The clinical signs of ileus include moderate to severe abdominal pain (colic), depression, dehydration, absent/scant passage of faeces and decreased or absent borborygmi.

Information on bowel sounds should be noted, together with the frequency and character of faeces passed. The normal horse defaecates 8–12 times in 24 h, and the faeces should consist of firm balls of excrement that break on hitting the ground. Reduced faecal production, diarrhoea or the production of hard tarry faeces may indicate gastrointestinal disease. The newborn foal should pass meconium (the dark tarry fetal faeces) within the first 6–12 h of life before normal foal dung (of a softer consistency) can be passed.

The horse is unable to vomit, so if gut stasis or blockage occurs large volumes of secretory fluid can build up in the stomach. Because the horse is designed to be a continual eater, the stomach is small and a build-up of fluid can rapidly cause intense pain and even rupture of the stomach. Horses with colic benefit from siphoning off this fluid (reflux) through a nasogastric tube (see How to . . . 8.1). This can give immediate pain relief and reduces the likelihood of gastric rupture.

Colic (abdominal pain) in the horse is potentially a serious emergency, which responds best to rapid treatment (see Chapter 7).

Other gastrointestinal diseases may cause *anorexia* (reduced appetite) or changes in the appetite. Liver disease in particular may cause the development of

How to . . . 8.1

Passage of a nasogastric (stomach) tube

Indications

- To decompress the stomach.
- To give nasogastric fluids/liquid feed.

Method

- Select an appropriate sized tube (generally foal, small, medium, large horse).
- Hold it up against the horse to estimate the length required to reach the stomach and mark it.
- Have an experienced handler hold the horse on strong headcollar and lead-rope.
- Restrain the horse adequately. This may necessitate twitching/sedation and the horse may need to be backed into a corner or put in stocks.
- Lubricate the fenestrated end of the tube and hang it over shoulders.
- With one hand over the nose, insert the fenestrated end of the tube ventromedially into the nasal passages using the other hand.
- Using the thumb of the hand on the horse's nose, keep the tube guided ventromedially and held in place.
- Advance the tube slowly but firmly; the horse will resent it for first 25 cm or so but then usually it is well tolerated. (If the tube will not go in, take it out and start again. It may have gone into the middle or lateral meatus, which is not wide enough to accommodate the tube. If the tube feels tight, change it for a smaller size.)
- At the larynx you may have to twist the tube and advance it and retract it a few times to induce swallowing. Blowing down the tube may help. Once through the larynx, watch/palpate the left-hand side of the neck to check that it goes down the oesophagus and not the trachea. Check that it is in place by feeling for breaths from the end of the tube. If it is intratracheal, pull it back out through the larynx and advance it again.
- When the tube is in the stomach gurgling can be heard at the end of tube and stomach contents can be smelt.
- Siphoning of stomach contents then may be possible or fluids may be administered if the stomach is not full.
- If the nasogastric tube is to be left in place it can be secured to the headcollar with sticky tape; care should be taken to ensure that it does not become dislodged and that damage to the nasal and oesophageal mucosa does not occur. A bung should be inserted to prevent air from entering the stomach via the tube.

Potential complications

- Incorrect tube placement (i.e. intratracheal) can cause aspiration pneumonia; avoid this by ensuring that the tube is in the oesophagus.
- Irritation or erosion of the oesophagus and nasopharynx can occur. Avoid this by gentle use of a well-lubricated tube with a smooth exterior. Nose bleeds are not uncommon, and are unlikely to represent a serious problem (will stop within 15 min), but if oesophageal damage is suspected it should be examined endoscopically to assess any injuries.
- Kinking or obstruction of the tube may complicate fluid delivery. If it is difficult to pump in fluids, try moving the tube a little and then pumping again. If in doubt, remove tube, unblock it and re-commence procedure.

After use, tubes should be flushed and cleaned with a dilute chlorhexidine solution and hung up to dry. They should be stored somewhere clean and dry, and abrasions of the surface, which can scratch the inside of the horse's nasal mucosa, should be avoided. If they become damaged, they should be replaced.

an abnormal appetite (pica) resulting in the ingestion of indigestible substances such as soil.

Musculoskeletal examination

See Chapter 16.

Care and nursing of patients

Sick horses require nursing care. At the most basic level this means the provision of a suitable environment and sufficient fluids and nutrition for their needs. These requirements depend on the age of the horse as well as on its type or breed and its medical condition. A horse that has had pneumonia, for instance, may well be able to eat and drink normally, whereas a horse that has had, say, oesophageal surgery may require total parenteral (intravenous) nutrition and fluids. As well as the provision of nutritional requirements, nursing may involve removal of waste (e.g. by catheterisation of the bladder (see How to . . . 8.2). In addition, nursing may constitute giving medication, cleaning and flushing catheters, dressing wounds and changing bandages.

General management

There are a variety of bedding materials on which horses can be stabled (see Chapter 1). While hospitalised, most horses will benefit from hand-walking or turnout for exercise and access to grass; access to grass can help to stimulate the digestive system but may be contraindicated in certain cases.

Managing the horse's food and water intake is a vital part of the nursing of a sick horse (see Chapters 5 and 13).

How to . . . 8.2

Catheterisation of the bladder

Indications

- To withdraw an uncontaminated urine sample.
- To empty the bladder if normal micturition is not possible.
- Prior to some types of bladder/penile surgery.
- During a general anaesthetic.

Method

Suitably restrain the horse using sedation/twitching/stocks.

Males

- Grasp and extrude the penis.
- Wash it thoroughly with dilute povidone iodine.
- Wearing sterile gloves, and without touching the tip of a sterile flexible urinary catheter (or foal stomach tube), lubricate it with a water-based lubricant (one containing a local anaesthetic, e.g. Xylocaine (Astra) can be particularly helpful).
- Insert into urethral orifice and feed it in from the packet (still not touching the actual catheter).
- Advance it until urine is voided (approximately 60 cm in an average 500-kg male). If no urine is voided, try moving the catheter slightly in or out or applying syringe pressure to the end.

Females

- Bandage tail and hold it to one side.

- Wash perineum in dilute povidone iodine.
- Insert sterile gloved hand into vagina approximately 10 cm (in an average 500-kg female), feeling for urethral orifice in floor of vagina.
- Once the urethra has been identified, use finger in this position to guide a sterile lubricated catheter (usually a semi-rigid one is used) into the urethra and advance it.

Potential complications

- Introduction of infection to the bladder is unlikely but iatrogenic cystitis could result from inadequate hygiene.
- Blockage of the catheter may occur. If no urine is voided, try moving the catheter slightly in case it is up against the bladder wall. Alternatively try flushing some sterile saline in through the catheter. If blockage with crystals occurs, the catheter may need to be removed and the procedure re-commenced.
- Damage to the urethral mucosa can result from poor technique or roughening of the outside of the catheter. Always use a well-lubricated catheter with a smooth surface.

After use, catheters should be flushed and cleaned with a dilute chlorhexidine solution. They may then be re-sterilised. If they become damaged or develop any surface abrasions that could cause injury to the horse's urethral mucosa, they should be replaced.

Patient care

Maintenance of body temperature

Sick horses may have a reduced ability to control their body temperature. Temperature monitoring is important. Rugs and blankets are used to reduce heat loss (particularly in clipped individuals), and heat lamps and heat pads may be used (particularly with foals) but care must be taken to avoid burns.

In rare cases when horses are acutely hyperthermic, cool water baths, ice packs and fans can be used to aid temperature reduction.

Care of the skin

Grooming is important both psychologically and to help to avoid sores developing in ill and recumbent horses. The coat should be brushed thoroughly at least once daily to remove any dirt or sweat, and the mane and tail may be combed out. Soiling of the skin can be avoided by prompt removal of any faeces passed and prompt cleaning of the perineum after defaecation or urination. Tail bandaging can be employed to prevent soiling but bandaging can cause pressure-related injuries and more often a loose rectal sleeve is used to keep the tail clean (see Fig. 1.8).

Soiled areas should be washed and dried daily. Clipping of surrounding hair with electric clippers or half-curved scissors is advisable so that adequate drying can be ensured. Where any body fluids (e.g. urine around the perineum, or wound discharge) fall on the skin, protection from scalding can be achieved by applying petroleum jelly (e.g. Vaseline®) twice daily after cleaning and drying of the affected area.

Cleaning should be carried out with a dilute solution of antiseptic. All damp areas then should be dried with soft towels. Hair dryers and heat lamps also may be used to aid drying, but care should be taken to avoid burns.

One of the complications of dealing with sores on horses is the potential for the colonisation of damaged tissue with blow-fly maggots within less than 24 h (fly strike). To avoid this, fly control in hospitals must be stringent and fly repellents may be required on individual horses.

Dressings

Wherever possible, wounds should be dressed in order to:

- Keep the wound clean
- Reduce inflammation and fluid loss from the wound
- Control swelling and encourage healing

Bandages also can be used to provide support to injured limbs. When a limb is injured, a support dressing should be applied to the contralateral limb because this will be bearing more weight and will be subject to increased stresses. In addition, frog support dressings may be applied to the feet (see Chapter 16) to reduce the chance of laminitis developing. Where possible, pressure sores should be prevented by the use of padded dressings over pressure points. When they do occur, soft padded non-adherent dressings should be used to assist healing and prevent exacerbation of the injury.

It is important to ensure that bandages are never applied too tight or they may cause damage to underlying tissues. They must be applied evenly.

Nursing the aged horse

The aged horse may have specific health problems that need to be taken into account. Ageing results in irreversible changes in many of the body's organs, and many old horses will have subclinical disease.

Diseases that become more common in old age include:

- Liver disease
- Musculoskeletal diseases, such as arthritis
- Some hormonal diseases, such as pituitary adenoma (equine Cushing's disease).

General management of the apparently healthy aged horse should include stringent monitoring for signs of disease. Twice yearly dental checks are advisable in order to check for gum disease and loose teeth, to ensure that the molars still form a good grinding surface and to rasp off any sharp molar edges. Regular farriery should be continued into old age to ensure good foot balance and thus minimise any joint pain that may accompany arthritic changes. Exercise may need to be reduced (although small amounts of regular exercise are usually better than no exercise at all) and feeding may need to be increased due to reduced efficiency of digestion (see Chapter 5)

Nursing the recumbent patient

Recumbency (the inability to stand) may follow injuries of the head, spine or limbs, neurological disease, old age and severe disease or debilitation. Horses do not cope well either physically or pschologically with recumbency (see Summary 8.1). Long-term nursing of recumbent horses is rare but recumbent foal care is more common. Nursing is aimed at providing the optimal environment for the horse to stand as soon as possible and, at the same time, avoiding complications. Regular turning (preferably at least every 4 h) is necessary (see How to . . . 8.3). Slinging of recumbent horses can be carried out and may help. Many horses do not tolerate slings well and sling-related sores can be a problem.

Where possible, recumbent horses should be encouraged to eat a normal diet, although they may have an increased risk of developing aspiration pneumonia. Food and water should be provided in low-edged buckets positioned so that they are easily accessible but not in danger of being knocked over or fallen into. Highly palatable food may be offered to tempt the horse (see Chapter 5).

Moving the recumbent or unconscious horse

Situations when unconscious or recumbent horses may need to be moved include the transport of anaesthetised animals between the induction or recovery room and the operating theatre and the transport of seriously injured animals to a place where they can be treated. Profound sedation, anaesthesia or unconsciousness is a prerequisite because horses are easily panicked by being restrained. Any injured areas should be dressed or supported prior to at-

---

Summary 8.1   The complications of recumbency

Hypostatic pneumonia

Hypostatic pneumonia occurs when pooling of blood in dependent lungs causes reduced aeration and secondary infection. Clinical signs include dyspnoea, rapid shallow breathing, moist respiratory noises and depression. Blood gas monitoring can allow early identification of this condition. If profound hypoxia (<60 mmHg p_aO_2) occurs, nasal insufflation of oxygen should be commenced; if profound hypercapnia (>60 mmHg p_aCO_2) occurs, mechanical ventilation may be necessary. Hypostatic pneumonia occurs in sick and debilitated animals, particularly if they remain in lateral recumbency for long periods. It can be avoided by turning at least every 4 h and encouraging sternal recumbency. Coupage may also be helpful in foals and miniature horses.

Decubital ulcers

These are pressure-related sores (bedsores) that follow prolonged recumbency. They are predisposed to by pressure, moistness of the skin and poor skin circulation. They most commonly affect boney prominences such as the distal limbs, elbows, hocks, tuber coxae and the head. They can be avoided

by careful padding of such prominences with dry soft pads. A thick, soft, dry bedding such as paper, auboise or shavings can be helpful, or foam mats, duvets and water beds may be used (particularly in foals). Careful positioning is of extreme importance. Pads should be changed daily to avoid the skin underneath becoming moist. In addition, the skin should be kept clean and dry. If any wounds occur, they should be treated promptly by washing and drying of affected areas and use of emollient creams. Periods of lateral recumbency can help to take pressure off the affected areas but may increase the likelihood of hypostatic pneumonia developing. Physiotherapy techniques that help to promote blood circulation to affected areas can be helpful.

Myopathies and neuropathies

Muscle and nerve damage can occur during or soon after anaesthesia and may prevent horses from being able to rise post-anaesthesia. In addition, horses that are recumbent for other reasons may develop myopathies and neuropathies if they are not positioned carefully on adequately padded bedding/matting (see Chapter 20).

How to . . . 8.3

Turning the recumbent horse

Indications

- Positioning during anaesthesia.
- Assisting the recumbent horse to rise.
- Turning the recumbent horse to avoid complications of recumbency.

Method

- This should never be attempted without a minimum of three experienced handlers.
- Extreme care must be taken at all times to avoid human injury.
- The horse should always have a headcollar on and one person should control head movements.
- If the horse is unconscious or deeply sedated, ropes may be applied to the pasterns (after padding) to aid control of the limbs; however, this is likely to cause panic in conscious animals and should be avoided.
- Easily accessible, quick-release, non-slip knots always should be used.
- A deeply unconscious horse may be moved from lateral recumbency on one side to the other by rolling it onto its back and over, with the limbs controlled by ropes; however, this should never be attempted in the conscious animal.
- A horse in lateral recumbency may be helped into sternal recumbency by having the hindlegs flexed at the hock and stifle and the front legs flexed at the knee to bring the limbs in towards the body. Pushing hard on its back, while the head is brought round towards the upper side, should allow the horse to be brought into sternal recumbency.
- A horse in sternal recumbency may need to be supported by bales or padded wedges at its back. The muscles of the lower hindlimb are subjected to pressure in this position, and the horse should be moved from one side to the other at least every 4 h.
- Short periods of lateral recumbency and passive movements of the limbs can help to maintain the limb circulation.

Potential complications

- Handler injury
- Horse injury

tempting to move the horse, and further injury should be avoided.

Whatever the method of moving horses, it is important to bear in mind the potential dangers to both handlers and horse. Sufficient handlers always should be present to deal with any eventuality. At least one person should be responsible for avoiding injury to the horse's head and eyes, and in some cases a hood or blindfold may be applied both to reduce stimulation of the horse and for its protection. All areas where ropes, hobbles and headcollars are in contact with the horse should be well padded to avoid injury. The cheek piece of a headcollar overlies the facial nerve, and particular care should be taken to pad this area in order to avoid nerve damage. Direct pressure in the pastern area can cause tendon damage, so the pasterns also should be well padded. All knots should be non-slipping, quick-release knots that can be undone rapidly.

Foals weighing up to 100 kg may be moved by stretcher or trolley, with sufficient staff present to restrain the foal. For larger horses the most common mode of transport in hospital situations is by a winch connected to pastern hobbles (Fig. 8.5). At least three staff members are required: one to control the winch, one to position the body and one to control the head. Some hospitals use drag mats or trolleys for moving horses, but these are more commonly used in field situations.

In the field, a horse can be moved (*with care*) using traction applied to strong soft ropes around the brisket, breech or withers. These ropes can be used to drag an injured horse onto a drag mat, which then can be used to move the horse, or may be connected to a winch to drag the horse onto an ambulance box or to a tractor or digger to move the horse. A rope also should be connected to a strong headcollar to allow control and movement of the head. Hobbles also can

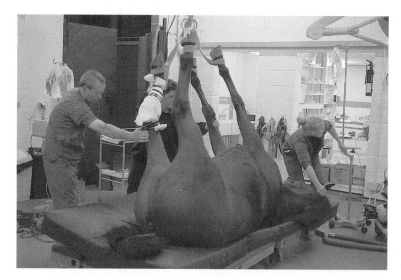

Fig. 8.5 Moving an anaesthetised horse into the operating theatre using hobbles and a winch. Any attempt to move a partially conscious animal should be avoided, if possible. General anaesthesia is safer when dealing with such large and potentially dangerous animals.

be applied to the pastern area to control the limbs. In partially conscious animals this can cause increased struggling and increase the likelihood of injury. In such situations, extreme care must be taken to avoid injury to either humans or the horse involved. General anaesthesia (using total intravenous methods) is usually the only safe solution.

Further reading

Spiers, V.C. (1997) *Clinical Examination of Horses*. WB Saunders, Philadelphia, PA.

CHAPTER 9

Safety Management in the Practice

A. Jones & E. R. J. Cauvin

The Health and Safety at Work Act (HSAWA) 1974 applies to all persons at work. The Act encompasses all areas of working practice by the use of 'enabling legislation', which allows for new regulations to be implemented quickly under the umbrella of the HSAWA. Serious breaches of health and safety legislation can lead to criminal charges. It is implemented by the 'Health and Safety Executive' (HSE), who produce a poster ('Health and Safety Law–What you should know') that should be available in all practices. Parts of it relate to *employees* (such as veterinary nurses) who must:

- *Take reasonable care* for the health and safety of themselves and of others who may be affected by their acts or omissions at work.
- *Cooperate* with the employer as far as is necessary to enable any duty or requirement under the Act to be performed or complied with.
- *Not interfere*, recklessly or intentionally, with anything provided in the interests of health and safety.

In general terms there is a requirement for the employer to:

(1) Provide a safe working environment.

(2) Carry out suitable *training* and *supervision* to ensure that employees are not likely to be a danger to themselves or colleagues.

(3) Provide *personal protective equipment* where the HSAWA or where a risk assessment indicates that it is required.

(4) Provide a *safety policy statement* of how the employer intends to ensure a safe and healthy environment. This need be in written form only when there are five or more persons in the practice.

(5) Provide a duty of care to employees. In a veterinary practice this could be extended to the clients, when they are on the premises or when visiting the patients.

(6) Safe systems of work should be established, written down and displayed.

(7) Maintain equipment in a safe working condition and to the manufacturer's specification.

(8) Keep the premises, including practice vehicles in a good state of repair.

(9) The working environment should be maintained to provide adequate facilities and arrangements for the employee's welfare at work. This should include the provision of suitable washing and toilet facilities. There should also be an area set aside for rest and refreshments.

Regulations and associated acts relating to the HSAWA are listed below:

(1) Management of Health and Safety at Work Regulations 1992 (amended 1996)

(2) Electricity at Work Regulations 1989

(3) Chemical Hazards Information and Packaging Regulations 1993

(4) Control of Waste Regulations 1992

(5) Misuse of Drugs Regulations 1985

(6) Reporting of Injuries, Diseases and Dangerous Occurrences Regulations 1995

(7) Control of Substances Hazardous to Health Regulations 1999

(8) Firearms Amended Act 1988*
(9) Environmental Protection Act 1989*
(10) Litter (Animal Droppings) Order 1991*
(11) Trade Union Reform and Employment Rights Act 1993
(12) Provision and Use of Work Equipment Regulations 1992
(13) Workplace (Health, Safety and Welfare) Regulations 1992
(14) Health and Safety (Display Screen) Regulations 1992
(15) Lifting Operations and Lifting Equipment Regulations 1998
(16) Manual Handling Operations Regulations 1992
(17) Personal Protective Equipment Regulations 1992
(18) Fire Precautions Act 1971* and Fire Precautions (Workplace) Regulations 1997
(19) Health and Safety (First Aid) Regulations 1981
(20) Health and Safety (Signs and Signals) Regulations 1996

Note that the Acts indicated by an asterisk are separate legislation that have a strong influence on the safety management of veterinary practices. This list is not exhaustive and is constantly being updated; it is therefore prudent to check with The Stationery Office to ensure that the latest guidelines and regulations are being followed.

Risk assessments

A risk assessment is a methodical investigation of the work to be performed, the hazards involved and the risks associated with those hazards. It can take many forms, depending on the nature of the work. The usual practice is to follow a series of questions that can be asked of the working procedure, e.g.: What if X happens? How can Y be done safely? Is there a suitable alternative? If not, what protective measures are needed?

A *hazard* is defined as something with the potential to cause harm. A *risk* is the probability of harm being caused resulting in injury. For example, the height of a tightrope, once established, could represent a hazard with known consequences (falls resulting in injury), however the risk of injury can be reduced

greatly by the use of a safety rope and a catch net. The decision to use a safety net is an example of the result of the thought process required in making risk assessments.

General *risk assessments* and *systems of work* or 'standard operating procedures (SOPs)' are of great importance in the maintenance of a safe working environment and good management practice. These also should contain information on the hazards and risks associated with a particular task, together with the relevant first aid instructions. This could be related also to chemical products that have either general or specific first aid measures included in the text of health and safety data sheets. Tables 9.1 and 9.2 give two examples of risk assessment forms.

Areas to be considered in an equine veterinary practice include:

(1) *Electrical safety*, particularly with use of mains-operated electric clippers.
(2) *Chemical safety*. Chemicals used in the workplace are subject to the Control of Substances Hazardous to Health Regulations (COSHH) 1999. The nature of the chemicals, their use and disposal need to be considered. Medicines and pharmaceutical preparations that carry a risk to persons handling them should be treated as hazardous chemicals for safety management purposes. Any spillages must be dealt with properly. The action to be taken in the event of a spillage or release of substances depends on what is spilt and where. This could range from a drop of blood on the worktop, easily mopped up with an absorbent swab, to widespread release of potentially harmful fumes. Generally, the areas to consider are:
- Liquid spills: if acids, alkalis, mercury, flammable or toxic solvents are spilt, then use a dedicated 'complete spillage kit', which will contain quick-acting absorbent material, appropriate neutralisers and bags to collect the waste in.
- Fumes: evacuate area and call emergency services.
- Eye contamination: sterile eye washes or a hand-washing sink should be used to flush the

Table 9.1 Example of a risk assessment form

Activity	Handling horses for examination
Hazard	Physical injury from kicks, bites, compression, rapid movement
Person involved	Veterinary nurses, surgeons and grooms in the practice
Precautions	Physically fit staff, stout footwear, overalls and appropriate handling equipment, e.g. Chifney bit
Emergency procedures	If a member of staff is injured, the horse must be secured and/or removed from the vicinity to remove the risk of further injury. Casualty to be assessed, carry out first aid required or call an ambulance
Training requirements	All staff handling horses in the practice or on the practice's business must be fully trained in the handling of horses in clinical situations. They must be aware of the warning signs and be able to control the horse to avoid accidents or be able to warn others of impending problems. They must have a good knowledge of the examination procedures so that some anticipation can be made
Waste disposal	Not applicable
Signed and dated by competent person	

affected eye copiously. Medical advice should be sought immediately.

(3) *Postage of pathological samples.* Packaging and sample handling will need to have a risk assessment that may be general in its format, indicating the packing process and labelling. The current legislation (guidelines available from main post offices) has specific legal requirements relating to the labelling and standard of packaging required (see Chapter 12).

(4) *Disposal of general waste, sharps and clinical waste.* The relevant regulations are:
- Control of Pollution Act (1974)
- Controlled Waste Regulations (1992)
- Environmental Protection Act (1990)

These are important to the correct segregation, storage, transfer and eventual destruction of waste products produced at the practice. Waste must be classified as:

- Clinical waste: anything that is, or is contaminated with, animal tissue/fluids/excretions, medicines or other pharmaceutical products, which may be hazardous to health. It needs to be collected into and stored in yellow plastic sacks, printed with 'clinical waste' on the outside.
- 'Sharps': includes used needles, scalpel blades and other sharp objects. These must be put immediately into the yellow plastic tubs, which are sealed when full.
- Special waste: bottles and vials contaminated with pharmaceutical products that should be put into specific plastic bins.
- Cadavers: these are technically clinical waste. Most equine practices have an arrangement with a licensed knackerman.

(5) *Mechanical and lifting equipment.*

(6) *Offices and reception areas*, including computer and general equipment safety.

(7) *Pressure systems, including transportable gas cylinders, autoclaves and pipelines.* The purpose of The Pressure Systems and Transportable Gas Containers Regulations 1989, with the asso-

Activity	Induction of anaesthesia (induction box)	**Table 9.2** Another example of a risk assessment form
Hazard	Sedated horse in an unfamiliar environment; horse may be in pain and/or anxious; weight of the horse; collapse of horse on induction	
Person involved	Grooms, veterinary nurses and surgeons	
Precautions	Preparation of equipment before horse arrives; quiet, calm atmosphere; shoes to be removed or covered with rubber protective overshoes; padded appropriate headcollar; staff to wear appropriate protective clothing. All equipment should be in position before the horse arrives to reduce the risk of the horse waking before it is settled on the operating table. i.e. hoists in position, intubation equipment ready, anaesthetic reservoir bag filled, spare syringes of induction agents drawn up and in close proximity to the induction box, hobbles laid out ready	
Emergency procedures	As per system of work instructions. Secure the safety of the casualty from further injury	
Training requirements	Professional qualifications and 'on the job' supervision and tutoring for staff inexperienced with horses in this situation	
Waste disposal	Not applicable	
Signed and dated by competent person*		

*The competent person would be a member of nursing or veterinary staff with a full understanding of the risks involved and behaviour of horses in this situation

ciated HSE guidance notes, are to prevent hazards to people and property by the inadvertent release of energy stored in a gas system under pressure.

(8) *Handling of horses* (see Chapter 1).

(9) *Pregnancy*: a member of staff who is pregnant should inform her supervisor in writing because a risk assessment of her working environment and work conditions will need to be made to protect her health and safety and that of her child. Risk areas that require assessment are:

- Radiation
- Night working
- Manual handling (including animals)
- Extremes of temperature
- Physical posture and prolonged standing
- Contact with some pathogenic organisms
- Contact with cytotoxic agents
- Pharmaceuticals that may cause harm to the mother, breastfed child or unborn child.

First aid management

One or more members of staff should be trained in basic first aid techniques and there should be a designated first aid officer. It is the responsibility of this person to keep the approved first aid box up to date.

First aid training is available from the St John Ambulance brigade or the Red Cross. There are also companies that will provide first aid training specifically tailored to the workplace and they are able to advise practices regarding the numbers of staff that it would be necessary to train. Manuals in first aid techniques can be provided by the above organisations and are often of most use in conjunction with a formal course. First aid manuals alone are not a substitute for training.

Detailed understanding and administration of human first aid is beyond the scope of this book. Readers are referred to the standard texts on the subject (see further reading list) or, better still, recommended to undergo proper first aid training.

Accidents

Accidents that occur at work or when on the employer's business must be recorded. This can be in an accident book approved by the HSE (form B1 510) or by forms produced in the practice. Practice-produced forms can have additional comments, such as remedial action taken as a result of the accident, and any changes in procedure that result from it. This is a useful addition in that the process to change a procedure, where an accident has occurred, is the basis of good health and safety management. Accident details should include:

- The full name, address and occupation of the injured person.
- A signature from the person reporting the accident, including the time and date of the injury and when the report was made. This must also include the address and occupation of the person reporting the accident if different from the casualty.
- A record of the accident, clearly stating the place, time, first aider and any witnesses. This information may be useful should an insurance claim be made.
- Details that may be required by the HSE if an injury warrants investigation by them.

Reporting accidents

The Reporting of Injuries, Diseases and Dangerous Occurrences Regulations require the employer to report serious accidents and occurrences directly to the HSE. There are three main categories described by the legislation:

(1) Major or fatal accidents, which include a fractured long bone, skull, spine or pelvis or loss of sight in an eye, plus any other injury that results in the injured person being admitted to hospital as an inpatient for more than 24 h, unless this is solely for observation. A *fatality* includes those accidents where the injured person dies within a year of the original injury sustained at work.

(2) Accidents where a person is off work for three or more days.
(3) Dangerous occurrences and near misses, e.g. uncontrolled release of a substance liable to be hazardous to health.

Major and fatal accidents must be reported by telephone as soon as possible after the event. A written report confirming the details (form F2508) must be sent within 7 days. *Dangerous occurrences* should be reported to the HSE (form F2508) whether or not a person has been injured.

Radiation safety and the law

It is essential to realise that radiation can have serious effects on the body. The risks must be understood so that appropriate protective measures are taken to minimise this, particularly by equine nurses who may be at risk in their work.

Radiation injuries

The effects of ionising radiation include:

(1) *Somatic effects*: direct effects of radiation due to the absorption of energy by the tissues. Very large amounts of radiation cause burns (erythema), inflammation and tissue destruction (necrosis). Rapidly growing cells, especially in the skin, bowel, blood-cell-forming marrow, embryos and reproductive organs, are most affected. These are directly related to the dose of radiation received. In the early days of radiology, the most recognised syndromes included eye cataract and thyroid gland insufficiency. Somatic effects are rarely a significant risk in modern diagnostic radiology.
(2) *Stochastic effects*: injuries that may or may not develop regardless of the radiation dose. They occur as a result of damage to the genome through ionisation. The higher the radiation dose and the more frequent the exposure, the more likely they are to occur. They are also cumulative, i.e. repeated exposure gradually increases the chance of disease. They are insidious because one does not feel the effect of radiation and lesions may develop years later.

(a) Genetic hazards: modification of the DNA (mutations) may not have any direct effects on the affected person but may lead to abnormalities in their children.

(b) Carcinogenic effects: probably the main concern associated with radiation is the risk of malignancy. Tumours may develop anywhere in the body and occur many years after exposure.

Monitoring radiation exposure

The amount of radiation that the personnel and patient are subjected to must be monitored constantly.

Methods of measurement

(1) Radiation counters: these devices are designed to measure the ambient radiation immediately. Geiger–Müller counters (see Chapter 17, Fig. 17.32) are the most commonly used and should be available when performing scintigraphy, to measure potential soiling of the workbench and equipment with radiopharmaceuticals. These must be calibrated for the right type of radiation and the appropriate wavelength.

(2) Personal dosimeters:

(a) The simplest dosimeters are special X-ray films placed in a *film badge*. These record the radiation as would a normal radiographic film. Filters in the badge help to differentiate between different types of radiation. They are usually worn for 4–6 weeks and then processed to give an exposure dose. Film badges should be worn under lead aprons to record the whole body exposure. Finger-ring badges are available to measure the exposure to non-protected areas and should be used for more risky procedures, including delivery of drug for scintigraphy and hand-holding of X-ray cassettes.

(b) Thermoluminescent dosimeters use special phosphor screens placed in dosimeter badges. The crystals are activated by radiation but require heat to produce a flash of light. They can, therefore, be used for a longer time to record radiation exposure and are sensitive to a wide range of radiations. They are re-usable.

(c) Pocket electronic dosimeters, similar to Geiger tubes, are also available for immediate monitoring of the exposure. These are particularly useful for occasional assistants or for risky procedures such as fluoroscopy. They are less accurate and not ideal for long-term monitoring.

Radiation regulations

Since radiation hazards were first appreciated, the law has gradually evolved to take into account the recognised risks and to protect workers. The current regulations in the UK are compiled in the *Ionising Radiation Regulations of 1999* (IRR 99) and appended *Approved Code of Practice*. These regulations complement the *Health and Safety at Work Act* and are based on the recommendations of the International Commission on Radiological Protection of 1977 (ICRP 77). The Code of Practice sets practical rules based on the interpretation of the law. It covers all aspects of radiation protection and work. A booklet entitled *Guidance Notes for the Protection of Persons Against Ionising Radiation Arising From Veterinary Use* is published by the HSE to provide guidance notes for veterinary workers. This booklet should be available to all personnel involved in radiology and should be read carefully by potential radiographers.

Principles of the Ionising Radiation Regulations 1999

There are three major principles:

(1) Radiography should be carried out only if absolutely required. This is largely a matter of interpretation and the law remains vague in this regard. Practically, it means that radiographs should be taken only if there is a definite clinical indication for it and the diagnosis cannot be obtained by any other means.

(2) All steps should be taken to keep radiation to personnel to a minimum. This rule spans from the ICRP 77's *ALARA* principle, namely that exposure must be kept *As Low As Reasonably*

Achievable. A major implication is that everything should be set up in order to prevent having to repeat exposures, including adequate exposure charts, trained personnel, etc. The Code of Practice gives detailed indications in this regard.

(3) The dose limits set by law must not be exceeded: the *dose limits* are based on what the legislator regards as an acceptable work-related risk. This has been based on high-risk industries and corresponds to a risk of cancer or other radiation injury of 1 in 1000 over a lifetime. These doses are arguably very high. A radiation worker should not be exposed to more than *50 mSv/year* and members of the public to no more than 5 mSv per year. Doses ten times less are actually recommended by the National Radiological Protection Board (the HSE advisory board). For veterinary use, the maximum dose is *10 mSv/year*, and it is stated that it should not normally exceed *3 mSv/year*.

Main points covered by the regulations

(1) The veterinary practice must notify the HSE prior to using radiography or nuclear imaging facilities, using a special form (F2522 9/99).

(2) The HSE may appoint a *radiation protection advisor* (RPA), usually a veterinary radiologist holding a specialist diploma (DVR or DipEAVDI). The role of the RPA is to advise on the necessary requirements and risks and provide practical help whenever needed. The RPA must be involved also in writing up the Local Rules.

(3) A *radiation protection supervisor* (RPS) must be appointed within the practice (usually a senior partner), whose responsibility it is to enforce the regulations and supervise the use of the equipment.

(4) Controlled areas: the area where radiation is used must be designated a *controlled area* (a special triangular sign and the words 'Controlled Area' must be displayed (Fig. 9.1). Practically, this corresponds to a distance of 2 m from the primary beam. Because horizontal beams are used routinely to radiograph horses, the whole room should be designated. This

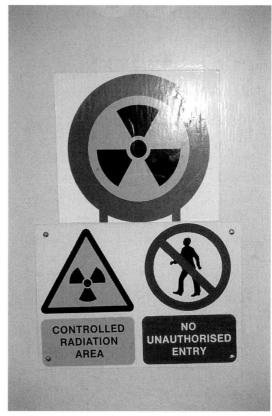

Fig. 9.1 Example of a sign placed at the entrance to a controlled radiation area.

implies the use of warning signs and limitation of access to the room when it is in use. Fixed units are often linked to a sign outside the room, which is lit when the machine is switched on.

(5) Written system of work: entry into a controlled area must be restricted to persons under a *written system of work* (WSW). This describes who is allowed into the room, the expected workload, the protocol used to monitor radiation exposure, the names of the RPS and RPA and the maximum dose accepted for the personnel. It must, by law, also state that the X-ray unit must be isolated from the mains after each use. Access to the room may be unrestricted when this is the case. A copy of the WSW is to be displayed in the X-ray and scintigraphy rooms.

(6) Local rules: these are a broader list of rules to be followed to use the radiation area (X-ray or scintigraphy). It encompasses the WSW. It describes the regulations and the names and details of the RPA and RPS. It sets standard procedures to follow to perform radiography, i.e. names of personnel allowed to enter the room and use the equipment (see below), protocols, maintenance protocol for the equipment and use of protective equipment. A basic contingency plan for faults, fire or accidents, should be included.

(7) Training: only adequately trained personnel should be involved in any procedure.

(8) Limitations for higher risk persons: with *pregnant women and persons under 18 years of age* it is not a legal requirement but it is advised that these persons should not be involved. This should be stated in the WSW.

(9) Dose assessment: it is a legal requirement that *dosimeters* be worn on the trunk during radiation work. If a significant exposure to unprotected parts of the body is expected, extremity dosimeters also must be used. The meters should be analysed every *1–3 months*, depending on the RPA's advice, and records must be kept for 2 years. The RPA also determines regular checks for the radiation levels in the relevant rooms. A list of local dosimetry services is available from the HSE.

(10) X-ray equipment: most requirements have been described above. All units must include tube filters and a beam collimator. It is the responsibility of the provider to ensure that the equipment is safe, but maintenance services must be carried out at least yearly. Regular controls of the radiation emanating from the tube (outside the primary beam) must be made (film badges may be used for this purpose).

Radiation protection

Protection against the effects of radiation should not be taken lightly. Mostly it relies on common sense but some guidelines should be followed.

Limiting exposure to radiation

Protection is never absolute, so limiting exposure to radiation is the best compromise. The principles are the same for all types of radiation, but concentrating on radiography primarily, one should:

(1) Limit the number of radiographs: radiography is not a localising technique, only an imaging method that is used once a problem is suspected. The number of X-rays should be limited to those absolutely required. However, a complete series of projections should be obtained to avoid missing any abnormalities. It is important to avoid having to repeat any views. An adequate technique chart and standardised processing are prerequisites. Each examination should be well planned, according to a routine:

(a) Prepare and label the cassettes

(b) Prepare the patient

(c) Ensure adequate restraint

(d) Position the tube head, then the cassette

(e) Always check the film focal distance (FFD).

It is important to reduce the risk of movement, the most common cause of wasted radiographs.

(2) Limit the amount of radiation produced: use the fastest cassettes providing sufficient quality; avoid unnecessary use of grids and filters.

(3) Avoid the path of X-rays: no personnel should be exposed to the primary beam. Evidence of a finger (even gloved) on a radiograph is an offence. The beam goes through the cassette, so no part of the body should be placed behind it. The farther from the beam, the less the exposure. It is generally considered that a distance of 2 m (2 yards) is safe, but only the people absolutely required should be in the room at all. The minimum number of operators and assistants should be used. The use of stocks or other restraining devices is helpful; self-standing cassette holders are ideal but not always practical. Cassettes should not be held directly by hand, even gloved, unless absolutely necessary (as in stifle projections). In the latter case, the largest possible cassettes should be used. Otherwise, long handles generally are recommended, although not so long that move-

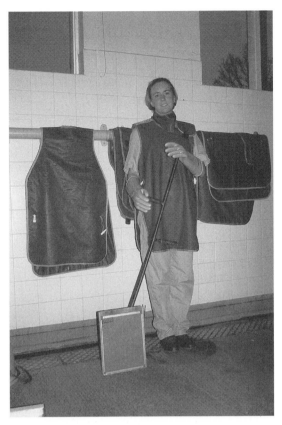

Fig. 9.2 Protective clothing used for radiography, including lead gown, gloves and thyroid shield and a long-handled cassette holder. The gowns are held on a rail to avoid damaging the lead fabric.

ment blur becomes likely. The regulations require that the exposure switch be on a wire at least 2 m long. A screen with at least 0.5-mm lead shielding must be fitted to protect the control area of fixed radiographic units. Virtually all X-ray tubes leak, so one should stay as far from the tube as possible.

Protection against radiation

No material can stop all the X-rays. Heavy metals such as lead and barium absorb the radiation well, but the proportion of the beam removed is related to the thickness of the metal.

Protective clothing (Fig. 9.2)

Most items include sheets of lead rubber between protective fabrics. Only very thin layers can be used to design practical clothing: gowns usually have a lead thickness equivalent of 0.25 mm. This is sufficient to reduce significantly the low-energy scattered rays but not the primary beam. Gloves and thyroid shields are slightly thicker (0.35 mm) to protect against higher scatter close to the beam. A thickness of 2 mm of lead or equivalent would be necessary to attenuate the primary beam adequately. Lead rubber is very fragile and protective clothing should be looked after carefully. Folding will break the lead, causing tears that let X-rays through. Aprons therefore should be hung carefully over thick bars or hangers, never folded or dropped on the floor. They should be checked for defects regularly by exposing a film through them.

Premises

Premises used should be shielded adequately to protect members of the public outside the X-ray room. Single brick walls and other materials equivalent to 0.5 mm of lead are sufficient to protect against scattered radiation. Equine radiography, however, involves the use of horizontal and oblique beams, so all the walls, floor and openings should be protected sufficiently to nearly stop the primary beam photons. This requires a double thickness of brick, 15 cm of solid concrete or an equivalent of 2 mm of lead. Doors and all wooden partitions, etc. should be lined with lead ply. Windows should be placed high enough or covered.

Field radiography

When performing radiographic examinations outdoors, it is virtually impossible to control adequately all the above parameters. The vet is responsible for the safety of the personnel. The controlled area is defined as the area located within 2 m of the centre of the beam. Whenever possible, the procedure should be performed within a walled area, ensuring that no members of the public are present behind insufficiently thick walls. If performed outdoors, the beam must be oriented away from any dwellings or areas where access cannot be controlled.

Summary

The local rules, risk assessments and staff training are important parts of the management of health and safety in the workplace, both for radiation and for all other issues. Each member of staff should be encouraged to take an active interest in the safe working environment and contribute positively to the maintenance of a safe working culture.

Further reading

British Red Cross (1998) *Practical First Aid.* British Red Cross, London.
St John Ambulance Association (1997) *First Aid Manual.* St John Ambulance Association, London.

Basic Hospital Practice

J. Masters

The duties of a receptionist

Reception skills are often given minimal training time, yet can prove hard to learn. Flexibility, tolerance and understanding need to be combined with excellent organisational and communicational skills. It is likely that an equine veterinary nurse (EVN) will have come into practice to work with horses, but it is their 'people' skills that may be tested most. Dealing with clients at emotional moments can be very difficult and should never be regarded as unimportant.

At reception

When a client firsts walks into the practice or telephones the office, the first point of contact will be with whoever is at reception. This person plays a key role. No-one in the practice should be left on reception without appropriate training.

A professional appearance should be adopted at all times (see Key points 10.1), ideally a practical uniform that is clean and tidy, together with an approachable demeanour. On arrival, clients should be acknowledged even if the receptionist is busy. This may mean excusing oneself from another task in order to say a quick hello, but clients should never be ignored.

Interpersonal skills are crucial. Greet the client in a friendly manner and use their name, if possible. Regular clients like to feel that the practice staff know them and will appreciate it if you can remember their horses' details too. Listen carefully to all the

> ### Key points 10.1   Uniform
>
> **What is a professional uniform?**
>
> In equine practice, a traditional uniform for a veterinary nurse is impractical. It is common nowadays for practices to supply their own personalised garments. It is important that this uniform is clean and presentable and this may mean keeping a change of uniform to hand. Badges are a common way of letting clients know to whom they are speaking and their role in the practice, e.g. receptionist, student nurse, head nurse.

information given by the client and make notes of any relevant details. Ensure that you are aware of the different specialisms of the vets at your practice (see Key points 10.2), the practice policies for procedures such as colt castration and vaccine regimes, as well as what exactly are classified as serious emergencies. It is a good idea to incorporate this information into a reception handbook for easy reference by all staff.

> ### Key points 10.2   Roles
>
> **Who does what?**
>
> You may have vets in your practice who specialise in certain procedures and not others. Some vets may be interested in surgery and others in medicine. Make sure you are aware of the special interests of all your colleagues; you will be very unpopular with both the practice and the owner if the wrong veterinary surgeon is sent to a visit!

If you do not know the answer to a client's question, ask them to wait while you find out. If an answer is still unavailable, offer to telephone the client back when the answer is available and remember to do so.

The reception area must be clean and tidy at all times. Posters and leaflets advertising products that are recommended and available at the practice are useful. Any reading materials should be up to date and appropriate. Comfortable seating should be provided, ideally with a view to outside parking for owners with horses in trailers.

Answering the telephone (Fig. 10.1)

All telephone calls should be answered promptly with the standard greeting used by the practice (see Key points 10.3). Firstly obtain details regarding who is calling and what it concerns. If the caller needs to speak to a vet or make an appointment, it is extremely important to obtain all their relevant details (see Key points 10.4), so that case notes can be retrieved or other arrangements made. The client may have an enquiry that you are unable to deal with at the present time. If you have to put the caller 'on hold', keep going back to apologise for any delay. If you know that there will be an unavoidable wait, it may be better for the client to be telephoned back. Ensure that a

> **Key points 10.3   Greeting**
>
> **Which greeting?**
>
> It is common today to answer with the name of the practice. It is important that clients are aware of where they have called once the telephone is answered and therefore all practice staff should answer calls in the same way. Some practices also add 'how may I help?' to the greeting, or you may be required to give your name, e.g. 'Jane speaking', when answering.

message reaches the person concerned. Many practices have a message book at reception or nearby, where messages can be recorded and ticked off when they are no longer outstanding. A reception handbook can help with practice policy, especially concerning information and advice that can be given out over the telephone. Client details are confidential; unless you have permission from the client to distribute them, then this information should *never* be given out to other callers. If a caller is trying to reach one of your clients, take their details and contact the client yourself.

Giving out advice over the telephone can be difficult, however experienced you are. You should never give out any advice without the full permission of a

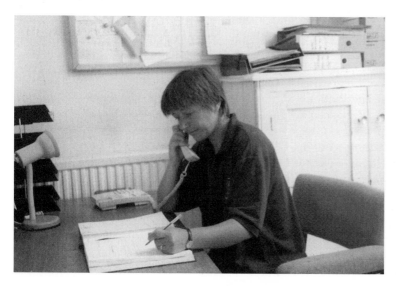

Fig. 10.1 Effective communication skills are of the utmost importance when dealing with telephone calls. (Photo: courtesy of Karl Holliman.)

Key points 10.4   Facts required

What information do I need?

When dealing with any enquiry it is important to obtain all the necessary information quickly and efficiently, especially in an emergency situation. Again, a reception handbook could contain a list to remind you of any areas you may otherwise omit.

Information should include:

- *Name of owner/keeper*: this may not be the caller; check under which surname the horse is registered.
- *Address of owner/keeper*: this may not be where the horse is kept, but it may be where the account will be sent.
- *Contact telephone number*: always take a contact number.
- *Details of horse*: more than just its name — you may have many animals with the same name on record.
- *Basic case history*: even in an emergency situation it can be vital to know if the horse is under any treatment or has had any similar problems in the past.
- *Condition*: a basic outline of the condition that the vet is going to treat. For example, 'it's bleeding' can mean anything from a minor ooze to a major haemorrhage.
- *Where is the patient?* Is it at home? If so, check the exact whereabouts; there can be several 'Church Farms' in any one area! Is it out on a hack? In this case, is the animal accessible by car? Is it at a show?, etc.
- *Is the animal registered at this practice?* If not, this will need to be clarified with the vets concerned according to the Royal College of Veterinary Surgeons (RCVS) code of conduct.

---

vet. If a vet is not available for advice or if you are in any doubt, the client should be given an appointment or at least arrange for a vet to call back.

First aid advice over the telephone

It is likely that any first aid or emergency situation will be brought to your attention over the telephone. Often the caller will be very stressed and it can be very difficult to obtain accurate and detailed information (see Chapter 7). Care always must be taken when trying to ascertain the degree of seriousness over the telephone. If you are unsure whether the

problem is an emergency, then refer to the vet (ideally the one who will see the case) as soon as possible. The client should be reassured that a vet will be contacted and sent to them as soon as possible, should it be required.

Once the vet has been reached, a call to let the client know that he/she is on the way, along with an approximate time, may be appropriate. Sending a vet out to an emergency call will undoubtedly make the remainder of the day's calls late. It is good practice policy to telephone these clients and warn them of an expected delay.

Arranging visits

The majority of cases will be seen on visits to the yard where the horse is kept. Some of these will be at large yards where the vet visits regularly. Others will be kept in a paddock with one or two ponies, which the practice visits only very occasionally. Familiarise yourself with all the main yards and contacts for regular visits because this can save time in collecting details. Keep this sort of information by the telephone for easy reference for everyone.

Remember that the owner's name and address are as important as the clinical details of the problem. A veterinary practice is a business and cannot function without accounts being paid. Make sure that the owner's details such as title, initial and address, including postcode, are on file for accounting purposes.

The horse's details obviously need to be taken, as does the reason for the visit, so that appropriate time can be allocated. In some practices, routine visits such as vaccinations may be booked in directly and a time given. For other cases a convenient day and time may be suggested by the client and confirmed by the practice later.

Getting clear directions to yards that are not visited regularly is crucial. If you are dealing with a new venue, it may be useful to find out exactly what facilities are available; some procedures can be impossible without the aid of electricity or a clean water supply.

Some visits may require more than one vet or the help of an EVN and therefore need to be arranged for a time that does not upset the smooth running of the remainder of the practice. Personal safety of practice staff on visits can be a concern and the attending vet may need the back-up of another member of staff for safety reasons. A newly qualified vet may benefit from the assistance of another member of the practice when he/she first starts. Some clients will bring horses to your clinic for examinations, particularly in the bigger equine hospitals.

Second opinions

Second opinion and/or referral cases are commonly seen in equine practices, either from non-specialist mixed practices or from practices that do not have the resources (such as an operating theatre) to treat the condition in question.

Second opinion cases are brought to your attention either by the referring vet or by clients who may be dissatisfied with the treatment they have received from their original practice. In the first case, it is relatively simple to organise: the original practice sends the case history to the second practice, where the animal is examined and the opinions of the examining vet are sent back to the original practice. When the client instigates the second opinion, the same rules need to be applied. The client may be under the impression that the patient can be examined by another practice without their usual vet needing to know. They may feel also that they do not wish to 'upset' their usual practice. However, it should be explained that the primary practice needs to be contacted *before* the animal is seen, both for reasons of professional ethics and good clinical practice. *Never* be seen to criticise another practice, its service or its treatment, this is extremely unprofessional.

If a client makes a booking to see a vet in your practice without notifying you of any previous treatment, not only are they putting their horse in possible danger but also your practice may be entering into *supersession*. Supersession occurs when a second vet takes over the case of another vet without their knowledge. This is an unethical situation; refer to the RCVS *Guide to Professional Conduct* for further information (see further reading list). It is safe to assume that all new animals registering with you will have seen another veterinary surgeon previously, unless they are newborn!

Contacting a previous veterinary practice may give you useful information on the client as well as the animals concerned. Debtors, for example, may try to move from practice to practice and you may find that you are taking on extra problems!

It must be remembered that in a *true emergency situation* animals can be seen at any practice. A vet *must* deal with any suffering animal and it cannot be turned away because it is not your client.

Second opinion or referral?

- A *second opinion* is when a vet or client seeks the opinion of another vet on a particular case. The second vet may be either in the same practice or at another clinic. For example, if a horse has been treated for a skin disease with certain drugs but seems to be getting no better, they another opinion on the case can be sought from another veterinary surgeon.
- A *referral* is instigated by a vet when it is felt that the condition needs specialist therapy. For example, if a horse has been diagnosed with a skin disease that requires specialist therapy, it is referred to a veterinary dermatologist.

Taking a case history

When dealing with second opinions, referral cases and new clients you may be required to take a case history from another practice. This information can be crucial to the correct continuation of treatment. The person taking the details should have a clear understanding of veterinary terminology. It can be useful to have any previous history faxed or e-mailed through to your practice; a typed case summary is most helpful. The case history as given by the client in a second opinion case may be misleading. Ensure that all records are available in the practice *before* the animal is examined.

Client communication

With each type of client, there are different points to consider. Difficult and emotional situations have to be handled diplomatically while always keeping a professional manner.

New clients

When new clients come into your surgery you have an ideal opportunity to promote the services of the practice. They should feel well informed with regard to how the practice is run and the services available. Some clinics have an information pack to hand out, which can be helpful if kept up to date. It is an opportunity to train your clients. Let them know important facts that help the practice to run efficiently, e.g. when to telephone to speak to a vet, book a visit, what to do with queries out of hours, when to settle their account and other key points. Providing an all-round service, especially for new owners, can be extremely rewarding. The client should feel that they can always approach the practice with queries regarding their horse.

Young clients

When dealing with very young clients, check that they are old enough to give their consent for procedures, to collect drugs and be responsible for their accounts. Usually this means that they have to be over 18 years of age. Certain procedures will have to be explained sympathetically and simply; young children often accept the euthanasia of their pony far better than do adults, but often will get distressed by the practicalities. It is often better to ask children to wait outside whilst their parents discuss procedures, and it may be useful to have some toys to distract clients with young families whilst they are in the practice.

Older or physically impaired clients

Older clients may be suffering from physical disabilities that sometimes are not obvious. Make sure that they have understood what has been said (they may be hard of hearing). Ensure that they are comfortable if they have to wait for long periods. Some older people find it difficult to talk to the vet and may feel more comfortable talking to nursing staff.

If a vet is to make a visit to an older or physically impaired client, diplomatically check to see if help may be needed. Remember that the vet may be liable if the client is put in danger. The key to managing the situation is to pre-empt any problems before they occur.

Customer care

All your clients should receive the same high standard of customer care. On leaving the practice, the owner should feel that they have had a good service from a professional organisation that cares about both them and their horse. Satisfied clients will promote your practice to other owners. This is the best form of advertising available!

Admitting and discharging patients

Admission

Adequate time should be allowed to admit patients to your clinic; it is always necessary to review the patient's history (see Key points 10.5) and a consent form *must* be signed before the animal is left. Although the vet may have taken an in-depth clinical history, a general history should be taken routinely on admittance.

Key points 10.5   Admitting a patient

- Check the condition of the animal: have there been any changes since its last examination?
- When did the horse have its last feed?
- Has it been taking any medication?
- Check the date of its last vaccination and particularly ensure that it is up to date for anti-tetanus prophylaxis
- Check with the owner if there is anything special or unusual relating to their horse, e.g. requiring soaked hay
- List and label the items that have been left with the horse, e.g. headcollar, rugs, etc., to ensure that these are returned to the owner on discharge

Owners / agents will often wish to unload and put the horse in a hospital stable or stall themselves, and this may be preferable in some cases. However, check the practice policy with regard to owners entering other clinic areas.

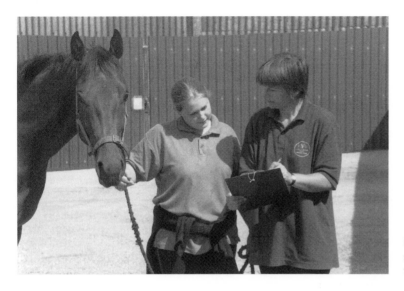

Fig. 10.2 A consent form should always be signed by the client before the patient is left at the clinic. (Photo: courtesy of Karl Holliman.)

Consent forms

The owner or their agent should always sign a form of consent before the patient is left at the clinic (Fig. 10.2), however minor the procedure or however well the practice may know them. This consent form should ensure that all parties understand the procedures that are about to take place and if completed correctly the form will protect the practice in the case of a future dispute.

It is likely that your practice will have its own personalised consent forms, which are either produced by computer from the client records or completed by hand. Remember that a consent form is only as good as the information it contains and therefore must be completed fully. The Veterinary Defence Society produce a form that lists all the relevant details required on a surgical consent form (Fig. 10.3) but your practice may have added items such as hospitalisation / treatment consent or euthanasia consent to its forms. It may be appropriate to add a statement enabling any of the vets working in the practice to perform the procedure, thus ensuring that the owner is aware that it may not be the vet they regularly consult performing the surgery.

On admitting the horse, read through the consent form with the owner and ensure that all the details are correct and understood by all parties.

Completion of a consent form

(1) Patient details should be described adequately:
   (a) Name: it may be appropriate to use a full name rather than a stable name.
   (b) Breed: a general description so that the horse is recognisable.
   (c) Colour: any distinguishing marks should be noted.
   (d) Age and gender: both may have a bearing on the treatment received by the patient. Check that there is no possibility of mares being pregnant.

(2) Details of the owner should be double-checked with your records and a contact telephone number (for the time the animal is with you) should always be noted.

(3) Details of the procedure should be described and explained clearly if complicated terminology is used.

(4) Informed consent must always be obtained and if any part of the treatment is not clearly stated on the consent form, i.e. the owner / agent has not signed for it, this could lead to later problems (Fig. 10.4).

(5) The form should be signed by the owner or a recognised agent acting on their behalf and by witnesses if considered appropriate. The person signing the consent form must be over 18 years old.

FORM OF CONSENT
FOR ANAESTHESIA AND SURGICAL PROCEDURES IN HORSES

Description of Patient

Name _____

Breed _____

Colour _____ Age _____ Sex _____

Owner / Agent

Name _____

Address _____

_____

_____

Telephone Home _____

Work _____

Operation_____

Any relevant clinical history / special precautions _____

_____

I hereby give permission for the administration of an anaesthetic to the above animal and to the surgical operation detailed on this form, together with any other procedures which may prove necessary, I understand that all anaesthetic techniques and surgical procedures involve some risk to the animal.

I have notified the insurers concerning the procedures planned for this animal.

Signature _____ Owner/Agent   Date _____

Name _____
(BLOCK CAPITALS)

Fig. 10.3 An example of a consent form.

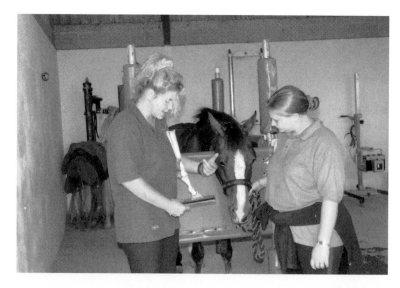

Fig. 10.4 An explanation of the procedure should be given to the client. (Photo: courtesy of Karl Holliman.)

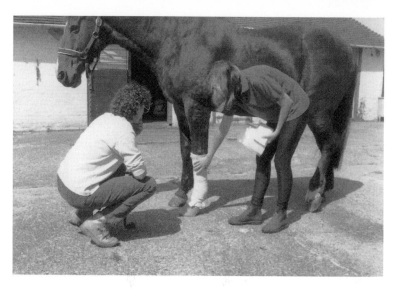

Fig. 10.5 A discharge form should be given to the client along with a verbal explanation of post-operative care. (Photo: courtesy of Karl Holliman.)

Discharging a patient

Arrangements for discharging a patient should be made only when the vet has confirmed that the horse is sufficiently recovered to leave the clinic. It may be that the vet has discussed further treatment with the owner prior to collection of the patient or they may be planning to discuss this at discharge. In either case it is good practice to complete a discharge form, outlining all aspects of aftercare, to be collected with the patient. It can be difficult for owners to remember all the advice given at one time, and having a discharge form to refer to can save phone calls to the practice or misunderstood directions. For horses returning to large yards, a discharge form can be used as a good method of communicating any further treatment required to all yard staff (Fig. 10.5).

A practice discharge form can be devised easily (Fig. 10.6), perhaps with the addition of who discharged the patient and to whom. Discharge instruc-

A   Veterinary Clinic;
Their address

DISCHARGE INSTRUCTIONS

HORSE:

OWNER:
ADDRESS:

VETERINARY SURGEON:

PROCEDURE:
DATE PERFORMED:

STABLING:

EXERCISE:

FEED:

DRESSINGS:

DRUGS TO TAKE HOME:

FOLLOW UP:

MISCELLANEOUS:

DATE OF DISCHARGE:

Signature _____ Owner/Agent   Date _____

Name _____
                          (BLOCK CAPITALS)

Fig. 10.6 An example of a discharge form.

tions should be discussed with the vet and a copy should be kept for practice records.

Practice administration

Patient records

Filing
Many practices have computer systems for client records but there will still be an amount of paper or electronic filing to be done on a daily basis. Radiographs, laboratory reports, insurance claims and other documentation need to be kept within a system that ensures that the information contained can be retrieved quickly and easily (see Key points 10.6). Filing that is mis-managed and not kept up to date can lead to wasted time spent searching for inaccessible documents.

There are legal requirements regarding the length of time some documents are stored. (Table 10.1)

Key points 10.6   Filing

General points of a filing system

- Enables easy and quick retrieval of files
- Applicable system of indexing (usually alphabetical or numerical)
- Secure (data protection)
- Colour coded: misfiled files are obvious; groups of files are easily identified
- Allowance for necessary expansion
- Easily accessed — i.e. placed where the file is needed, e.g. patient records in reception area

---

Table 10.1 Document storage time

Type of document	Legally required storage time
VAT records	6 years
PAYE records	3 years (after the pertaining year)
Accident records	3 years

Specific practice-generated documents, such as consent forms and diagnostic reports, do not carry any statutory obligations but the Veterinary Defence Society advises that they be kept for at least 2 years. The RCVS recommends that records be kept for a minimum of 6 years, especially where there may be a dispute about a particular case.

Computers in the practice

There are many different types of computer systems used in practice with differing programs to suit practice needs. Computers are generally used in five main ways:

(1) Patient records
(2) Client accounts
(3) Appointment systems
(4) Stock control
(5) Business analysis

Your practice also is likely to use its system for word processing, and some practices also will rely on their computer systems for areas such as budgets, salary systems and desktop publishing. Employers who keep data such as personnel records on their computer systems should be aware of the *Data Protection Act 1984*. If the practice keeps data such as personnel records on its computer system, it needs to register as a 'data user' with the Data Protection Registrar.

Money control systems

If your clients do not pay their bills or if money is habitually lost to the practice as a result of accounting errors, then business budgets will suffer, the services you are able to offer your clients will suffer and your wages will suffer. A veterinary practice is a business like any other, and even if you are the target for clients complaining about the practice prices, it is worth remembering that they are paying private medical fees for large expensive animals!

Practice policies must be adhered to when dealing with client payments. The person dealing with each payment should be responsible for it being entered either onto the computer or in a cashbook. At each change of shift, the till should be reconciled to check for inaccuracies, although many equine payments will be settled by monthly account. Costs outstanding and estimates of future treatments may require discussion with the owner. If the client advises you that 'it's being paid by insurance', check that they have informed their insurance company and that this has been confirmed before large accounts start mounting up.

Insurance claim forms should always be handed directly to the vet in charge of the case, or whatever system your practice has, to ensure that they are completed promptly. Often in a busy practice where there seems to be mountains of paper, an insurance form can 'disappear', which almost certainly will mean a delay in receiving payment for the practice.

Taking payment (Table 10.2)

The most immediate type of payment to the practice is in cash. However, mistakes can be made easily, both in counting the money received and in the change given. Care should be taken in looking for possible forged notes. Some practices will have a 'forgery pen', which can be used at the time of payment. Cheques often are sent to the practice by post

Table 10.2 Advantages and disadvantages of different types of payment

Type of payment	Advantages	Disadvantages
Cash	• Instant method of receiving payment • It is the only type of payment that cannot be refused	• Mistakes can occur in counting/giving change • Large amounts of cash in the practice lead to a security risk
Cheque	• Easily posted after receiving account • Safer than cash • No change to give *NB*: Always take the number of the guarantee card	• Delay in the practice receiving monies into its account due to bank clearing systems • Charges for clearing cheques and for 'bounced' cheques
Credit cards and debit cards	• If the practice has an electronic transfer, same-day credit can be paid into the practice account • The vast majority of clients will carry their 'cards' at all times and will therefore be able to make prompt payments	• A flat fee is charged to the practice for debit card transactions and a percentage of the transaction made by a credit card

but the details should be checked thoroughly before they are entered as payment. The date, numbers and amount in words should be correct and of course the cheque must be signed. If the cheque is in a name other than the registered name of the client, then note this on the client records because this will save time if the cheque is returned to the practice uncleared and the client needs to be contacted. If the client is present while writing the cheque, ask to take the number of the cheque guarantee card.

Debit cards have taken the place of cheques in that they mean same-day payments to the practice if you have an electronic terminal, unlike cheques, which usually require a few days to clear. Credit cards also will mean prompt payments to the practice and are useful for those clients who cannot afford the whole payment at once, even though there is a charge to the practice. It is better for practice turnover if the client owes money to the credit card company rather than to the practice. Check that the signature given by the client matches the signature on the card.

Invoicing

Invoices request money to be paid and are usually either computer generated or hand written. If they are the latter, ensure that they are clear and that the addition is correct. Value-added tax should be added to veterinary fees and should be shown as a separate figure.

Further reading

Lane, D.R. & Cooper, B. *Veterinary Nursing*, 2nd edn, pp. 152–162. Butterworth–Heinemann, Oxford.
Royal College of Veterinary Surgeons. *Guide to Professional Conduct*. RCVS, London.

Medicines and their Management

R. J. Baxter & R. D. Jones

Pharmacology is the study of the actions of medicines on living things; *medicines* are chemical substances that modify the functions of living things; and the subject of *pharmacy* relates to the practical preparation and dispensing of medicines.

Legal requirements in veterinary pharmacy

There are over 30 legal requirements and codes of practice that relate to veterinary pharmacy. The principal ones governing the sale and supply of veterinary medicinal products are the Medicines Act (1968), the Misuse of Drugs Act (1971), the Misuse of Drugs Regulations (1985) and the Medicines (Veterinary drugs)(Pharmacy and Merchants' List) Order (1992).

The British Veterinary Association runs pharmacy courses and produces a Code of Practice on medicines to ensure best pharmacy practice. There are also regulatory bodies, such as the Veterinary Medicines Directorate (VMD), which is an executive agency of the Ministry of Agriculture, Fisheries and Food, and the European Medicines Evaluation Agency (EMEA). Both have an active role in the licensing and regulation of veterinary medicines. In the UK, veterinary medicines are classified into the legal categories shown in Table 11.1.

Currently only a vet may prescribe medicines for animal use, and vets may dispense medicines only for animals under their care. Equine nurses need to be able to understand and administer the correct

doses of such medication, as well as to store such medicines appropriately. When medicines are prescribed that could cause ill-effects to the owners, they must be made aware of the risks and be suitably informed of a safe method of administration and waste disposal.

Storage of medicines

Organisation of a pharmacy should be based around security, careful stock control (especially with respect to expiry dates) and correct storage of all medicines according to the manufacturers' recommendations. The pharmacy should be in a room that is insulated from extremes of temperature and humidity, any windows should be screened to prevent direct sunlight from falling on medicines and adequate ventilation should be ensured. Most medicines that can be affected by light are kept in brown glass bottles. A fridge should be available for the storage of those medicines that require low temperatures (such as vaccines, antisera, certain reconstituted antibiotics and certain hormonal products). The fridge must be kept at 2–8°C and a maximum–minimum thermometer must be kept in the fridge and checked daily to ensure that medicines are not exposed to higher or lower temperatures.

If multidose vials are opened they should be marked with the date of opening. Previously dispensed medication should never be accepted back into the pharmacy, because it may have been stored incorrectly or contaminated.

Table 11.1 Legal categories of medicines

Legal category	Definition
GSL	*General sales list* medicines, which may be sold without prescription or restriction
P	*Pharmacy* medicines, which may be supplied by a vet for administration to animals under their care, or over the counter by a pharmacist. Very few veterinary medicines fall into this category
PML	*Pharmacy and merchant's list medicines*; these can be supplied by a vet for administration to animals under their care. They also can be sold in pharmacies under the supervision of a pharmacist and supplied by an agricultural merchant who has the appropriate registration, e.g. sale of equine anthelmintics
POM	*Prescription-only medicines*; these may be supplied by a vet for administration to animals under their care or supplied by a pharmacist on a vet's prescription
CD	*Controlled drugs*; substances controlled by the Misuse of Drugs Act 1971 (see text)
STA	*Special treatment authorisation*; where there is no suitable product available in the UK to treat a particular condition in a specific animal, a vet may apply for an STA from the VMD. This allows the supply of a medicine on a named patient basis under certain conditions, e.g. virginiamycin for laminitis control in ponies

Particular care must be taken with controlled medicines under the Dangerous Drugs Act. These are substances that are capable of being abused, e.g. cannabis and ketamine. Controlled medicines are divided into five schedules in decreasing order of stringency of control. A vet has the authority to supply drugs in Schedules 2, 3, 4 and 5 under the Misuse of Drugs Regulations 1985. Some Schedule 2 and 3 controlled medicines, which include medication such as pethidine, are relatively commonly prescribed for equine use. There are specific controls ensuring that they are used safely and responsibly. These include the requirement for any prescription to be in the vet's *own handwriting* to minimise the risk of forgery.

Certain Schedule 2 and 3 controlled medicines must be kept in a locked receptacle, the key of which should be kept by an appropriate vet or authorised person. A locked car is not deemed to be a lockable receptacle. If controlled medicines are to be carried in a car they should be in a locked metal container bolted to the chassis.

Details of all controlled medicines used should be recorded in a bound ledger at the time of receipt and at each time of use. The records must be retained for inspection for a period of at least 2 years after the last entry.

Recording of medicines supplied

The Medicines (Restrictions on the Administration of Veterinary Medicinal Products) Regulations (1994) and the Medicines (Exemptions for Merchants in Veterinary Medicines) Order (1998) demand that all vets should keep permanent records after administration of medicines to food-producing species (which can include horses, according to European Union legislation). A detailed audit of stock should be taken annually and this should include any medicines stored outside the pharmacy, e.g. in vets' cars.

Medicines prescribed for use by the client should be recorded in this manner by the vet, and where large numbers of horses are present the owner/handler also should keep records of the details of those animals that are treated. The National Office of Animal Health in conjunction with the Animal Health Distributors Association produce a book for such records, as do the National Trainers Federation.

All medicines must be labelled, prior to dispensing, with:

- The animal's identity
- The owner's name and address
- The date
- The name and address of the prescribing veterinary practice
- The quantity and strength of medication prescribed
- The dosing instructions

Labels should also state:

(1) For animal treatment only
(2) Keep out of reach of children

(3) The withdrawal period of the drug in food-producing animals and competition horses

Medicines dispensed within the practice need not carry all this information but should be identified clearly. Unlabelled syringes of medication are not acceptable. The use of cytotoxic drugs in the equine practice requires the same precautions as their use elsewhere. Guidance Note MS21 from the Health and Safety Executive gives precise guidance on the precautions needed for the safe use of these drugs.

Safety

The Royal College of Veterinary Surgeons (RCVS) recommends that each practice have a Practice Safety Officer, ideally a vet. They should be responsible for overseeing the legal and ethical requirements for the sale and supply of veterinary medicinal products (VMPs). All medicinal products must be treated as potentially harmful. Accidental exposure to all medicines should be carefully avoided, particularly those that may affect humans. If in doubt, gloves should be worn when handling medication and additional protective clothing where necessary. Needle caps always should be kept on, and some medicines should never be handled by certain personnel, e.g. griseofulvin/prostaglandins should not be handled by pregnant women (see Chapter 9).

Sharps, unused medication and clinical waste should be disposed of in separate sealable yellow plastic tubs that should be incinerated by a licensed company in order to comply with the Collection and Disposal of Waste Regulations 1988 and the Environmental Protection Act 1990. The recycling of certain items such as syringes and urinary catheters is possible. First they should be dismantled and soaked in enzymatic solutions to dissolve blood and then cleaned with dilute antiseptics (such as chlorhexidine), sterilised and re-used. Such re-use is rarely economical.

Use of medicines in competition animals

Restrictions apply to the use of certain medicines that may affect performance in competition animals. Owing to the difficulty in testing some of these medi-cines, the use of other medicines that may leave similar residues is also restricted. For the purposes of the Jockey Club Rules such restrictions apply to antipyretics, analgesics, anti-inflammatories, cytotoxic drugs, antihistamines, diuretics, local anaesthetics, muscle relaxants, respiratory stimulants, sex hormones, anabolic steroids, corticosteroids and substances affecting blood coagulation. Vaccines and most antibiotics can be used, but care must be taken not to use medicines that may leave residues in the blood, e.g. procaine penicillin, which can leave procaine (another local anaesthetic) residues for up to a month or more. Care should be taken also when using topical products, particularly if the skin is damaged, because significant amounts may be absorbed.

Regulations regarding vaccinations should be followed. The majority of UK competition horse organisations, e.g. the Jockey Club, recommend vaccination against equine influenza (and sometimes tetanus). Records of when vaccines were given are kept on the horse's passports, which may be brought with the horse into a hospital. The Jockey Club Rules for equine influenza vaccination are as follows:

- *Primary course*: two injections 21–92 days apart
- *First booster*: booster 150–215 days after 2nd injection of primary course
- *Annual boosters*: within 365 days of first booster

Calculation of dosages

Correct calculation of a dosage is vital for the safety of the animal for which a medicine is prescribed, as well as ensuring the medicine's efficacy. If insufficient is given it is unlikely to work, and an excessive dose may have toxic side effects. It is the vet's responsibility to prescribe the correct dose and for this specific reason dosages are not included in this textbook for equine nurses. However, it is important for nurses to understand how a correct dose is calculated.

The active ingredients of most medicines are expressed in terms of their weight, using metric measurements of kilograms (kg), grams (g), milligrams (mg) and micrograms (which is not routinely abbreviated). With liquids containing a solution or suspension of medicine, measurements are made in litres (L) and millilitres (ml).

Most medicines have stated dose rates in the literature, which are usually expressed in terms of the dose/kg bodyweight. Knowledge of the horse's weight is therefore essential, and in hospitals a weighbridge may be available for monitoring and recording of bodyweight. If unavailable, approximations of bodyweight can be made by a combination of an experienced eye and a weight tape (this is used to measure the horse's girth, which then is compared with the height and an approximate weight is given). As a rough guide:

- The average foal weighs around 60 kg when born
- The average 12 hh child's pony might weigh about 250 kg
- The average lean 15.2 hh thoroughbred weighs around 500 kg

The formula for calculating a horse's approximate weight is as follows:

$$\text{Weight (kg)} = \frac{\text{Girth (cm)} \times \text{Length (cm)}}{11900}$$

where girth is the measurement around the horse's thorax behind the withers and front legs, and length is the measurement from the point of the shoulder to the point of the buttocks (tuber ischii).

Many medicines are not available in a pure form; some are extracted from animal tissues, e.g. insulin and oxytocin. The concentration of such medicines is provided in terms of international units (IU). If the active ingredient is presented in a solid base, the strength will be stated in terms of weight of the medicine per weight of the medication (w/w). If a medicine is presented as a solution, the strength of the solution is usually expressed as weight of the medicine per volume of the solution (w/v), or it may be expressed as a percentage. To convert a percentage solution to mg/ml, multiply by 10 (e.g. a 15% solution contains 150 mg/ml).

Once the dose rate of the medicine and the weight of the patient are known, the quantity of medication that needs to be administered can be calculated (see How to . . . 11.1).

How to . . . 11.1

Calculation of dosages

- Dose in mg/kg/day × bodyweight of horse = amount of dose to give daily.
- Take care to calculate the amount of medication that needs to be given based on its percentage of active ingredient and not the total weight or volume.

Example

- If 0.7 mg/kg of a medicine needs to be given to a 450-kg horse, then 0.7 × 450 = 315 mg or 0.315 g of the medicine needs to be given.
- In the imaginary case above, if an injectable solution of 50 mg/ml of the medicine is available, then 1 ml of solution will contain 50 mg of the medicine. The number of millilitres of the medicine needed to give the correct dose of 315 mg is therefore 315/50 = 6.3 ml.
- If, however, the medicine was available as 10 mg drug/1 g of powder, the amount of powder that would need to be given would be 315/10 = 31.5 g.

NB

- microgram × 1000 = mg
- mg × 1000 = g
- g × 1000 = kg

A minority of doses are expressed in terms of the quantity of medication needed per square metre of body surface area. Such medicines are uncommon, but this type of dosing allows for increased dose rates in smaller animals. A surface area to weight (depending on size) conversion chart is needed to calculate the doses of such medicines.

Directions on a pharmacy label or prescription should be in clear English without abbreviation but some Latin abbreviations are used (see Table 11.2).

Administration of medicines

There are several types of medication used in horses (see Summary 11.1) and these may be given by a variety of routes to achieve either local or systemic effects.

Table 11.2 Abbreviations in common use in the pharmacy

Abbreviation	Latin	Translation
b.d.	bis die	Twice daily
b.d.s.	bis die sumendus	Twice daily
b.i.d.	bis in die	Twice daily
p.o.	per os	By mouth
q.i.d.	quarter in die	Four times daily
q.s.	quantum sufficiat	Sufficient
s.i.d.	semel in die	Once daily
t.i.d.	ter in die	Three times daily

Other abbreviations used include e.o.d. (every other day) and n.t.g. (not to be given).

Summary 11.1

Types of medication most commonly used in horses (see Chapter 20 for futher information)

- Analgesics: used as painkillers
- Anthelminitics: used in the treatment of endoparasites
- Antibiotics: compounds produced by microorganisms or synthesised to kill or inhibit bacterial growth
- Bronchodilators: used to increase airway width, commonly by reducing smooth-muscle spasm
- Corticosteroids: used for their anti-inflammatory action
- Diuretics: used to increase urine output
- Non-steroidal anti-inflammatory drugs (NSAIDs), e.g. phenylbutazone, used to inhibit inflammatory mediators and to help reduce the pain and swelling of inflammation
- Vaccines: antigenic material, e.g. tetanus toxoid designed to stimulate an immune response

Administration of medicines locally/topically

Local and topical administration of medicines includes the application of medicines to the skin and eyes, as well as the internal surface of the lungs, rectum, uterus and joints. Delivering a high concentration of medication locally can reduce the quantity of medicine that otherwise would be required systemically to achieve the same effect. In some cases, local administration is the only way of achieving efficacious quantities at the site of action.

Eye conditions may necessitate medicines being applied directly to the surface of the eye. Care should be taken to avoid allowing the tip of the nozzle to touch the eye or eyelids because this can result in bacteria being transferred onto the end of the tube. Alternatively, medication may be delivered through an indwelling lavage system, or subconjunctival injections may be given to provide high local levels of injectable medication.

Skin conditions may be treated with a variety of types of medication, including creams (semi-solid emulsion in oil, fat or water that penetrates the skin well), ointments (semi-solid, greasy and does not penetrate the skin), powders (that usually only penetrate the skin poorly), lotions and aerosol sprays. Particular care should be taken if the skin is broken. Intradermal injections are used occasionally to provide a local dose of a substance within the skin. Most commonly they are used for injecting potential allergens as part of an intradermal skin test.

Administration of medication directly to the lungs can be achieved by connecting a nebuliser or a metered dose inhaler to an equine facemask (Fig. 11.1). Delivering medicines in this manner can allow rapid onset of activity with comparatively low dose rates of medicines and can be very useful in some cases.

Some medicines are given rectally (e.g. enemas, which can be given via rubber tubing inserted into the rectum); this is an act of veterinary surgery in the horse. Particular care must be taken to avoid rectal tears. Administration of medicines to the interior of the female reproductive tract also must be carried out with care; this is a common method for the treatment of endometritis in the mare.

Intra-articular injections may need to be given as part of a diagnostic procedure in lameness investigation, or to medicate joints. Surgical clipping and preparation of the site prior to injection is necessary to reduce the risk of sepsis.

Administration of systemic medicines enterally (orally)

Administration of medicines by mouth (see How to ... 11.2) avoids the risk of iatrogenic infection following penetration of the skin by injection and

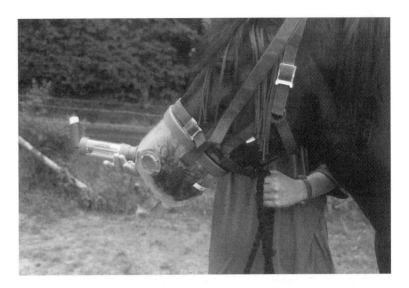

Fig. 11.1 Horse inhaling steroids for respiratory condition via an aeromask.

How to . . . 11.2

Administration of oral medication

Indications

- Veterinary medical products that are only licensed for oral use.
- Use of licensed oral alternatives in cases where parenteral administration is contraindicated.

Method

- Oral medicine can be mixed into feed: try feeding the powder or granules in food that is highly palatable; molassed food helps to hide flavours, as does the addition of peppermints. Titbits such as chopped carrots can increase palatability. Alternatively, medication may be hidden within an apple or carrot by coring out a portion, introducing the medication and then plugging the hole through which it was introduced.
- Horses that will not take medicine in feed may be forced to take it directly by mouth using an oral dosing syringe.
- Some medicine also is available in a paste form, and those that are not may, in some cases (check first with the vet), be mixed with water to form a paste and then given by syringe.
- An experienced handler may be needed to hold the horse's head down.
- Nose twitching the horse may aid control of the head.
- After checking that the mouth is empty, the tip of the syringe should be inserted at the side of the mouth, pointing up towards the back of the tongue.
- The medication should be introduced directly onto the tongue.
- Holding the horse's head up and trying to keep its mouth shut may help to prevent him spitting it out.

Potential complications

- Difficulty in ensuring that the complete dose is ingested.
- Aspiration of medication, causing aspiration pneumonia (this is unlikely to happen).
- Less efficacy of medication compared with parenteral routes.
- Injury to fractious horses or their handlers.

How to . . . 11.3

Subcutaneous and intramuscular injections

Indications

- Administration of medications licensed for use by these routes.

Method for subcutaneous injections

- Subcutaneous injections are given usually on the side of the neck, just in front of the leading edge of the shoulder blade.
- An appropriate size (e.g. 21-gauge) of sterile hypodermic needle attached to a luer-mounted syringe can be slid into a fold of skin lifted by hand.
- After drawing back on the syringe plunger to ensure that inadvertent puncture of a blood vessel has not occurred, the medicine can be injected.

Method for intramuscular injections

- Intramuscular injections can be given in many sites, but the most commonly used are the brisket, the neck and the rump.
- A (40-mm) sterile hypodermic needle attached to a luer-mounted syringe is suitable in most horses.
- The site on the rump is approximately halfway along an imaginary line between the point of the hip and the tail base. When using it, stand as far forward as possible to avoid being kicked.
- In the neck, a needle can be introduced about a hands breadth back from the front of the shoulder, halfway between the under side of the neck and the upper side of the neck.
- On the brisket, a needle can be introduced to either of the large masses of muscle medial to the upper front legs.
- Fine-gauge (e.g. 21-gauge) needles can be used to inject solutions of medication. These may be slid in at right angles to the skin with little response, but larger needles (e.g. 18- or 19-gauge) that are used to inject thicker suspensions of

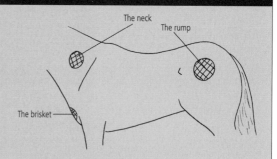

medication may need to be inserted quickly and deftly. The site should be thumped once or twice and the needle then introduced rapidly and firmly perpendicular to the skin, right up to the hub. Alternatively, the skin may be pinched and the needle slid in.

- A firm connection between the syringe and the needle should be made before withdrawing the plunger of the syringe, to ensure that venepuncture has not occurred, and then giving the injection.

Potential complications

- Injury to fractious horses or their handlers, including accidental self-injection; should this occur, take details of the medicine involved and seek medical attention.
- Inadvertent puncture of structures other than muscle, e.g. venepuncture (see above) or damage to the vertebral column/nuchal ligament in the neck or the sciatic nerve in the hindlimb. Adherence to the method advised should ensure that these structures are avoided but if damage to them is suspected then immediate veterinary attention should be sought.
- Pain/stiffness/abscessation at the injection site: seek veterinary attention.
- Anaphylaxis, i.e. acute allergic reaction: seek veterinary attention.

reduces the risk of being injured by the horse. It also enables owners to treat their horse more easily. Absorption of medicines from the gastrointestinal system is, however, slow and relatively unpredictable and accidental aspiration of medicines can occur, so parenteral routes may be preferred, particularly when horses may be reluctant to eat their medication.

How to . . . 11.4

Intravenous injection

Indications

- Administration of intravenous medication.

Method

- Intravenous medication may be given by injection into the vein using a needle (a 19- or 20-gauge, 25-mm or 40-mm needle is usually ideal) and syringe, or may be given via a catheter (see Chapter 13). The jugular veins are normally used but other sites (such as the lateral thoracic and cephalic veins) can be used if necessary.
- The jugular vein can be located on either side of the neck by palpation.
- If it is difficult to see, it can be located by raising it (occluding it close to the thoracic inlet) and watching it fill with blood.
- Before injection is carried out, the area should be clipped and prepared surgically and then swabbed with surgical spirit.
- For injection, the vein is raised and the needle inserted deftly at an angle of 45° to the skin pointing upwards.
- If the needle was removed from the syringe, blood should be seen immediately issuing from the needle. If the needle

and syringe are still attached, the plunger will need to be withdrawn to ensure that blood flows into the syringe.
- Once the needle is located in the vein, the medicine is injected slowly, with intermittent drawing back of the plunger to ensure that the needle remains in the vein.
- For catheter insertion, see Chapter 12.

Potential complications

- Injury to fractious horses or their handlers, including accidental self-injection: should this occur, take details of the medicine and seek medical attention.
- Inadvertent puncture of other structures: e.g. intra-arterial injections can occur by accident when a needle is inserted too deeply during attempts to find a vein. Blood usually flows into the syringe/spurts out of the needle under pressure. Intravenous medication should not be given into an artery because adverse reactions such as acute collapse may occur. Immediate veterinary attention should be sought.
- Extravascular injection may cause pain/infection at the injection site or may even cause tissue sloughs in the case of irritant substances: seek veterinary attention.
- Anaphylaxis: seek veterinary attention.

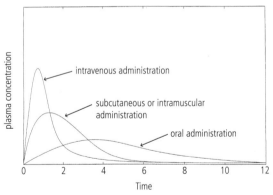

Fig. 11.2 Relative plasma concentrations of medicines given by different routes: intravenous administration gives an immediate high peak followed by an exponential fall in plasma concentrations; intramuscular administration gives a peak plasma concentration after about 15 min followed by a more gradual reduction in plasma levels, as does subcutaneous administration; oral administration gives lower peak plasma concentration about 4 h after administration of the medicine. The speed of reduction of the plasma concentration of the medicine depends on its half-life within the individual.

Administration of systemic medicines parenterally (by injection)

Medicines administered by injection rapidly give more predictable levels in the body systems (Fig. 11.2) than do medicines given orally. The route of parenteral administration adopted i.e. subcutaneous, intramuscular (see How to . . . 11.3) or intravenous (see How to . . . 11.4) usually depends on the formulation and the routes for which it is licensed. Where medicines may be given by several routes, the intravenous route is often chosen initially by the clinician so that optimal plasma concentrations can be achieved. In some cases, however, the intramuscular or subcutaneous routes may be chosen because they may give a longer duration of effect.

Horses are often uncomfortable at the site of injections (particularly intramuscular injections) for 24–48h and so repeat injections should be given at another site, or the site should be rotated on a daily basis. If swelling occurs at the site of a neck injection, food and water may need to be provided at a raised level. Occasionally such a swelling develops into an abscess, even with good technique. This may require veterinary attention. Other complications include allergy to the medication used, which can result in signs ranging from pain and swelling at the injection site to sweating, colic and collapse. The latter signs necessitate veterinary attention and cessation of treatment with the medicine that caused them. The prescribing vet must report suspected adverse reactions to the manufacturer and the VMD on Form MLA 252A under the Suspected Adverse Reaction Surveillance Scheme. This is a legal requirement.

Further reading

Bishop, Y. (2001) BVA Code of Practice on Medicines and BVA Guidelines on the Prudent Use of Antimicrobials. In: *The Veterinary Formulary*, 5th edn., pp. 1–29. The Pharmaceutical Press, London (also available direct from the British Veterinary Association as two separate documents).

Jones R.D. & Taylor P.M. (1998) Medicines for the millennium? *Equine Vet. Educ.* **10**, 328–333.

Laboratory Diagnosis

L. L. Hillyer & M. H. Hillyer

Laboratory health and safety

There are various legislative Acts and Regulations that affect any work carried out in a laboratory. These are covered in Chapter 9.

Laboratory apparatus

Care and cleaning

Equipment and work surfaces are best cleaned 'as you go along'. You need to know how to care for the basic laboratory apparatus.

Glassware

There is an efficient 'five-point' way to clean glassware while wearing gloves:

(1) Soak in detergent
(2) Remove surface material with soft bristle brush
(3) Soak in disinfectant (often when a 'batch' of equipment is ready to clean)
(4) Rinse two or three times in distilled/deionised water
(5) Drain and dry.

Microscope

This is an important piece of precision equipment that should be kept in one place and not moved unnecessarily. It must be:

- Kept away from vibrating objects (e.g. washing machine, centrifuge)
- Kept covered when not in use
- Kept with the lowest power objective in position when not in use
- Cleaned (lenses and eyepieces) only with special lens paper that will not scratch
- Cleaned of oil, when used with the oil immersion objective, straight after use.

Centrifuge

Proper use of the centrifuge should limit its contamination. As a general rule, the inner bowl should be cleaned and disinfected regularly. In addition, routine servicing needs to be carried out and someone must be responsible for this.

Incubator

Potentially dangerous bacteria may be grown in an incubator, so it is important that there is a set procedure for its care. This should be set out by the practice using advice from the manufacturer.

Equipment

Pipettes

These are used to transfer fluids and measure quantities. The meniscus of the fluid in the pipette must be level with the mark required. There are five different types:

(1) *Graduated pipettes* are inscribed with divisions to indicate volume, e.g. a 10-ml pipette is divided into 1-ml divisions.

(2) *One-mark volumetric pipettes* only have a single mark on them where a specific volume is measurable.

(3) *Micropipettes* usually come with disposable pipette tips and are used for measuring very small volumes.

(4) *Automatic pipettes*: 'single-shot', where you dial the volume required, which is then dispensed from a reservoir; and 'multi-head', which usually have eight tips so that eight wells may be filled at once (e.g. used for enzyme-linked immunosorbent assay work).

(5) *Pasteur pipettes*: either glass with a rubber bulb at the end, or, more often now, all plastic; these are not graduated (e.g. used to draw serum from a clotted blood sample).

Microscope

Most practices will have a *compound binocular microscope*, which has the following components:

- *Foot* (*base*); the part contacting the work surface that houses the light source.
- *Light source*; intensity altered via a dial. This should be turned down before turning the microscope off, or if the light is left on when the microscope is not in use.
- *Limb*; upright part between foot and *body*. The microscope must be held by foot and limb if moved.
- The light passes from the source through a lens to a mirror. This directs the light via the *iris diaphragm* to the *sub-stage condenser* (altered by the condenser knob). The iris diaphragm determines how much light passes through the condenser; the condenser focuses the light onto the slide.
- The *stage* holds the slide and is moved about by the *mechanical stage*.
- The stage is racked up and down by both *coarse* (outer knob) and *fine* (inner knob) *adjustment*.
- Above the stage is the *nose piece*, with a rotating turret that holds the *objective lenses* (usually three or four).
- Light passes through the objective lens in use, up

to the *eyepiece lenses*. These can be adjusted to suit the individual.

- The *Vernier scales* are like map coordinates on each side of the stage; the location of something on the slide therefore may be recorded precisely.

For a step-by-step guide to the use of a microscope, see How to . . . 12.1.

How to . . . 12.1

Use of the microscope

- Have lowest objective in place and light intensity down low
- Slide on stage, placed centrally
- Switch on and turn light dial up as required to be able to see
- Adjust distance between eyepieces so that you view both fields as one
- Focus on subject using first coarse then fine focus
- Adjust condenser and diaphragm to have optimal illumination
- Examine field on slide logically (e.g. top to bottom, left to right)
- To look at an area in more detail, rotate in the next objective lens 'up' and adjust the fine focus (may need more light; adjust condenser and diaphragm)
- To use oil immersion, first locate spot of interest using the lowest power. Then place a drop of oil on the slide at that spot and rotate the oil immersion lens into place. The lens should be in touch with the oil but not the slide! Adjust using fine focus. When finished, lower stage and clean lens immediately

Centrifuge

A centrifuge is used to separate cells/debris (sediment) from fluid (supernatant). There are three different types of centrifuge:

(1) *Swing out*: rotor with specimen buckets suspended vertically from the arms of the rotor. When rotor slows they fall into a vertical position, slightly remixing samples.

(2) *Angle-head*: has holes drilled round rotor at set angles. Deposit is laid down at a fixed angle and may be disturbed when tubes are placed vertically in test tube racks. Samples are placed in *buckets* with rubber cushions at the bottom that must be balanced. The inner *guard bowl* of the centrifuge is very solid for safety. A further safety feature of most centrifuges is a lid lock (prevents opening while still spinning).

(3) *Microhaematocrit*: used particularly for separating whole blood in capillary tubes to obtain a packed cell volume (PCV). A *safety plate* is screwed down on top of the balanced samples, which are placed on a horizontal bed, and a *rubber cushion* seals the outside lip of the rotor. Both of these should be replaced regularly.

For safe use of a centrifuge, see How to . . . 12.2.

How to . . . 12.2

Safe use of a centrifuge

- Keep it on a flat solid surface away from the edge (they can 'walk'!)
- Keep it regularly cleaned, lubricated and serviced (maintain a log of use)
- Place samples opposite each other (i.e. balanced); if only one, use a blank tube as ballast
- Screw down safety plate securely once samples are in place; then close lid properly
- Use bucket lids to prevent aerosolisation of samples
- Remember that it is electrical! Keep cables and plug out of water

---

Incubator

Incubators are sealed units used to culture bacteria. They are very well insulated so that the internal temperature is maintained at a set temperature, usually 37°C. This is the ideal temperature for most pathogenic bacteria. A daily record of the temperature should be kept.

Laboratory analysers

For biochemistry

Various machines are used to assess biochemical parameters in different fluid samples, such as serum or peritoneal fluid. A *colorimeter* measures the light absorbed or transmitted by a solution at a particular wavelength, via filters. A *spectrophotometer* does the same thing but via prisms or monochromatic gratings. Both are *wet* chemistry systems as distinct from *dry* systems, where a sample is put onto a reagent strip and the reflective light is analysed as the reaction occurs (e.g. 'Vet test' machines).

For haematology

Samples are frequently submitted for a 'CBC' (complete blood count, i.e. white cell count and various red cell parameters). Electric cell counters are used widely to assess cell numbers. The drawback of these compared with manual counting is that there is no distinction between types of cells, i.e. it does not give a 'differential count'. Thus, for example, in a thoracocentesis sample the epithelial cells would be 'seen' as leucocytes, giving a spuriously high white cell count.

Blood—haematology

Blood forms about 10% of bodyweight and comprises *cells* in *plasma*. Plasma is the liquid part of blood and differs from serum; serum is what is left when a clot has formed (i.e. plasma without clotting factors).

Cells

Normal blood cells include erythrocytes (red blood cells), leucocytes (white blood cells) and thrombocytes (platelets).

Plasma

Plasma comprises the following components:

- Water
- Plasma proteins (albumin, globulin, fibrinogen, prothrombin)
- Mineral salts
- Nutrients (amino acids, carbohydrates, fatty acids)
- Gases (carbon dioxide and, less so, oxygen, as free gases in solution)
- Waste products (urea, creatinine)
- Hormones
- Enzymes

- Antibodies
- Antitoxins

Functions of blood

Blood is used to transport:

- Oxygen to and carbon dioxide away from tissues
- Digested nutrients to tissues
- Waste products from tissues to kidneys for excretion
- Water to tissues
- Hormones and enzymes around body

Blood is used to regulate:

- Body temperature by heat distribution
- Haemorrhage via clotting mechanism
- pH
- Against infection via the cells it contains
- Against infection via the antibodies and antitoxins it transports

Collection of blood

Blood is usually collected from veins (venepuncture), notably the

- Jugular vein (most often used, readily accessible in adults and foals)
- Cephalic vein on forelimb
- Saphenous vein on hindlimb
- Transverse facial vein (small volume only)

It is most easily collected using a 'Vacutainer' tube (see How to . . . 12.3) with needle and holder (yellow), but an ordinary hypodermic needle and syringe also may be used. There are various types of 'Vacutainer', depending on the anticoagulant they contain:

- Red top: plain, no anticoagulant
- Purple top: ethylenediaminetetraacetic acid (EDTA)
- Green top: heparin
- Grey top: oxalate fluoride, for assessing glucose concentration
- Yellow top: acid citrate dextrose, for crossmatching or blood typing
- Blue top: citrate, for coagulation studies

How to . . . 12.3

To collect blood

- Restrain the horse properly before blood sampling is attempted.
- Adult horses should be wearing a headcollar or bridle no matter how quiet they seem.
- Foals must be held properly around the head and body (e.g. 'tail and ear' hold).
- Have 'Vacutainer' ready assembled.
- Raise vein by applying gentle pressure at its base (usually use left vein).
- Clip hair over vein one-third of the way down the neck, with scissors perpendicular to the direction of the vein. Here, should avoid the carotid artery, which is more superficial in the caudal neck.
- Clean with spirit-soaked swab.
- Gently sink needle, bevel up and parallel with vein, into skin over vein until a lack of resistance is felt. Blood should drip from the other end of the needle.
- Clip 'Vacutainer' onto needle and hold steady (EDTA tube first if >1 tube).
- Remove needle from neck and apply pressure to vein for 2 min while inverting the tube.

Foals will often struggle violently and their veins are smaller, more 'corded' and harder to sample. They are also very susceptible to infection and so an aseptic technique is essential (see Chapter 15).

Some people prefer a 'stab' technique whereby the needle is quickly pushed into the vein without the sinking technique. It is important to develop what works best for you and it may vary depending on the horse and its temperament.

Blood also may be required from arteries, most commonly for blood gas analysis. Sites include the:

- Facial artery (heavily sedated/anaesthetised horse)
- Transverse facial artery (heavily sedated/anaesthetised horse)
- Dorsal metatarsal artery (preferred in recumbent foals)
- Carotid artery (conscious horse)
- Median artery (safer if anaesthetised/sedated)

Haematology

Packed cell volume

The packed cell volume (PCV) is estimated (see How to . . . 12.4) and describes the percentage of whole blood made up of cells. This is *not* the same as the microhaematocrit, which is *calculated* in an analyser.

How to . . . 12.4

To estimate a PCV

- Take whole blood in an EDTA tube
- Ensure that it is mixed adequately
- Fill plain capillary microhaematocrit tube three-quarters full by capillary action
- Plug end with plastic while finger is on other end
- Use microhaematocrit centrifuge for 5 min
- Place in haematocrit reader with bottom of tube contents at zero and top of plasma meniscus at 100
- Read off number level at top of red column; this is the PCV that must be recorded
- The *buffy coat* is the grey layer on top of the red cells
- The plasma is above the buffy coat
- If a fresh blood sample is collected directly from the horse by a lancet puncture, then a *heparinised microhaematocrit capillary tube* must be used in the centrifuge

---

The normal PCV in a horse varies with age, fitness and breed, and the 'normal' value varies between laboratories, but generally the values are: Thoroughbred, 40–46%; hunter type, 35–40%; pony, 33–37%. Greater values are found in 'hot-blooded' breeds such as Arabians and Thoroughbreds, fitter horses and excited horses (splenic contraction). Neonates have a PCV of 40–52%, which decreases to 29–41% by 6 months of age. Interpretation of samples from foals must take this into account.

An increased PCV may be due to:

- Dehydration
- Stress, excitement (splenic contraction)
- Endotoxic shock

A decreased PCV may be due to:

- Blood loss anaemia, e.g. haemorrhage

Table 12.1 Normal values of haematology parameters

	Thoroughbred	Hunter	Pony
RBC ($\times10^{12}$/L)	7.2–9.6	6.2–8.9	6.0–7.5
Hb (g/dL)	13.3–16.5	12.0–14.6	11.0–13.4
MCHC (g/dL)	34–36	34–36	33–36
MCV (fl)	48–58	45–57	44–55
MCH (pg)	14.1–18.1	15.1–19.3	16.7–19.3
WBC ($\times10^9$/L)	5.4–14.3	6.0–12.0	6.0–12.0
Platelet count ($\times10^9$/L)	100–350	200–350	200–350

RBC, red blood cells; Hb, haemoglobin; MCHC, mean corpuscular haemoglobin concentration (an index of the haemoglobin concentration per 100 ml of packed RBCs); MCV, mean corpuscular volume (average volume of each RBC); MCH, mean corpuscular haemoglobin (average haemoglobin content of a single RBC); WBC, white blood cells.

- Haemolytic anaemia, e.g. isoimmune haemolytic anaemia in foals
- Decreased erythrocyte production, e.g. secondary to chronic inflammatory disease, nutritional deficiency, neoplasia or toxicity

Red blood cells

The normal ranges for red blood cell-related parameters vary according to the type of horse, similar to the PCV. Refer to the range given for the laboratory used but as a general guide see Table 12.1.

Red blood cell production

Red blood cells are produced from stem cells in the bone marrow. They divide and commence haemoglobin synthesis, which is stored in the cytoplasm. Once haemoglobin production is complete, the nucleus is extruded and the cells are called *reticulocytes*. These do not usually leave the bone marrow and are rarely seen in the peripheral circulation except in cases of severe anaemia. At this time the cells have a variable blue–grey appearance, which is known as polychromasia. Once mature, the cells have a uniform appearance and are released into the peripheral circulation.

Red blood cell morphology

Spikey or irregular margins of red cells seen on a smear is termed crenation and usually results from cell shrinkage during slow air drying of the blood film. The basophilic remnants of the nucleus may be visible in an immature red blood cell and are called Howell–Jolly bodies. Supravital stains are useful to detect the presence of abnormal inclusions in a red blood cell, such as *Babesia* spp.

Erythrocyte indices in the horse are *not* as useful as in small animals for showing regenerative changes where big cells reflect regeneration. However, a moderate increase in the mean corpuscular volume can reflect a regenerative anaemia, as can *anisocytosis* (cells of differing sizes).

Haemoglobin concentration is measured by assessing the degree of a chemical reaction by colorimetry or spectrophotometry. This may be performed manually or by an automated analyser.

White blood cells

There are a number of different white blood cells:

- Neutrophils (= polymorphs): neutrophilia if inflammation, stress or corticosteroid use. May be mature with lobed nucleus or immature with band-shaped nucleus and foamy cytoplasm.
- Lymphocytes: lymphopenia in early viral infection, stress or corticosteroids. Large rounded nucleus that dominates the cell.
- Monocytes: monocytosis in chronic inflammation. Large bean-shaped nucleus.
- Eosinophils: eosinophilia, possibly with hypersensitivity or parasite infection. Covered in granules, appears raspberry-like with 'Diff-Quik' stain.
- Basophils: also covered in granules but basophilic as distinct from eosinophils.

The resting ratio of neutrophils to lymphocytes is 60 : 40. Normal values for white blood cells in the adult horse are summarised in Table 12.2.

Blood smears

To make a blood smear, see How to . . . 12.5. Generally, if submitting smears elsewhere send two or three unstained slides with two or three Romanowsky-type stained slides in proper slide carriers, correctly labelled.

Common faults in blood smears include:

How to . . . 12.5

To make a blood smear

- Prepare slide as soon as possible after blood collection. Cells are alive and start to degenerate immediately after collection, which will affect their morphology.
- Take a clean smear-free microscope slide.
- Place a small drop of well-mixed EDTA and whole blood at left end of slide.
- Place spreader slide edge on right side of drop at an angle of 30° to the main slide.
- Draw spreader towards left; blood will fill join between spreader and main slide.
- Briskly push spreader to the right, drawing out film of blood across whole of main slide.
- Allow to air dry (clean spreader slide while drying).
- Ready to stain! Follow manufacturer's directions for each type of stain. Generally flood slide with stain for set time and rinse.
- Most common stains are Romanowsky type (combination of basic and acidic stains dissolved in methyl alcohol).
- Example stains are Leishman's, Giemsa stain and quick polychromatic stains such as 'Diff-Quik'.

Table 12.2 The normal values for white blood cells in the adult horse

Cell type	Normal range ($\times 10^9$/L)
Total leucocyte count (white cell count)	6.0–12.0
Neutrophils	2.7–6.7
Lymphocytes	1.5–5.5
Eosinophils	0.1–0.6
Monocytes	0.0–0.2
Basophils	0.0–0.3

---

(1) Thickness: too thick (individual cells cannot be seen) or too thin (insufficient cells)
(2) Unequal distribution, leaving thin and thick bands
(3) Crenation due to too slow air drying of the smear
(4) Streaks and spots, which make interpretation difficult
(5) Incorrect staining: may need several different stains per sample

Faults (1), (2) and (4) are avoidable with good technique in spreading the drop of blood; but it takes practice!

Blood smears should be examined logically, e.g. using the 'battlement technique': the slide is covered by repeatedly moving two fields up, two fields along and two fields down until 100 cells have been counted to give a percentage of each cell type. In this way a *manual differential count* can be performed. Alternatively, automated counters will give a differential count.

Equine haematology differs from that in other species. The difficulty in assessing regenerative anaemias from the red blood cell parameters has been mentioned already. Rouleaux formation describes the stacking of red cells in columns and is readily seen on a blood smear. This may occur in association with increased plasma protein concentrations in other species but is a normal feature of equine blood.

Platelets

Platelet counts are routinely performed on EDTA samples from smears or by electronic cell analysers. The EDTA may cause platelet clumping, and more accurate counts can be obtained from blood collected into tubes containing sodium citrate.

Blood—biochemistry

Serum biochemistry analysis

Most biochemical assays are performed by automated machines. High-throughput diagnostic laboratories use 'wet' analysers where liquid reagents are added to samples and the chemical reaction is measured by a spectrophotometer. Smaller laboratories may use 'dry' analysers; these are more expensive per test but give instant results from a small number of tests or samples. With all laboratory tests, but particularly biochemistry, it is important to check normal values according to the laboratory you use.

Serum proteins

The total serum protein concentration (g/L) consists of the combined concentrations of albumin and globulins (see Table 12.3). These may be estimated by colorimetry in automated machines or the total serum protein concentration may be estimated manually using a refractometer. Serum protein electrophoresis may be used to quantify the individual components of the total globulins. This is useful when the total globulin concentration is abnormal.

Table 12.3 Normal values of serum proteins and common causes of abnormalities

	Total serum protein	Albumin	Globulin
Normal value	60–70 g/L	25–40 g/L	20–35 g/L
Increased value	• Dehydration • Secondary to increased globulins	• Dehydration	• Dehydration • Acute inflammation • Chronic inflammation • Parasitism • Liver failure
Decreased value	• Secondary to decreased albumin	• Protein losing enteropathy • Massive exudate production • Protein losing nephropathy • Liver failure	• Immune dysfunction

Laboratory Diagnosis

211

Specific globulin estimations

Acute-phase proteins form one group of the total globulins (alpha-globulins). They are produced by the liver in response to inflammation and include fibrinogen and haptaglobin. These are useful as sensitive indicators of inflammation. The immunoglobulins (gamma-globulins) include the antibodies. Specific measurement of antibody levels (immunoglobulin G) is useful to determine the immune status of an animal and is commonly used to assess the efficacy of transfer of maternal immunity to a newborn foal via the colostrum.

Electrolytes

Sodium, potassium, chloride, calcium, magnesium and phosphorus can all be measured in the blood (see Chapter 13).

Acid–base balance

Normal tissue metabolism results in the production of hydrogen ions whose concentrations are closely controlled by homeostatic mechanisms. Hydrogen ion concentrations are measured on pH scale 1–14. In the normal horse, blood is slightly alkaline (pH 7.35–7.45). Processes leading to a rise or fall in blood pH are known as alkalosis and acidosis, respectively (see Chapter 13).

Muscle enzymes

If muscle cells are damaged, enzymes leak into the blood and may be measured. The two important enzymes are:

- *Creatinine phosphokinase* (CPK): highest concentrations are found in skeletal muscle, cardiac muscle and brain tissue.
- *Aspartate aminotransferase* (AST), which is found in skeletal muscle, cardiac muscle and the liver.

The most often damaged of these is skeletal muscle, e.g. in exertional rhabdomyolysis, myositis or post-anaesthetic myopathy. The plasma concentration of CPK peaks within 6 h and rapidly decreases, whereas AST concentrations peak at 24 h and remain high for 7–10 days. The values reached are in the thou-

sands rather than hundreds. Dehydration may result in AST and CPK concentrations of a few hundred more than normal.

Liver enzymes

These include:

- AP (*alkaline phosphatase*): not liver specific but may reflect chronic damage to the hepatobiliary tract. Can check the isoenzyme intestinal AP in order to see if increased value is of liver origin. Normal range is 86–285 IU/L.
- AST (*aspartate aminotransferase*): not liver specific (also released from muscle) but is released in acute liver disease. Normal range is 138–409 IU/L.
- GGT (*gamma-glutamyl transferase*): technically not liver specific because it is also increased if there is renal or pancreatic disease. These are, however, rare so it is in fact a very useful indicator in both acute and chronic liver disease. It reflects damage to the biliary tract. Normal range is 0–44 IU/L.
- GLDH (*glutamate dehydrogenase*): liver specific and reflects current damage ('acute' enzyme) but is unstable in transit and so requires assay shortly after collection. Normal range is 0–11.8 IU/L.
- LDH (*lactate dehydrogenase*): need to look at the isoenzyme related to liver because it is a widespread enzyme. It is not particularly useful. Normal range is 162–412 IU/L.
- SDH (*sorbitol dehydrogenase*): liver specific and released early in damage ('acute' enzyme). It is not stable therefore as GLDH. Normal range is 0–8 IU/L.

Remember: dehydration mimics increased serum concentrations of liver enzymes.

Serum bilirubin concentrations are of limited use in the horse compared with other species. They are often not increased in equine liver disease but increases may be seen with biliary disease. The most common physiological reason for an increase in bilirubin concentration is anorexia.

If liver failure is suspected then a liver *function* test such as the total serum bile acid estimation (TSBA) should be carried out. This is an extremely useful test to monitor the progression of liver disease. Blood *ammonia* concentrations also may be increased in cases of liver disease, especially those showing encephalopathy. However, ammonia is not stable in plasma and needs to be assayed rapidly after collection. Other analytes may be altered in hepatic disease, such as triglyceride levels. These are particularly significant in hyperlipaemia, a metabolic disorder seen in ponies, particularly Shetlands, where increased triglyceride concentrations will be encountered.

Blood glucose

The normal range for blood glucose concentration is 3.5–6.0 mmol/L (60–100 mg/dl). It can be estimated using dipsticks or, better, a biochemistry analyser. Transient increases in blood glucose concentration are common and may be due to insulin resistance (stress, pregnancy, obesity or breed related, e.g. Shetland ponies), corticosteroid administration or α_2-agonist administration (sedative). Prolonged hyperglycaemia is uncommon in the horse but if it occurs it is usually due to hyperadrenocorticism ('Cushing's disease'). Hypoglycaemia is extremely uncommon in horses but may be associated with anorexia or liver failure.

Foals have an increased blood glucose concentration compared with adults: 108–190 mg/dl in the neonate, decreasing to 105–165 mg/dl by 12 months. Monitoring glucose concentrations is important in sick foals.

Renal function

Assessment of urinary function may be made from:

- Creatinine
- Blood urea
- Blood urea nitrogen (BUN).

Although an increase in the circulating concentrations of urea and creatinine (*azotaemia*) indicates renal failure, 75% of renal function will have been lost already by this point (see Chapter 14). Azotaemia is therefore an insensitive indicator of the onset of failure. However, further changes in the concentrations can be used to assess progress, so they are then useful as monitors. Small increases in urea and BUN are often found in dehydration, diseases with tissue catabolism and if the horse is on a high-protein diet. Increases in creatinine occur in severe acute myopathies. If urea, creatinine and BUN are all increased, then a nephropathy (renal disease) should be suspected.

Intestinal function

Intestinal disease may result in the release of cellular enzymes from the damaged enterocytes. Typically those used clinically are:

- AP: released following damage to the intestinal epithelium; intestinal AP is the gut-specific isoenzyme.
- LDH: release of the intestinal isoenzyme reflects gut damage.

Anything that invades the mucosa lining of the intestine will damage it and result in increased serum concentrations of these isoenzymes. Broadly, this divides into:

- parasites, e.g. cyathostomes
- cellular infiltrates, e.g. lymphosarcoma, eosinophilic enteritis.

An assessment of intestinal function may be made with the *oral glucose tolerance test*. This test measures the absorption of glucose from the small intestine into the bloodstream. Any condition affecting the small intestine may disrupt the glucose absorption and result in a decreased glucose absorption (malabsorption).

Urinalysis

Urine collection

Urine may be collected as a free-flow sample collected during normal micturition. It is usually most useful to collect a mid-stream sample. Alternatively, urine may be collected by catheterisation. This is a simple technique in both the mare and the male horse. Samples collected by catheterisation are often more appropriate for bacteriological examination because contamination from the external genitalia is avoided. However, catheterised samples will often have increased red cell, transitional epithelial cell and protein concentrations.

Urine samples should be collected into clean sterile containers. Ideally the sample will be analysed immediately but preservatives, such as boric acid, may be used if there is going to be a delay before analysis.

Urine appearance

Normal horse urine is yellow and may range from clear to cloudy in appearance. The colour may vary from light to dark, depending on the hydration status of the animal. It may froth when shaken, due to the normal high protein content. Crystals are often visible in the urine and result from the high concentration of calcium carbonate in normal equine urine. These may settle out as a sludge if the sample is allowed to stand.

Red discolouration of urine may be a result of haematuria, i.e. blood in the urine. The red blood cells, and therefore the colour, will settle out if the sample is left to stand and, in addition, the red blood cells will be seen during microscopic examination of the urine deposit. Haemoglobinuria, with a pink to red appearance, may be distinguished from haema-

turia, because the discolouration will not settle out if the sample is left to stand. Also, in cases of haemoglobinuria the plasma usually will have an abnormal orange/red discolouration. Rarely, drug administration may cause abnormal urine discolouration (e.g. rifampicin may result in orange urine). Brown to red/black discolouration of the urine is associated with myoglobinuria. (Note: myoglobinuria, unlike haemoglobinuria, will not be associated with any visible discolouration of the plasma.)

Specific gravity

Specific gravity is a measure of the density of a fluid. It is measured with reference to distilled water (which has a reference value of 1.000) by refractometer or, less reliably, on a dipstick.

Normal equine urine may have a specific gravity in the range 1.020–1.050.

Chemical tests

A variety of biochemical tests may be performed on equine urine (see Table 12.4). These are commonly performed on a dipstick for ease of measurement,

Table 12.4 Biochemical tests on equine urine

Test	Normal range	Disease that may cause an abnormal result
pH	7.0–9.0	Acidic with concentrate feeding or metabolic acidosis
Protein	<100 mg%	Massive concentrations seen with glomerular disease; slight increases seen with lower tract inflammation
Glucose	None usually present	Glucosuria can be seen with hyperadrenocorticism, stress or excess glucose administration
Ketones	None usually present	Ketosis is rarely seen in horses
Bilirubin	None usually present	Bilirubinuria may be rarely seen with obstructive jaundice or haemolysis
Haemoglobin	None usually present	Haemoglobinuria seen with severe intravascular haemolysis
Myoglobin	None usually present	Myoglobinuria is seen with extensive muscle cell degeneration

but where abnormalities are detected it is sensible to confirm these by other more accurate methods.

Urine deposit

Examination of the urine deposit or sediment by microscopy is an important part of the examination of a urine sample (see Table 12.5).

Biopsy techniques

Tissue biopsies are collected for histopathological examination. This usually allows definitive diagnosis where other techniques such as fine-needle aspirates and smears are limited. Biopsies may be taken from a number of sites in the horse:

- *Skin*: should not be prepared surgically because this would destroy the microscopic features. Following local anaesthetic administration at the site, a punch biopsy, elliptical biopsy or excisional

biopsy is taken. The horse usually would be sedated for this simple procedure.

- *Liver*: site should be prepared surgically and a sample taken using a Tru-cut technique with the needle introduced through the skin and intercostal muscles, which have been infiltrated with local anaesthetic. The horse should be sedated.
- *Endometrium*: taken using a special instrument introduced through the cervix. The tail should be bandaged out of the way and the perineum and vulva should be clean.
- *Rectal biopsy*: similar to endometrial biopsy, although cleaning of the region is not required.
- *Neoplasm*: the preparation required depends on the location of the neoplasm.

Samples are submitted for histopathology (need to be placed in formol saline; see below) and/or to bacteriology for culture (need to be collected aseptically and usually placed on a sterile isotonic saline-soaked swab in a sterile container). Handling of the tissue

Table 12.5 Examination of equine urine deposit

Content	Normal finding	Disease that may cause an abnormal result
Red blood cells	None usually present	Red cells may be seen following catheterisation or may indicate inflammation, trauma or neoplasia
White blood cells	None usually present	Marked numbers associated with inflammation
Transitional/epithelial cells	Few usually present	Marked numbers may indicate inflammation, trauma or neoplasia of the bladder
Bacteria	None usually present	Presence only significant if accompanied by inflammatory cells
Crystals (may be distinguished by their morphological appearance)	Calcium carbonate crystals are commonly seen; triple phosphate and calcium oxalate crystals are rarely seen	Increased numbers of triple phosphate crystals may indicate infection
Casts	Cellular casts are rarely seen; hyaline (protein) casts may be seen occasionally	Tubular damage may result in increased numbers of cellular casts

sample must be done with care and as atraumatically as possible (e.g. use a hypodermic needle point to transfer liver biopsy from Tru-cut needle to sample pot). If facilities allow, samples may be submitted for frozen section or immunofluorescence; advice should be sought from those assessing the samples as to sample size and fixative requirements.

Faecal analysis

Faecal samples need to be as fresh as possible. This sometimes may necessitate collection directly from the horse. There are very real risks associated with this, including damage to personnel and the rectal mucosa tearing, which may result in life-threatening peritonitis. A rectal examination is an act of veterinary surgery to be undertaken by a qualified clinician with proper restraint of the horse.

Equine faecal samples may be assessed for number and type of parasite ova or larvae (see Fig. 12.1). Ova are counted using faecal flotation (see How to . . . 12.6) or sedimentation, usually followed by the McMaster technique, which uses a special counting chamber.

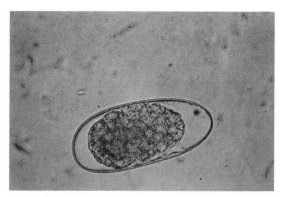

Fig. 12.1 Example of a nematode egg (magnification × 680).

may be seen but only sporadically (a serum test is now available for the more accurate diagnosis of tapeworm infection).

Larvae are separated from a faecal sample via sedimentation using the Baermann apparatus. This is suitable for looking at larvae from a patent lungworm (*Dictyocaulus viviparous*) infection or a case of cyathostomosis. Cyathostomes are a major cause of parasitic disease in the UK at this time.

Skin and hair

Collection of specimens

Horses undergo dermatological investigation frequently, because there is a vast expanse of hair and skin to sample and skin conditions are relatively common. Various techniques are used:

- *Hair plucks*: e.g. for dermatophyte ('ringworm') culture. The area to be sampled should be wiped with 70% isopropyl alcohol (to reduce contaminants) and allowed to dry. Hair plucks should be taken with sterile forceps from the edge of a suspected lesion (e.g. hairless area) and placed into a sterile container.
- *Hair brushings*: rarely performed in horses but may be used to investigate dermatophytosis.
- *Acetate tape preparations*: usually used to identify *Oxyuris equi*, or 'pinworm', infections in the perianal region. The tape should be pressed on a number of areas around the anus and placed on a microscope slide prepared with mineral oil.

How to . . . 12.6

Use of flotation to examine a faecal sample

(Based on differences in specific gravity: water at 1.000 compared with most ova at 1.100–1.200 and certain 'solutions' (e.g. zinc sulphate) at 1.200–1.250.)

(1) Mix faeces and 'solution' and sieve through a fine gauze.
(2) Collect draining sample into test tube so that it is *full* and seal with a cover slip.
(3) Leave for 20 min.
(4) Lift coverslip off vertically and place on microscope slide, with fluid trapped between them.
(5) Using a low-power objective, examine microscopically.

Large strongyle and small strongyle (cyathostome) eggs may be identified. It is also possible to identify tapeworm eggs (*Anoplocephala* species) but they rarely float out of the solution and so may be missed. Whole adult tapeworms or their segments

• *Skin scrapings*: e.g. for mite identification, especially *Chorioptes*. Any hair should be mostly clipped away before mineral oil is rubbed into the site. A scalpel blade then is held at right angles to the skin and gentle pressure applied as it is stroked to and fro until capillary ooze is seen. The sample then should be placed in a sterile container or applied directly to a microscope slide.

If a sample is being taken from a horse suspected to have a zoonotic infection (one transmissible to man) such as dermatophytosis ('ringworm'), extra care must be taken in sampling. Gloves should be worn and disposed of safely after use and any equipment used must be considered similarly. No other part of the body (horse or human) should be touched so that contact contamination is avoided. Any personnel involved with the handling of the samples or equipment used must be informed of the risk, either directly or through correct labelling of the samples.

Collection of body fluids

A number of body fluids may be collected for diagnostic purposes (see Table 12.6 for normal features). In all cases the collection should be performed using as sterile a technique as possible. In the field, surgical asepsis often is not possible but adequate preparation of the site of sampling (usually an area 15 cm × 15 cm) together with sterile equipment and gloved hands should be employed. Effective restraint of the horse is also essential to avoid injuries and a break in the aseptic technique.

Samples should be collected into sterile containers and split between plain vessels (biochemistry, bacteriology, limited cytology) and an EDTA vessel (cytology). In specific cases other vessels may be required, such as oxalate fluoride for glucose estimation or selective culture media. Depending on the sample collected, a variety of tests may be performed; usually these consist of total protein estimation and cytological examination. Most fluids collected normally would be relatively acellular with a low protein concentration. Increases in either of these parameters may occur with disease and are most marked when inflammation is present. Occasionally a specific diagnosis may be reached, e.g. with the identification of neoplastic cells in a sample.

Peritoneal fluid collection

Peritoneal fluid is most easily collected in the standing animal from a site 10–15 cm behind the xiphister-

Table 12.6 Normal features of fluid samples

Feature	Peritoneal fluid	Pleural fluid	Synovial fluid	Cerebrospinal fluid
Colour	Pale yellow/yellow	Yellow	Pale yellow	Colourless
Turbidity	Clear	Clear	Clear	Clear
Viscosity	Not tacky	Not tacky	Tacky (will form a string)	Not tacky
Nucleated cell count	$<5 \times 10^9$ cells/KL	$<10 \times 10^9$ cells/L	$<0.5 \times 10^9$ cells/L	$<0.01 \times 10^9$ cells/L
Predominant cells present	Large mononuclear cells and neutrophils	Large mononuclear cells and neutrophils	Mononuclear cells	Mononuclear cells
Protein concentration	<20 g/L	<40 g/L	<15 g/L	<1.0 g/L
Other				CPK: <25 IU/L Glucose: 1.7–4.2 mmol/L

num in the ventral midline. In this place the needle will pass through the linea alba at the most dependent point of the abdomen. After adequate restraint and preparation of the site, a needle is placed through the skin and into the linea alba. It is then slowly advanced into the abdomen until peritoneal fluid drips out. In most horses an 18-gauge 1.5-inch needle is suitable, but longer needles may be needed in obese animals. In the neonate the technique may be performed in the recumbent animal but extra care must be taken to avoid inadvertent puncture of the intestine.

Pleural fluid

Pleural fluid is collected by thoracocentesis through an intercostal space. In normal horses only a small volume of pleural fluid is present in the dependent part of the thorax. In cases of pleural disease an increased volume of fluid may be present. Thoracic ultrasonography is invaluable in identifying the site for pleural fluid collection.

After preparation of the site, local anaesthetic is infiltrated into the intercostal tissues. A needle then is inserted immediately cranial to the rib and into the pleural space. The pleural space usually contains a negative pressure so entry will be accompanied by an influx of air. Once this is recognised, the needle should be closed to prevent the creation of a pneumothorax. In most horses a 19-gauge 2-inch needle is most suitable for diagnostic thoracocentesis. If excess pleural fluid is present then it will usually appear from the needle under pressure. If therapeutic pleural drainage is indicated then a large intravenous catheter, bitch urinary catheter or human chest drain is more suitable.

Synovial fluid

Selection of the most suitable anatomical site for synovial fluid collection varies with the horse and the fluid to be collected. Following adequate preparation, a small bleb of local anaesthetic may be used to reduce movement of the horse as the needle is inserted. The most suitable needle will vary with the size of the horse and the synovial cavity under investiga-

tion. Once the needle is inserted, synovial fluid usually will flow freely from the hub and can be collected. Occasionally aspiration with a syringe may be used.

Cerebrospinal fluid

Cerebrospinal fluid (CSF) may be collected from the lumbosacral space in the standing horse or from the atlanto-occipital space in the recumbent animal. Following adequate preparation of the site, a bleb of local anaesthetic is placed under the skin at the point of needle entry. For the lumbosacral puncture a long needle is required and a bovine paravertebral needle with a stylet is most useful. For atlanto-occipital puncture a 19-gauge 3.25-inch spinal needle with stylet is appropriate. In each case, as the needle is inserted an appreciable loss of resistance is felt as the needle enters the space and the stylet then should be removed to allow fluid collection. Bilateral jugular vein occlusion may help the collection by increasing the CSF pressure.

Submission of pathological samples

After collection, all samples deteriorate. To minimise this, the samples should be placed in a suitable preservative, where appropriate, and transported to the analysing laboratory as soon as possible. Samples should arrive at the laboratory ready for immediate analysis and not at the weekend.

Records, labelling and request forms

Any sample collected from an animal must be identified suitably and accompanied by a completed request form prior to submission to an internal or external laboratory for analysis. Information that is needed on a request form includes:

- Owner's name
- Animal's name or identification
- Animal's details: age, gender and breed
- Date and time of sample collection
- Relevant clinical history of the animal (including previous samples submitted)

- List of samples (and their type) to be submitted
- Details of samples and the sample sites
- Details of the tests or investigations required.

Packaging of samples

All samples, even those being transported to an internal practice laboratory, need to be packaged suitably to ensure that they arrive safely and securely. In addition there must be no risk of leakage if a rigid container is broken and no risk to personnel handling the package. Those samples being transported by the postal service must comply with United Nations Packing Instruction 602. This can be obtained from the Post Office and includes the following:

- Samples should be placed in a labelled, watertight and leak-proof primary container made of glass, metal or plastic.
- Specialised leak-proof seals are available or alternatively a screw cap may be used with additional waterproof tape wound around the way the thread tightens the cap.
- The primary container with suitable padding and enough absorbent material to absorb all its contents is placed in a secondary container.
- The secondary container should be durable, watertight and leak-proof. If enough padding and absorbent material is included it may contain several primary containers.
- An itemised list of contents, the identity of the shipper and receiver (with contact numbers) and any additional paperwork (request forms) should be attached to the secondary container.
- The secondary container and attachments are placed in an outer shipping package.
- The outer shipping package, usually cardboard, should protect its contents from external damage and be labelled with the sender and receiver details and contact numbers and appropriate hazard designation.
- It is best to obtain packaging and or practical instructions from the laboratory to which samples are being sent.

In addition, the following Post Office regulations should be complied with:

- Packages should be sent First Class or Data Post.
- They should be labelled 'PATHOLOGICAL SPECIMEN–FRAGILE. HANDLE WITH CARE'.
- Primary containers should be sealed securely and have a maximum volume of 50 ml.
- Secondary containers may be a leak-proof plastic bag placed within a rigid container such as a plastic clip-down tub, screw-to-metal cylinder or two-piece polystyrene box.
- It is recommended that a padded (Jiffy) bag is used as the outer shipping package.

Sample deterioration/loss

Gross damage, loss or contamination of a sample is uncommon and can be avoided with suitable packaging and handling. However, even mild deterioration of a sample can render it unsuitable for analysis or contribute to erroneous results being produced.

Autolysis
Autolysis is the process of cell membrane breakdown leading to destruction and lysis of cells. It is an inevitable process once samples are collected, but is accelerated by increased temperatures and humidity. The use of preservatives and cooling help to slow down the rate of autolysis.

Haemolysis
Haemolysis is the process of degeneration of blood cells. It is most apparent in red blood cells and is exacerbated by extremes of temperature and physical shock. It is clinically important because haemolysis causes discolouration of the serum or plasma, which then may distort any subsequent colorimetric or photometric analysis. Where possible, serum or plasma should be harvested from a blood sample soon after collection and before transport to the laboratory.

Necrosis
Necrosis is the process of cell death and lysis that occurs in tissues after death or in tissue samples after collection. It begins immediately and, especially at high temperatures, may rapidly render a sample

219

unsuitable for histopathological examination. To reduce this deterioration, fresh tissue samples should be transferred immediately into a fixative. Most commonly 10% formol saline is used. This is made by diluting formalin (a concentrated 40% solution of formaldehyde in water) in a buffered saline solution as a 1 : 10 solution. Samples should be placed in ten times their volume of the 10% formol saline in a wide-mouthed container that allows easy retrieval at the laboratory.

Virology

Submission of samples

Virus detection may be carried out using swabs, body fluids or tissues. A special transport medium is usually required (containing proteins to support the virus and antibodies to inhibit bacteria) and the sample needs to be collected early in the course of disease. Transport to the laboratory should not be delayed and the samples may need to be sent packed with ice. Details like this are important; the laboratory always should be consulted if there is doubt about the type of sample required and way in which it should be sent.

Samples required

Where viral disease is suspected, samples may be collected and submitted in order to make a diagnosis. With a more epidemiological perspective, samples are used to assess vaccine efficacy and to eradicate disease. Some important notifiable diseases are caused by viruses, e.g. equine viral arteritis (EVA) and African horse sickness. Samples may be assayed for:

- Virus isolation (*VI*)
- Viral antigens (*AG*), by a variety of techniques such as enzyme-linked immunosorbent assay (ELISA), polymerase chain reaction (PCR), immunofluorescence or radioimmunoassay (RIA)
- Antibody titre (*AB*), e.g. an agar gel immunodiffusion test ('Coggins test') if equine infectious anaemia is suspected.

Serial samples may be required to demonstrate a rising antibody titre. Samples frequently required include:

- Blood: e.g. equine influenza (*AB, VI, AG*), equine herpes virus (*AB, VI, AG*)
- Tissues: e.g. fetal tissues for equine herpes virus (*AG, VI*)
- Swabs: e.g. nasopharyngeal swabs for equine influenza (*VI*), conjunctival swabs for EVA (*VI*)
- Body fluids: e.g. semen for EVA (*VI*).

Microbiology

Microorganisms (or microbes) are living organisms, namely bacteria, fungi, viruses and protozoa (see Table 12.7), that are too small to be seen with the naked eye. Those that cause disease are termed *pathogens*. Pathogens are almost invariably *parasites*, living in or on the horse as a host. Not all of these harm the host: those that neither benefit nor harm the host are *commensal* and those that benefit the host are *mutualistic*. Commensalism, parasitism and mutualism are all examples of *symbiosis*, where different organisms live closely together. Another group, *saprophytes*, are free-living microbes in the soil that derive their nutrients from dead plants and animals. Microorganisms are measured in micrometres (μm, i.e. 1000th of a millimetre). For example, most bacteria are between 0.5 and 5μm long.

Microorganisms and disease

If a microbe invades and replicates within an animal then that animal is infected. An infection may be *clinical* (overt) or *sub-clinical* (occult), depending on whether there are signs of disease. A disease may be *endemic* if it is constantly present in an animal population but only clinically recognisable in a few individuals. Endemic diseases are usually less severe (low morbidity). An *epidemic* is a disease of high morbidity that is present infrequently in the population. When it occurs, an epidemic usually is rapidly spreading and present in many individuals. *Zoonotic* disease is a disease of animals that is transmissible to man. Examples of zoonoses with respect to

Table 12.7 Comparison of microorganisms

Feature	Bacteria	Viruses	Fungi	Protozoa
Size	0.5–5 μm	20–300 nm	3.8 μm	10–200 μm
Number of cells	Unicellular	Non-cellular	Multicellular	Unicellular or multicellular
Cell wall	Yes	No	Yes	No
Reproduction	Asexual or conjugation	Replicate within cells	Asexual and sexual by spores	Asexual and sexual
Motility	Some motile	Not motile	Not motile	Motile
Nucleus	No membrane-bound nucleus	No	Membrane-bound nucleus	Membrane-bound nucleus
Nucleic acids	DNA and RNA	DNA or RNA	DNA and RNA	DNA and RNA
Toxin synthesis	Some produce toxins	No	Some produce toxins	Some produce toxins

horses include dermatophytosis ('ringworm') and salmonellosis.

The development of disease from infection in any animal is the result of an imbalance between the animal's immune system and the microorganism challenge to which it is exposed. This challenge is determined by the amount of microbe present and its virulence. The virulence of a microbe is its degree of *pathogenicity* (i.e. ability to cause disease) and depends on factors individual to it, such as its ability to gain access to the host cells and whether it can produce toxins to damage host physiology.

For a microbe to cause disease it must be able to:

- Enter the host
- Overcome or avoid the host defences
- Replicate and establish a presence
- Damage the host tissues.

Some microorganisms do this by secreting or releasing toxins that have deleterious effects on the host cells. Others, such as viruses, may directly invade the host cells and cause damage or cell death.

Toxin synthesis is a significant factor in the development of disease in any animal; in horses, both endotoxins and exotoxins are of major significance. *Exotoxins* are synthesised by the living microbe (bacteria or fungus), e.g. tetanus toxin is an exotoxin produced by *Clostridium tetani* causing tetanus, which is often fatal in horses. *Endotoxins* are part of the bacterial cell wall of some Gram-negative bacteria and are only released when it dies. Although not as immediately life threatening as exotoxins, they exert a devastating effect on the horse's health if not addressed, e.g. in horses with severe gastrointestinal compromise 'endotoxic shock' may occur. This is where the

gut wall becomes 'leaky', allowing bacteria and endotoxins across it, which then trigger a cascade of inflammatory reactions resulting in potentially fatal endotoxic shock.

Toxaemia describes the presence of toxins in the blood. Using similar terminology, *viraemia* indicates viruses in the blood, *bacteraemia* denotes bacteria in the blood, *septicaemia* refers to the active replication of bacteria in the blood and *pyaemia* suggests pus in the blood.

Basic bacterial cell structure

Bacteria are generally encased in a *cell wall*, which varies in thickness and in composition; this variety accounts for why some are Gram positive and some Gram negative. Around this there is usually a *capsule* that protects the cell and may contribute to its virulence. Inside the cell wall is the *cell membrane*, which surrounds the fluid cytoplasm. Within this floats the bacterial *chromosome*, which is the genetic material of the cell. There also may be one or more *plasmids*; these are important in the development of antibiotic resistance. Some bacteria possess other structures outside the cell wall, including *flagella* (to help movement), *pili* (important in cell reproduction) and *fimbriae* (involved in adherence of the bacteria to host cells).

Classification of bacteria

Three shapes are recognised:

(1) *Bacilli* (rod shaped)
(2) *Cocci* (spherical)
(3) *Spirilla* (spiral shaped)

Curved bacilli are termed *vibrios*. Paired cocci are described as *diplococci* whereas a chain of them are called *streptococci* (e.g. *Streptococcus equi* subspecies *equi*, which causes 'strangles') and a cluster of cocci are known as *staphylococci* (e.g. *Staphylococcus aureus*, which is a common equine commensal bacteria).

Bacteria are further classified as:

- Gram-stain positive, e.g. *Clostridium* species
- Gram-stain negative, e.g. *Salmonella* species

This depends on the cell wall characteristics.

Acid-fast bacilli are another group differentiated on the basis of a staining technique. They are stained red with carbol fuchsin before being heated. They are then resistant to decolourisation with acid alcohol and so retain the red colour when counter-stained with methylene blue. This is known as a Ziehl–Neelsen stain; examples of acid-fast bacilli are the Mycobacteria.

There is a distinction between *aerobic* bacteria, which can only grow when oxygen is present (e.g. those found on the skin) and *anaerobic* species. *Obligate anaerobes* cannot withstand oxygen in the environment whereas *facultative anaerobes* will grow with or without it. *Microaerophilic* bacteria favour conditions when the concentration of oxygen is lower than in atmospheric air.

Bacterial reproduction

Bacteria reproduce by:

(1) *Binary fission*, where the cell simply divides into two identical daughter cells (asexual).
(2) *Conjugation*, which involves the transfer of DNA from one bacterial cell to another, via a pilus. Conjugation is important because the recipient cell acquires new genetic material, e.g. resistance to an antibiotic.

Gram-positive bacteria tend to reproduce by fission but Gram-negative species favour conjugation. Spore production occurs when environmental conditions are unfavourable; the endospore forms within the bacterium. Spores are extremely resistant to destruction and can survive for years. *Clostridium* species, which cause botulism and tetanus, are examples of spore-forming organisms. Spores are destroyed by autoclaving, dry heat (160° for >2 h!) and Tyndallisation (repeated steaming).

Bacterial culture

Bacteria may be grown in the laboratory in a culture medium; this is a solid or liquid that contains the nutrients for a particular species in the correct proportions. Solid media are usually found in flat-lidded clear petri dishes. There are a number of media commonly available to veterinary practice laboratories (see Table 12.8) and the type of media used depends on the bacteria suspected to be present.

Additionally, biochemical media may be used to differentiate between different species of bacteria by demonstrating the way in which the species react with the media, shown as an indicator colour change.

Once a plate has been selected appropriate to the bacteria suspected, then the sample must be 'plated out' onto it (see How to . . . 12.7). This is done to disperse the sample so that colonies grow thinly and may be identified, e.g. by the 'streaking method'.

Viruses

Viruses comprise a *capsid* made of protein encasing *nucleic acid*, which may be RNA or DNA. A number

---

How to . . . 12.7

To plate out a bacterial culture

- Place a small sample of the culture (e.g. one drop) onto the medium at the edge of the plate
- Flame a platinum bacterial loop until it is red hot, allow to cool and touch onto agar somewhere distant from the sample
- Streak from the sample in a zigzag across one-third of the plate
- Use a hooded Bunsen flame to heat the loop again to red hot
- Cool loop and repeat streaking, going from the zigzags already there to form a new patch over another one-third of the plate
- Repeat again to cover the last one-third of the plate and lid the plate before it is incubated

Table 12.8 Media commonly used in veterinary practice laboratories

Medium	Plate (P) or broth (B)	Type	Will grow . . .
Nutrient agar	P	Simple (basal)	Any
Chocolate agar	P	Enriched	Certain pathogens
Blood agar	P	Enriched	Most pathogens
MacConkey's agar	P	Selective (for enteric species) and differential	Enteric species: lactose fermenters vs. non-lactose fermenters
Deoxycholate citrate agar	P	Selective	*Salmonella* species
Sabouraud's agar	P	Selective	Fungi
Nutrient broth	B	Simple (basal)	Any
MacConkey's broth	B	Selective	Enteric species
Selenite broth	B	Enrichment	*Salmonella* species

of shapes are recognised, including helical, icosahedral, complex and composite. Additional variety is provided by the presence or absence of an *envelope* around the capsid. Viruses replicate by attaching to a host cell through recognition of a particular receptor on that cell. The virus then discharges its genetic material into the host cell. This genetic material is reproduced by the host cell, forming new viral parts. These are then released either by rupture of the cell membrane or by passing through it without destruction of the host cell.

Fungi

Horses may be infected by both of the two main types of fungi: multicellular moulds (e.g. dermatophytes, 'ringworm'); and unicellular yeasts (e.g. *Candida* sp.), seen in furring of the tongue in sick foals.

Bacteriological examination

Bacteriological examination of samples may be performed within a practice laboratory or sent away, e.g. testing for contagious equine metritis swabs (CEM) should be sent to a laboratory approved by the Horserace Betting Levy Board. Some fungal samples will be dealt with internally compared with a viral assay, which usually requires specialist laboratory work.

Bacteria are examined by making a smear on a microscope slide. The smear may be made:

- Directly from a swab that is rolled onto the slide (e.g. from open wound or vesicle)
- From a liquid using a sterile wire loop or pipette to transfer one drop (e.g. from an abscess)
- From an agar plate with a sterile wire loop, picking off a colony and mixing with sterile saline.

The smear then must be heat fixed once it has air dried by passing it through a Bunsen flame (sample facing up!) two or three times. Once cooled, it can then be stained.

A simple stain is methylene blue, which should be used to cover the slide for 3 min before it is rinsed with tap water and examined for bacteria. An idea of the number of bacteria and their shape may be obtained. Alternatively, a Gram stain may be used (see How to . . . 12.8), which will both reveal the bacteria present and help to classify them.

It is important to note that swabs taken for bacteriology, as with any pathological sample, need to be collected and processed as quickly as possible. Labelling must be correct to both identify the sample and avoid unnecessary delay in processing. They may be taken from a variety of sites and should be taken aseptically to avoid contamination, which will give spurious results. In equine practice, swabs are routinely taken from:

- The nasopharynx (in investigating, for example, suspected 'strangles' caused by *Streptococcus equi* subspecies *equi*)

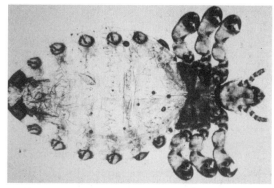

Fig. 12.2 Example of a sucking louse (magnification × 44).

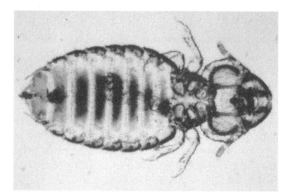

Fig. 12.3 Example of a biting louse (magnification × 60).

- The clitoris (to detect the presence of *Taylorella equigenitalis*, the causative organism in contagious equine metritis)
- The uterus (to detect the presence of infectious endometritis)
- Abscesses and wounds
- During surgery (e.g. from a septic tendon sheath)
- The conjunctiva.

Ectoparasites

Ectoparasites affect the horse externally, as distinct from endoparasites that are internal parasites. A wide variety of ectoparasites affect equines; some are host specific and some have the potential to affect other species, including humans (zoonotic).

Lice

A common ectoparasite in the horse is the louse, leading to lice infestation (pediculosis), which often occurs in groups of horses when housed in the winter months. Both biting lice (*Damalinia equi*) and sucking lice (*Haematopinus asini*) are found (see Figs 12.2 and 12.3). Lice are six-legged and about 2 mm in length.

The biting species have obvious mouthparts when compared with the sucking species. The eggs (nits) may be seen attached to the mane and tail hairs and sometimes the adult lice can be seen in the mane, tail, along the dorsum or anywhere else. Other clinical signs can include pruritus (this may cause secondary self-induced trauma), alopecia and anaemia if the infestation is severe. Lice are host specific and only survive a few days off the horse. Transmission is by direct contact or fomites (e.g. grooming equipment, rugs or tack). A cure may be effected by synthetic pyrethroids, e.g. permethrin.

Mites

Chorioptic mange

Chorioptic mange in horses is caused by *Chorioptes equi* (see Fig. 12.4). These host-specific eight-legged

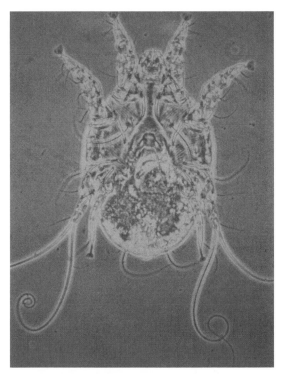

Fig. 12.4 Example of a *Chorioptes* mite (magnification × 150).

mites live on the skin surface for their entire lifecycle and cause local irritation. They are typically found in the long hair (feathers) of the distal limb of heavy horses and cobs, where their presence causes stamping and self-trauma and is often complicated by secondary bacterial infection. Clinical disease is more common in the winter. Transmission is by direct or indirect contact.

The mites may be identified from skin scrapings, which should be collected from new lesions after excess hair has been clipped off. They are superficial, unlike *Psoroptes equi* (see below), and so only chew skin debris rather than penetrating the skin. Treatment for all mites is as for lice, and topical ivermectin or fipronil (unlicensed) is also effective.

Psoroptic mange

Psoroptes equi and *Psoroptes communis* are host-specific mites that are less common (and not found in the UK, where the disease is notifiable). They live on the skin surface, typically around the mane and tail,

where they cause intense pruritus. Diagnosis is by identification of the mite on skin scrapings. The mites are very similar to *Chorioptes equi* but in *Psoroptes* the mouthparts are less round and the pedicels (parts at the ends of all eight legs to which the cup-shaped suckers are attached) are longer and jointed. They measure about 0.75 mm in length.

Sarcoptic mange

Sarcoptes scabiei are burrowing mites that affect domestic mammals and man. The condition is extremely rare in the horse. They induce marked pruritus and often there is severe self-trauma with excoriation and skin damage. Deep skin scrapings are required to identify the mites, which can be difficult to find. Sarcoptes mites are smaller than the other types, measuring up to 0.4 mm in length. They are more rounded and notably are covered in distinctive ridges and scales in their dorsum.

Ticks

Ticks may be found on horses, particularly in known tick areas such as moorland. The species involved is the castor bean tick, *Ixodes ricinus*, which will affect birds and mammals, including man. It is readily identified attached to the horse by its mouthparts and the tick's body enlarges as it feeds. The pale grey female measures up to 1 cm in length, compared with the male that is 2–3 mm. They are usually found on the lower parts of the horse and care must be taken when removing them to avoid leaving the mouthparts embedded in the skin. Their significance is not yet fully understood, but it is suspected that they are important vectors for the transmission of blood-borne disease such as babesiosis, borreliosis and ehrlichiosis in horses.

Harvest mites

Larvae of the 'harvest mite' *Trombicula autumnalis* may be seen on the lower limbs of horses in the late summer and autumn. They will also affect other mammals, including man. The nymph and adult stages are free living. Large numbers of ovoid orange-brown larvae about 0.6 mm long may be seen clustered together. They may be associated with local irritation and have been reported to be associated with 'headshaking' in horses when found uncommonly in the ears. Treatment is as for lice.

Culicoides

These are very small flies ('midges'), the adult females of which bite and feed on blood. They are irritating, are vectors for disease (e.g. for African horse sickness) and cause a hypersensitivity reaction in sensitised horses ('sweet itch'). They affect all mammals, including man.

Stomoxys calcitrans

This is the stable fly and looks similar to a housefly. It is a very irritating ectoparasite because it causes painful bites. It may bite other domestic mammals and man. It is also implicated in insect hypersensitivity and is a vector for *Habronema*.

Habronema muscae/microstoma

These species affect horses and donkeys and are pathogenic in terms of their effect in the skin and eyes. This is how the infestation is generally recognised; the appearance of reddish-brown non-healing areas ('summer sores') on the skin, prepuce, penis or, in the eye, conjunctivitis with ulcers. Larvae may be seen in samples submitted for microscopy. Treatment is aimed at reducing the inflammation and preventing re-infestation.

Onchocerca cervicalis

This equine nematode is widespread in the UK but rarely causes clinical disease. The larval stage is transmitted via *Culicoides* species as vector to the preferred site, the ligamentum nuchae at the withers. There it causes a painless swelling, which forms a defined lump. Unless this becomes secondarily infected, it does not break open to the surface. Once developed to adults, fresh microfilariae are produced that migrate predominantly to the skin of the ventral midline but also to the face, neck and lower limbs. Alopecia, ulceration and scaling with possible pruritus may be observed, which are thought to re-

sult from hypersensitivity to the nematode rather than direct pathogenic effects. Ivermectin is an effective treatment.

Endoparasites

Horses are potential hosts to a range of endoparasites, including:

- Nematodes: *Parascaris equorum*, *Strongyloides westeri*, *Oxyuris equi*, *Cyathostome* species, *Strongylus* species, *Dictyocaulus arnfieldi*
- Cestodes: *Anoplocephala* species, *Echinococcus* species
- Protozoa: *Sarcocystis neurona*, *Ehrlichia* species
- *Gastrophilus* species

Nematodes

The use of faecal examination for the detection of various life stages of different types of nematodes is described earlier in this chapter: the limitations of this in assessing the presence or degree of parasitism cannot be overestimated. In addition, changes may be noted on blood haematology/biochemistry and histopathology may be used. The most clinically significant nematodes are the cyathostomes (small strongyles, about eight significant species) and large strongyles (three main species).

Cyathostomes

These have a direct, non-migratory life cycle. Eggs in faeces on pasture develop to third-stage larvae. These are ingested and invade the large colon wall where they develop to fourth-stage larvae. These emerge and moult to adults, which lay eggs that are passed in the faeces. The larvae in the gut wall are able to hypobiose (arrest development) for months to years. The prepatent period (i.e. development time from egg to an egg-laying adult) is 6–20 weeks. Clinical signs of cyathostomosis include weight loss, diarrhoea, colic and ventral oedema.

Large strongyles

These have a direct migratory life cycle and do not hypobiose. The adult stages are in the large intestine but the larval stages may migrate to damage certain arteries (the cranial mesenteric artery is the main site), the liver and the peritoneum. Clinical signs of strongylosis (mixed small and large strongyles) include weight loss, possibly diarrhoea, colic and anaemia.

Cestodes

There are two important species of tapeworm relevant to equines: *Anoplocephala perfoliata* and, less commonly, *A. magna*. They have an indirect life cycle via the oribatid mite as an intermediate host. *Anoplocephala perfoliata* is found in the distal small intestine and caecum where it may cause colic. Tapeworm eggs and segments may be identified in the faeces and a blood test is also available to detect infestation.

There are two main strains of *Echinococcus granulosus* in domestic species: *E. granulosus granulosus* and *E. granulosus equinus*. They are both found in Europe. The life cycle of *E. g. granulosus* involves ruminants and dogs or foxes, whereas in *E. g. equinus* equines are the specific intermediate host as opposed to ruminants. Following ingestion of an infective segment from dog or fox faeces, the larval stage develops in the liver (usually rarely in the lung) giving a 'hydatid cyst'. These rarely seem to cause a clinical problem for the horse and are often found incidentally at post-mortem examination.

Protozoa

Sarcocystis neurona is the causative organism in equine protozoal myelitis, which is confined largely to North America. It must be borne in mind, therefore, when dealing with neurological disease in imported horses.

Ehrlichia risticii is the causative organism of Potomac horse fever in North America. *Ehrlichia equi* is the cause of tick-borne fever in ruminants transmitted by ticks and is suspected to cause disease in equines, but this has not yet been assessed fully.

Gastrophilus species

There are four important species of this insect, of which *Gastrophilus intestinalis* and *G. nasalis* are most often identified. The adult flies lay yellow sticky eggs, which are attached to the hairs on the forelegs or head. These are licked during grooming and hatch to larvae, which are ingested. These attach to the stomach mucosa and persist for 10–12 months before being passed in the faeces, where they pupate and adult flies emerge. The red-brown larvae may be identified in the stomach during gastroscopy or at post-mortem examination, where they are seen attached to the mucosa.

Control measures

Endoparasite control may be achieved by management of the grazing pasture and the horse. It is important to remember that most of the parasite burden exists on the pasture and not in the horse. Although several groups of anthelmintics are readily available, these will only treat the parasites in the animal. Hence, except in the case of a clinically parasitised animal, these products should be used only to reduce future contamination of the pasture. For this to be effective, all animals should be treated at the same time, all newcomers should be treated on arrival and, if possible, animals should be moved to a clean environment after treatment. Over-use of wormers has already led to anthelmintic resistance in other animals and this has been recognised also in horses.

It should be emphasised that simple pasture management techniques can be as effective and more economical than the use of anthelmintics. Such techniques are based on regular removal of faeces (and the worm eggs) from the pasture. Depending on circumstances, this may be performed effectively by hand or with mechanical devices.

Further reading

Duncan, J.R., Prasse, K.W. & Mahaffey, E.A. (1994) *Veterinary Laboratory Medicine*, 3rd edn. Iowa State University Press, Ames.

Lane, D.R. (1991) *Jones's Animal Nursing*, 5th edn. Pergamon Press, Oxford.

Lane, D.R. & Cooper, B. (1999) *Veterinary Nursing*, 2nd edn. Butterworth-Heinemann, Oxford.

Mair, T.S., Love, S., Schumacher J. & Watson, E.D. (1998) *Equine Medicine, Surgery and Reproduction*. WB Saunders, London.

Taylor, F.G.R. & Hillyer, M.H. (1997) *Diagnostic Techniques in Equine Medicine*. WB Saunders, London.

CHAPTER 13

Fluid Therapy

J. C. Boswell & M. C. Schramme

Fluid therapy is an integral part of supportive care, required in nursing many clinical conditions. Disorders of fluid, electrolyte and metabolic status can arise from:

- The inability to eat or drink
- Loss of fluids or electrolytes
- Trapping of fluid within the body (e.g. pooling within the gut)
- A consequence of shock

The aims of fluid therapy are to:

(1) Replace and correct any imbalances.
(2) Restore the effective circulating volume and blood pressure.
(3) Provide the body's maintenance requirements of water and electrolytes.

To do this, it is necessary to understand the normal physiological processes that control body water, electrolyte and acid–base balance and the pathophysiological processes that disrupt these homeostatic mechanisms.

Electrolytes are molecules that, when dissolved in water, dissociate into positively (*cations*) and negatively (*anions*) charged ions. A *solution* is a liquid that comprises water and dissolved substances. A solution is *isotonic* if it has the same concentration of dissolved substances as another solution, e.g. plasma. A solution with a higher concentration of dissolved substances is *hypertonic*, whereas a solution with a lower concentration is *hypotonic*. If solutions of different concentrations are mixed, then they equilibrate to a new concentration. This process is called *diffusion*.

Water and electrolytes

Water is the most abundant molecule in the horse's body and represents approximately 65–70% of an adult horse's bodyweight. The total body water (TBW) varies between individuals, depending on:

- Age
- Gender
- Nutritional status
- Environmental factors.

Fat contains almost no water, therefore lean animals and neonates have more body water than older or obese animals. The TBW of foals is proportionately higher than in adult animals (almost 80% of bodyweight) and gradually decreases as the animal ages.

Distribution of body fluids (Table 13.1)

The TBW is divided between:

(1) *Intracellular fluid* (ICF): approximately 30–40% of bodyweight.
(2) *Extracellular fluid* (ECF): approximately 20–30% of bodyweight, divided into:
    (a) *Interstitial fluid* (10–12% bodyweight),
    (b) *Intravascular fluid* or plasma (4–6% of bodyweight),

Table 13.1 Fluid compartments in adult horses (NB: 1 l of water weighs 1 kg)

Fluid	Proportion of bodyweight	Approximate volume (L) in a 500-kg horse
Total body water	65–70%	325–350
Intracellular fluid	30–40%	150–200
Extracellular fluid	20–30%	100–150
Interstitial fluid	10–12%	50–60
Intravascular fluid	4–6%	20–30
Transcellular fluid	8–10%	40–50

(c) *Transcellular fluids* (8–10% bodyweight). Transcellular fluids are fluids that have been produced by transport across glandular cell walls. In the horse these are primarily fluids within the gastrointestinal tract but also include cerebrospinal fluid, bile, saliva and semen.

Although the *osmolality* (concentration of dissolved solutes) of the ICF and ECF is the same, there is a marked difference between the ionic compositions of the two compartments. The ECF has:

- High concentrations of sodium (Na^+) and chloride (Cl^-) ions.
- Low concentrations of bicarbonate (HCO_3^-), potassium (K^+), inorganic phosphate (PO_3^-), calcium (Ca^{2+}) and magnesium (Mg^{2+}) ions.

The ICF has:

- High concentrations of K^+ and PO_3^- ions.
- Low concentrations of Na^+, Cl^- and Ca^{2+} ions.

Exchange of water between compartments

Water is constantly moving between the different body compartments. The movement of water is governed by *osmotic* and *hydrostatic pressure gradients*. If a semi-permeable membrane (e.g. a cell membrane) separates two solutions, water will move from the lower concentration solution to the higher concentration solution down a concentration gradient (*osmosis*).

The body compartments are separated by cell membranes that allow free passage of water but are selectively permeable to dissolved solutes. Movement of water along an *osmotic pressure gradient* is the most important determinant of water movement in the body.

Cell membranes act as barriers to some solutes but not to others. Only those dissolved solutes that are unable to move across cell membranes between adjacent compartments are able to exert an osmotic pressure and cause water to move between compartments.

Movement of water between the ICF and the ECF

Movement of water between the ICF and the ECF depends on osmotic pressure differences between these two compartments. If water is added to the ECF compartment, the osmoconcentration of the ECF decreases and an osmotic pressure gradient between the ECF and the ICF causes water to move into the cells until the osmoconcentrations are equalised. If water is lost from, or a strong salt solution is added to, the ECF, the osmoconcentration of the ECF will be higher than that of the ICF, resulting in movement of water out of the cells.

Movement of water between the plasma and the interstitial fluid

Both osmotic pressure and hydrostatic pressure determine the movement of water between the plasma and the interstitial fluid across the capillary walls. The capillary walls (unlike the cell membranes) are permeable to electrolytes and other dissolved solutes (e.g. glucose) that are important in providing osmotic forces between the ICF and the ECF. These molecules do not exert an osmotic pressure gradient at this interface. In the healthy horse, the capillary wall is essentially impermeable to protein macromolecules and therefore the plasma protein represents the major osmotic pressure difference between the plasma and the interstitial fluid. Plasma proteins therefore tend to 'hold' water within the capillaries because the protein concentration of plasma is much higher than that of the interstitial fluid. In sick, shocked (e.g. endotoxic) horses, changes in the capillary walls result in leakage of protein out of the plasma and consequently loss of water from the circulation into the interstitial space, resulting in peripheral oedema and a loss of circulating blood volume.

The tendency for water to be drawn from the interstitial space into the circulation is offset by *hydrostatic pressure*. As the heart contracts, the pressure in the capillaries increases, tending to force water out of the circulation.

Regulation of total body water (TBW)

Water is lost from the body in:

- Urine
- Faeces
- Sweat
- Expired breath
- Milk (in the lactating mare).

The amount of water lost will be affected by environmental factors, including ambient temperature, humidity and the horse's workload. In the diseased horse, additional water losses may occur due to haemorrhage, diarrhoea, nasogastric reflux or sequestering (i.e. trapping) of abnormal quantities of fluid in one part of the body.

Water is gained by:

- Drinking
- Ingestion of water in food
- Generation of water by protein, fat and carbohydrate metabolism.

On average, a healthy 500-kg horse will drink approximately 12–40 l of fluid each day (or 25–80 ml/kg/day).

Normally, gains and losses of water are kept in balance by regulatory mechanisms. The amount of water in the body is monitored by osmoreceptors in the brain, which detect changes in the concentration of water in body fluids, and by stretch receptors in blood vessels, which detect changes in the circulating blood volume. This sensory information is relayed to the hypothalamus in the brain, which controls the intake of water by influencing thirst and regulating loss of water by the release of antidiuretic hormone (ADH), which acts on the kidneys and controls the amount of urine produced (Fig. 13.1).

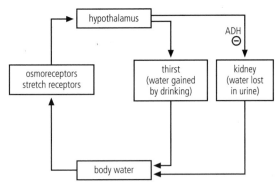

Fig. 13.1 Feedback control of body water content.

Disturbances of water balance

Dehydration is defined as a reduction in TBW and occurs because of water deprivation (either through lack of access to water or the inability to swallow) or because of excessive fluid loss.

The effective circulating volume is a term used to refer to the fluid in the circulation. If the circulating volume is adequate the horse is said to be *normovolaemic*. States of inadequate or excessive circulating volume are termed *hypovolaemia* and *hypervolaemia*, respectively.

Hypovolaemia may occur as a result of dehydration, although if the onset of dehydration is insidious the effective circulating volume may be maintained despite a reduction in TBW. Hypovolaemia may also occur as a result of haemorrhage, shock or sequestration of abnormal quantities of fluids in the body.

Hypovolaemia is associated with:

- Reduction in circulatory fluid volume
- Reduced venous return to the heart
- Decreased cardiac output
- Inadequate tissue perfusion
- Development of metabolic acidosis due to poor tissue perfusion.

The end result of these responses is circulatory shock, which if untreated may result in death.

Definition of shock: profound physiological changes to the body causing circulatory collapse and consequently inadequate tissue oxygenation and perfusion. Basically treatment involves re-establishing tissue blood flow, so fluid therapy is vital. It is also important to treat the underlying cause. Shock may be initiated by many things, including:

- Allergic reactions
- Blood loss
- Dehydration
- Infection, including endotoxic or septic shock, when bacterial infection results in toxin release
- Trauma.

Assessment of hydration status and effective circulating volume

Clinical examination

Clinical examination is the first, and most important, means of assessing fluid deficits. The clinical signs of *dehydration* include:

- Decreased skin elasticity
- Sunken eyes
- Dry mucous membranes.

Clinical signs of *hypovolaemia* include:

- Tachycardia (increased heart rate)
- Pale mucous membrane colour
- Prolonged capillary refill time
- Poor pulse quality
- Cool extremities
- Delayed jugular refill time.

Although it is not possible to make an accurate assessment of percentage dehydration on the basis of clinical signs alone, a subjective assessment of mild, moderate or severe dehydration is possible and an estimation of the percentage fluid deficit can be made (see Table 13.2).

Packed cell volume (PCV) and total plasma protein concentration

Packed cell volume and total plasma protein concentration are invaluable for assessing fluid deficits and monitoring the response to fluid therapy. These can be performed easily and quickly, requiring only a small centrifuge, a microhaematometer and refractometer (see How to . . . 13.1).

Table 13.2 Estimation of water loss and dehydration based on clinical signs

Dehydration	Water loss (% bodyweight)	Clinical signs
Mild	5–7	Slight decrease in skin elasticity, dry mucous membranes, prolonged jugular venous filling time (12 s)
Moderate	8–10	Decreased skin elasticity, dry mucous membranes, prolonged capillary refill time (>2 s), prolonged jugular venous filling time (>12 s)
Severe	>10	Depression, decreased skin elasticity, sunken eyes, pale, dry mucous membranes, prolonged capillary refill time, weak pulse quality, increased heart rate (>40 bpm), prolonged jugular venous filling time, cool extremities

How to . . . 13.1

Technique to measure PCV and total plasma protein concentration

- Venous blood should be collected into a vacutainer or blood collection tube containing either heparin or ethylenediaminetetraacetic acid (EDTA).
- If measurements are being taken from a horse with an indwelling intravenous catheter, then blood may be withdrawn through the catheter. The first 20 ml of blood should be discarded to ensure that a representative blood sample is collected.
- Blood is transferred to small capillary tubes and the ends of the tubes are sealed.
- The tubes are placed in a centrifuge and spun for 3 min at 1500 rpm to separate the blood cells from the plasma.
- The capillary tube is placed in the microhaematometer and the PCV can be measured as a percentage of the total blood volume.
- To measure total protein concentration of plasma, the capillary tube is snapped carefully above the packed cells and a drop of plasma is placed onto the refractometer. The total protein concentration of the sample may be measured in units of g/L.

Table 13.3 Interpretation of PCV and total plasma protein concentration

	PCV	Total protein
Dehydration	↑	↓
Splenic contraction (e.g. with pain, fear or excitement)	↑	N
Dehydration with protein loss	↑	N or ↓
Acute blood loss	↓	↓
Chronic blood loss	↓	N
Dehydration with anaemia	N	↑

↑, Increased; ↓, decreased; N, within reference range.

Interpretation of PCV and total plasma protein concentration

The normal PCV range is 32–52% and the total plasma protein range is 5.9–8.4 g/L. Both PCV and the total protein concentration should be interpreted together and guidelines for their interpretation are given in Table 13.3. An elevation of both PCV and total protein concentration occurs in dehydration. As a rough guide they increase by approximately 5–10% and 10 g/L, respectively, for each 2–3% increase in percentage dehydration above 5%. An anaemic animal that has become dehydrated may show a PCV within the normal range but with a concurrent elevation in the total protein concentration.

Urine specific gravity

Urine specific gravity is a measure of the concentration of urine, which is easily measured by refractometry. In adult horses, the urine specific gravity ranges from 1.020 to 1.050, whereas in foals the urine is more dilute and therefore has a lower specific gravity. As a horse becomes dehydrated, the kidneys attempt to conserve water, therefore the amount of urine produced decreases and the concentration of the urine (and urine specific gravity) increases. If a dehydrated horse has a urine specific gravity of less than 1.020, this suggests renal impairment, which should be investigated.

Central venous pressure

Central venous pressure is dependent on the cardiac output and venous return. It is influenced by:

- Blood volume
- Vascular tone
- Heart rate
- Ventricular contractility.

Central venous pressure falls in association with hypovolaemia and is elevated with hypervolaemia. Measurement of central venous pressure may be used to assess cardiac function and to monitor fluid therapy. Normal central venous pressure ranges from between −3 to +7 cmH$_2$O.

How to . . . 13.2

Procedure to measure central venous pressure (see Fig. 13.2)

- Advance a long, saline-filled intravenous catheter into the right atrium via the jugular vein (18–24-inch catheter in adult horses or 12-inch catheter in foals).
- Attach a saline-filled extension tube to the intravenous catheter (patient line).
- Connect a water manometer to the extension tube via a three-way tap.
- Attach a saline-filled syringe to the remaining inlet of the three-way tap.
- Position the manometer so that the baseline (0 cm) is at the level of the right atrium, using the shoulder as a landmark.
- Ensure that the horse's head is in a normal position.
- Close the manometer and flush the patient line.
- Close the patient line and flush the water manometer with saline.
- Turn the three-way tap so that the patient line is open to the water manometer.
- The fluid column in the water manometer will fall to the level of the central venous pressure.

Arterial blood pressure

Hypovolaemia will result in a fall in arterial blood pressure and in many clinical situations the goal of fluid therapy is to restore the arterial blood pressure. Arterial blood pressure may be measured directly via an intra-arterial catheter or indirectly

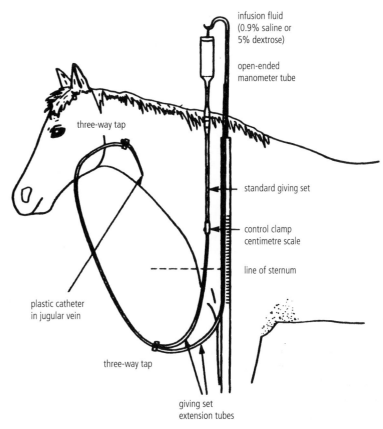

infusion fluid
(0.9% saline or
5% dextrose)

open-ended
manometer tube

three-way tap

standard giving set

control clamp
centimetre scale

line of sternum

plastic catheter
in jugular vein

three-way tap

giving set
extension tubes

apparatus for the measurement of central venous
pressure

Fig. 13.2 Central venous pressure line.

Table 13.4 Normal values of arterial blood pressure

	Direct measurement	Indirect measurement
Mean	80–110 mmHg	82–110 mmHg
Systolic	110–160 mmHg	100–135 mmHg
Diastolic	70–90 mmHg	70–97 mmHg

using Doppler or oscillation techniques (see Table 13.4). In the standing horse, intra-arterial catheters are maintained most easily in the transverse facial artery for direct arterial blood pressure monitoring. Indirect arterial blood pressure monitoring is usually achieved by applying a cuff around the tail to measure the pressure in the middle coccygeal artery.

Serum urea and creatinine concentrations

Serum urea and creatinine concentrations are elevated in acute dehydration. Significant increases in both urea and creatinine reflect prerenal failure associated with hypovolaemia. Restoration of effective circulating blood volume with fluid therapy should produce a rapid response in serum creatinine in these horses. If serum creatinine concentrations remain persistently increased, the presence of primary renal dysfunction should be considered.

Electrolyte imbalances (see Table 13.5)

Sodium

Sodium is the major cation within the ECF and is

Table 13.5 Conditions associated with electrolyte and metabolic imbalances

Electrolyte/metabolic imbalance	Condition
Sodium	
Hyponatraemia	Oesophageal obstruction
	Enterocolitis
	Intestinal obstruction
	Polyuric renal failure
	Urinary tract disruption
	Inappropriate ADH secretion
Hypernatraemia	Enterocolitis
	Excessive sweating
	Water deprivation
Potassium	
Hypokalaemia	Enterocolitis
	Intestinal obstruction
	Anorexia
	Renal tubular acidosis
	Polyuric renal failure
	Diuretic administration
	Bicarbonate administration
	Insulin administration
Hyperkalaemia	Muscle necrosis
	Urinary tract disruption
	Anuric renal failure
	Hyperkalaemic periodic paralysis
Chloride	
Hypochloraemia	Intestinal obstruction
	Ileus
	Proximal enteritis
	Exhausted horse syndrome
	Equine rhabdomyolysis syndrome
Hyperchloraemia	Excessive salt intake
	Renal dysfunction
Calcium	
Hypocalcaemia	Stress/transit
	Lactation tetany
	Acute renal failure
Hypercalcaemia	Chronic renal failure
	Hypercalcaemia of malignancy
	Vitamin D toxicosis

NB: hypo = low levels; hyper = raised levels.

important in the development of plasma osmotic pressure and therefore in maintaining the fluid volume of the ECF. Alterations in sodium concentrations may lead to clinical signs associated with cerebral oedema or dehydration, namely depression, seizures, blindness and ataxia. Sodium is ingested with food and water and lost from the body in urine, sweat and faeces.

Hyponatraemia (i.e. low blood sodium) is usually the result of excessive loss of sodium, as occurs with oesophageal obstruction, enterocolitis, intestinal obstruction, polyuric renal failure or urinary tract disruption, and rarely may be due to a reduced intake of sodium.

Hypernatraemia (i.e. raised blood sodium) is rare but can follow acute dehydration or excessive sodium replacement in fluid therapy.

Potassium

Potassium is the primary intracellular cation. The normal intracellular potassium concentration is 145–150 mmol/L, whereas its extracellular concentration is 2.4–4.7 mmol/L. Serum potassium concentrations are useless in estimating total body potassium levels. Total body potassium levels may be low and yet the serum potassium concentrations may be normal.

Potassium has a central role in the maintenance of cell membrane electrical potentials. Its distribution between the intracellular and extracellular compartments is influenced by the acid–base status. Potassium ions leave or enter the cells in exchange for hydrogen ions so that serum or plasma potassium levels rise during acidosis and fall during alkalosis.

Potassium is lost from the body in gastrointestinal secretions, sweat and urine. Hypokalaemia (i.e. low blood potassium) may occur in anorexic horses due to rapid depletion of potassium levels, or due to loss of potassium ions in horses with diarrhoea.

Hyperkalaemia (i.e. raised blood potassium) is unusual in the horse unless associated with severe acidosis, haemolysis or impaired renal function. Hyperkalaemia should be considered as a medical emergency because it frequently leads to cardiac arrhythmias.

Chloride

Chloride ions are present in high concentrations in the ECF and therefore changes in the plasma concentrations tend to reflect changes in the total body levels. At most sites within the body, chloride tends to follow sodium passively by diffusion across the cell membrane so that regulation of the chloride concentration within the ECF is related directly to the sodium concentration. In the ECF, the chloride concentrations are inversely related to the bicarbonate concentrations. The amount of chloride excreted in the urine is dependent on the body's need for bicarbonate.

Hypochloraemia (i.e. low blood chloride) usually occurs as a result of loss of chlorine ions in gastro-intestinal secretions and therefore occurs with oesophageal obstruction (choke), reflux due to ileus, proximal enteritis or intestinal obstruction. Hypochloraemia is usually accompanied by metabolic alkalosis.

Primary hyperchloraemia (i.e. raised blood chloride) due to excessive salt intake is uncommon but hyperchloraemia may accompany renal dysfunction and dehydration due to water loss only.

Calcium

Calcium is abundant throughout the body. It has an intergral role in multiple physiological processes, including nervous, skeletal muscle and smooth-muscle function and blood clotting.

Hypocalcaemia (i.e. low blood calcium) may be associated with lactation, particularly if the mare is stressed by transport. Mild hypocalcaemia frequently is observed in horses with colic and may contribute to postoperative ileus.

Hypercalcaemia (i.e. raised blood calcium) is usually due to chronic renal failure but rarely may be due to paraneoplastic syndromes or vitamin D toxicosis.

Assessment of electrolyte imbalances

The assessment of electrolyte disorders must be based on laboratory evaluation of serum concentrations of electrolytes (see Table 13.6).

Serum concentrations of sodium are accurate in assessing sodium deficits or relative excesses because sodium is an extracellular ion, whereas measurement of serum potassium concentration does not re-

Table 13.6 Reference values for plasma electrolyte ranges in mature horses

Electrolyte	Reference range (mmol/l)
Sodium	132–146
Potassium	2.4–4.7
Chloride	99–109
Calcium	2.7–3.2

flect the whole body content of potassium because this is primarily an intracellular ion. Acid–base status further complicates the interpretation of serum potassium ion concentrations.

Estimates of sodium and potassium deficits for the purpose of replacement therapy are made by considering the difference between the measured and desired serum concentrations, the horse's body weight and the distribution of the ion within the body, as follows:

$$\text{Na deficit (mmol/L)} = (\text{Desired [Na]} - \text{Actual [Na]}) \times \text{bodyweight (kg)} \times 0.6$$

$$\text{K deficit (mmol/L)} = (\text{Desired [K]} - \text{Actual [K]}) \times \text{bodyweight (kg)} \times 0.3$$

where [electrolyte] = concentration of electrolyte.

Measurements of calcium are affected by serum protein concentrations because 40–50% of calcium is protein-bound. Protein-bound calcium decreases as the concentration of albumin decreases, and ionised calcium increases with acidosis. Therefore, the total calcium deficit cannot be calculated accurately. Measurement of ionised calcium concentration is preferable because this is the physiologically active form.

Acid–base balance

Definition of pH: a scale used to measure acidity and alkalinity, with zero being most acidic, 14 being most alkaline and 7 being neutral.

Blood pH is dependent on the respiratory system and the function of a variety of buffering systems. The clinically important variables that contribute to the metabolic component of acid–base balance are sodium, chloride and other unidentified anions and plasma proteins. Metabolic disturbances are buffered by the carbonic acid/bicarbonate system and therefore disturbances can be manifested by a change in bicarbonate. The bicarbonate buffering can be represented by:

$$CO_2 + H_2O \leftrightarrow H_2CO_3 \leftrightarrow H^+ + HCO_3^-$$
$$\text{carbonic acid} \quad \text{bicarbonate}$$

Acid–base imbalances are conventionally classified as respiratory or metabolic in origin. Failure of ventilation results in the inability to remove carbon dioxide, producing *respiratory acidosis*, whereas hyperventilation results in removal of excessive carbon dioxide causing *respiratory alkalosis*.

Metabolic acidosis is the most common acid–base disorder in horses. Metabolic acidosis can be the result of excessive production of organic acids, particularly lactate, due to poor perfusion of tissues, or the excessive loss of bicarbonate ions. Metabolic acidosis is associated with shock, hypovolaemia, diarrhoea, sepsis, enterocolitis, intestinal obstruction or renal disease.

In metabolic acidosis, the increased H^+ (number of hydrogen ions) in the plasma causes the equilibrium equation above to shift to the left, so that H^+ combines with HCO_3^- (bicarbonate), which in turn increases the plasma pCO_2 (carbon dioxide), which may be excreted as CO_2 from the lungs. Therefore, metabolic acidosis results in a decrease in plasma HCO_3^- and an increased respiratory rate.

Metabolic alkalosis is uncommon in horses and is usually associated with hypochloraemia. This may occur in conditions resulting in the production of high volumes of gastric reflux (e.g. grass sickness, ileus, proximal enteritis or intestinal obstruction), exhaustion or exertional rhabdomyolysis. In addition, metabolic alkalosis may be associated with hypoalbuminaemia, because albumin is a weak acid, and may occur with severe enterocolitis, renal disease or severe parasitism.

In metabolic alkalosis, the equilibrium is shifted to the right, so that more bicarbonate is produced.

Mixed metabolic acidosis and alkalosis may be present in horses with gastrointestinal disease. This occurs when fluid is sequestered in the proximal gastrointestinal tract, leading to chlorine and hydrogen ion loss and metabolic alkalosis, with a concurrent reduction in effective circulating volume, producing shock, poor tissue perfusion and lactic acidosis.

Assessment of acid–base balance

Although a venous blood sample is adequate for assessment of the metabolic contribution to acid–base balance, an arterial blood sample is used for assessment of the respiratory component. Arterial samples may be obtained in the standing horse from the transverse facial artery, which runs over the temple, lateral to the eye. In foals it may be easier to take samples from the dorsal metatarsal artery, which lies on the lateral aspect of the third metatarsal (cannon) bone, just distal to the tarsus. The infiltration of a small volume of local anaesthetic subcutaneously over the artery may make sampling easier. Ideally the blood sample should be processed immediately but samples may be stored on ice for up to 4 h if necessary.

Acid–base status is assessed by measuring:

- Blood gases
- Serum bicarbonate ion concentrations
- Anion gap
- Base deficit.

Normal values for arterial and venous blood analysis are shown in Table 13.7.

Assessment of the pH and pCO_2 in arterial blood will provide an indication of whether respiratory acidosis or respiratory alkalosis is present (see Table 13.8):

- In respiratory acidosis the pH will be decreased and pCO_2 will be increased.
- In respiratory alkalosis the pH will be increased and pCO_2 will be decreased.

Metabolic disorders are reflected as an alteration in bicarbonate ion concentration in both the venous and arterial samples.

Table 13.7 Reference ranges for blood gas analysis in mature horses

	Arterial	Venous
pH	7.347–7.475	7.345–7.433
pO_2 (mmHg)	80–112	37–56
pCO_2 (mmHg)	36–46	38–48
HCO_3^- (mmol/L)	22–29	22–29
Base excess (mmol/L)	−1.7 to +3.9	−2.7 to +4.1
Anion gap (mEq/L)	10–20	

Table 13.8 Interpretation of blood gas analysis and acid–base abnormalities in arterial blood samples

	pH	pCO_2	$[HCO_3^-]$	Anion gap
Respiratory acidosis	↓	↑	N	N
Respiratory alkalosis	↑	↓	N	N
Metabolic acidosis	↓	N	↓	N or ↑
Metabolic alkalosis	↑	N	↑	N
Mixed metabolic acidosis/ alkalosis	N	N	N	↑

↑, Increased; ↓, decreased; N, within reference range.

The *anion gap* is the calculated difference between measured cations and anions and is represented by the equation:

$$\text{Anion gap} = ([Na^+] + [K^+]) - ([Cl^-] + [HCO3^-])$$

The anion gap is increased in horses in which metabolic acidosis is due to lactic acidosis secondary to endotoxaemia or hypovolaemic shock. It is unchanged in horses with metabolic acidosis due to loss of bicarbonate ions. Assessment of anion gap may be useful to identify horses with mixed metabolic acidosis and alkalosis (see Table 13.8), which might otherwise go unnoticed, because in these horses the pH and bicarbonate concentration may be normal due to the two conflicting processes counteracting each other.

Principles of fluid therapy

In most clinical situations, the goals of fluid therapy are:

(1) Replacement of existing deficits.
(2) Supplying maintenance fluid requirements.
(3) Matching ongoing losses.

Occasionally overhydration (administration of fluid in excess of the horse's requirements) may be indicated, e.g. in the treatment of horses with colonic impaction.

Basic considerations

There are four essential questions for practical fluid therapy:

- What type of fluid does the animal need?
- How much fluid does the animal need?
- Which route of administration should be used?
- At what rate should the fluid be given?

Types of fluid used for fluid therapy

Crystalloids

Hartmann's solution or lactated Ringer's solution
- These are *isotonic fluids*, which means that their effective osmotic pressure is the same as intracellular fluid and therefore they do not cause a net movement of water into or out of the cells but remain in the ECF.
- Hartmann's or lactated Ringer's solution contains sodium, potassium, chloride and lactate in concentrations similar to ECF.
- These fluids are excellent for replacement therapy because they are restricted to the ECF compartment due to their high sodium content. However, the high sodium content also means that they are unsuitable for maintenance therapy.

Normal saline (0.9% sodium chloride, NaCl)
- Isotonic.
- Normal saline has a high sodium content and does not contain lactate. Therefore administration of large volumes can produce a dilutional acidosis and hyperkalaemia. Consequently, normal saline should not be used for volume replacement but to correct specific sodium or chloride deficits and as an acidifying solution.

Hypertonic saline (7.2% NaCl)
- This is a *hypertonic* fluid that causes movement of water out of the ICF compartment into the ECF compartment and therefore is used to expand the circulating volume.
- Hypertonic saline is extremely useful in the treatment of animals in shock where the aim of therapy is to restore an effective circulating volume as quickly as possible.
- Because hypertonic saline does not replace fluid but rather causes a redistribution of fluid in the body, it is essential that large quantities of isotonic

fluids are given following the administration of hypertonic saline.

- Hypertonic saline is contraindicated in exhausted horses, horses suffering heat stress and renal disease. There are reservations about its use in haemorrhagic shock because increasing the blood pressure may promote further bleeding. It should not be used in horses with ongoing, uncontrolled bleeding.

5% Dextrose

- Isotonic.
- Used for maintenance therapy.

Colloids (e.g. Gelofusin, Haemaccel, Hespan starch, dextrans)

- These fluids contain large molecules that are maintained in the intravascular fluid compartment, thereby increasing the colloid osmotic pressure and causing movement of water into the circulation from the interstitium.
- Colloids are useful if the total protein concentration falls below 35 g/l, to increase the colloidal osmotic pressure and 'hold' fluid within the circulation.
- Colloids are widely used in other species to restore the effective circulating volume in the treatment of shock. However, the large volumes required in the adult horse mean that their use is usually prohibited by cost.
- Colloids may be used in the management of shock in foals when rapid improvements in cardiovascular function are necessary. They should be infused together with isotonic, polyionic fluids (e.g. Hartmann's solution) for the best results.
- Some colloids have been associated with anaphylactic reactions in horses.

Plasma

- Plasma may be considered to be another form of colloidal fluids.
- It is used primarily in the treatment of hypoproteinaemia and hypogammaglobulinaemia in foals (see below).

Whole blood

- Whole blood is rarely indicated except for cases of acute, severe haemorrhage or severe anaemia.
- Blood transfusions are discussed below.

Replacement therapy

Replacement of fluid and restoration of an effective circulating volume is the first priority in the treatment of horses presenting with signs of shock and cardiovascular collapse. Intravenous fluid therapy is necessary to provide sufficient volumes of fluid quickly. Effective circulating volume can be restored using crystalloid, colloidal solutions or plasma, although crystalloid solutions are most commonly used in horses because the volumes of colloidal solutions and plasma required tend to be very expensive.

Isotonic crystalloids

For most conditions, isotonic polyionic fluid is the most appropriate and safest choice. If no electrolyte abnormalities are suspected or identified, Hartmann's or lactated Ringer's solutions are most commonly used.

The volume of fluid required to replace the fluid deficit can be calculated easily using the equation:

Litres of fluid needed = Bodyweight (kg) × % Dehydration

That is, a 500 kg horse, at 5% dehydration, requires 2500 L. Any evidence of continued fluid loss (e.g. nasogastric reflux, diarrhoea) also must be taken into consideration.

The rate of administration depends on:

- Severity of the fluid loss
- Type of fluid needed
- Disease being treated
- Route of administration
- Presence or absence of electrolyte abnormalities requiring correction.

It is usually recommended that half the required volume of fluids should be given over the first 6 h and the remainder given over the next 12 h. In adult horses with cardiovascular collapse, fluids may be administered safely at rates of up to 30 L/h.

Fluid may be administered as a continuous infusion (either by gravity flow or with an infusion pump) or alternatively in boluses whereby the total volume of fluid to be administered in 24 h is divided into aliquots, that are then administered intermittently at a faster rate.

Overzealous administration of fluids will result in diuresis before adequate expansion of the ECF compartment can occur. Fluid overload produces signs of pulmonary oedema and therefore the respiratory rate and effort should be monitored if large volumes of fluid are being administered quickly. Fluid overload is rare in adult horses but care must be taken when administering fluids to young foals. Monitoring the central venous pressure is the most objective means of monitoring the rate of fluid administration.

Hypertonic (7.2%) saline

Hypertonic (7.2%) saline is a valuable alternative to isotonic crystalloids for the treatment of horses with endotoxic, haemorrhagic or hypovolaemic shock. In the presence of shock, the volume of isotonic fluids required to achieve an obvious improvement in cardiovascular signs may be more than 50 l. This amount of fluid may take several hours to administer. Attempts to administer isotonic fluids more quickly may result in complications such as pulmonary oedema, hypoproteinaemia and oedema.

The administration of hypertonic saline results in increased cardiac output, increased arterial blood pressure, increased plasma volume and a reduction of PCV and total protein concentration. Hypertonic saline should be given at a dose of 4–6 ml/kg (2–3 L for a 500-kg horse) over a period of approximately 10–20 min. Hypertonic saline is indicated in emergency situations where rapid restoration of effective circulating volume is needed to preserve life. It is also particularly useful in the pre-anaesthetic stabilisation of horses with strangulating bowel lesions. It provides rapid improvement in cardiovascular status, which allows anaesthesia and surgery to be performed sooner. It is an initial resuscitative

measure and large quantities of isotonic fluids must be given subsequently.

Correction of acid–base abnormalities

Although the ultimate goal in acid-base disorders is to resolve the underlying condition, stabilisation of the disturbance is often required. It is important to appreciate that respiratory acid–base disorders cannot be alleviated by fluid therapy and require modification of respiratory function.

Metabolic acidosis

The most important part of treatment for metabolic acidosis is restoration of the circulating volume with either Hartmann's or lactated Ringer's solutions. These buffered solutions have a mild alkalising effect but, more importantly, restoration of renal blood flow allows the kidneys to excrete the excess anions and correct the acid–base balance.

The use of sodium bicarbonate in the treatment of metabolic acidosis is controversial. Sodium bicarbonate increases the plasma sodium concentration, thereby alkalising the blood, and excess bicarbonate is excreted as carbon dioxide by the lungs. Administration of bicarbonate will decrease serum potassium and ionised calcium concentrations. Paradoxical cerebral acidosis may occur if metabolic acidosis is corrected too rapidly. Sodium bicarbonate should be used with caution in the following circumstances:

- Respiratory dysfunction: if the lungs are unable to excrete excess bicarbonate as carbon dioxide there will be an increase in pCO_2, therefore exacerbating acidosis. For this reason, sodium bicarbonate should be used with care in anaesthetised horses.
- Hypocalcaemia: administration of sodium bicarbonate may result in tetany.
- Severe hypokalaemia: sodium bicarbonate may worsen hypokalaemia.
- Congestive heart failure: large sodium loads may exacerbate fluid retention.

Sodium bicarbonate should be supplemented only when the serum base deficit is greater than 10–15 mmol/L (or serum bicarbonate is less than 15 mmol/L). The amount to be given can be calculated as:

$$HCO_3^- \text{ deficit (mmol)} = 0.4 \times \text{Bodyweight (kg)}$$
$$\times \text{Base deficit (mmol/L)}$$

It is common practice to replace half the deficit initially over a 1–2 h period and to replace the remaining deficit over the next 12–24 h. Bicarbonate is available as 5% and 8.4% solutions. Both of these are hypertonic and should be diluted with sterile water before use. Bicarbonate should not be added to solutions containing calcium because precipitation may occur.

Metabolic alkalosis

Metabolic alkalosis is uncommon in horses but may be associated with heat stress, exertion or in horses with nasogastric reflux, when it is usually associated with hypochloraemia and hypokalaemia. Therapy is primarily aimed at replacement of chloride and promotion of renal excretion of bicarbonate by restoring the effective circulating volume. Normal saline supplemented with potassium is the fluid of choice for the treatment of metabolic alkalosis.

Correction of electrolyte abnormalities

Sodium

Hyponatraemia

Normal saline, Hartmann's or lactated Ringer's solutions are generally appropriate for the treatment of asymptomatic hyponatraemia. Hypertonic (7.2%) saline should be used only for symptomatic hyponatraemia.

Hypernatraemia

Hypernatraemia indicates a relative water loss. Replacement of water can be achieved using 5% dextrose, because at this concentration dextrose is metabolised to water and carbon dioxide. Alternatively an infusion of 0.45% saline in 2.5% dextrose may be used to supply additional fluid without lowering the serum sodium concentration too rapidly. Extreme caution should be exercised in the treatment of hypernatraemia because cerebral oedema may develop if the plasma osmolarity is reduced too rapidly.

If hypernatraemia is associated with a normal or increased extracellular fluid volume, as in water-retaining renal failure, then treatment also involves salt restriction and the administration of diuretics.

Potassium

As discussed previously, it is difficult to assess accurately the total body stores of potassium.

Hypokalaemia

Hypokalaemia is very common and potassium should be supplemented when serum potassium falls below 3 mmol/L, especially if the animal is anorexic. Potassium chloride may be added to intravenous fluids (5–40 mmol K^+/L). Care should be taken not to administer potassium at rates of more than *0.5 mmol/kg/h* because cardiac dysrhythmias may occur. Alternatively, potassium may be safely given to horses orally at 5–40 g every 6–12 h.

Hyperkalaemia

Hyperkalaemia is life-threatening because it causes cardiac dysrhythmias and should be considered a medical emergency. The concentration of potassium in the ECF can be reduced by promoting the uptake of potassium into the cells. This can be achieved by administration of sodium bicarbonate or insulin (0.1–0.5 u/kg) or enhancement of the secretion of insulin by dextrose infusion (6 ml/kg of 5% dextrose) and sodium bicarbonate administration. Administration of calcium chloride (0.5 ml calcium borogluconate/kg by slow intravenous infusion) also has been advocated for its cardioprotective effects.

Calcium

Replacement of calcium in horses requires caution. It is impossible to calculate calcium deficits accurately and therefore treatment is generally given to effect. A 23% calcium gluconate solution (0.25–1 ml/kg) should be diluted and administered slowly to effect over a period of 12–24 h.

Maintenance fluid therapy

The maintenance fluid requirement is the volume of fluid required to replace the normal ongoing losses and additional losses that occur as a result of the clinical problem. The normal ongoing losses are made up of:

(1) Sensible losses: representing fluid lost in the urine that can be adjusted according to the body's overall water balance.

(2) Insensible losses: these are inevitable and include fluid lost in faeces, during cellular metabolism, breathing and sweating. The normal maintenance requirement for an adult horse is approximately *40 ml/kg/day* (i.e. a 500-kg horse needs at least 20 l of fluid each day). However, diarrhoea or nasogastric reflux can considerably increase this figure.

Maintenance fluid therapy may be provided either with oral or intravenous fluids.

Intravenous maintenance fluid therapy

Fluids for maintenance therapy are predominantly needed for the ICF compartment, which has very different sodium and potassium concentrations compared with the ECF compartment. The net sodium concentration of normal urine is much less than that of the ECF (40 mmol/L) whereas that of potassium is much higher (20 mmol/L). Although Hartmann's or lactated Ringer's solutions are often used for short-term maintenance, these solutions provide too much sodium and insufficient potassium. If renal function is normal, the excess sodium can be excreted; however, if these solutions are used for maintenance in the long term then hypokalaemia will result. It is therefore preferable to use either 0.18% sodium chloride (N/5) and 4% dextrose solution with 20 mmol/L of potassium chloride added, or a mixture of 1 part Hartmann's solution and 2 parts 5% dextrose solution with 15 mmol/L of potassium chloride added.

Ideally maintenance fluids should be administered as a constant infusion (approximately 5 drops/s for a 500-kg horse using a giving set delivering 20 drops/mL). However, if necessary, the daily requirement may be divided into 4–6 aliquots and administered as boluses. This is an inefficient method because some fluid is lost by urination following rapid bolus administration.

Routes of fluid administration

When selecting a route of administration for fluids several factors should be considered, including the volume of fluid to be administered, the type of fluid required, the specific condition being treated and the expense.

In horses, fluids are most commonly administered by oral (voluntary drinking or nasogastric intubation) or intravenous routes.

Oral administration of fluids

The oral route should be used if possible because it is more physiological, obviates the need for sterile fluids and catheters, carries a low risk of infection and is cheap. If this route is to be used the horse must be able and willing to drink and swallow fluids, must be able to tolerate fluids (i.e. this route should not be used if horses are refluxing) and must be able to absorb fluids (i.e. may be unsuitable for animals with diarrhoea).

If the horse is unable or unwilling to drink, fluids may be administered via a nasogastric tube. The average adult horse can tolerate approximately 8 L of fluid by nasogastric intubation, which can be repeated every 2–4 h as required. Whenever fluid is administered by intubation it is important to ensure that there is no gastric reflux prior to administration of fluids, to prevent overdistension of the stomach.

The disadvantages of nasogastric intubation are that some horses will not tolerate passing of a stomach tube and that repeated intubation may cause trauma to the nasal passages, pharynx, larynx or oesophagus. If repeated fluid administration is required, in-dwelling stomach tubes may be used. However, these may cause pharyngitis and oesophageal stricture formation. Fluids should not be administered by nasogastric intubation to recumbent horses.

The oral route for administration of fluids is unsuitable in the following circumstances:

- If large volumes of fluids are required.
- In emergency situations, when fluid needs are immediate.

• When the horse is refluxing or unable to absorb water from the gastrointestinal tract.

In these conditions fluids should be administered intravenously.

Intravenous administration of fluids

Intravenous catheters and their management

Catheter selection

The choice of which catheter system to use and which vein to access for fluid and medication depends on several factors, including:

• The volume and rate of fluid to be administered
• The type of fluid administered
• The potential for thrombosis
• The duration of catheterisation required
• Costs.

Catheters are available in a number of materials, including polypropylene, polyethylene, PVC, polytetrafluoroethylene (Teflon), nylon, silicone (silastic) and polyurethane. All catheter materials incite varying degrees of inflammation and thrombus formation but some materials are more thrombogenic than others. The softer materials tend to cause less inflammation and are therefore less thrombogenic. Silastic and polyurethane catheters are the softest, least thrombogenic, most flexible and least likely to kink and therefore most appropriate for long-term use. Polypropylene and teflon catheters tend to be the most thrombogenic and are prone to kinking and cracking with long-term use.

Various techniques are available for the introduction of a catheter into a blood vessel. The basic *'over the needle'* technique relies on the advancement of the catheter into the vessel over a stylet, which is withdrawn once the catheter is in position (Fig. 13.3). Problems associated with this basic design have included excessive venous trauma, carotid puncture, catheter laceration, air embolism, limited catheter length and shorter catheter durability.

Alternative designs have been used to minimise these problems and allow the placement of catheters of greater length. The Seldinger technique for percutaneous catheterisation allows the introduction of a long catheter over a flexible guide wire (Fig. 13.4).

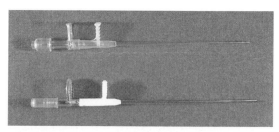

Fig. 13.3 Braunule MT® polypropylene catheters hubbed with thumb support are introduced using an 'over-the-needle' technique.

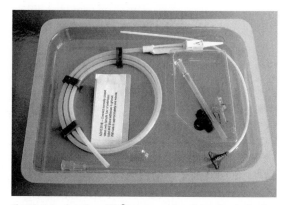

Fig. 13.4 A polyurethane Mila® long-term catheter is introduced using the 'Seldinger' over-the-wire technique.

This *'over-the wire'* technique allows entry into a vein without a cut-down and results in minimal trauma to the surrounding tissues because small-gauge needles are used to seat the stainless-steel wire inside the vascular lumen. This technique is rather cumbersome and requires some experience. Wire breakage and wire embolism are potentially serious complications of this technique.

The *'catheter-through-catheter'* principle is also used in the horse. These polyurethane catheters are introduced through a polypropylene cannula, which is inserted into the vein over a stylet. The catheter is packed in a sterile plastic sleeve that fits tightly into the cannula, so the catheter can be fed into the vein without being touched. Following this, the cannula should be backed out of the vein and the catheter fixed in place. Although asepsis is more easily maintained with this technique, the cannula cannot be removed completely because its diameter is smaller than the hub of the catheter. Therefore, it must remain attached to the extravenous part of the catheter. This is not only impractical but makes it difficult to fix the catheter to the skin. As a compromise in horses, the cannula is usually left in the vein as a protective sheath around the proximal part of the catheter. However, this increases the rate of thrombosis and decreases the longevity of the catheter. In some catheter designs this cannula can be split and therefore can be removed totally, regardless of the size of the catheter hub.

The standard catheter design consists of a catheter with a hub for connection of an extension, a fluid line or an injection cap. The presence of the hub at the level of the insertion site has several disadvantages (kinking, irritation, contamination). Alternative catheter designs with an integrated or 'swaged-on' extension, continuous with the intravascular part of the catheter, are now available in most brands.

Different designs are utilised for fixation of the catheter to the skin at the insertion site. There are catheters with simple hubs, hubs with 'wing' supports for suture fixation and 'thumb' supports on cannulae that can be incorporated into a skin suture.

Some recent catheter designs contain haemostatic valves. If a catheter becomes disconnected, retrograde flow of blood or normograde flow of air through the catheter is impossible.

Large-gauge (10G and 12G) catheters permit rapid administration of large volumes of fluid but are more thrombogenic and unsuitable for long-term use. Smaller gauge polyurethane catheters (16G) should be used for long-term intravenous catheterisation for the administration of medications and can be maintained for up to 30 days with minimal complications.

How to place a catheter
Intravenous catheters are usually placed in one of the jugular veins. The jugular veins are large and easy to catheterise and allow for easy access to and maintenance of the catheter. The disadvantage of using the jugular veins are that if thrombosis and/or thrombophlebitis occur they can have severe and life-threatening consequences (e.g. oedema of the head). Alternatively the cephalic (Fig. 13.5) or lateral thoracic veins can be used. These veins are less easy to

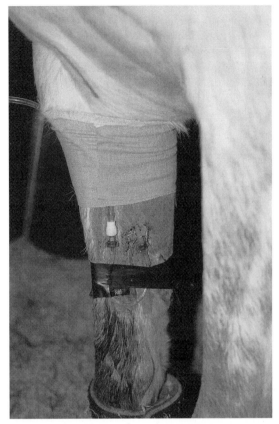

Fig. 13.5 A Teflon Angiocatheter® placed in the cephalic vein.

access but the sequelae of thrombophlebitis are less severe in these locations. Although the saphenous vein of the hindlimbs can be used, catheter placement and handling may be dangerous and it is often difficult to maintain a catheter in this location for any length of time.

The following is a list of materials required for venous catheterisation in the horse:

- Catheter of choice for given purpose
- Clippers
- Zinc oxide tape
- Surgical scrub and surgical spirit
- Sterile gloves
- Local anaesthetic agent
- Scalpel blade (optional)
- 20-Gauge hypodermic needle
- Suture material or Superglue

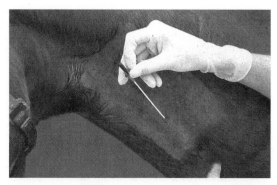

Fig. 13.6 Introduction of a polyurethane Mila® catheter in normograde fashion into the left jugular vein using an 'over-the-needle' technique. Note that the surrounding area has been clipped, aseptically prepared and sterile gloves are worn.

- Extension piece with zinc oxide tape wings (T-piece)
- Injection cap or three-way tap
- Fluid line coil for fluid replacement
- Heparinised saline (10 IU/ml).

Technique (Fig. 13.6)
- It is essential that catheters are placed using an aseptic technique. The operator should wear sterile gloves.
- A wide area of skin should be clipped over the cranial two-thirds of the jugular vein and then aseptically prepared. Catheters should not be placed in the distal one-third of the neck because inadvertent puncture of the carotid is more likely.
- A subcutaneous bleb of local anaesthetic solution should be deposited subcutaneously over the vein.
- A small stab incision can be made through the skin at the catheterisation site. However, this may lead to unnecessarily large or deep incisions in inexperienced hands.
- The direction of catheter placement is controversial. Some clinicians argue that catheters should be placed against the direction of blood flow (retrograde), to minimise the risk of air embolism should the catheter become disconnected (this argument obviously does not apply to catheters with haemostatic valves). Others argue that catheters placed in an antegrade manner result in decreased turbulence of blood flow and consequently decreased irritation of the endothelium. Antegrade catheter placement also allows for easier recognition of inadvertent penetration of the carotid artery and more rapid fluid administration.
- The catheter should be advanced through the skin into the vein at a reasonably acute angle (about 70°) until blood wells up in the hub. If inadvertent puncture of the carotid artery occurs, blood will spurt from the hub of the catheter. If this occurs then the catheter and stylet should be withdrawn immediately and firm pressure applied to the site for at least 5 min. Once blood is observed in the hub, the angle of advancement is reduced so that the catheter comes to lie almost parallel with the skin (20–30°) and the catheter and stylet are advanced together into the vein until the hub reaches the skin. The stylet must be held firmly together with the catheter so that the stylet cannot back out of the catheter during the procedure. Some clinicians prefer to withdraw the stylet partially from the catheter once blood is seen in the hub, before the catheter is advanced, to minimise the risk of puncturing the medial wall of the vein. This should be done only with caution because it may cause the catheter to kink; and attempts to reintroduce the stylet once it has been backed out should be avoided because this may result in cutting the catheter.
- Once the catheter has been placed within the vein, its hub should be secured to the skin with Superglue or sutures. These sutures should minimise the movement of the catheter into and out of the vein as the horse moves its neck. An extension piece or injection site with a flexible extension should be attached to the catheter and also sutured to the skin. These facilitate frequent manipulation, decrease direct handling of the catheter parts close to the skin and prolong the life of the catheter. The use of 'swaged-on' or 'integrated extension' catheters in which the intravenous part is continuous with the external part of the catheter reduces the risk of kinking or irritation of the skin. These catheters avoid the need for any connecting pieces and prevent concentration of bending forces at the level of the skin portal.

• The inclusion of a coiled fluid line that stretches as the horse moves around its box is essential if horses are left unattended as fluids are being administered (see Fig. 1.1). The coiled line helps to minimise tension on the catheter and therefore reduce the possibility of catheter problems. The fluid line should be fixed to the patient's mane or halter to avoid undue tension on the catheter and its connections.

• It is advisable to apply a protective bandage over the catheter in foals to prevent contamination, because they spend considerable amounts of time lying down, and to prevent interference by the mare.

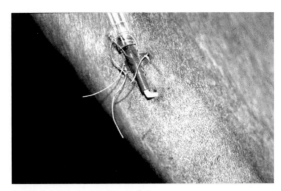

Fig. 13.7 A kinked polyurethane catheter.

Monitoring and maintenance

A catheterised vein should be checked several times each day for increased firmness, heat, pain, discharge or swelling. If any of these signs arise, the catheter should be removed *immediately*.

Proper disciplined management of the catheter is indicated, especially at the level of the hub where movement is greatest and where the catheter connections (three-way taps, extensions, fluid lines, injection caps) are attached. Any manipulation of the catheter or its connections should be performed, with care, as aseptically as possible.

Prior to injection into the catheter, the injection cap should be cleaned with antiseptic or spirit and allowed to air dry before introduction of a needle. Narrow-gauge (23 or 21 G) needles should be used and the number of times the cap is penetrated should be kept to a minimum. Different drugs administered at the same time should be injected through the same needle.

Every time a catheter is used for drug administration, it should be flushed with 10–20 ml of heparinised saline (10 000 IU heparin to 1 l of Ringer's solution or saline, giving a final concentration of 10 IU/ml). This ensures that all of the potentially irritating drug is flushed into the vein and prevents occlusion of the catheter by blood clots. During intravenous fluid administration, fluid bags should be checked regularly to ensure that they do not run empty, because the catheter may rapidly become obstructed by a thrombus. Stiff catheters or wide-bore catheters should not be left in the vein for more than 3

days. It is always preferable to replace a catheter and to use a different venous access site rather than leave the same catheter in the one vein for too long.

Catheter-related complications

Kinking/backing out/catheter movement (see Fig. 13.7). The degree of catheter kinking is dependent on the movement, softness and construction of the hub of the catheter.

It is essential that the catheter is carefully secured to the skin to prevent kinking of the catheter as the horse moves its neck. The softness of the material also will affect its tendency to kink. Very soft materials are so flexible that they cannot kink and the very rigid materials are sufficiently stiff not to do so. Materials of intermediate softness (e.g. Teflon) tend to kink most frequently.

Catheters usually kink at the transition between the catheter and the hub. The newer catheter designs with integrated extensions are superior because they do not contain this weakness.

Kinking may result in irritation and thrombosis, blocking of the catheter, leakage of the fluid subcutaneously and catheter breakage.

Breaking/leakage. Foreign body embolism as a result of a broken catheter can result from catheter laceration with the stylet during insertion or from frequent bending and kinking of the catheter at the hub. A broken catheter usually lodges in the heart or the lungs, from where it is virtually impossible to retrieve.

245

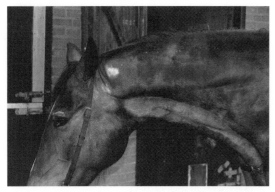

Fig. 13.8 Thrombophlebitis following intravenous catheterisation of the jugular vein. The vein is occluded and hard, warm and painful on palpation.

Disconnection. Disconnection of the catheter from a fluid line or injection cap may lead to death of the patient. It remains unclear whether this is due to massive air embolism or exsanguination. The use of catheters with haemostatic valves obviously eliminates the occurrence of these complications.

Thrombosis. All catheters are thrombogenic. Thrombus formation usually occurs as a result of trauma during catheter placement (puncture or cut-down), excessive catheter movement or excessive duration of catheterisation. Thrombus formation is more common in horses that are excessively dehydrated, endotoxaemic or septicaemic and therefore extra vigilance should be taken in very sick animals.

Thrombophlebitis (Fig. 13.8). Thrombophlebitis occurs when thrombosis is complicated by catheter contamination. The most common source of catheter contamination is the skin. Skin bacteria are introduced during catheter placement, following contamination of the hub from the surrounding skin or from manipulation of the intravenous line. Thrombophlebitis may result in abscessation of the vein and can cause septicaemia.

Jugular occlusion. Unilateral jugular occlusion will not impair blood drainage from the head significantly, although it may result in external signs of unilateral venous congestion. Bilateral occlusion, however, may result in marked nasal oedema

and life-threatening dyspnoea, requiring emergency tracheostomy.

Embolism. Embolism can occur secondary to air leakage, catheter breakage or laceration, breakage of the introduction wire, thrombosis or thrombophlebitis.

Blood transfusion

Indications

The objectives of a blood transfusion are to expand the circulatory volume and to supplement red blood cells to improve the oxygen delivery to the tissues. The benefits from a blood transfusion are temporary, providing supplemental blood until the recipient's bone marrow responds and produces new red blood cells.

Whole blood transfusion may be indicated following acute and severe blood loss (e.g. during surgery, accidental trauma, guttural pouch mycosis or parturition accidents), after chronic blood loss or in the treatment of anaemia resulting from red blood cell destruction (haemolysis) in neonatal erythrolysis or other haemolytic anaemias.

In general, a blood transfusion is indicated after an acute haemorrhage if more than one-third of the total blood volume has been lost (~15 L in a 500-kg horse with a total blood volume of ~45 L) or if the PCV falls below 15%. It should be considered, however, that after acute blood loss significant changes in PCV and total protein may not be evident until 12–24 h after the haemorrhage, due to release of red blood cells from the spleen. Therefore, the absolute PCV is not as important an indicator of the need for a blood transfusion as the rate at which the PCV falls. Following acute and severe haemorrhage, the effective circulating volume will be depleted and the horse will show signs of hypovolaemia. It is important that the circulating volume is restored by administration of crystalloids or hypertonic saline in addition to the administration of whole blood.

In horses with chronic blood loss or haemolytic anaemia, the gradual onset of the condition means that the effective circulating volume is maintained and therefore lower PCVs may be tolerated. Transfusion should be considered if the PCV falls below 8%.

Selection of a donor

Potential blood donors should be identified locally before the need for blood arises. A suitable donor should: be a stallion, gelding or maiden mare, be healthy and vaccinated, weigh at least 450 kg and have a normal PCV and total plasma protein concentration. At least 30 blood factors, such as red blood cell antigens and alloantibodies, have been identified in horses. The antigens have been classed into the seven blood systems: A, C, D, K, P, Q and U. As there are over 400 000 possible equine blood types, a true 'universal donor' does not exist and a totally compatible blood transfusion is unlikely. If screening is possible, Aa and Qa negative horses that are also negative for alloantibodies offer the best choice for donors to recipients of unknown blood type.

For a summary of the various factors involved in choosing a donor for blood transfusion, see Summary 13.1.

Summary 13.1 Blood transfusion

- Ideally the donor and recipient blood should be cross-matched before transfusion to prevent problems with either agglutination or lysis of the donor or recipient red blood cells during transfusion. However, this requires laboratory work and a time delay. A simple screen for agglutination can be carried out by mixing donor serum with recipient red blood cells and looking for agglutination (clumping) of the red blood cells.
- Most horses share dominant blood groups and a serious transfusion reaction is unlikely provided that the donor and recipient horses have not been transfused before.
- Ideally choose a previously untransfused gelding of the same type/breed as the donor.
- Bleed the donor horse using a strict aseptic technique via a wide-gauge jugular catheter into blood collection bags (commercially available) containing ACD (acid citrate dextrose) as the anticoagulant. These should be gently agitated periodically during collection to ensure adequate mixing of the blood and anticoagulant. Blood can be collected into bottles with an ACD/blood ratio of 1:15.
- Up to 10 l of blood can be collected from a healthy 500-kg donor horse.

Volume of blood to transfuse

The transfusion should not exceed 20% of the total blood volume, calculated as 8% of bodyweight. Volume overload should be considered in smaller patients, especially foals. A more precise estimate of the volume required can be obtained from the following calculation:

Litres of blood required

$$= \frac{(\text{Desired PCV} - \text{PCV of recipient})}{\text{PCV of donor}} \times \frac{(\text{Bodyweight in kg} \times 0.08)}{\text{PCV of donor}}$$

Storage of blood

Whole blood is usually administered immediately, although whole blood in ACD may be stored in a refrigerator at 4°C for up to 3 weeks.

Administration of blood

Blood is delivered through an administration set with an in-line filter. An intravenous catheter should be placed in the recipient. Blood is delivered slowly at 0.1 ml/kg (slow drip) for 10 min while the horse is closely monitored for signs of increased heart rate, increased respiratory rate, trembling, restlessness, urticaria or collapse. If no adverse reactions are seen in the first 10 min, blood may be administered at a rate of 20 ml/kg/h. If signs of an adverse reaction occur, flunixin meglumine (1.1 mg/kg) should be administered. If signs improve, transfusion can be continued but at a slower rate. In cases of severe reaction, administration of adrenaline, high-volume intravenous polyionic fluids and prednisolone sodium succinate should be considered.

Plasma transfusion

Indications

Plasma transfusion is indicated in:

(1) Foals with failure of passive transfer and immunoglobulin G levels less than 400 mg/dl in order to boost the levels of circulating immunoglobulins and reduce the risk of sepsis.

(2) In adult horses with severe hypoalbuminaemia (usually secondary to protein loss from the gastrointestinal tract) to support the plasma colloidal osmotic pressure. Plasma transfusion should be considered in horses with signs of peripheral oedema and a total protein concentration of less than 40 g/dl.

(3) Horses with disseminated intravascular coagulation, to supply additional clotting factors.

Sources

Either commercially available plasma or plasma collected from another horse (e.g. the foal's dam) may be used. If plasma is collected from another horse, whole blood should be collected as described above and the bags left to hang for several hours to allow for sedimentation of the red blood cells. The supernatant plasma then may be siphoned or decanted from the settled red cells, with an expected plasma yield of 40–50% of the total blood volume collected. Plasma may be stored frozen at 0°C for at least 1 year.

Administration of plasma

It is not possible to calculate the precise volume of plasma required due to individual variation in redistribution from the vascular space and loss of protein. As a general rule, foals with complete failure of passive transfer need 2–4 l of intravenous plasma over a 2–4-day period. The foal's immunoglobulin G levels should be monitored daily and further transfusions performed as required. Adult horses will generally require a minimum of 6–8 l of plasma to increase their plasma protein by 5–10 g/dl.

Further reading

Durham, A.E. (1996) Blood and plasma transfusion in the horse. *Equine Vet. Educ.* **8**(1), 8–12.

Ecker, G.L. (1995) Fluid and ion regulation: a primer on water and ion losses during exercise. *Equine Vet. Educ.* **7**(4), 210–215.

Seahom, T.L. & Comick-Seahom, J. (1994) Fluid therapy. *Vet. Clinics N. Am.: Equine Practice* **10**(3), 517–525.

Medical Nursing

J. D. Slater

Infectious and non-infectious disease

Definitions

- *Infectious diseases* are caused by bacteria, viruses, fungi and protozoa.
- *Contagious diseases* are transmissible between animals or between animals and people (these are zoonotic diseases). Many, but not all, infectious diseases are therefore also contagious.
- Some horses become *carriers* of infectious disease and may shed the organism continuously or intermittently. In *persistently infected* carriers the organism is shed continuously (e.g. *Streptococcus equi* carriers). In *latently infected* carriers, the organism is shed intermittently during periods of reactivation (e.g. equine herpes virus carriers).
- *Transmission* of contagious disease can be *direct* (from animal to animal by physical contact) or *indirect* (via aerosols, discharges or via grooms, nurses or veterinary surgeons). Some infectious agents can survive in the environment for long enough to infect the horse indirectly via feed bowls, water troughs or bedding. Objects that transmit pathogens are called *fomites*.
- Some infectious diseases are transmitted by *vectors*, e.g. mites and midges.
- *Non-infectious diseases* are diseases that are not caused by bacteria, viruses, fungi or protozoa.

Infectious and contagious disease

Infectious and contagious diseases are extremely important in horses. Contagious diseases are especially important in groups of young horses, e.g. in training yards. Controlling the spread of infectious and contagious diseases in yards and in equine veterinary hospitals is a fundamental goal of management and nursing strategies. Infectious diseases can be controlled in yards by:

- Isolation and testing of new horses
- Isolation and testing of horses with clinical signs of disease
- Strict hygiene precautions
- Vaccination

In equine veterinary hospitals precautions must be taken to recognise and isolate infectious disease cases to prevent spread to other hospitalised horses (see Chapter 1).

Vaccination is possible for some of the equine infectious diseases, notably tetanus and influenza. Vaccines aim to produce an effective and appropriate immune response against that microorganism by stimulating the effector cells of the immune system: the lymphocytes (see Table 14.1). There are essentially two types of vaccine: *killed* or *live*. Killed vaccines are the most common and consist either of whole bacteria/viruses or of part ('sub-units') of the

Table 14.1 Types of vaccines and their action

Lymphocyte type	Function	Required in	Stimulated by
B Lymphocyte	Produces antibody	Virus infections Bacterial infections	Killed vaccines Live vaccines
T Lymphocyte	Kills infected cells	Virus infections Certain bacteria, e.g. *R. equi*	Live vaccines

bacterium/virus, e.g. surface proteins. Live vaccines are modified versions of the living bacterium/virus that do not cause disease but produce immunity. There are no live vaccines for use in horses in the UK at present, but other countries do have live equine vaccinations available, e.g. there is a live intranasal equine influenza vaccination in the USA. Vaccines can be given systemically (by intramuscular injection) or mucosaly (orally or intranasaly). All currently licensed equine vaccines in the UK are given by intramuscular injection.

Respiratory system diseases

Respiratory diseases are the most common and important group of medical diseases affecting horses. Along with colic they account for the majority of equine medical consultations. There are many different equine respiratory diseases but they can be grouped into four broad categories:

(1) Infectious upper respiratory tract disease (IURD)
(2) Non-infectious upper respiratory tract disease (NIURD)
(3) Infectious lower respiratory tract disease (ILRD)
(4) Non-infectious lower respiratory tract disease (NILRD)

The most important respiratory diseases are in the IURD group (e.g. equine influenza virus infections) and the NILRD group (e.g. chronic obstructive pulmonary disease).

These four groups of respiratory disease have the following characteristics:

- IURD: mainly young horses, often occurs as outbreaks, depression, pyrexia, nasal discharge, coughing, lymphadenopathy; no dyspnoea, no abnormalities on lung auscultation.
- NIURD: any age of horse, usually single cases only, nasal discharge, epistaxis, possibly facial swelling.
- ILRD: any age of horse, coughing, nasal discharge, depression, dyspnoea, tachypnoea, pyrexia, abnormal lung auscultation, ± pleural effusion.
- NILRD: often older horses, coughing, nasal discharge, dyspnoea, tachypnoea, exercise intolerance, lung auscultation abnormal; no depression, no pyrexia, no lymphadenopathy.

Although coughing is a specific clinical sign for respiratory disease, in horses it is not (in contrast to small animals) a sensitive indicator of respiratory disease.

Flexible endoscopes are used frequently in the investigation of respiratory disease in the horse. Proper care and disinfection of these instruments is an important nursing duty to avoid spread of infection from horse to horse, damage to the instruments or to the personnel using them (see How to . . . 14.1).

Infectious upper respiratory tract disease (IURD)

- Equine influenza virus (EIV)
- Equine herpes virus (EHV)
- Equine viral arteritis (EVA)
- Equine rhinovirus (ERV)
- Adenovirus
- *Streptococcus equi* (S. equi)
- Sinusitis
- Guttural pouch empyema
- Guttural pouch mycosis

Equine influenza virus (EIV)

Aetiology

The EIV is a virus that undergoes frequent genetic changes to produce different virus strains. This is called 'antigenic drift' and is responsible for frequent outbreaks of disease that may spread globally. The Far East is implicated as the main source of new virus strains.

The EIV is classified into two groups (A equi 1 and A equi 2) based on its surface proteins: A equi 1 viruses

How to ... 14.1

Cleaning an endoscope

- The endoscope should be cleaned as soon as possible after use to prevent mucus drying within the instrument.
- The endoscope should be wiped over with a prorietary cleaning solution such as 'Endoscope dettol'.
- The biopsy channel then should be flushed with the same solution and a cleaning brush put down the channel to remove debris.
- The channel should be flushed again.
- The instrument should be connected to the power unit and a disinfectant solution aspirated through the flushing channel. This should be rinsed using water.
- Air and water buttons should be depressed to blow out all remaining water from the system.
- The outside of the endoscope may be wiped over with a solution of 70% alcohol.
- The endoscope then should be hung up to dry.
- Some endoscopes are now fully immersible and a leak test should be performed before immersion to ensure that fluid will not enter the optic system.
- Wherever possible, endoscopes should be sterilised using ethylene oxide at the end of the day because this is a more effective means of sterilisation than chemical solutions. Like arthroscopy equipment, this type of fibre-optic equipment would be damaged by heat sterilisation.
- Care must be taken not to coil the endoscope excessively prior to gas sterilisation because this will damage the optical fibres.
- Always check the exact protocol with the manufacterer (see further reading list) (see Fig 14.1).

have not been isolated in the UK for 15 years. Vaccines generally contain a mixture of both A *equi* 1 and A *equi* 2 viruses.

Pathogenesis

Infection is acquired mainly by inhalation of virus via aerosols from other infected horses or via virus-containing droplets in the horse's environment. Indirect transmission via feed buckets or grooms/handlers/nurses/veterinary surgeons is possible. However, virus survival outside the horse is limited.

The virus replicates mainly in the upper respiratory tract (nasal cavity, pharynx and proximal trachea), causing epithelial destruction. Clinical signs are due to local epithelial damage and the systemic inflammatory and immune response to infection. The virus generally does not cause viraemia (virus particles in the blood stream).

Clinical signs

- Short incubation period
- Clinical signs usually appear within 1–5 days of exposure
- Generally transient, self-limiting disease resolving within 3–6 weeks provided that horses are well managed
- Pyrexia (up to 42°C)
- Depression
- Inappetence
- Conjunctivitis and ocular discharge
- Nasal discharge, initially serous but becoming mucopurulent after 4–5 days
- Lymphadenopathy, especially the submandibular lymph nodes
- Coughing
- Generally no lower respiratory tract signs
- Horses may experience chronic poor performance syndromes after the initial acute phase of infection

Diagnosis

- History.
- Clinical signs.
- *Haematology* may reveal reduced total white blood cell counts (leucopenia) with reduced lymphocytes (lymphopenia) within the first 7–14 days after infection. This may be followed by an increase in total white blood cell counts (leucocytosis) with associated increase in lymphocyte numbers (lymphocytosis) between 14–28 days after infection. At this stage the numbers of lymphocytes may exceed the number of neutrophils. This is referred to as a 'reverse ratio' and is usually taken as evidence of virus infection (in the normal horse there are more neutrophils than lymphocytes, i.e. the neutrophil/lymphocyte ratio is 2:1). Note that this is not a specific change for EIV infections but rather a non-specific change seen with most virus infections.

- *Virology*: demonstration of virus antigens in nasal or nasopharyngeal swabs collected early in infection (within 7–10 days of exposure) confirms the diagnosis. This is done using the quick (same-day) and reliable fluorescent antibody test.
- *Serology*: demonstration of rising antibody titres on paired serum samples taken 10–14 days apart confirms exposure to virus. A high titre on a single sample is also considered diagnostic. The assay used is the single radial haemolysis (SRH) assay.

Treatment and nursing
- Isolate.
- Rest for at least 3 weeks.
- Improve stable management: switch to dust-free bedding and feed-soaked hay, or better still haylage. Palatable short feed should be offered to promote food intake. Water intake should be monitored, although inadequate water intake is seldom a significant nursing problem with EIV cases.
- Broad-spectrum antibiotics (e.g. potentiated sulphonamides) are generally used to prevent secondary bacterial infection.
- Other drugs are used occasionally to improve removal of discharge from the airway (e.g. mucolytics).
- In the USA, immunomodulators ('immuno-stimulants') are used by some, although none are licensed in the UK.

Prevention
The EIV is difficult to control by management alone because horses are kept for competition and so are routinely transported and mixed extensively. Vaccination is therefore the means by which EIV is controlled. Vaccination is compulsory under Jockey Club and Federation Equestre Internationale (FEI) rules in the UK. Most vaccines are whole killed virus vaccines (e.g. 'Duvaxyn' from Fort Dodge Animal Health; 'Prevac' from Intervet) but a 1 sub-unit 'Iscom' vaccine is also available ('Equip', from Schering-Plough Animal Health). All currently available EIV vaccines are administered intramuscularly (see Chapter 11).

Equine hepes virus (EHV)

Aetiology
- Of the nine herpes viruses identified to date, EHV-1 and EHV-4 are the most important in the UK.
- Both viruses cause respiratory disease.
- EHV-1 also causes abortion, neurological disease and ocular disease and is consequently regarded as the more significant of the two viruses.
- Both viruses establish latent infections in which the carrier horse is normal but sheds infectious virus intermittently and usually asymptomatically when stressed, e.g. while at race meetings, events, shows or when hospitalised.

Pathogenesis
Infections with EHV-1 and EHV-4 are acquired by the respiratory route, mainly by aerosols. Indirect transmission is also important, especially from abortions where uterine fluids may contain large amounts of virus. There is some potential for indirect transmission although virus survival outside the horse is limited. After inhalation, both viruses replicate in the upper respiratory tract and cause epithelial destruction and associated clinical signs. The EHV-1 invades through the epithelium and causes viraemia, which can persist up to 21 days after infection. Viraemia distributes virus to the uterus, nervous system and eye. Abortion usually occurs in the last one-third of pregnancy. Neurological and ocular disease occur during or shortly after the viraemic phase of infection

Clinical signs
- Short incubation period
- Clinical signs usually appear within 1–5 days of exposure
- Pyrexia (up to 42°C)
- Depression
- Inappetence
- Conjunctivitis and ocular discharge
- Nasal discharge, initially serous but becoming mucopurulent after 4–5 days
- Lymphadenopathy, especially the submandibular lymph nodes
- Coughing
- Pneumonia may occur in foals with both EHV-1 and EHV-4

- Abortion in the last third of pregnancy (EHV-1)
- Paresis or paralysis affecting mainly the hindlimbs within 7–21 days after infection (EHV-1)
- Retinal lesions (EHV-1).

Diagnosis
- History.
- Clinical signs.
- *Haematology*: initially leucopenia with lymphopenia followed by leucocytosis with lymphocytosis 14–28 days after infection.
- *Virology*: demonstration of virus antigens in nasal or nasopharyngeal swabs collected early in infection (within 7–10 days of exposure) by fluorescent antibody test.
- *Serology*: demonstration of rising antibody titres on paired serum samples taken 10–14 days apart confirms exposure to virus. A high titre on a single sample is also considered to be diagnostic. The assay used is the complement fixation test (CFT).

Treatment and nursing
- Isolate; this is especially important with aborting mares where barrier nursing provides the best means of controlling spread.
- Aborting mares should be monitored for signs of metritis.
- For respiratory disease, take horses out of training for at least 4 weeks and improve stable management: switch to dust-free bedding and feed-soaked hay, or better still haylage. Palatable short feed should be offered to promote food intake. Water intake should be monitored although inadequate water intake is seldom a significant nursing problem.
- For respiratory disease, broad-spectrum antibiotics (e.g. potentiated sulphonamides) are generally used to prevent secondary bacterial infection. Other drugs are occasionally used to improve removal of discharge from the airway (e.g. mucolytics).
- In the USA, immunomodulators ('immunostimulants') are used by some practitioners, although none are licensed in the UK.
- Horses with paresis or paralysis require careful nursing to prevent self-inflicted injury or becoming cast. Recumbent horses should be supported carefully to prevent skin ulceration and muscle or nerve injury. Bladder catheterisation may be required and slings may be needed to support horses with hindlimb paralysis. Some horses will warrant euthanasia on humane grounds. The use of corticosteroids in neurological cases is controversial because they may reduce inflammation in the central nervous system (CNS) but may allow increased virus replication and thus potentially cause more injury (see later section on nervous system diseases).

Prevention
As for EIV, control is based on vaccination. Vaccination is not compulsory and this, coupled with the alleged poor efficacy of current vaccines, means that a minority of horses in the UK are vaccinated. The vaccine currently available in the UK is a combined EHV-1 and EHV-4 whole-virus killed vaccine administered intramuscularly (Duvaxyn 1,4, Fort Dodge Animal Health). Vaccination is recommended every 6 months or, in pregnant mares, at months 5, 7 and 9 of pregnancy.

Equine viral arteritis (EVA)
Equine viral arteritis virus is a notifiable disease in the UK. The virus is transmitted mainly by stallions because it establishes persistent infection in some stallions, known as 'shedders', with virus shedding in semen. The virus is prevalent in Northern Europe. The UK is at risk of EVA infection via imported breeding stallions. The recommended procedures for EVA monitoring and prevention are described in a code of practice issued by the Horserace Betting Levy Board, which covers the testing, hygiene, isolation and barrier measures that should be taken. Monitoring of EVA is carried out by serology and virology on stallion genital swabs and semen. The EVA virus is transmitted by both venereal and respiratory routes and so causes respiratory disease resembling that seen for EHV-1 and also abortion. The virus may cause marked vasculitis (more than occurs with EHV infections) and thus corneal and ventral oedema can be obvious additional clinical signs. The principles of therapy are the same as for EHV-1. Vaccination can be carried out only under licence from the Ministry for Agriculture, Fisheries and Food because vaccination

produces antibodies that complicate the EVA monitoring programme. Therefore, horses that are vaccinated must be blood tested first.

Equine rhinovirus (ERV)

Equine rhinoviruses are extremely common but generally only cause mild, self-limiting upper respiratory tract disease resembling, but not as severe as, that seen for EIV with marginal pyrexia, nasal discharge, lymphadenopathy and some coughing. Diagnosis is as described for EIV, although serology is carried out using a complement fixation test. Management is also as described for EIV. There is no vaccine in the UK.

Equine adenovirus

Adenovirus infections are usually subclinical. However, adenoviruses can cause significant respiratory disease in immunocompromised foals, especially colostrum-deprived foals or Arabian foals with immunodeficiency conditions.

Streptococcus equi (strangles)
Aetiology

Strangles is caused by *Streptococcus equi* (*S. equi*). This is a Gram-positive bacterium. It is not normally found in the respiratory tract and its isolation from any horse is significant and is associated either with disease or long-term carriage of the organism. *Streptococcus equi* is an extremely common respiratory infection that affects all types of horse worldwide.

Pathogenesis

Streptococcus equi infection occurs directly from infected horses via aerosol spread and droplets. The bacteria can live for a limited time (possibly up to 3 weeks in moist conditions) in the environment and so transmission indirectly via feed utensils and personnel is a significant risk. After infection the bacteria cause local damage to the epithelium lining the upper respiratory tract but also invade to reach local lymph nodes, causing abscesses. In some cases bacteria may cause systemic infections and produce abscesses at other sites in the body, e.g. the abdomen and thorax, producing the condition known as 'bastard strangles'. Persistent infections can be estab-

lished in the guttural pouches and this appears to be the main site for long-term carriage of bacteria.

Clinical signs
- Affects mainly young horses, and clinical signs are more severe in young animals.
- *Streptococcus equi* is highly contagious: there is usually rapid spread through a group of horses, with most animals becoming infected (i.e. high morbidity).
- Initially clinical signs resemble those seen for the virus infections (EIV and EHV) with pyrexia, depression, inappetence, mucopurulent nasal discharge, lymphadenopathy and coughing.
- In classical strangles the disease progresses with abscesses developing approximately 3 weeks after infection in the submandibular and retropharyngeal lymph nodes. Other lymph nodes in the head region, e.g. the parotid lymph node, can also develop abscesses. Retropharyngeal lymph node abscesses may become sufficiently large to obstruct the airway and pharynx, producing dyspnoea and dysphagia, hence the name 'strangles'.
- Bacteria may spread into the blood and lymphatic circulations to produce metastatic abscesses in other lymph nodes or in other organs. The two main sites affected are the thorax and the abdomen. This is a chronic syndrome known as 'bastard strangles' that may have a duration of 6–9 months. It is difficult to diagnose and treat and the majority of horses with bastard strangles do not survive. Symptoms of bastard strangles are often vague but include depression, weight loss, intermittent pyrexia, colic, coughing and exercise intolerance.
- Up to 10% of cases may develop chronic abscessation of the guttural pouch (guttural pouch empyema) with persistent unilateral purulent nasal discharge, coughing and possibly dyspnoea and dysphagia if there is significant compression of the airway and pharynx. In long-standing infections the pus may become inspissated to form hard, pebble-like masses known as *chondroids*. In this case there is no nasal discharge but the horse is still infectious to others, because viable bacteria will be present in the pouch. Bacteria may persist

in the pouch for many months, with shedding possibly continuing for over 3 years in some cases.

- Some horses develop immune-mediated vasculitis ('purpura haemorrhagica'). This causes urticaria-like swellings over the proximal limbs, head and trunk, with petechial haemorrhages in mucous membranes, and is often fatal.
- Many cases do not develop abscesses or other sequelae and merely develop a transient self-limiting respiratory disease. This syndrome is referred to as 'atypical strangles' and often goes undetected.

Diagnosis
- History.
- Clinical signs, especially if abscesses are present, are suggestive although early cases are difficult to differentiate from virus infections.
- *Bacteriology* on nasal and nasopharyngeal swabs confirms the diagnosis.
- *Endoscopy* is required to identify guttural pouch empyema.
- *Radiography* and *ultrasonography* are useful to confirm the presence of retropharyngeal lymph node abscesses.

Treatment and nursing
The treatment of strangles with antibiotics provokes strong and conflicting opinion amongst clinicians. The bacteria are usually sensitive to penicillins but there is concern that antibiotic treatment may promote abscess formation and delay recovery. Many practices do not use antibiotics at any stage of infection whereas others treat with antibiotics in the early stages of infection to improve welfare and to reduce shedding of bacteria from infected horses. There is agreement that antibiotics should not be used once abscesses are developing. Abscesses should be managed by hot compresses to encourage maturation and bursting; large abscesses may require needle or surgical drainage. Compression of the airway may require placement of a temporary tracheotomy tube until the abscess matures and bursts or is drained. Guttural pouch empyema can be treated successfully by placing a Foley catheter into the pouch via the nose. Leaving it in place and lavaging with 1–3 L of saline/water/dilute (0.1%) povidine iodine twice

daily until the pouch is clean. Chondroids usually can be removed endoscopically using a polyp basket.

Prevention
Although strangles vaccines are widely used in the USA and Australia, there are no vaccines licensed in the UK. Control therefore relies totally on management precautions. A code of practice has been released by the Horserace Betting Levy Board that establishes standard protocols for controlling the spread of *S. equi*. The principles of control are:

- Isolate all newly arrived horses
- Collect nasal or nasopharyngeal swabs at weekly intervals
- Only allow new arrivals to join the group once they have had three negative swabs
- Investigate suspected cases promptly
- Isolate clinical cases immediately and maintain strict barrier nursing
- Confirm that recovered cases are bacteriologically negative before re-entering the herd.

Sinusitis
The important sinuses clinically are the maxillary and frontal sinuses. In the horse the frontal sinus drains into the maxillary sinus, which in turn drains into the nasal cavity. The sinuses connect to and are extensions of the nasal cavity (see anatomy section, Chapter 2).

Aetiology
Sinusitis can develop secondary to any of the viral or bacterial upper respiratory tract infections but clinically apparent sinusitis is associated with bacterial infection of the sinuses. The most common bacterium involved is *Streptococcus zooepidemicus*, although a variety of other Gram-positive as well as Gram-negative bacteria can be involved. The most common presentation is maxillary sinusitis secondary to cheek tooth abscessation, because the caudal four cheek teeth (premolar 4–molar 3) have their residual crown in the maxillary sinus.

Clinical signs
- Chronic, foul smelling, unilateral nasal discharge

- The affected sinus is dull on percussion and may be painful
- There is usually little or no facial swelling
- If the primary problem is dental there will be quidding
- Ipsilateral submandibular lymphadenopathy.

Diagnosis
- History and clinical examination are useful
- Radiography will confirm the presence of pus in the sinus and dental disease
- Sinoscopy can be used to visualise the sinus directly.

Treatment and nursing
- Remove the diseased tooth by surgical repulsion via the maxillary sinus
- Lavage (5–10 L of water or dilute (0.1%) povidone iodine) the sinus via an indwelling Foley catheter to remove accumulated pus (this may take 2–3 weeks)
- If the sinusitis is primary then treat by lavage
- Systemic antibiotics are not useful.

Guttural pouch empyema

This is usually secondary to strangles infection (see above) although other bacteria, especially *Streptococcus zooepidemicus*, can be the cause. In *S. equi* infections bacteria may enter the pouch directly from the nasopharynx or may enter via rupture of retropharyngeal lymph node abscesses into the pouch (see Example 14.1). Clinical signs are:

- Persistent mainly unilateral purulent nasal discharge
- Ipsilateral retropharyngeal lymphadenopathy
- Possible swelling in the retropharyngeal region
- Occasionally compression of the airway and pharynx, producing dyspnoea and dysphagia

Treatment by guttural pouch lavage via a Foley catheter is generally successful.

Guttural pouch mycosis

This is an uncommon but life-threatening condition that is due to fungal infection (usually *Aspergillus fumigatus*) in the guttural pouch. The fungus colonises and erodes through the wall of the internal carotid artery in the pouch and may also damage the cranial nerves (numbers IX, X and XII) supplying the larynx and pharynx that travel through the pouch. This results in:

- Large-volume epistaxis, which may be fatal
- Dysphagia
- Dyspnoea.

All suspected cases should be investigated promptly (although investigation during an epistaxis episode is difficult) by endoscopy of the pouch to confirm the presence of fungi and damage to the arterial wall. Treatment is surgical and involves ligation of the internal carotid artery and inclusion of an angioplasty balloon proximal to the haemorrhage site.

Non-infectious upper respiratory tract disease (NIURD)

- Recurrent laryngeal neuropathy (RLN)
- Dorsal displacement of the soft palate (DDSP)
- Epiglottic entrapment
- Fourth branchial arch defects

These are conditions of the larynx and pharynx. They all cause inspiratory noise during exercise and are important causes of poor performance.

Recurrent laryngeal neuropathy

Recurrent laryngeal neuropathy (RLN) occurs mainly in horses over 16 hands, especially thoroughbreds. It is due to degeneration of the nerve (recurrent laryngeal nerve) that supplies the abductor muscle of the larynx. This results in the horse being unable to open its larynx fully during exercise, causing obstruction to airflow and inspiratory noise during exercise. This varies from whistling sounds through to harsh, loud, roaring noises. Signs are unusual in young horses (<5 years old). History and clinical examination (palpation of the larynx may reveal muscle wastage and reduced movement) are useful pointers but definitive diagnosis requires endoscopy. Treatment is surgical: ventriculectomy and chordectomy (Hobday procedure), prosthetic laryngoplasty ('tie back' procedure) or nerve-muscle pedicle grafts. Although permanent tracheostomies have been used in some horses, it is now less common.

Example 14.1 Strangles

A pony that had strangles 3 months ago is in your hospital because it now has difficulty breathing and swallowing. The pony makes inspiratory noise and has some food material at its nostrils while eating. It does not have a purulent nasal discharge.

This pony almost certainly has a large retropharyngeal lymph node abscess that is compressing the larynx and pharynx. It presents two nursing problems:

(1) It should be regarded as contagious and must be isolated.
(2) The laryngeal and pharyngeal obstruction may become life threatening.

The pony should be housed in a separate area of the hospital. A limited number of staff, ideally one staff member, should deal with the pony and only after attending to their other cases. Feed, utensils and headcollars should not leave the stable or be used on other horses. All people entering the stable should wear overalls dedicated to that stable, change into wellington boots or put on overshoes and wear gloves. Theatre caps should be considered. Disinfectant should be available outside the stable to clean footwear on leaving the stable. The abscess should be managed by twice-daily hot compresses to encourage the abscess to mature and burst. In the meantime the pony should be monitored carefully and a temporary tracheostomy tube may need to be placed to relieve the dyspnoea. The pony also should be monitored for signs of aspiration pneumonia. Antibiotics should not be used on this pony. Soft, palatable feed should be offered, e.g. soaked cubes to facilitate swallowing. The pony should be fed from the ground to minimise the risk of feed inhalation while swallowing.

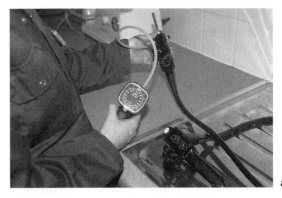
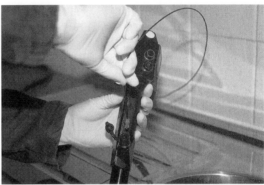
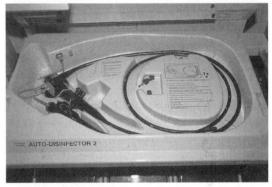

Fig. 14.1 A video endoscope. (a) Before the endoscope is immersed, it must be pressure tested for leaks. (b) After rinsing the biopsy channel it should be cleaned thoroughly with a brush. (c) The endoscope should be placed in a washing bath for disinfection once the exterior has been wiped down, the channels have been rinsed and the biopsy channel has been brushed.

Dorsal displacement of the soft palate

Dorsal displacement of the soft palate (DDSP) causes acute obstruction of the airway because the soft palate is displaced from its normal position below the epiglottis and is sucked into the airway during exercise. This produces loud choking noises and the horse usually will stop running until the palate repositions itself. Diagnosis is difficult and requires video endoscopy (see Fig. 14.1) on a high-speed treadmill.

Treatment requires identification and elimination of any underlying respiratory disease and possibly surgical modification of the soft palate.

Epiglottic entrapment

Epiglottic entrapment describes a condition where the epiglottis becomes trapped in a fold of soft tissue that runs between the base of the epiglottis and the tongue. Diagnosis is by endoscopy. Treatment is surgical and involves sectioning the soft-tissue fold.

Fourth branchial arch defects

Fourth branchial arch defects are congenital defects in which some regions of the larynx and pharynx fail to develop properly from the fourth branchial arch. Diagnosis is by endoscopy and there is no effective treatment.

Infectious lower respiratory tract disease (ILRD)

- Pleuropneumonia
- *Rhodococcus equi*
- *Dictyocaulus arnfieldi*
- *Parascaris equorum*

Pleuropneumonia

Aetiology

Pleuropneumonia is a serious, potentially fatal, bacterial infection of the lungs and pleura causing pneumonia and pleural effusion/pleuritis (fluid in the pleural space). Although it is uncommon in UK it is very important to recognise and treat this condition promptly, because it can be rapidly fatal (see Example 14.2). Affected horses often have a history of recent stress, e.g. lengthy transport or surgery. A wide range of bacteria may be involved, although *S. zooepidemicus* is a common isolate.

Clinical signs
- Pyrexia
- Depression
- Tachypnoea
- Dyspnoea
- Thoracic pain
- Weight loss

> ## Example 14.2 Pleuropneumonia
>
> *A 9-year-old sport horse had a lengthy arthroscopy procedure in your clinic 2 days ago. This morning when you carry out your routine assessment of the inpatients you find that it is depressed and has pyrexia, nasal discharge and difficulty breathing. What do you do?*
>
> This horse is very likely to have pleuropneumonia. You should record the clinical parameters in the case notes and get help immediately. The vet may suspect pleuropneumonia on the basis of the clinical examination (decreased breathing sounds in the ventral thorax and demonstration of a fluid line on thoracic percussion). An ultrasound examination will confirm the presence of pleural fluid. The horse will require intensive therapy and nursing: pleural drainage and lavage, intravenous antibiotics, intravenous fluids (to replace fluid lost into the pleural space) and systemic non-steroidal anti-inflammatory drugs (to provide pain relief and protect against endotoxaemia). The horse should be monitored closely and handled carefully and quietly throughout treatment. It should be offered soft, palatable feed and free access to water. These cases are a major challenge but treatment is worthwhile because recovery is usually complete.

- Coughing
- Foul-smelling (often bloody) nasal discharge
- Rapid deterioration
- Decreased breathing sounds ventrally, with abnormal lung sounds dorsally
- Percussion reveals loss of resonance ventrally and this delineates the level of pleural fluid.

Diagnosis
- Radiography and ultrasonography are helpful for confirmation
- Collect pleural fluid and nasal discharge for bacteriology.

Treatment and nursing
- Aggressive treatment is needed
- Drain pleural fluid (insert the drain in intercostal spaces 7, 8 or 9 on either left or right sides) and lavage with large-volume sterile saline
- Broad-spectrum antibiotics i.v., e.g. penicillin, gentamycin and metronidazole

- Non-steroidal anti-inflammatory drugs (NSAIDs), e.g. flunixin
- Intravenous fluids.

Rhodococcus equi

Rhodococcus equi is a soil-borne bacterium and in some regions is an important cause of pneumonia in older foals (up to 6 months old). Dense stocking and dusty, dry weather are important predisposing factors. Two main syndromes occur:

(1) The acute form: foals develop acute, severe, diffuse pneumonia and die within a few days.
(2) The chronic form: localised abscesses develop in the lungs and cause depression, ill thrift (i.e. poor bodily condition) and coughing.

Occasionally gut infections occur, producing colic and diarrhoea. Tracheal lavage, bacteriology and thoracic radiography are diagnostic. Treatment is difficult and requires antibiotic treatment with erythromycin and rifampicin for 3–4 months.

Dictyocaulus arnfieldi (lungworm)

The reservoir of infection and asymptomatic host is the donkey. Infection in horses/ponies causes clinical signs but infected horses usually do not produce eggs. Clinical signs are due to migrating larvae ± adults in the lungs and resemble the signs seen with chronic obstructive pulmonary disease (COPD). Diagnosis is by demonstrating eosinophils and larvae in tracheal lavage samples. Treatment is by anthelminthics (e.g. ivermectin or fenbendazole).

Parascaris equorum

This causes disease in yearlings/young horses during their first full season at pasture. Clinical signs are due to migrating larvae through the lungs. Clinical signs are depression, coughing, nasal discharge, tachypnoea and dyspnoea. Diagnosis is by demonstrating eosinophils and larvae in tracheal lavage samples. Treatment is by anthelminthics (e.g. ivermectin or fenbendazole).

Non-infectious lower respiratory tract diseases (NILRD)

- Chronic obstructive pulmonary disease (COPD)/heaves
- Summer-pasture-associated obstructive pulmonary disease
- Foreign bodies
- Neoplasia.

Chronic obstructive pulmonary disease/heaves

Aetiology

Chronic obstructive pulmonary disease (COPD), or heaves, is very common in the UK and is the most common cause of respiratory disease in older horses. It is a pulmonary hypersensitivity to spores of fungi and moulds that are commonly found on straw and hay and are present in large concentrations in most stables, especially in stables with poor ventilation. The most common allergens associated with this disease are *Aspergillus fumigatus* and *Micropolyspora faeni*, although many other types of fungus and mould can be involved. Other allergens in stables, e.g. forage mites, also may be involved.

Pathogenesis

The disease is likely to have a genetic basis although this is not proven. When horses with COPD are exposed to allergens a complex inflammatory cascade is initiated, which results in:

- Airway inflammation
- Increase in the volume and viscosity of airway discharge
- Increased numbers of inflammatory cells (neutrophils) in the airway
- Bronchospasm
- Changes in airway and alveolar epithelium, resulting in loss of specialised cells (e.g. ciliated cells and surfactant-producing cells).

These changes occur throughout the lower respiratory tract but are particularly marked in the small airways (the bronchioles). The net result of these changes is difficulty in moving air in and out of the lung: decreased ventilation due to increased resistance to airflow along the airway and decreased compliance (elasticity) in the lung. Most of the pathology is reversible, except in end-stage disease where extensive pulmonary fibrosis may be present.

Clinical signs

Chronic obstructive pulmonary disease affects older animals, with peak age at onset being 9–10 years old. Ponies are more commonly affected than horses but all breeds and males and females are susceptible. Clinical signs initially appear slowly and are associated with stabling. Generally there will be improvement with turn out, at least in the early stages of the disease.

- Affected animals are bright, alert and usually in good condition
- There is a history of poor performance/exercise intolerance
- Tachypnoea
- Dyspnoea, particularly expiratory with double expiratory effort
- May develop a 'heave line' (hypertrophy of abdominal muscles due to chronic and severe dyspnoea)
- Nostril flare
- Nasal discharge
- Coughing is not always present
- Auscultation reveals crackling and wheezing in caudodorsal lung field in around 50% of cases.

Diagnosis

- History is extremely useful, especially one of chronic disease and an association with stabling where stables contain straw and/or hay.
- Clinical findings are also useful but many affected horses have only subtle symptoms at rest.
- *Endoscopy* is extremely valuable because it allows direct visualisation of the lower airway as well as enabling easy collection of airway lavage samples. A standard 1-m endoscope will allow examination of the cervical trachea but will not allow visualisation of the distal airway (carina and bronchial tree). A minimum length of 1.8 m is required for examination of the lower airway. Affected horses have moderate to copious quantities of mucopus in the trachea and distally with pools of discharge collecting at the thoracic inlet.
- *Tracheal lavage* (TL) and *bronchoalveolar lavage*

(BAL) are the most important samples to collect and are used for cytology and bacteriology. Affected horses have an increase in neutrophils in both locations. Tracheal lavage can be carried out with most practice endoscopes and is quick, easy and suitable for group investigations. Bronchoalveolar lavage, on the other hand, requires a long endoscope (minimum length 1.8 m) and so is often carried out using a BAL catheter. Bronchoalveolar lavage is less well tolerated than TL and horses often require sedation. It is more time consuming than TL and is less suitable for group investigations. In most situations TL samples are diagnostic but BAL samples (which provide a better quality sample) are required in some cases to establish a diagnosis.
- Simple *lung function tests* can be carried out by assessing the response to an intravenous or inhaled dose of a bronchodilator, e.g. clenbuterol (Ventipulmin®, from Boehringer Ingeheim). Measuring arterial oxygen levels at rest is usually not diagnostic unless the horse has very severe disease.
- Radiography, ultrasonography and haematology are less useful because these are usually normal in cases of COPD.

Treatment and nursing

The aims of therapy are to remove the source of allergens from the horse's environment and to reverse the changes in the airway and lung. Therapy is usually approached in a stepwise fashion:

- *Step 1: environmental management*. Turn the horse out 24 h per day or if this is not possible improve the stable environment by increasing ventilation and improving drainage. Do not use straw bedding but substitute with dust-extracted wood shavings (not sawdust), paper or rubber. Shavings and paper beds must be maintained as shallow litter because deep-litter beds promote heavy fungus and mould growth. If hay is fed it should be soaked (a 20–30-min soak for a loosely packed hay net is perfectly adequate) before use and the hay net should be eaten before it dries out again. Haylage is a better dust-free source of forage than hay. Complete cube diets provide a temporary means of achieving low dust levels in stables.

- *Step 2: bronchodilators and mucolytics.* Bronchodilators are used to reverse bronchoconstriction and improve ciliary clearance. Clenbuterol given in-feed is the most commonly used drug, although other less-potent bronchodilators are also available (e.g. theophylline, aminophylline, etamphylline).
- *Step 3: oral corticosteroids.* Corticosteroids (dexamethasone and prednisolone) are a useful adjunct to bronchodilators and mucolytics because steroids block the inflammatory cascade. However because of the risk of inducing laminitis, corticosteroids are not used routinely.

Some horses experience acute exacerbations of disease and present with severe symptoms. These should be managed by either intravenous or inhaled bronchodilators (e.g. clenbuterol) and not by intravenous corticosteroids (see Example 14.3). Inhalation therapy can be carried out using:

- Solutions of drugs and either ultrasonic or compressed air nebulisers attached to a nose bag-like face mask.

Example 14.3   Respiratory distress

You have a COPD horse in your clinic that suddenly develops acute dyspnoea and respiratory distress. What do you do?

Make a note of the respiratory rate and your assessment of its breathing effort in the case notes and contact a vet. The horse is probably having an acute bronchospasm episode and requires immediate treatment with either intravenous clenbuterol or nebulised clenbuterol. The horse should not be moved from its stable until its breathing has improved following treatment. However, you do need to examine the stable environment and find the source of allergen challenge, either in this stable or in adjacent stables, to prevent further acute episodes. You should turn the horse out if possible once you are happy that the episode is under control. The horse should not be treated with corticosteroids instead of clenbuterol to control the episode and it should not be sedated because this further reduces breathing effort.

- Dry powder drug formulations with delivery using metered dose inhalers (as used in asthma patients), using a spacer device or a rubber bulb that fits into the horse's nose (see Chapter 11).

Prevention

If the horse is not exposed to allergens then the disease will not return. In practice this is impossible to achieve but stable management should be approached with the aim of achieving zero exposure to allergens, dust or irritant gases. Sodium cromoglycate by inhalation may be useful to reduce the severity of disease in horses where exposure cannot be avoided. Control should be regarded as a failure if the horse requires frequent treatment with bronchodilators to alleviate its symptoms.

Summer-pasture-associated obstructive pulmonary disease

This is a COPD-like disease that occurs in late spring/summer. It is also a pulmonary hypersensitivity but is associated with plant and tree pollens. Oil seed rape has been implicated but not proven as a key allergen agent. Most cases are older horses with previous histories of COPD whereas some are younger horses with no history of COPD. Clinical signs resemble COPD closely, although the symptoms are often more severe. Diagnosis and treatment are as for COPD but aggressive drug management is needed and corticosteroids are usually included in therapy for this reason. Preventing exposure to pollen allergens is difficult, but stabling during the day may help.

Treatment

Sodium cromoglycate or steroids (by inhalation) are used, starting in early spring to prevent/reduce symptoms during the risk period.

Foreign bodies

Although uncommon, foreign bodies (e.g. brambles, blackthorn hedging) have been found in horse lungs. Foreign bodies present like COPD cases on clinical examination except that there is often marked coughing. Definitive diagnosis is only possible by endoscopy.

Neoplasia

Pulmonary tumours are rare in horses but these also present like COPD cases.

Circulatory system diseases

Heart murmurs and changes in rhythm (*arrhythmias*) are extremely common in horses. However, in contrast to small animals, the majority of murmurs and arryhthmias are not clinically significant. The challenge is to identify the small proportion of horses that have clinically significant murmurs or arrhythmias (see Summary 14.1). However, because most horses are kept for athletic use, clinically significant cardiac abnormalities will present much earlier than in small

animals. In stark contrast to small animals, equine cardiology is primarily a diagnostic and prognostic exercise: horses with heart failure are seldom treated unless they are in-foal brood mares or breeding stallions. The list of commonly occurring cardiovascular disorders is comparatively short for horses:

- Ventricular septal defect
- Patent ductus arteriosus
- Valvular regurgitation
- Pericardial effusion
- Arrhythmias

Ventricular septal defect

This is the most common congenital cardiac defect in horses and is more common in certain breeds, e.g. Welsh Mountain ponies. There is a defect in the septum between the right and left ventricles, which results in blood flow through the septum when the ventricles contract in systole. This results in a loud, coarse systolic murmur on the right side of the chest and also a loud coarse systolic murmur on the left side of the chest. Large defects result in heart failure and death in early life but horses with small defects may live for many years and even work.

Patent ductus arteriosus

The ductus arteriosus connects the pulmonary artery to the aorta and is a fetal structure that allows blood to bypass the lungs. In most thoroughbred foals there is a delay in closure of the ductus and it may remain patent for up to 5–7 days after birth, producing a continuous (systolic and diastolic) murmur on the left side of the chest. If the ductus does not close the horse will not grow properly and most will present for investigation before they reach the yearling stage.

Valvular regurgitations

Valvular regurgitation results in heart murmurs. Regurgitation occurs for a number of reasons:

- Congenital dysplasias (failure of the valves to form properly)
- Endocarditis (bacterial inflammation of the inner lining of the heart valves)

Summary 14.1

Clinical summary: examination of the cardiovascular system

- General appraisal of the horse for oedema, dyspnoea or tachypnoea.
- Assess the peripheral arterial pulse at the facial or transverse facial (the median or digital arteries can also be used).
- Normal pulse rate: 25–42 bpm.
- Normal pulse rhythm: regular (sinus arrhythmia is usually not present), although many horses have regular pauses in rhythm at rest associated with second-degree atrioventricular block.
- Assess mucous membranes for colour, hydration and capillary refill time.
- Assess the jugular pulse height and jugular filling time.
- Normal jugular pulse height is in the lower one-third of the neck.
- Normal jugular filling time is 12–15 s.
- Auscultate the heart.
- Heart failure initially results in poor performance, with few other clinical signs apart from a raised resting heart rate (50–60 bpm). This is *compensated* heart failure.
- This progresses to *decompensated* failure with obvious clinical signs, including exercise intolerance, lethargy, ventral oedema, tachypnoea and dyspnoea with raised resting heart rate, weak pulses and arrhythmias.

- Endocardiosis (non-infectious, progressive, age-related, thickening and degeneration of the inner lining of the heart valves)
- Chordae tendinae rupture (these are the chords that support and tense the heart valves and are essential for normal valve function).

In the majority of horses with quiet murmurs there is no apparent valve pathology and the regurgitation appears to be spontaneous or functional and non-progressive.

Regurgitation commonly occurs in the mitral valve (between the left atrium and left ventricle) and the tricuspid valve (between the right atrium and right ventricle). Quiet murmurs from these two valves are extremely common in horses in training; they do not appear to have any clinical significance and are non-progressive. In contrast, endocarditis (caused by bacteria that enter the circulation, e.g. from an intravenous catheter site, and lodge on the heart valves) and chord rupture (this usually occurs during exercise) result in loud, progressive murmurs that lead to heart failure. In young horses, aortic valve regurgitation occurs less commonly but this murmur is very common in older horses because it is usually due to endocardiosis of the valve. This murmur is generally progressive and eventually results in left ventricular failure.

Pericardial effusions

These are uncommon in horses and are often non-infectious effusions, rather than due to bacterial infection in the pericardium. Pericardial effusions prevent proper filling of the right ventricle during diastole and produce signs of right-sided output failure. The heart sounds are muffled on auscultation and there may be a quiet murmur, but murmurs are not a consistent finding.

Arrhythias

Although horses develop a range of arrythmias the most commonly encountered are:

- Second-degree atrioventricular block
- Atrial fibrillation

- Atrial premature contractions
- Ventricular premature contractions.

Second-degree atrioventricular block

Second-degree atrioventricular block is a normal phenomenon in fit horses at rest. The heart rate is normal and has regular pauses consisting of missed or 'dropped' beats. Typically the rhythm consists of one dropped beat in every four to six beats but this is variable. The phenomenon disappears with exercise or excitement once the heart rate increases above 60 bpm.

Atrial fibrillation

Atrial fibrillation is the most common pathological arrhythmia. Usually it occurs spontaneously (i.e. without any underlying heart disease), mainly in large horses, and causes poor performance, specifically fading during strenuous exercise. It will also appear during decompensated heart failure as one of the symptoms of heart failure. Atrial fibrillation results in an irregular heart beat and peripheral pulse. In some, but not all, horses with spontaneous atrial fibrillation the condition can be treated successfully with quinidine sulphate given by stomach tube. Quinidine has a number of unwanted effects and can result in dangerous tachycardia, hypotension and even death. Horses therefore require careful monitoring and nursing during treatment. It is important to watch the horse carefully for signs of toxicity: depression, tachycardia, hypotension, sweating and muscle tremors, diarrhoea, colic, nasal mucous membrane oedema, urticaria, ataxia and death. Treatment should be stopped if:

- Six doses have been given and the horse still has atrial fibrillation
- Tachycardia develops (>100 bpm)
- Other electrocardiogram abnormalities develop.

If toxicity develops the horse requires urgent treatment. The role of the nurse is to assist with the following treatments:

- Keep the horse calm and do not take it out of the stable
- Give digoxin (1 mg/450 kg i.v.)

263

- Fit large-gauge intravenous catheters to one or both jugular veins and give 40–50 L of Hartmann's (lactated Ringer's) solution as quickly as possible or give 2 L of hypertonic saline followed by 40–50 L of Hartmann's solution
- Give bicarbonate (1 mg/kg i.v.)
- The horse may require phenylephrine (2% solution i.v. to effect)
- Give activated charcoal or mineral oil by stomach tube to reduce absorption of quinidine from the gut.

Atrial premature contractions

Atrial premature contractions are often found after exercise in horses in training. Isolated atrial premature contractions are usually not significant but frequent contractions may indicate myocardial disease and usually are significant, particularly if there is a history of poor performance.

Ventricular premature contractions

Ventricular premature contractions are commonly seen in horses with surgical colic that have hypovolaemia, electrolyte and acid–base disturbances. Such contractions associated with colic cases usually resolve spontaneously once the circulatory disorders are corrected post-operatively.

Diagnosis of heart disease

- History
- Clinical examination
- Electrocardiography
- Echocardiography

Electrocardiography

Electrocardiography records the electrical activity of the heart on the surface of the horse. The way in which the electrical impulses travel through the equine heart means that, in contrast to small animals, equine electrocardiography can be used only to determine the heart rate and rhythm and is therefore restricted to the investigation of arrhythmias.

Using electrocardiography

(1) There is no advantage in using complex lead arrangements.

(2) The horse should not be sedated because this affects the heart rate and rhythm.
(3) The simple, practical lead position used is the base–apex lead, which requires three electrodes: a positive, a negative and an earth:
   (a) The negative electrode is positioned on the left neck (close to the heart base).
   (b) The positive electrode is positioned over the cardiac apex region.
   (c) The earth electrode can be positioned anywhere but usually is positioned behind the scapula to make a triangle with the other two electrodes.
(4) By using large-diameter (55-mm) adhesive electrodes there is usually no need to clip the horse unless it has a long winter coat.
(5) Most recordings are made in the stable with a static machine.
(6) Radiotelemetry is useful for detecting arrhythmias at exercise (e.g. exercise-induced atrial fibrillation) and also for determining the exercise capacity of the heart.
(7) Twenty-four-hour monitors (e.g. Halter monitors) are useful for identifying infrequent rhythm changes.

Echocardiography

Ultrasound examination of the heart (echocardiography) is the most useful investigation for murmurs; it allows identification of the type of murmur, and measurements of the heart chambers and walls can be made to assess the significance of murmurs. A sector machine equipped with a 2.25-MHz probe and M-mode and Doppler systems are required to carry out a full echocardiographic examination (see Chapter 17).

Imaging is carried out from both right and left sides of the chest wall and an area approximately 15 cm × 20 cm should be clipped behind the point of the elbow.

Haematopoietic system diseases

- Anaemia
- Lymphoma
- Neonatal isoerythrolysis

Definitions
- Leucopenia: decreased total white blood cell count
- Leucocytosis: increased total white blood cell count
- Neutropenia: decreased neutrophil count
- Neutrophilia: increased neutrophil count
- Thrombocytopenia: decreased platelet count
- Anaemia: decreased red blood cell count.

For normal values, see Chapter 12.

Anaemia

Aetiology
- Haemorrhage
- Immune-mediated haemolysis
- Chronic disease
- Bone marrow depression

Diagnosis
Establishing the cause of anaemia can be difficult and time consuming. A range of investigations may need to be carried out, including:

- Assess patient for signs of haemorrhage externally or from the gut (melaena), kidney (haematuria) or into the thorax or abdomen (haemothorax and haemoperitoneum).
- Immune-mediated destruction of red blood cells in the circulation will result in jaundice.
- Leakage of red blood cells through damaged blood vessel walls (vasculitis) will result in oedema, focal haemorrhages in mucous membranes (petechiation) or subcutaneous haematomas.
- Total and differential white and red blood cell counts as well as platelet counts should be tested; also the horse's iron status may be worth checking, although few horses become iron deficient.
- Laboratory assessment of clotting parameters.
- Check for immune-mediated haemolysis (Coomb's test).
- Bone marrow biopsy from the sternum or rib may be required to establish a diagnosis.

Clinical signs
- Weakness and depression
- Weight loss (if chronic)
- Pale mucous membranes
- Tachycardia and weak pulse
- Possibly jaundice

Treatment
Treatment depends on establishing the underlying cause. Blood transfusions may be required for emergency therapy for severe anaemia with packed cell volume (PCV) <12% (see Chapter 13).

Lymphoma

The symptoms of lymphoma vary depending on the sites in which these solid lymphoid tumours develop. Leukaemia (neoplastic lymphocytes in the circulation) is rare. Lymphoma in horses occurs as:

(1) *Multicentric lymphoma* with multiple lymph node enlargements and variable other clinical signs, depending on which other organs are involved. This is the most common type of lymphoma.
(2) *Intestinal lymphoma* with thickening of the gut wall by tumour, producing malabsorption (see later section on weight loss).
(3) *Cutaneous lymphoma* with multiple subcutaneous tumours.
(4) *Mediastinal lymphoma* with tumours in thoracic lymph nodes and thymus causing respiratory signs and pleural effusion.

Treatment is usually impossible, although corticosteroids may provide temporary amelioration. Radiotherapy has been attempted on localised masses.

Neonatal isoerythrolysis

Aetiology
This describes a condition where the neonatal foal's red blood cells are destroyed by antibodies in the mare's colostrum directed against the foal's red blood cells. This occurs when the mare does not have major red blood cell antigens (A and Q) that are present on the stallion's red blood cells, i.e. A–Q– mares covered by A+Q+ stallions producing A+Q+ foals. The red blood cells from the foal possess the stallion's A and Q antigens and its red blood cells are recognised as foreign antigens by the mare, which induces antibody production against the

foal's red blood cells. The mare becomes sensitised at the first foaling because this is when there is mixing of blood between the foal and mare. This syndrome therefore develops on second and subsequent pregnancies. When the foal suckles, antibodies against its own red blood cells are absorbed, which result in destruction of the foal's red blood cells.

Clinical signs
- Signs develop over the first 2–3 days after birth
- Weakness, jaundice, anaemia, tachycardia
- If untreated, may progress to collapse and seizures and death

Treatment
Transfuse the foal with blood from the mare that has been washed three times to remove antibody (see Chapter 15). The foal also may require plasma to correct failed passive transfer.

Prevention
The condition can be prevented in future pregnancies by either blood-typing mares and avoiding A+Q+ stallions with A–Q– mares, or muzzling the foal (and providing colostrum and milk from another mare by bottle) for the first 4 days of life.

Alimentary system diseases

The alimentary system in horses is fundamentally different from that of dogs and cats. Horses are herbivores and their gut is specialised for the digestion of forage (see Chapter 5).

Alimentary tract diseases cause three main syndromes:

- Weight loss
- Diarrhoea
- Colic (abdominal pain)

Weight loss (Table 14.2)

Anorexia
Anorexia is the loss of the desire to eat. The horse is able to eat but does not want to because it feels unwell. This may be because of pain or infection in the mouth (e.g. dental disease), the oesophagus (e.g.

Table 14.2 Causes of weight loss

Anorexia
Dysphagia
Malabsorption
Protein loss
Increased metabolic requirements
Pathological changes in metabolic activity
Lack of food

ulceration), the stomach or duodenum (e.g. ulceration or neoplasia, especially squamous cell carcinoma) or elsewhere in the abdomen (e.g. peritonitis or abdominal abscess).

Dysphagia
Dysphagia is the physical inability to pick up, chew or swallow food and can be due to compromised oral cavity, pharynx or oesophagus. In horses pharyngeal and oesophageal problems always result in the reflux of food and saliva from the nostrils rather than the mouth. Dropping of food from the mouth (called 'quidding') is associated with dental or other oral cavity disorders. Dysphagia may result from local problems with these regions or may be due to: neurological disorders, e.g. grass sickness, guttural pouch mycosis; compression of these regions by guttural pouch swellings or retropharyngeal lymph node abscesses; or part of generalised diseases, e.g. tetanus and botulism. The management and nursing of dysphagia thus depends on the underlying cause.

Choke
Choke is the classic cause of oesophageal obstruction in horses. Choke is due to obstruction of the oesophagus with dry feed, especially short feeds and particularly poorly soaked sugarbeet pulp. Greedy horses or horses with poor teeth are particularly prone to choke and may experience repeated episodes (see Example 14.4). Protracted or repeated choke episodes may result in oesophageal injury with permanent loss of function and dysphagia, e.g. strictures.

Clinical signs
- Variable degree of distress

You are nursing a horse that has had an oesophageal food impaction ('choke') relieved by the veterinary surgeon yesterday. The horse has been allowed to resume eating and now has food and saliva at its nostrils. What do you do?

This horse has further problems with oesophageal obstruction. The immediate priority is to remove the food and water from its stable before getting assistance to reduce the risk of aspiration of food into the airway. The horse will require sedation and re-examination by endoscope to establish what the problem is with the oesophagus. When food is re-introduced it would be prudent to offer small quantities of feed and perhaps to put some large stones in the feed to make the horse search for its feed so that it takes longer to eat.

- Drooling saliva and reflux of food and saliva from the nose
- Coughing
- Repeated swallowing or retching movements.

Diagnosis
- History and clinical examination
- Endoscopy (a 3-m endoscope is required to reach the stomach in adult horses).

Treatment
- Sedate and give spasmolytic
- Remove impaction by gentle, small-volume warm-water lavage by stomach tube, taking care to keep the horse's head down to avoid aspiration
- If this is unsuccessful, repeat under general anaesthetic with endotracheal tube fitted to prevent aspiration
- The horse should be treated with broad-spectrum antibiotics because of risk of aspiration pneumonia.

Nursing care after the impaction is cleared
- Withhold food for at least 12 h
- Feed small quantities of well-soaked pellets initially
- Ideally start feeding with grass rather than hay
- Allow free access to water
- Observe carefully for signs of choke reappearing.

Malabsorption

Malabsorption describes conditions in which there is reduced ability of the gut to absorb nutrients after food has been digested. Malabsorption occurs mainly in small intestinal disease but is also a feature of some large intestinal diseases. All diseases that cause malabsorption do so by reducing the blood supply to or damaging the gut wall and reducing its ability to absorb nutrients. Unless the large intestine is affected, malabsorption in horses usually does not cause diarrhoea, in marked contrast with small animals. The main causes of malabsorption are:

- Parasitism: mainly due to the migrating larval (rather than adult) stages of the large redworms (*Strongylus vulgaris*, *S. edentatus* and *S. equinus*) which cause damage and thickening of the gut wall. The small redworms (cyathostomes) also can cause malabsorption. Tapeworms (Anoplocephala) do not seem to cause malabsorption.
- Chronic salmonellosis: note that this is a zoonosis and strict barrier nursing is required of these cases.
- Granulomatous enteritis: this is due to inflammatory cell infiltration into the gut wall, possibly as a result of bacterial infection.
- Lymphosarcoma.
- Idiopathic: in approximately 50% of malabsorption cases a diagnosis is not made.

Nursing a malabsorption case
- Corticosteroids (prednisolone) may help to reduce gut wall thickening and improve function.
- Feed good quality hay or haylage *ad libitum*.
- Avoid cereals but if the horse is still losing weight feed cereals little and often, or try adding oil to the diet (see Chapter 6).

Protein loss

Protein (albumin) loss occurs in association with intestinal disease due to leakage of protein through damaged gut wall and also in renal disease due to protein loss through damaged glomeruli.

Increased metabolic requirements

Increased requirements for nutrients due to work, pregnancy or lactation cause weight loss if the diet is not adequate.

Pathological changes in metabolic activity

Pituitary adenoma (Cushing's disease), liver disease, hyperlipaemia and grass sickness (dysautonomia) all result in weight loss.

Diarrhoea (Table 14.3)

Diarrhoea is extremely common in foals and is usually benign, associated with:

- The mare's first oestrus after parturition ('foal heat scours')
- Dietary changes, e.g. introducing creep feed

Foal diarrhoea can be due to viral (e.g. Rotavirus) and bacterial infections (e.g. *Salmonella* and *Campylobacter*), especially on large studs or where hygiene is poor. *Salmonella* and *Campylobacter* are both zoonoses and care must be taken to protect spread to handlers. Control of viral and bacterial diarrhoea in foals relies on improving hygiene in foaling pens and reducing stocking density. A killed virus vaccine is available for prevention of rotavirus diarrhoea (Duvaxyn R, from Fort Dodge Animal Health) by vaccinating the mare in late pregnancy. The parasite *Strongyloides westeri* can be the cause of diarrhoea in young foals. This parasite is transmitted to the foal from the mare via the mare's milk.

Nursing the diarrhoeic foal
- Keep the foal's perineum and hindlimbs clean and coated with petroleum jelly to prevent burning and excoriation of the skin
- Monitor the foal closely for signs of depression or dehydration, because these require immediate investigation and management with intravenous fluids

- Administer simple kaolin-based absorbents by mouth
- Do not use antibiotics
- If the diarrhoea continues, consider muzzling the foal to limit milk intake. In this case the foal will need bottle feeding with electrolytes to prevent dehydration or sometimes intravenous fluids (see Chapter 15)

Diarrhoea in adult horses

Diarrhoea in adult horses is uncommon and is always associated with large intestinal disease, either as the primary or secondary problem. It is not possible to differentiate small and large intestinal disease in horses on the basis of the nature of diarrhoea, as can be done for small animals. Diarrhoea in adults is usually severe and can be life threatening.

Salmonella

Salmonella infections produce a spectrum of disease from peracute, haemorrhagic diarrhoea through to mild chronic diarrhoea. All salmonella cases should be barrier nursed to prevent spread and hygiene precautions must be taken, because this is a zoonosis.

Cyathostomiasis

Cyathostomiasis is a well-recognised cause of severe, possibly fatal diarrhoea in horses in the spring. Diarrhoea is due to mass emergence of overwintered 'hypobiotic' larvae from the wall of the caecum and ventral colon causing extensive damage to the gut wall. Treatment of this disease is difficult because severe, possibly fatal, gut damage has occurred by the time clinical signs appear. Hypobiotic cyathostome larvae are resistant to anthelminthic treatment and control is based around elimination of larvae from

Table 14.3 Causes of diarrhoea

In foals	In adults
• Dietary changes	• Bacterial infections e.g. *Salmonella*
• Virus infections, e.g. Rotavirus	• Parasitic infections, e.g. Cyathostomiasis
• Bacterial infections, e.g. *Salmonella*, *Campylobacter*, *Escherichia coli*	• Haemorrhagic oedematous colon
• Parasitic infections, e.g. *Strongyloides westeri*	• Peritonitis
	• Drug-induced diarrhoea, e.g. antibiotics and non-steroidal anti-inflammatory drugs

the gut in the autumn using either increased doses of fenbendazole or routine doses of ivermectin or moxidectin. Severe cases of acute diarrhoea in adult horses require hospitalisation and treatment with intravenous fluids.

Colic

The term *colic* refers to abdominal pain and is not a specific diagnosis. The various causes of colic are listed in Table 14.4 and initial assessment of the colic case aims to separate the alimentary causes from the non-alimentary causes.

Most colics are due to alimentary disease and the majority (approximately 90%) of colics do not require surgical intervention, in other words they are medical colics that require only medical management. With medical colics, the clinical signs are usually, but not always, less severe.

The common medical colics are:

- spasmodic colic
- tympanic colic
- colonic impactions.

The medical colics have four predisposing factors in common:

(1) Exercise and excitement.
(2) Diet:
  (a) Too little fibre.
  (b) Poor quality fibre.
  (c) Eating bedding or sand.
  (d) Changes in diet, especially increases in cereals.
  (e) Sudden access to lush grazing.
(3) Inactivity, e.g. stabling in the autumn or being hospitalised.
(4) Parasitism: especially large strongyle (*Strongylus vulgaris*) larval damage to the blood vessels supplying the gut wall.

Management and nursing of medical colics

The horse should not be allowed to become too violent or to roll frequently because this may result in injury and perhaps may predispose to gut torsion.

Spasmodic colic is probably the most common cause of colic. The pain is due to intestinal spasm and horses have intermittent bouts of moderate to severe pain and are often normal or quiet between episodes. Treatment is by analgesics and spasmolytics and diet restriction (hay and bran mashes only for 24 h).

Tympanic/flatulent colic is due to gut distension with gas, usually the caecum and colon, after feeding on highly fermentable feeds. The pain is intermittent to moderate, becoming more severe and continuous. There may be flatulence. Treatment is the same as for spasmodic colic.

Colonic impactions usually occur at the pelvic flexure and are predisposed to by situations that result in decreased gut motility, such as:

Table 14.4 Causes of colic

Alimentary tract causes	Non-alimentary tract causes	Conditions that resemble colic
• Spasmodic colic	• Peritoneal pain (peritonitis, abdominal abscess)	• Myopathies (rhabdomyolysis)
• Tympanic colic	• Liver disease (ragwort poisoning, cholelithiasis)	• Laminitis
• Colonic impactions	• Urinary (renal calculi, pyelonephritis, bladder calculi)	• Other orthopaedic conditions, e.g. bilateral flexor tendon rupture
• Small intestinal obstruction (e.g. torsion, herniation, intussusception, pedunculated lipoma)	• Reproductive (uterine torsion)	
• Large intestinal obstruction (e.g. torsion, displacement, entrapment)		
• Gastroduodenal ulcers and neoplasia		
• Grass sickness		
• Proximal enteritis		
• Other causes of severe enteritis, e.g. *Salmonella*		

- Decreased water intake
- Eating bedding or sand
- Diet change in autumn when the horse is stabled for the winter
- Poor dentition
- Inactivity, especially stable rest when unwell
- After general anaesthetic
- Parasitism.

The pain is progressive: initially vague and intermittent, becoming mild/moderate and continuous. Horses lie quietly, occasionally rolling and get more active as gut distends. There are reduced faeces or no faeces produced at all. Treatment includes:

- Stomach tubing laxatives (liquid paraffin or Epsom salts)
- Analgesics
- The horse being turned out or lunged to promote gut activity and relieve the impaction
- Restriction of further feed intake
- Intravenous and oral fluids
- Occasionally surgery for severe cases.

Grass sickness (equine dysautonomia)

This is a diffuse nervous system disease that presents with mainly alimentary signs. It was first described in Scotland but now occurs all over the UK, although it is still more common in the North and East. It affects mainly young adults (2–7 years old) at grass between April and July. Usually the horse will have moved recently (<6 months ago) to the farm. The disease closely resembles dysautonomias of cats (Key–Gaskell syndrome) and hares.

Clinical signs

There are three forms of grass sickness:

(1) Acute grass sickness:
  (a) Rapid death (within 3 days).
  (b) Profound depression, unrelenting colic, silent abdomen, tachycardia, salivation, dysphagia, nasogastric reflux, muscle tremors.
(2) Subacute grass sickness:
  (a) Death occurs in approximately 7 days.
  (b) Signs similar to acute but there is spectacular weight loss with severe dysphagia and nasogastric reflux when stomach-tubed.

(3) Chronic grass sickness:
  (a) Chronic disease (lasting weeks to months) with progressive weight loss without gastric reflux.
  (b) Depression, tremors, sweating, tachycardia, dysphagia, decreased gut sounds.

Diagnosis
- Based on clinical signs
- Ileal biopsy is currently the only ante-mortem diagnostic aid
- Research is looking for non-invasive simple tests, e.g. use of phenylephrine eye drops

Treatment
- Chronic cases that are bright, can swallow and are not emaciated can be nursed to recovery. The importance of human contact to keep the horse stimulated and interested is critical (see further reading list)
- Keep stabled and rugged
- Offer palatable high-energy feeds
- Treatment with cisapride helps to restore gut motility.

Liver disease

Aetiology

The liver has a large capacity for regeneration and a large functional reserve. This means that:

- Mild liver damage does not result in clinical signs: this is liver *disease*.
- Clinical signs only appear after more than 75% of the liver has been destroyed and thus the prognosis is poor whatever the aetiology: this is liver *failure*.
- Clinical signs appear abruptly (once the hepatic reserve has been destroyed), although most aetiologies, in particular ragwort poisoning, involve gradual, progressive destruction of hepatocytes.

There are many different causes of liver disease and failure in horses. Liver damage may be caused by (in decreasing order of likelihood):

- Plant toxicities (e.g. ragwort, St John's Wort)
- Non-differentiated cirrhosis
- Other toxicities (e.g. mouldy corn, causing leucoencephalomalacia)

- Cholangiohepatitis (infection and inflammation of biliary tract)
- Haemochromatosis (abnormal uptake of iron)
- Hyperlipaemia (assessed using serum triglyceride concentration)
- Cholelithiasis ('stone' in biliary tract)
- Serum hepatitis ('Theiler's disease', due to administration of an equine product, e.g. tetanus antitoxin)
- Parasitism (rare, possibly liver fluke but many question that it clinically affects horses)
- Tyzzer's disease (in foals, caused by *Clostridium piliformis*).

Ragwort poisoning. This is caused by eating ragwort (*Senecio jacoboea*) plants and is mainly due to ingestion of small quantities of plants over a long (usually a few weeks) period. Ragwort is not palatable and horses usually only eat the plant when it is wilted, although in starvation the fresh green plant may be eaten. The main means by which horses become poisoned is therefore via hay made from pasture with ragwort contamination and most owners thus will be unaware that their horse has eaten ragwort.

The liver-toxic compounds in ragwort plants are pyrrolizidine alkaloids. These are compounds that prevent liver cells from dividing and forming new daughter cells, resulting in an increase in size of hepatocytes ('hepatic megalocytosis') followed by death of hepatocytes and replacement of these cells by fibrous tissue ('cirrhosis'). This is most obvious around the biliary tree because this area experiences the highest concentrations of alkaloid toxins.

Although this is a chronic poisoning, clinical signs appear abruptly, usually several months after the ragwort was eaten, after more than 75% of the liver has been destroyed.

Non-differentiated cirrhosis. This is the other main cause of liver disease although it is less common than ragwort poisoning. These horses have a similar presentation to ragwort poisoning. There is extensive liver cirrhosis but without the megalocytosis seen in ragwort cases. The cause of this syndrome is unknown but may be an alternative presentation for ragwort poisoning.

Liver disease *secondary* to a number of other diseases:
- Hyperlipaemia
- Pituitary adenoma
- Abdominal abscess
- Secondary neoplasia (metastatic spread from other sites)

Pathogenesis
The pathogenesis of liver disease involves loss of hepatocytes and, in the case of cirrhotic liver diseases, obstruction to bile flow. Loss of hepatocytes results in disruption of the many metabolic functions of the liver. The liver is central to the metabolism of carbohydrates, lipids and proteins. It is responsible for the production of almost all of the plasma proteins and clotting factors. It eliminates toxic nitrogen waste from protein metabolism by converting ammonia to urea in the liver before it is transported to the kidney for excretion. Aromatic amino acids arriving from the large intestine are converted into branched-chain amino acids before entering the circulation. The liver metabolises and excretes phylloerythrin, the photodynamic intermediate breakdown product of chlorophyll. The liver is responsible for the conjugation and excretion of bilirubin and bile acids. Vitamins A, D, E, K and B12 are stored in the liver.

Clinical signs
Clinical signs all relate to loss of the liver's metabolic functions and consist of:

- Weight loss and anorexia
- Depression
- Abdominal pain (mild/moderate and intermittent)
- Hepatic encephalopathy with depression, ataxia, tremors, circling and head pressing. Note that seizures are unusual and horses generally become comatose
- Photosensitisation, with lesions on the white regions of skin, e.g. the muzzle and distal limbs
- Ventral oedema
- Jaundice
- Petechiation of mucous membranes is a potential sign but is rarely seen

Diagnosis
Diagnosis is based on history and clinical signs but relies heavily on blood biochemistry (see Chapter 12):

- Prolonged bromsulphalein clearance (this test measures the ability of the liver to remove an exogenous dye from the circulation)
- Definitive diagnosis of liver disease requires ultrasound examination and liver biopsy
- Ultrasound is useful to examine liver for homogeneity and is valuable for biopsy guidance (especially if focal lesions are detectable).

Treatment
- Liver *disease* cases are worth treating (some survive), although there are no specific therapies for ragwort poisoning
- Consider welfare carefully before treating liver *failure*.

Nursing horses with liver disease. Dietary management is the only practical/affordable option:

(1) Low protein:
  (a) Avoid most cereals (barley, wheat and oats).
  (b) Avoid early-cut hay.
  (c) Avoid clover or alfalfa hay.
  (d) Feed oat hay *ad libitum* or (less satisfactory) feed meadow hay *ad libitum*.
(2) High carbohydrate:
  (a) Feed molassed sugarbeet pulp plus maize (2:1 ratio) little and often, to appetite, at a rate of up to 2 kg/100 kg bodyweight.
  (b) Maize is also rich in branched-chain amino acids.
(3) Supplement vitamins A, D, E and B12.

Nursing horses with liver failure (see Example 14.5)

(1) Sedation (xylazine, detomidine or romifidine is better than acepromazine because this may precipitate seizures).
(2) Maintain plasma glucose levels (intravenous dextrose as continuous infusion of 5% solution in 0.9% saline; or oral glucose) and add potassium chloride as required.

Example 14.5 Liver disease

A horse presents with depression, anorexia and ataxia. The owner reports that the horse has been circling in its stable. How would you manage this horse until a diagnosis is made?
This type of case presents a significant nursing challenge. The horse is very likely to be in liver failure. The main concerns are to encourage food intake and to prevent the horse from injuring itself. The horse should be offered oat hay and molassed sugarbeet pulp with maize mix, with palatable additional feeds like carrots or apples to encourage appetite. Intravenous dextrose saline and treatment with oral neomycin or lactulose might improve the CNS signs. The horse should be kept in a well-bedded or ideally padded box with built-up bedding at the edge of the box to help prevent the horse becoming cast. Stable bandages should be applied to protect the legs. The horse may need sedating to allow safe handling but this should be done with care. The horse's welfare should be forefront in the nursing priorities and early, rather than later, decisions about euthanasia must be taken.

(3) Decrease ammonia production in the gut by oral neomycin or oral lactulose:
  (a) Supplement vitamins A, D and E.
  (b) Feed high-carbohydrate, low-protein diet.
  (c) Diet as for liver disease management: oat hay with maize/molassed beet pulp (2:1).

Prevention
Ragwort should be removed from pastures used for grazing or for making hay. Pulling them up and burning best controls the plants. Herbicides can also be used. Mowing and leaving the plants in the field will not control ragwort, as horses will eat the wilted plant and it will leave the young plantlets behind.

Renal system diseases

- Prerenal azotaemia
- Acute renal failure
- Chronic renal failure

Definitions
- *Azotaemia*: elevated blood concentrations of the nitrogen waste products that the kidney excretes

(urea and creatinine). In most situations azotaemia in horses is due to endotoxaemia and other causes of hypovolaemia ('shock') causing decreased renal perfusion. This is referred to as prerenal azotaemia.

- *Renal disease*: a reduction in kidney function that is not sufficient to cause azotaemia (i.e. is not detectable using routine biochemistry tests). More sophisticated tests of renal function, e.g. fractional clearance of electrolytes, need to be used to detect renal disease. There are generally no clinical signs associated with renal disease.
- *Renal failure*: occurs when more than 75% of kidney function has been lost. Failure is associated with clinical signs and increased concentrations of urea and creatinine in the blood.

See Chapter 12.

Prerenal azotaemia

This is the most common reason for elevated blood urea and creatinine levels in horses. It occurs secondary to hypovolaemia induced by endotoxaemia, e.g. in surgical colic cases or peracute salmonellosis, diarrhoea or severe haemorrhage. Diagnosis is made by demonstrating azotaemia with well-concentrated urine (specific gravity >1.030). Provided that the condition is recognised and treated promptly with intravenous fluids to restore the circulating volume, the condition is completely reversible and does not result in damage to the kidney.

Acute renal failure

This can be a consequence of untreated hypovolaemia (i.e. a progression from prerenal azotaemia). It may also result from damage to the kidney by nephrotoxins, especially aminoglycoside antibiotics (e.g. gentamycin, neomycin and amikacin) and NSAIDs (e.g. phenylbutazone and flunixin). Diagnosis is by demonstrating azotaemia with poorly concentrated urine (specific gravity <1.020) and proteinuria. Treatment relies on removal of the nephrotoxin (if possible) and intravenous fluid therapy to restore the circulating volume.

Chronic renal failure

Aetiology

This occurs as:

(1) An end result of acute renal failure (called tubulointerstitial disease).
(2) An immune-mediated disease (called chronic glomerulonephritis).
(3) A consequence of bacterial infection (called pyelonephritis).

Clinical signs

- Depression and anorexia
- Weight loss
- Polyuria and polydipsia (normal horse drinks 5 L water/100 kg/day and urinates 15–20 L urine/day)
- Oedema
- Mouth ulcers and excessive tooth plaque.

Diagnosis

- Urinalysis: specific gravity = 1.008–1.014; protein (beware false positives if blood or myoglobin present, and trace false positives using dipsticks in alkaline urine); protein casts; white blood cells and bacteria (pyelonephritis only)
- Azotaemia
- Hyponatraemia and hypochloraemia
- Hypercalcaemia (cf. dogs) and hyperkalaemia.

Treatment

Treatment is difficult and is supportive rather than curative only:

- Offer *ad libitum* water and salt
- There is usually no need to restrict protein intake
- Encourage the horse to eat (see Chapter 5)
- Anabolic steroids may help

Nervous system diseases

- Spinal cord trauma
- Cervical vertebral stenosis (CVS)
- EHV-1 myeloencephalitis
- Tetanus
- Botulism

Definitions

- *Ataxia* describes loss of proprioception (awareness of the position of the limbs, joints and feet). Horses with ataxia have a swaying, unstable gait and may trip. Their limb and foot placement is erratic. They often fall in the stable or field and injure themselves by striking into themselves and treading on themselves.
- *Paresis* describes more marked abnormalities where there is reduced ability to move the limbs, resulting in dragging of the limbs and stumbling.
- *Paralysis* is more severe still and the horse cannot move its limbs or use them for weight bearing. Paralysis usually results in recumbency.

Spinal cord trauma

Spinal cord diseases are the most common neurological problems in horses and cause ataxia and, if severe enough, paresis or even paralysis (see Table 14.5).

Trauma to the spinal cord, especially the cervical cord, is common. The severity of the clinical signs depends on the degree of trauma. The neck should be radiographed for signs of fractures because these carry a poor prognosis.

Cervical vertebral stenosis

Cervical vertebral stenosis (CVS) is also known as

Table 14.5 Regions affected by spinal cord trauma

Region affected	Clinical signs
Head	Depression
	Seizures
	Forelimb and hindlimb ataxia
Neck	Forelimb and hindlimb ataxia (or forelimb and hindlimb paresis or paralysis if severe)
Thoracolumbar	Hindlimb ataxia/paresis/paralysis
	Forelimbs normal
Sacral	Hindlimb ataxia/paresis/paralysis
	Loss of tail tone
	Incontinence

'wobbler syndrome'. It occurs in well-grown, young (less than 3 years old) thoroughbreds and is more common in males. It is a developmental disease where there are abnormalities in the formation and/or articulation of one or more vertebrae in the neck that cause compression of the spinal cord. These abnormalities include:

- Static lesions: abnormal formation and shape of vertebrae.
- Dynamic lesions: abnormal movement of vertebrae relative to one another.

The severity of the signs varies from subtle ataxia through to paresis or possibly paralysis. Most cases present with progressive ataxia, which is not symmetrical and the hindlimbs are more severely affected than the forelimbs. Plain radiography of the neck may be useful but definitive diagnosis requires a myelogram (see Chapter 17). Treatment is very limited, although surgery can help some cases or sometimes specific restrictive diets are attempted. Corticosteroids may provide temporary amelioration but are not curative. Cases of CVS present a nursing challenge because they are prone to self-injury and casting and can be difficult to handle safely.

EHV-1 myeloencephalitis

EHV-1 myeloencephalitis occurs after EHV-1 viraemia and is due to virus-mediated damage to blood vessels in the spinal cord. The clinical signs are mainly caudal with hindlimb ataxia and flaccid tail and anus with urinary and faecal incontinence. Some horses develop paresis or even paralysis and in a few cases this may affect all four limbs. Pregnant mares that have aborted are particularly susceptible to developing myeloencephalitis but non-pregnant mares, geldings and stallions also can be affected. If the horse does not require euthanasia on humane grounds, these cases can be rewarding to nurse and many make a slow and complete recovery:

- Provide deep bedding
- Turn the horse every 4–6 h to prevent muscle and skin necrosis
- Consider using slings to assist standing
- Catheterise the bladder
- Corticosteroids may help.

Tetanus

Horses and ponies are very susceptible to tetanus, although vaccination generally provides protection. Most cases of tetanus occur in unvaccinated animals.

Aetiology

Tetanus is caused by toxins produced by the soil-borne bacterium *Clostridium tetani*. The bacteria are anaerobic (i.e. they prefer environments without oxygen) and grow in deep puncture wounds, especially on the distal limbs, and also in the umbilicus or retained placenta.

Pathogenesis

The toxin is produced in wounds and travels to the spinal cord where it binds irreversibly to motor neurones and causes spasticity.

Clinical signs

- Tetanus progresses rapidly once signs appear
- Early signs are stiff, slow gait, hyperaesthesia to sound and touch, spasm of third eyelid if stimulated
- Later signs are marked hyperaesthesia to touch and sound, anxious expression, sawhorse stance, dysphagia, regurgitation
- Terminal signs are lateral recumbency, death from pneumonia, dehydration, cardiac and respiratory arrest

Diagnosis

Diagnosis is based on clinical signs only.

Treatment and nursing

- Early cases can be nursed but recumbent horses are a major welfare issue
- Reduce stimulation by keeping in a dark, quiet box away from other horses
- Handle carefully and considerately
- Feed soft food from elevated troughs
- Sedation may help to decrease hyperaesthesia
- Antibiotics (penicillin) help to remove bacteria at the wound site
- Tetanus antitoxin given intravenously or intrathecally will neutralise unbound toxin

Prevention

- All horses with wounds (or after surgical procedures) should be treated with tetanus antitoxin irrespective of vaccination status
- Routine vaccination with tetanus toxoid starting from 4 months old, with boosters every 18–24 months for life

Botulism

This is an uncommon but highly publicised paralysing disease caused by toxins from the anaerobic soil-borne bacterium *Clostridium botulinum*. Most cases have been associated with feeding poor-quality baled silage but other conserved feeds also have been implicated. Baled silage should be considered high risk for botulism if:

- The bag is not intact
- The outer layers of the bale are moulded
- The silage is too wet (>75% water)
- The pH is not low enough (optimum pH is 4.5 or less)
- The silage contains soil

Bales fitting the above profile will support the growth of botulinum bacteria producing botulinum toxin. When the silage is eaten, the toxin is absorbed and binds irreversibly to nerve/muscle junctions causing flaccid paralysis.

Clinical signs

- Progressive weakness, first noticed in the limbs
- Tongue paralysis
- Pupillary dilation
- Dysphagia
- Decreased gut activity

Treatment and nursing

- Take care to consider the horse's welfare at all stages
- Offer soft, palatable, easily swallowed food
- Consider stomach tubing if unable to swallow
- Intravenous fluids may be necessary
- Consider supporting recumbent horses in slings
- Botulinum antitoxin will neutralise unbound toxin but not toxin bound to neuromuscular junctions

Cutaneous system diseases

- Dermatophilus
- Ringworm
- Chorioptic mange mites (see Chapter 12)
- Lice (see Chapter 12)
- Sarcoids
- Melanoma
- Sweet itch
- Collagen granuloma

Dermatophilus

Dermatophilus is a very common equine bacterial skin pathogen that causes *rain scald* on the trunk and *mud fever* and *cracked heels* on the distal limbs. The bacteria are found on the skin of most horses and cause disease when skin defences are compromised by skin getting wet from rain or mud or damaged by stubble, long grass, coarse bedding or is otherwise traumatised. Disease is thus more common in horses and ponies kept outside in the winter or in animals that are worked in muddy areas. White areas of skin appear to be more susceptible and often become affected by mud fever or cracked heels before coloured limbs.

Clinical signs
- Extensive exudation and thick crust formation through which the hairs protrude
- Unlike ringworm the hairs do not break off
- Lifting off scabs reveals a shallow skin erosion with a raw surface
- The lesions are not pruritic but are usually painful and horses with extensive lesions may be difficult to examine and treat
- There may be leg swelling because of cellulitis (infection in tissues).

Diagnosis
- Demonstration of bacteria on an impression smear of the underside of the scab
- Bacterial culture in the laboratory.

Treatment
- Remove all scabbing (this may require a sweat wrap overnight or sedation and lengthy gentle washing)
- Remove hair by clipping
- Clean the area with Hibiscrub®(chlorhexidline) shampoo to reveal a fresh, pink, skin surface
- Apply topical antibiotics
- Systemic antibiotics may be useful.

Prevention
- Keep the horse rugged if it is overwintered outside and groom the coat regularly to control rain scald
- For mud fever, keep the legs clean and dry by washing off mud after exercise
- Regular washing with Hibiscrub® shampoo may help to reduce bacterial numbers on the leg
- Apply waterproofing (e.g. Lanolin) to the leg before turnout or exercise during the winter.

Ringworm

Ringworm is a fungal infection caused by *Trichophyton* and *Microsporum* species of fungi and is common where horses are kept in groups (e.g. racing stables and livery yards). The fungi are transmitted via shared tack and grooming equipment. Ringworm is a zoonosis and so infected horses must be handled wearing disposable examination gloves. Most cases occur over the winter because of closer contact between horses when stabled and damper conditions that encourage fungal growth.

Clinical signs
- Multiple, raised, roughly circular lesions, particularly in tack areas
- Hair loss with broken hairs at the periphery of the lesion
- Affected skin has a scaly or sometimes corrugated, thickened appearance
- Usually not pruritic.

Diagnosis
- Demonstrate fungi on hair plucks from the edge of the lesion
- Fungal culture is slow and unreliable.

Treatment and control

- Infection usually self-limiting. Most cases resolve in 1–3 months
- Topical antifungals, e.g. enilconazole or natamycin are used. Tack and fomites also should be treated
- Systemic antifungals (not suitable for pregnant mares), e.g. griseofulvin, are not proven to be effective in horses
- Direct and indirect contact with infected horses should be prevented, if possible.

Sarcoids

Sarcoids are fibroblastic skin tumours and are the most common tumour of horses. There is almost certainly a genetic predisposition to sarcoids. A papillomavirus has been implicated as a possible causal agent. Sarcoids usually appear in young adult horses and susceptible animals usually develop multiple sarcoids over a period of months to years. Sarcoids may appear anywhere on the horse but predilection sites are the head (especially around the eye), the axillae, ventral abdomen, udder, sheath, inner thigh and distal limbs. There are three main types of sarcoid:

(1) *Verrucose* (flat, slowly progressive tumours)
(2) *Nodular* (subcutaneous, slowly progressive tumours)
(3) *Fibroblastic* (aggressive tumours that may ulcerate).

Treatment is difficult and may involve surgery, cryosurgery, cytotoxic agents, immunotherapy (BCG) or radiation treatment. Combinations of treatments may be required.

Melanoma

Melanomas are the other common skin tumour affecting horses. They are more common in grey horses and may be benign or malignant. These tumours most commonly develop in the perineal area under the tail and around the anus but also develop in the parotid region. The tumours may cause welfare problems because of interference with the anus and rectum or because of compression of the larynx and pharynx. Treatment is difficult: surgery is usually unsuccessful. Medical management with cimetidine may slow tumour progression but is not curative.

Sweet itch

Sweet itch is a hypersensitivity to the saliva of biting midges. It is seasonal and occurs during the summer in temperate areas and all year round in warmer climates, where the midges continue to bite in winter. It is most common in ponies and donkeys. Midge bites cause severe pruritus along the mane and tail head. The pony rubs at these regions, causing extensive self-inflicted damage and hair loss. Occasionally the lesions occur ventrally. Treatment is by topical application of benzyl benzoate and pyrethroid fly repellents. Occasionally steroids are required and special rugs have been developed to protect against the midges during turnout. Stabling during the cool parts of the day may reduce exposure to midges.

Collagen granuloma

Collagen granuloma (also called nodular skin disease) describes non-painful and non-pruritic, firm, small, skin nodules along the dorsum. The cause is unknown but insect bite hypersensitivity or trauma from tack has been suggested.

Eye diseases

- Conjunctivitis
- Corneal ulceration
- Uveitis

Conjunctivitis

Aetiology
- Irritants, e.g. stable dust, ammonia in stables
- Bacterial and viral infections
- Foreign bodies, e.g. straw, hay, thorns, splinters
- Part of other diseases of the eye, especially corneal ulceration and uveitis.

Clinical signs
- Pain and partial/complete closure of the eyelids
- Eyelid swelling ('chemosis')

- Reddening of the conjunctiva ('pink eye')
- Excessive tear production and/or discharge from the eye

Treatment
- Clean discharge from around the eye using dilute antiseptic, e.g. Hibiscrub® (chlorhexidine)
- Underlying problems (corneal ulceration, uveitis, foreign bodies) should be identified and treated
- Topical (ophthalmic) antibiotics

Corneal ulceration

Aetiology
Corneal ulceration is common in horses because their eyes are prominent and positioned laterally. When operating, care must be taken to protect the cornea in anaesthetised horses by padding the periorbital area to prevent contact between the cornea and the floor. Most ulcers are the result of trauma to the cornea and may also have a foreign body associated with the ulcer. Superficial ulcers respond well to medical management. However, deep ulcers exposing the basement membrane of the cornea (Descemet's membrane) require surgical treatment (suturing or covering with a conjunctival pedicle flap). Care must be taken to prevent bacterial infections in the damaged area of the cornea because bacteria can induce total destruction of the cornea with potentially catastrophic consequences for the eye.

Clinical signs
- Pain and partial/complete closure of the eyelids
- Swelling and reddening of the conjunctiva
- Excessive tear production and/or discharge from the eye
- Corneal opacity with an irregular surface that stains green with fluorescein dye
- The eye may have secondary 'reflex' uveitis associated with the ulceration

Treatment
- Stable the horse in a dust-free stable and avoid strong light
- Clean discharge from around the eye

- Topical antibiotics, e.g. gentamycin (for Gram-negative bacteria) and fucidic acid (for Gram-positive bacteria)
- Therapy to inhibit destructive bacterial enzymes, especially collagenase enzyme, e.g. fresh serum, ethylenediaminetetraacetic acid (EDTA) or acetylcysteine
- Therapy for uveitis (if this is present)

Uveitis

Aetiology
Uveitis (inflammation of the uvea) is an extremely important condition because the uvea contains most of the blood supply to the eye. Uveitis can result in degeneration in most layers of the eye and chronic or recurrent uveitis can result in blindness.

Recurrent uveitis (also known as periodic ophthalmia and moon blindness) is an immune-mediated disease that occurs after a variety of infections, e.g. leptospirosis, salmonellosis and *Streptococcus equi*. Horses experience recurrent episodes of disease that eventually result in blindness.

Reflex uveitis is a transient form of uveitis that occurs secondary to corneal inflammation, especially corneal ulcers. This form of uveitis is less serious, is not recurrent and does not result in blindness, although there may be damage to the iris and lens.

Clinical signs
- Pain and partial/complete closure of the eyelids
- Resentment of bright light
- Swelling and reddening of the conjunctiva
- Excessive tear production and/or discharge from the eye
- Corneal oedema (opacity but with a regular corneal surface)
- Pupillary constriction (miosis)

Recurrent uveitis cases may develop other chronic changes in the eye:

- Adhesions between the iris and the lens (synechiae)
- Cataract (lens opacities)
- Retinal degeneration
- Blindness

Treatment

(1) It is important to recognise and treat both forms of uveitis because:
  (a) Reflex uveitis is painful and makes the horse more difficult to nurse, as well as delaying recovery.
  (b) Recurrent uveitis is painful and can eventually result in blindness.
(2) Stable the horse in a dust-free stable and avoid strong light.
(3) Clean discharge from around the eye.
(4) Recurrent uveitis cases may need to have a palpebral lavage system fitted to allow easy application of drugs onto the eye.
(5) Mydriatics to dilate the pupil, e.g. atropine.
(6) Corticosteroids to reduce inflammation, e.g. prednisolone.
(7) Antibiotics to prevent secondary bacterial infection.
(8) Systemic NSAIDs.

Muscular diseases

• Myopathies/equine rhabdomyolysis

Equine rhabdomyolysis syndrome (ERS)

Aetiology

Equine rhabdomyolysis syndrome (ERS) is a common problem in all types of performance horse, especially racehorses and sport horses. It is also known as:

• Tying up
• Azoturia
• Exertional rhabdomyolysis
• Paralytic myoglobinuria
• Recurrent equine rhabdomyolysis

Classic management triggers for the diseases are:

(1) Fit horses in full work that are rested for 1–2 days on full feed and then returned to work.
(2) Sudden increases in intensity/amount of work.

Electrolyte imbalances/deficiencies (especially sodium and calcium) in the diet have been implicated, as have deficiencies in vitamin E and or selenium. Although supplementing these can be

of value in some horses, there is no evidence that ERS is directly due to mineral/electrolyte/vitamin deficiencies.

Clinical signs

(1) All types of horse and pony can be affected.
(2) Any age, both sexes but female more than male and younger more than older horses.
(3) More common in nervous/excitable individuals.
(4) Often, but not always, triggered by exercise.
(5) Very variable from mild to severe:
  (a) *Mild*: slight stiffness (hindlimbs mainly) with shortened stride; muscles appear normal.
  (b) *Moderate*: reluctance/inability to move, muscles firm and painful, sweating and tachycardia/tachypnoea, myoglobinuria, possible circulatory compromise.
  (c) *Severe*: recumbent, severe pain, profuse sweating, apparent muscle wasting, myoglobinuria, dehydration, hypovolaemia and renal failure.

Diagnosis

• History and clinical signs
• Raised muscle enzymes on biochemistry: creatinine kinase and aspartate aminotransferase
• Urine may be dark, chocolate-coloured due to presence of muscle protein (this is called myoglobinuria).

Treatment

• Do not walk the horse or force it to walk
• Feed at maintenance levels only (hay and water + electrolytes)
• Give pain relief: NSAIDs (e.g. flunixin or phenylbutazone)
• Sedation may be required if the horse is very distressed
• Oral or (for severe cases) intravenous fluids.

Prevention

This is the most difficult aspect on which to advise but is the area on which all owners want information. Lack of understanding of the precise aetiology makes prevention difficult but the following are sensible precautions:

- Provide adequate warm-up before strenuous exercise
- Match feeding with exercise (see Chapter 6).

Foal diseases (also see Chapter 15)

- Colostrum deficiency
- Septicaemia
- Prematurity and dysmaturity
- Neonatal maladjustment syndrome (NMS)/ perinatal asphyxia syndrome (PAS)

Colostrum deficiency

Failure to receive enough good-quality colostrum (see Key points 14.1) is the most important predisposing factor in the development of bacterial infections and septicaemia in foals. Foals depends entirely on maternal antibody via colostrum for immunity up to the age of 6–12 weeks old when their own immune system matures.

Key points 14.1 Colostrum

Good-quality colostrum

Thick and sticky
Specific gravity > 1.060
Protein content > 30 g/L
Contains antibodies against pathogens in the foal's environment

Normal colostrum intake for a foal is at least 1 L within the first 18 h after birth, with most foals consuming 2 l. There is little absorption of colostral antibodies after 18 h old and almost none after 24 h old. A normal foal should achieve serum antibody levels of >8 g/L (most reach 12–16 g/L) by 24–26 h old. Failure to achieve a level of 8 g/L is referred to as 'failure in passive transfer' and should be corrected to prevent the foal from developing septicaemia.

Passive transfer of colostral antibodies can be assessed by taking a blood sample when the foal is between 18 and 30 h old and estimating the amount of antibody in plasma by:

- Zinc sulphate turbidity (semi-quantitative)
- Glutaraldehyde precipitation (semi-quantitative)
- Immunoassays, e.g. Cite® (quantitative)

If a foal fails to drink enough colostrum, this should be corrected by giving:

- Plasma from the mare (or use proprietary plasma). Give at least 20 ml/kg (40 ml/kg is optimum) of the mare's plasma by slow intravenous infusion or give 200 mg/kg of proprietary plasma.
- Broad-spectrum antibiotics.
- Tetanus antitoxin.

Septicaemia

Aetiology
Septicaemia occurs when bacteria enter the circulation from the respiratory tract, gastrointestinal tract or umbilicus and establish devastating, rapidly developing multi-organ infections that are rapidly progressive and often fatal. The main organs to become infected are the lungs, joints and CNS.

Clinical signs
Initially the clinical signs are vague, but they progress rapidly from 24 to 48 h old:

- Lethargy, poor suck reflex
- Initial pyrexia then hypothermia
- Pneumonia ± respiratory distress
- Diarrhoea and colic
- Painful, swollen joints
- Swollen, painful navel (omphalitis)
- Uveitis
- Progressive dehydration
- Recumbency
- Convulsions, coma, death.

Diagnosis
- History and clinical signs
- Positive bacterial blood culture
- Neutrophil count normal, then falling total white blood cell count
- Increased fibrinogen
- Hypoglycaemia, hypoxia, acidosis
- Low plasma antibody levels.

Treatment

Treatment is difficult and foals with septicaemia (see Example 14.6) require intensive nursing effort (see Chapter 15):

Example 14.6   Foal septicaemia

A 4-day-old foal has had diarrhoea and now appears depressed and is unwilling to suck. (The mare's udder is distended.) You take the foal's temperature and you find that it has pyrexia. What do you do?

The foal may be developing septicaemia. This is a rapidly progressive, ultimately fatal condition if untreated. Other findings on clinical examination in septicaemia include signs of pneumonia, swollen umbilicus, swollen joints and uveitis. The major nursing problems that this foals presents are dehydration and hypovolaemia (because it is not suckling and because of bacterial endotoxins) and hypothermia (because it is not suckling and therefore has no energy intake). These should be addressed by giving the foal intravenous fluids (Hartmann's solution), keeping the foal in a warm, draught-free room, putting on a rug and limb bandages and giving milk by stomach tube. The foal also will require treatment with antibiotics. The perineum should be cleaned and the skin protected from damage by the diarrhoea by petroleum jelly. If the foal becomes recumbent it will need constant attention, keeping it on plastic-covered mats and turning every 4 h with intensive nursing care (see Chapter 15).

- Intensive drug therapy will also be used including plasma from the mare, antibiotics (usually gentamycin or amikacin)
- Intravenous fluids, see foal nursing (15) and fluids (13) chapters.

Prematurity and dysmaturity

These terms are used to describe foals that are smaller and weaker than expected:

- *Prematurity* refers to weak, small foals, that are delivered after less than 320 days of gestation.
- *Dysmaturity* refers to weak, small foals that are delivered close to or at full term, i.e. after more than 320 days of gestation.

Premature foals are at more risk than dysmature foals but both groups may show some or all of the following: delay in standing and suckling, soft and silky and possibly 'respiratory distress syndrome'. Severely affected foals may deteriorate rapidly resulting in lateral recumbency, opisthotonus, paddling, convulsions and death.

Neonatal maladjustment syndrome (NMS)/perinatal asphyxia syndrome (PAS)

The cause of this is not well understood but is associated with variable severity of hypoxia, cerebral oedema and haemorrhage following either apparently normal births or problem births, e.g. dystocia, premature cord rupture postpartum or poor pulmonary function. Affected foals are also known as 'dummies', 'wanderers' and 'barkers'. Generally NMS foals are full term and normal birthweight (i.e. they are not premature/dysmature foals).

Clinical signs

The foal may be normal at birth and passes meconium normally. Clinical signs develop at approximately 24 h old. Mild cases lose their suck reflex, appear blind (wander aimlessly around and do not follow mare) and have an exaggerated response to handling (hyperaesthesia). Severe cases cannot suck or stand, may have respiratory distress, hypothermia, jerky (clonic) convulsions (may be violent), may develop opisthotonus and may make expiratory barking or yapping noises.

Treatment

These foals are worth treating in many cases. Their main requirement is diligent and patient nursing and many will make a full recovery. Medications such as diazepam or phenobarbitone may control convulsions.

Endocrine system diseases

- Pituitary tumour (equine Cushing's disease)
- Hyperlipaemia

Pituitary tumour (equine Cushing's disease)

Aetiology
Pituitary tumours are common in aged ponies and cause equine Cushing's disease. The tumour causes disease via altered hormone production from the pituitary gland and the adrenal glands, as well as effects due to compression of the base of the brain and optic nerves.

Clinical signs
Old pony mares are mainly affected, but the tumour can occur in horses and ponies of any age and in both males and females. The tumour causes a wide range of clinical signs, although the four most common signs are:

(1) Hirsuitism
(2) Weight loss
(3) Lethargy
(4) Laminitis.

A pony or horse that has this profile of clinical signs is very likely to have a pituitary tumour (see Fig. 14.2).
  Other clinical signs include:

- Polyuria/polydipsia
- Excess sweating
- Tachycardia/tachypnoea
- Skin and other infections
- Oral and colonic ulceration
- Bulging supra-orbital fat pads.

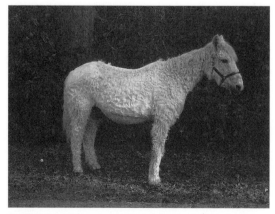

Fig. 14.2 Pony with long curly coat typical of equine Cushing's disease.

- Neurological signs
- Irregular oestrus
- Lactation (without pregnancy).

Diagnosis
Haematology and biochemistry may be helpful:

- Leucocytosis with neutrophilia, lymphopenia and eosinopenia
- Hyperglycaemia and glucosuria
- A persistently raised serum insulin is a good indicator of the disease.

A definitive diagnosis requires dynamic hormone testing. The two most frequently performed tests are:

(1) Thyroid-releasing hormone (TRH) stimulation test: if a pituitary tumour is present there is an increase in plasma cortisol levels after intravenous injection of TRH.
(2) Dexamethasone suppression test: if a pituitary tumour is present there is less than normal reduction in plasma cortisol levels following intramuscular injection of dexamethasone.

Management
Pituitary tumour cases can be managed successfully although this is expensive and requires commitment. Treatment is not curative but will prolong the animal's life. Treatment with drugs that inhibit the metabolic activity of the tumour are helpful:

- Pergolide 'Celance©' (a dopaminergic agonist): daily treatment
- Cyproheptadine 'Periactin©' (a serotonin antagonist): daily treatment
- The coat should be kept clipped and groomed
- The feet require regular farriery; if laminitis is present this will need specific treatment (see Chapter 16).

Hyperlipaemia

Aetiology
Hyperlipaemia is a serious (usually fatal) metabolic disease of fat native ponies where there is excessive mobilisation of lipid from fat stores resulting in hepatic and renal failure because of fatty infiltration of these organs.

Pathogenesis

Hyperlipaemia occurs mainly in fat ponies when there is uncontrolled mobilisation of fat in response to:

- Energy demands in late pregnancy and early-peak lactation (see Example 14.7)
- Stress (transportation or illness, especially laminitis or severe alimentary disease)
- Malnutrition (poor teeth) or following underfeeding, e.g. to prevent laminitis

---

Example 14.7   Hyperlipaemia

A fat, pregnant pony mare suddenly becomes depressed, lethargic and inappetent. A blood sample reveals that the plasma is cloudy.

This pony almost certainly has hyperlipaemia. The metabolic demands of late pregnancy and peak lactation are important trigger factors in fat, native pony breeds. The nursing priority is to maintain energy intake to reduce the demand for fat mobilisation. The pony should be given glucose (1 g/kg four times daily) by stomach tube and 5% dextrose saline intravenously. The pony probably will be treated with insulin and possibly also heparin. The pony should be offered a selection of palatable feeds to encourage it to eat and as soon as it starts eating glucose should be added to the diet to avoid the need for repeated stomach tubing. It may be necessary to abort the foal but this is not straightforward in mares, it is stressful and may lead to further deterioration.

Native ponies are predisposed to this disease because of an inherent resistance to insulin.

Clinical signs

- Progress rapidly, with death in 6–21 days
- Initial signs are depression, anorexia, weakness and mild abdominal pain
- Later signs are profound depression and hepatic encephalopathy; diarrhoea, progressive dehydration, acidosis and hypokalaemia

Diagnosis

- History and clinical signs
- Plasma may appear cloudy or fatty
- Increase in plasma lipid levels (triglyceride levels >5 mmol/L)
- Raised liver enzymes

Management

(1) Remove the precipitating cause:
   - (a) Wean lactating mares.
   - (b) Abort pregnant mares.
   - (c) Treatment of all cases with anthelminthics is sensible.
   - (d) Treat any underlying disease, especially laminitis.

(2) Prevent further lipid mobilisation:
   - (a) 5% Dextrose saline (5 L/100 kg/24 h).
   - (b) Oral glucose (1 g/kg by stomach tube four times daily) may be sufficient in early cases.
   - (c) Feed slurry of complete pony cubes by stomach tube if it will not eat.
   - (d) Insulin therapy may help.
   - (e) Corticosteroids should not be used.

(3) Promote movement of lipid into fat stores by using heparin, but use with caution because of the risk of haemorrhage.

(4) Treat dehydration and acidosis:
   - (a) Advanced cases become dehydrated with associated acidosis and azotaemia.
   - (b) Use Hartmann's (lactated Ringer's) solution to correct before moving on to glucose saline for maintenance.

(5) Hepatic encephalopathy:
   - (a) Consider welfare and prognosis before treating.

Further reading

Mair, T., Love, S., Schumaker, J. & Watson, E. (1998) *Equine Medicine, Surgery and Reproduction*, 1st edn. WB Saunders, London.

Millar, B. (1998) Care and disinfection of endoscopes. *Equine Vet. Educ.* **10**, 278–280.

Milne, E. & Wallis, N. (1994) Nursing the chronic grass sickness patient. *Equine Vet. Educ.* **6**, 217–219.

Foal Nursing

S. J. Stoneham

Nursing the neonatal and young foal

Why are foals different?

At birth the foal leaves the protected uterine environment and during the first few days of life (i.e. the *neonatal period*) the body systems must develop and mature (see Key points 15.1 for initial reflexes and adaptive behaviour). A healthy foal grows rapidly, and by 3 months old is far more like the mature horse. There are certain diseases to which foals remain particularly susceptible due to their immaturity and continuing growth.

Immune system

The foal is born without circulating antibodies (agammaglobulinaemia) because the epitheliochorial equine placenta prevents the transfer of antibodies (immunoglobulins) from mare to fetus. The foal is totally dependent on ingestion and absorption of colostral immunoglobulins.

The mare concentrates antibodies in the colostrum during the last 3–4 weeks of gestation. If the mare suffers premature lactation ('runs milk') the colostrum will be lost. The foal absorbs the immunoglobulins via specialised cells throughout the length of the small intestine and they pass via the lymphatics to the systemic circulation. This process is at its most efficient immediately after birth and declines rapidly to be ineffective by 24 h after birth. It is important that

Key points 15.1   The newborn foal

Normal adaptive behaviour and reflexes of the newborn foal

- Within moments of birth the foal starts gasping respiration and exhibits a righting reflex sitting in sternal recumbency.
- The suck reflex develops within 5–10 min of birth.
- The foal starts struggling attempts to stand; most foals will stand within 1–2 h.
- Foals should be suckling from the mare within 3 h of birth; many foals will stand and suck far more rapidly.
- Foals will suck 5–7 times an hour, although the frequency of nursing may be decreased during periods of sleep.
- Foals should begin to produce large quantities of dilute urine within 12 h.
- Meconium is usually passed within 12 h and then paler milk dung is observed.
- Young foals are bright and inquisitive: they explore the environment and interact with the mare; they are very reactive to external stimuli.

the best-quality colostrum is ingested in the first few feeds.

When nursing neonatal foals, it is vital to ensure that they receive adequate quantities of high-quality colostrum. Standards of nursing and hygiene must be high to reduce the risk of infection.

Table 15.1 Normal heart and respiratory rates and rectal temperature of the neonatal foal

Age	Heart rate (bpm)	Respiratory rate (bpm)	Temperature °C (°F)
1 min	60–80	Gasping	37–39 (99–102)
15 min	120–160	40–60	37–39 (99–102)
12 h	80–120	30–40	37–39 (99–102)
24 h	80–100	30	37–39 (99–102)

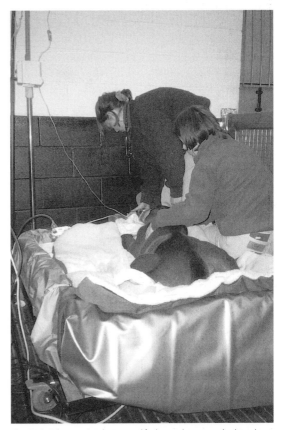

Fig. 15.1 When nursing the neonatal foal, sternal as opposed to lateral positioning can increase arterial oxygen tensions by up to 20 mmHg.

Cardiovascular system

There are dramatic changes in the cardiovascular system during the first few hours of extra-uterine life: closure of the ductus arteriosus and foramen ovale and reduction of pulmonary vascular resistance. Normally the foal receives up to 1.5 L of blood from the placenta prior to separation of the cord. Premature cord separation can produce significant hypovolaemia and anaemia. During the rest of the neonatal period there is a gradual increase in cardiac reserve and mean systemic arterial pressure. The heart rate changes over the neonatal period (see Table 15.1).

Respiratory system

The first few gasping breaths at birth open up the alveoli and expand the lungs (see Table 15.1). The chest wall of the neonate is very compliant and body position has a significant effect on blood oxygen levels. The equine neonatal lung is very prone to collapse or failure to expand (atelectasis). By the end of the first week the foal's respiratory reserve has increased significantly (Fig. 15.1).

Renal system

The neonatal kidneys are less able to respond to volume depletion by increasing urine concentration. Immature renal function also must be considered when using potentially nephrotoxic drugs such as aminoglycosides.

Gastrointestinal system

There are only small liver glycogen reserves in the newborn foal and unless it rapidly ingests colostrum it will start to break down other body tissue to meet its energy demands.

The foal is dependent on continuous ingestion of colostrum and milk to maintain blood glucose levels within the normal range. Foals consume large quantities of milk: a 50-kg 3-day-old foal will consume 12–15 L daily.

Thermoregulation

The newborn foal's ability to thermoregulate is poor. The foal must maintain body temperature by shivering, muscular activity and food intake. Foals, particularly those born in cold weather, are prone to hypothermia when food intake and muscular activity are reduced.

Nutrition

During the first few weeks of life the nutritional needs of the foal are met by mare's milk. Foals consume large quantities of milk (20–28% of bodyweight daily) and this continues to increase for the next 6–8 weeks until peak lactation. Digestion of mare's milk by the foal is very efficient, e.g. a Thoroughbred foal will have an average daily weight gain of 1–1.5 kg/day.

Young foals start to nibble mare's feed and hay at a few days of age, however 'solids' only make a significant contribution to their nutrition at 2–3 months old. Digestion in a young foal of less than 3 months is principally small intestinal. Large intestinal digestion and function develop gradually during this period. Some foals, particularly those on box rest, may ingest quantities of hay, which may contribute to a change in faecal consistency due to their inability to digest fibre.

Lactation

The mammary gland is made up of two mammae, each with two or rarely three lobes. There is one opening for each lobe at the end of the teat. Milk is secreted by specialised epithelial cells in response to complex action of many hormones, including prolactin, oestrogens, progestagens, adrenal steroids, insulin, growth and thyroid hormones.

During the last part of pregnancy a watery secretion is produced that gradually becomes thicker and whiter as parturition approaches. The electrolyte composition changes as well. Immunoglobulin concentrations in individual mare's colostrum vary considerably. Quality can be assessed easily using a sugar refractometer to evaluate specific gravity: levels above 23% are considered good; below 20% are inadequate. The nutritional needs of the mare increase during lactation and peak lactation occurs at about 2 months postpartum. Most mares in average body condition will require approximately 1.5 times maintenance during lactation, but every mare should be

fed according to individual needs. Owners tend to overestimate the nutritional needs of the mare during pregnancy but may not appreciate the increased demands of lactation.

Problems of lactation

Agalactia (failure of the mare to secrete colostrum or milk)

This condition should be distinguished from the more common problem of restricted milk let-down in first foaling mares or those with painful udders. In these cases careful management, the use of low doses of oxytocin (5 IU) and sedation usually resolve the problem in a few days. Some mares that foal early in the year may not increase milk production as rapidly as the foal's demands increase.

True agalactia is rare in the UK; fescue toxicity causes agalactia in the USA. Occasionally when a mare is ill the milk supply will fall, but as long as the foal remains with the mare and is allowed to suckle, production will usually return as the mare recovers. It is important to supplement the foal with milk replacer during this period.

It is also important to milk out the mare regularly if the foal is unable to suckle for any length of time to ensure that milk production does not stop.

Mastitis

This most commonly develops post-weaning, particularly when flies are prevalent. It occasionally develops during lactation, when the foal fails to suckle and this goes untreated. Signs of mastitis include a hot, painful udder, often with marked oedema and pyrexia. Some mares may become reluctant to move. Treatment is based on frequent stripping of the udder, the use of local antibiotics, if practical or systemic antibiotics and non-steroidal anti-inflammatory drugs (NSAIDs).

Weaning

Foals are usually weaned at about 6 months of age. Occasionally they may be weaned earlier (ideally more than 3 months old) if the foal has growth-related problems or if the mare dies.

They become increasingly independent of the

mare and ingest significant quantities of grass, hay or feed. It is usual to ensure that the foal is eating foal rations and the digestive system has adapted to this prior to weaning. Foal creep rations (feed for foals) are designed to be palatable and provide the proteins, mineral and trace elements necessary for healthy growth and development. Most large feed companies produce two types of foal ration:

(1) A concentrated ration providing appropriate levels of high-quality proteins, vitamins, minerals and trace elements for musculoskeletal growth and development. Energy levels are low and a small amount is fed. This feed is used for individuals in good or excess body condition.

(2) A more traditional ration that provides significant energy levels in addition to appropriate levels of proteins, minerals and trace elements.

Studs tend to wean foals by removing one mare from a group of suitably aged foals and mares at pasture every few days, leaving the quietest and most amenable mare until last. The mare should be moved to a distant site where she should receive reduced rations and adequate exercise to hasten drying up of the milk. There will be some passive loss of milk from the udder. Active stripping of the udder should be discouraged unless the mare develops mastitis; the increased pressure of milk in the udder helps to reduce milk production.

Weaning stresses foals and they frequently succumb to recurrent respiratory tract infections. It is particularly important that the foal's health and condition is carefully monitored during this period.

After weaning, the foal's nutrition can be regulated more carefully. Individual requirements vary considerably and the ration should be formulated by taking the following into consideration:

- The condition of the foal (important that growing foals should *not* become overweight)
- Any pasture and forage analysis
- The ration should meet the requirements for essential amino acids, minerals and trace elements
- Any developmental problems
- Method of feeding.

Regular monitoring of weight and height is important to ensure a steady growth rate.

The orphan foal

A foal may be orphaned by:

- Death of the mare
- Rejection by the mare
- Illness of the mare
- Disease of the foal
- Management reasons.

Orphans are difficult to rear and frequently develop behavioural problems later in life. Long term, it helps to foster a foal rather than to hand rear it.

Foals usually can be trained to feed from a bucket or bowl from a young age. It is important to avoid the foal becoming humanised. Some form of equine company, e.g. an old pony, is vitally important for the foal to develop normal equine behaviour patterns.

During the first 2 days a healthy 50-kg foal will consume 5–7 L of mare's milk and should be fed every 1–2 hours. The foal's intake will rise rapidly over the next week, rising to 12–15 L/day and then steadily increasing at about 23–28% bodyweight/day.

A good-quality milk replacer should be used. Calf and lamb milk replacers are *not* suitable. Some milk manufacturers recommend low volumes of more concentrated replacer.

There are several practical points to remember when feeding a young foal:

- Follow specific instruction for concentration of replacer
- Keep all utensils used for mixing and feeding foals scrupulously clean
- Record quantities of milk consumed
- Store any unused replacer to be fed later in the fridge until required
- Weigh or weigh tape the foal regularly to ensure appropriate daily weight gain. Growth should be plotted on a curve and compared to a standard growth curve for animal's expected mature weight
- A foal's bodyweight increases rapidly and so will milk consumption
- Note changes in faecal consistency.

It is advisable to feed a special mineral, vitamin and trace element supplement. Foals should be offered a creep ration from about 1 week of age. Although they are not able to digest it completely, it encourages the foal to eat concentrates and stimulates the gut to adapt.

Routine management of the foal/weanling

Foot care

It is best to start handling foals' limbs from a few days of age, so they become used to the handling and they pick up their feet. Foals are usually first seen by the farrier at 4–6 weeks and then should have their feet trimmed at approximately 4-week intervals, depending on the rate of horn growth and wear. Foals with congenital limb deformities may require corrective trimming and surgical farriery earlier on.

Worming

On well-managed premises, foals should be treated first with anthelmintics at about 1 month. An ivermectin preparation is most effective against the intestinal parasites affecting foals. The dosing interval is short in this susceptible group; they should receive an ivermectin preparation every 4–6 weeks. It is important to assess bodyweight each time and dose accordingly. Moxidectin should not be given to foals under 4 months old. Weanlings should receive a double dose of pyrantel in the autumn to treat for tapeworms. It is important also to recommend suitable paddock management, e.g. picking up droppings, plus strategic use of anthelmintics.

Vaccination

If the mare has not been vaccinated correctly for tetanus (including a booster 4–6 weeks prior to foaling,) the foal should receive prophylactic tetanus antitoxin soon after birth.

Maternally derived immunity interferes with early vaccination. Influenza vaccination should not be started until 6 months, although tetanus can be started much earlier. The vaccination schedule should follow vaccine manufacturers' recommendations. Vaccination against respiratory disease caused by equine herpes virus 1 and 4 (EHV-1 and -4) is also available.

Blood typing, microchipping and markings

All thoroughbreds and non-thoroughbreds to be registered with Weatherbys in the UK require a veterinary surgeon to take blood samples for typing, to insert a specific microchip and to record a certificate of markings. Other breed societies have slightly different requirements.

Sick foals

Common conditions affecting the neonatal foal

The common conditions that affect neonatal foals are listed in Table 15.2. It is important to remember that neonates may suffer multiple problems and that further complications often develop during the course of a condition. Many are unique and related to the adapting physiological status and poorly developed homeostatic mechanisms of the foal.

Clinical signs are often similar and subtle. Careful observation and recording of serial findings is

Table 15.2 Common conditions affecting the neonatal foal (after Rossdale, 1972)

Type of condition	Disease
Group 1 Infective conditions	• Septicaemia, bacterial or viral • Focal infections, e.g. septic arthritis, diarrhoea, pneumonia
Group 2 Disturbances in adaptive processes	• Neonatal maladjustment syndrome (hypoxic ischaemic encephalopathy) • Prematurity/dysmaturity • Meconium retention
Group 3 Developmental conditions	• Rupture of bladder • Patent urachus • Limb deformity • Congenital deformity
Group 4 Immunological conditions	• Failure of passive transfer • Neonatal isoerythrolysis • Combined immunodeficiency • Fell pony syndrome

important to allow trends rather than absolute changes to become apparent. Further diagnostic procedures are usually necessary to establish a diagnosis (see later section on common diagnostic procedures). Frequently the pregnancy and parturition provide a useful history. Clinical signs and specific therapy are well described (further reading list and Chapter 14).

Stabilisation of the sick neonatal foal

Many sick neonates present as dull, depressed and 'off suck', rapidly progressing to collapse and coma. Disease processes rapidly destabilise the maturing homeostatic mechanisms in the neonatal foal. The immediate care of these individuals, regardless of diagnosis, is vital in increasing their chance of recovery. It is important to assess and attend to the immediate needs of the foal and closely monitor their progress.

Fluid therapy

Neonatal foals are susceptible to hypovolaemia and severe electrolyte disturbances, because the immature kidney is less able to compensate for fluid and electrolyte losses. Foals have a relatively large extracellular fluid (ECF) and plasma volume compared with the adult horse. It is important to assess hydration and electrolyte levels at regular intervals and tailor a fluid therapy plan accordingly.

Initially a collapsed neonate may need a rapid infusion of fluids to support the circulation. One litre of fluid can be administered over 20 min to a 50-kg foal. In the absence of laboratory data, either 1 L of 5% dextrose saline or 1 l of Hartmann's spiked with 100 ml of 50% dextrose to give a 5% dextrose solution should be used. In most cases the foal is hypothermic, so fluids should be warmed.

The rate then should be reduced, the fluid requirement over 24 h calculated and fluid given continuously over this period. Maintenance requirements, when there are no excessive losses, have been estimated at 80–120 ml/kg/day. It is important not to overload the circulation or overhydrate the foal. It may be necessary to correct specific electrolytes, e.g. hypokalaemia or hypocalcaemia, or acid–base deficits. It also may be necessary to provide partial or total parenteral nutrition in foals with compromised gastrointestinal function.

It is important to monitor urine output (usually 3–4 L/day). Anuria or oliguria suggests renal compromise or disruption to the urinary tract.

Nutritional support

It is important to assess the foal's suck reflex. An indwelling nasogastric tube will be necessary if it is poor. Ileus is a common complication in sick recumbent foals, therefore gut function should be evaluated before large volumes of milk are given. If ileus is a problem and the foal is supported via the parenteral route, small volumes (5–10 ml/h) of milk should be given to allow normal maturation of gut function.

Sick neonatal foals are prone to severe hypoglycaemia (blood glucose levels <4 mmol/L); if this remains uncorrected, irreversible damage is inevitable. Intravenous 5–10% dextrose saline solution can be given to correct this, ideally administered by slow continuous infusion to avoid wide swings in blood glucose levels. Hyperglycaemia (blood glucose levels >10 mmol/L) occurs due to inappropriate administration of glucose solution, sepsis, prematurity or insulin insensitivity.

It is difficult to meet the requirements for maintenance and growth in sick neonates (see further reading list).

Respiratory support

Inadequate lung function is a common problem in recumbent neonatal foals. Lateral recumbency results in poor ventilation of the lower lung. Concerted efforts therefore should be made to keep sick foals in a sternal position.

It may be necessary to provide intranasal oxygen therapy (Fig. 15.2) as follows:

- Use soft intranasal tubing
- Place end of tubing to level of medial canthus
- Secure in place using tape or sutures
- Ensure there are no kinks in oxygen tubing
- Use of clear tubing allows monitoring of tubing
- Set flow rate (2–10 L/min); almost 100% oxygen is provided by a flow rate of 10 L/min
- Check oxygen tank and tubing regularly
- Change all tubing daily

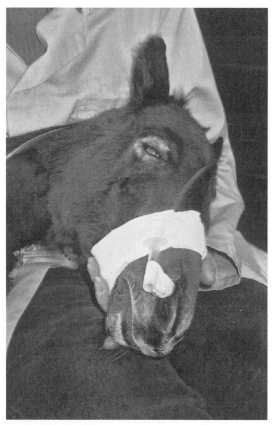

Fig. 15.2 Intranasal oxygen therapy.

If oxygen is to be used for more than 1 h, it must be humidified (using sterile water).

Regular arterial blood gas samples are taken to monitor respiratory function and the oxygen flow rates are altered accordingly.

Maintenance of body temperature

Hypothermia is common in sick neonatal foals and may be severe. Sick foals should be rugged and limbs bandaged to prevent further heat loss. In the initial stage, temperature should be monitored at least hourly. Fluids should be warmed. Once dehydration and hypoglycaemia have been corrected, more rapid warming can proceed. Environmental temperatures should be controlled and overheating avoided. Care must be taken when applying heat to the skin,

because foals are very susceptible to thermal burns. Foals with high temperatures (>39°C) should be 'unwrapped' and the environmental temperature reduced.

Management of pain or neurological signs

It can be difficult to assess pain in sick foals and difficult to distinguish neurological signs from those of pain, particularly in the recumbent foal. However, a complete evaluation of the foal and stabilisation may not be possible without the use of sedation and/or analgesia. Short-acting drugs, such as diazepam, often are used in the first instance in foals exhibiting neurological signs. Analgesics such as butorphanol additionally may produce significant sedation. Non-steroidal anti-inflammatory drugs (NSAIDs) should be used with caution.

Common diagnostic procedures used in foals

Blood sampling

Blood samples frequently are required from foals. It is usual to collect them by venepuncture of the jugular vein and it is important that the foal is adequately restrained to do so (Fig. 15.3). If the jugular is to be used for frequent blood sampling and drug administration it is useful to place an intravenous catheter. Samples may be required for haematology, biochemistry, serum proteins (particularly immunoglobulin G), serum electrolytes and blood glucose.

Blood samples should be taken for culture from all neonates with any signs of sepsis. Ideally samples should be taken prior to the administration of antibiotics. Samples for blood culture must be obtained aseptically, as follows:

- Clip site
- Prepare with surgical scrub and spray with surgical spirit
- Use surgical gloves
- Take 10 ml of blood using sterile needle and syringe
- Place directly in blood culture bottle using a clean needle.

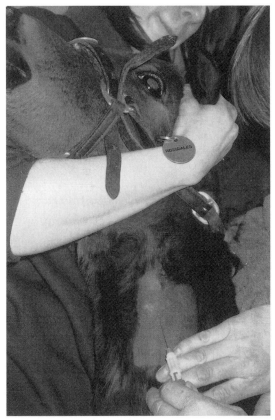

Table 15.3 Normal blood gas parameters for a foal in lateral recumbency

Parameter	Normal range
pH	7.3–7.4
P_aO_2	70–90 mmHg
P_aCO_2	42–45 mmHg
Base excess	+6 mmol/L
HCO_3^-	26–30 mmol/L

Fig. 15.3 Foal restrained for collection of a blood sample.

Synoviocentesis

Collection of samples from suspected septic synovial structures in the foal is performed as follows:

- The foal must be restrained adequately; often the use of sedatives facilitates this.
- Be well prepared with all the necessary equipment, including blood culture bottles, ethylenediamineltetraacetic acid (EDTA) and plain tubes, surgical gloves, syringes and needles, close at hand.
- Clip the site.
- Prepare the site with surgical scrub.
- It is usual to collect samples for cytology and proteins; place as much synovial fluid as possible directly into the blood culture bottles.
- When introducing synovial fluid into the blood culture bottle it is important to use a fresh needle and do so in an aseptic way to prevent contamination of the culture, only removing the cap from the bottle immediately prior to injecting the synovial fluid.

Ultrasound evaluation

Ultrasound evaluation of the chest, abdomen and umbilical remnants is often carried out in the foal. Useful diagnostic information can be obtained by this well-tolerated procedure, performed as follows:

- The neonate may be evaluated standing or in lateral recumbency; often only minimal, calm restraint is required. It may be necessary to hold the mare at a safe distance.
- In many cases clipping is not required and the liberal application of surgical spirit to the appropriate site is all that is necessary.

Blood gas samples

Arterial samples may be required because these provide useful information on lung function. Regular sampling can monitor blood gas levels and pH (Table 15.3). The procedure is as follows:

- Usually samples are collected from the metatarsal or brachial artery
- The foal is restrained in lateral recumbency
- Use a microsampler for collection
- The site may require clipping
- Apply surgical spirit to the site
- Sample is collected for immediate analysis or transported on ice
- Pressure must be applied over the site of arteriopuncture to prevent haematoma formation.

- Abdominocentesis often is performed with ultrasound guidance, in which case the ventral abdomen will require clipping and a surgical scrub prior to sample collection.

Radiography

Radiography of chest, abdomen and limbs can be carried out with a portable machine and rapid screens as follows:

- Chest and abdomen are usually radiographed in lateral and sternal recumbency in the neonate and standing in the slightly older foal.
- Radiography of the limbs often is performed to assess congenital deformity, in which case the foal must be weight-bearing on the limb.
- Serial radiography is particularly useful in evaluation of response to treatment of pneumonias, in which case it is important to record settings and distances so that films will be comparable.

Blood pressure

Blood pressure can be monitored indirectly in the conscious foal or a direct arterial line may be used in the anaesthetised or semi-conscious recumbent foal, as follows:

- Indirect measurement is simple to perform using an appropriately sized tail cuff (4 or 5 cm in a 50-kg foal).
- It must be carefully positioned and movement should be avoided.
- It is often helpful to repeat the procedure and compare the pulse rate to make sure that the reading is valid. It is more useful to monitor trends rather than absolute values.
- Direct measurement usually is performed using an arterial line in the facial or metatarsal artery. It is difficult to maintain patency of the line in a foal that is moving vigorously.

Pulse oximetry

This can be of limited use in the conscious foal, although provided that the rectum is empty a rectal probe may provide useful information in a foal with poor peripheral pulse that makes collection of repeated arterial samples difficult.

Bladder catheterisation

It may be necessary to catheterise a foal to collect a sample for urinalysis and fractional excretion of electrolyte or to monitor urine outflow. It may be necessary to collect urine continuously in a recumbent foal to prevent sores. The procedure for catheterisation is as follows:

- Essential to perform catheterisation aseptically to avoid introducing infection.
- Foal should be well restrained or sedated if necessary.
- Gloves must be worn and the vulva or end of the penis cleaned. The catheter should be inserted gently to avoid unnecessary trauma to the delicate tissues. A small amount of blood (1+) is usual in catheterised samples.
- If continuous urine collection is required, a bag is attached to the open end of the catheter. The open end always should be plugged or attached to a collection bag to avoid ascending infection.

Drugs commonly used in the treatment of sick foals

Antibiotic therapy

Aggressive antibiotic therapy often is essential. Usually a combination of penicillin and an aminoglycoside, either amikacin or gentamycin, is used in the first instance. Antibiotics usually are administered for a minimum of 1 week and in many cases, when there is secondary focal infection, they may be given for up to 1 month.

It is important to weigh the foal to dose it accurately. Foals gain weight rapidly once they start to recover, so drug doses should be reassessed on a weekly basis. In most sick neonates muscle mass is small, making intramuscular injections less appropriate. A long-term intravenous catheter, placed aseptically and maintained carefully, often is useful. Trimethoprim–sulphur combinations and erythromycin can be used orally. Fluroquinolones are *contraindicated* in growing horses due to their damaging effect on maturing cartilage.

Plasma

Intravenous plasma is a useful treatment to boost the foal's immune system and provide a source of specific antibodies. Plasma also increases the oncotic pressure, thus supporting the circulatory system. Commercially available frozen plasma with high immunoglobulin G content is readily available; plasma containing antibodies to the J-5 antigen is appropriate in cases where Gram-negative organisms are likely to be involved.

One litre can be administered intravenously over $\frac{1}{2}$ h. Thereafter, plasma should be administered at 10–20 ml/kg/h. All plasma and blood products must be administered via a blood-giving set containing a filter. The foal should be monitored during transfusion for any signs of an adverse reaction, including raised heart and respiratory rate, muscle tremors, restlessness, hypotension and collapse. Should these signs occur, then transfusion should be halted immediately. If they are mild, it may be restarted with caution at a slower rate.

Non-steroidal anti-inflammatory drugs (NSAIDs)

Low doses of flunixin meglumine can be used for its anti-endotoxic effect, but NSAIDs are known to produce gastric ulcers in foals. It is essential, if the foal is to receive NSAIDs, that it also receives anti-ulcer medication.

Anti-ulcer medication

Should be given routinely to all sick neonatal foals. Omeprazole can be given orally once daily, or ranitidine can be given orally three times daily. In a neonate intolerant to enteral feeding, it can be given intravenously.

Whole blood

Whole blood is administered in severe cases of neonatal isoerythrolysis (haemolytic anaemia). The dam's red cells, washed three times and resuspended in 0.9% sodium chloride as a 50% solution, can be administered. It is essential to monitor the foal closely during transfusion and there must be an in-line filter in the giving set.

Anticonvulsants

Phenytoin, phenobarbitone, pentobarbitone and diazepam are used to control seizures in neonatal maladjustment syndrome. They are usually given at the lowest effective dose to control convulsions. It is usual to make an assessment of the foal as the drug wears off. It is important to differentiate attempts to right and stand from neurological signs. If repeated doses of barbiturates are used, there may be a prolonged period of 'awakening'.

Practical points: nursing of young foals

In general terms, foals less than 2 weeks of age should be considered to be in a period of adaptation and require the greatest level of care. Their homeostatic mechanisms are poorly developed and they have fewer reserves to compensate for environmental challenges. A key feature is their naive immune system and dependence on colostral transfer of immunoglobulins, which makes them particularly susceptible to overwhelming infection. This is of particular concern when nursing them in a hospital environment.

Positioning

Rapidly deteriorating lung function and hypoxaemia are life-threatening complications in foals that are recumbent for prolonged periods. Maintaining recumbent foals in a sternal position plays a vital role in maximising blood oxygenation. This is facilitated by the use of wedges, bags and a suitable bed. Often, with struggling or convulsing foals, having someone sitting with the foal and propping up its chest is the only option. When this is not possible, the foal should be turned every 1–2 h. A record should be kept of position.

Skin

Pressure sores are a common complication that develops unless preventive measures are taken. Pressure relief and keeping the skin clean and dry are essential. The use of a soft synthetic fleece (vetbed) has proved beneficial. It is important that it is kept dry, either by changing the bed regularly or using disposable absorbent liners under the hind end of the foal. Mattresses, inflatable beds or waterbeds provide a soft surface and also raise the foal off the ground. These should be covered with a waterproof sterilisable sheet and the washable bed placed on top of this.

Limb bandages may be applied to help maintain body temperature, for protection or to cover dressings. Special care must be taken when applying these and they must be changed frequently to prevent pressure sores from developing.

If it is necessary to apply casts to correct flexural limb deformities, even padding should be applied beneath the casting material and the casts must be changed frequently (every 2–3 days). The limb should be massaged and physically stretched and manipulated at each change.

Cleanliness

The young foal is uniquely susceptible to infection. High standards of cleanliness and hygiene are essential to reduce the risk. It is important also to remember that some organisms causing infection in neonates may pose a risk to other patients, e.g. *Salmonella*, *Clostridium difficile* or EHV-1. The following steps should be taken:

- Use foot dips outside the box and wear special overalls when attending the foal to help reduce the contamination taken into the box.
- Thorough hand washing before and after attending the foal is important.
- Keep the box regularly skipped out and use plenty of clean bedding.
- Wash and disinfect the feeding utensils.
- Store milk in a fridge between feeds and discard any milk that has been warmed and unused.
- Use an aseptic technique for any invasive procedure.

- Keep the foal's ventral abdomen as clean and dry as possible.
- Clean and tidy the foal unit daily.
- Select a disinfectant appropriate to the organisms involved.
- Pay careful attention to cleaning, disinfecting and air drying of boxes between patients.
- Patients with highly contagious infections (*Salmonella* or *Clostridia* infections) should be isolated.

Umbilicus

Frequent evaluation and care of the umbilicus is important. Complications such as umbilical abscess or patent urachus are common. This area is a particular problem with recumbent foals, especially colts, because urine tends to soak the ventral abdomen. Catheterisation of the bladder may be required.

Eyes

Corneal ulcers can develop as a result of entropion, which may be congenital or secondary to dehydration or physical trauma. Careful monitoring and nursing care avoids the problem developing. The eyes should be check regularly and it is frequently appropriate to instil lubrication into the eyes several times a day as a preventive measure. Entropion should be treated without delay to prevent corneal ulcers from developing.

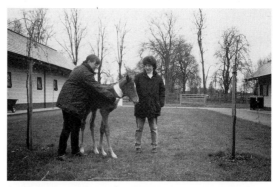

Fig. 15.4 During convalescence it is important to encourage the foal to increase physical activity outside.

Name: Page:
Date:
Clinician:

Time				
Position				
Attitude				
Temp. (°C)				
Resp. Rate (breaths/min)				
Pulse (bt/min)				
Mucous Membs.				
Lung Sounds				
Gut Motility				
Abdominal Distension				
Urine Output				
Faeces				
Blood Pressure (mmHg)				
Comments				
Signature				

Fig. 15.5 Critical care monitoring sheet.

Name: Page:
Date:
Case no.   Clinician:

Replacer strength:

Date	Time of feeding	Amount (ml)	Route and type of feed

Fig. 15.6 Protocol sheet for enteral feeding.

Hypopyon (pus in the front of the eye) may develop in the course of septicaemia.

Bodyweight

It is important to weigh the foal daily to monitor changes. A sick neonate will lose weight rapidly. Weight gain during the recovery phase is a good prognostic sign. It is important also to be aware of changes in bodyweight for calculating drug doses.

Physical therapy

An important part of the recovery phase involves spending time manipulating and mobilising foals. It is important to assist the foals to stand and encourage them to move as soon as possible. They also should be taken for short walks in the fresh air (Fig. 15.4).

Once foals start feeding from a bottle, they should be fed standing as soon as possible and then gradually encouraged to nurse from the mare.

Record keeping

Careful clear records are essential when nursing sick foals. Changes in various parameters are often insidious, and trends are as important as absolute changes.

Special record sheets should be kept for routine monitoring (Fig. 15.5), feeding (Fig. 15.6), fluid therapy (Fig. 15.7), drug dosing and laboratory results.

Foal handling

It is important to be confident when handling and restraining foals because they can react suddenly and unpredictably.

Name:
Date:
Case No.
Page:
Clinician:

Date and Time	Type of fluids	Vol. Fluid Started	Additives and amounts	Rate (ml/hr)	Initials

Fig. 15.7 Protocol sheet for fluid therapy.

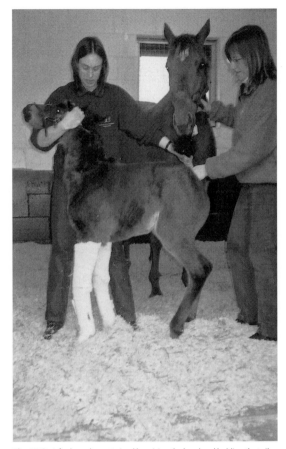

Fig. 15.8 A foal may be restrained by raising the head and holding the tail.

Catching your patient

Healthy foals, unless accustomed to being handled, are best approached slowly and quietly. It is often useful to let the foal come to you because they have a curious nature. It is usual to catch them by the headcollar but then they should be held with one arm around the chest and the other round the hindquarters. With larger lively foals it is often necessary to have a second person on the hindquarters. You should not restrain them by the headcollar because foals have a tendency to pull away and flip over backwards.

If the foal is reluctant to be caught, the mare can be used to make a V with the wall and the foal then is caught under the mare's neck.

Restraint

The general rule is to use the minimum restraint necessary but to be firm enough so that the foal feels secure. Temperament and experience of foals vary considerably and, together with the procedure to be carried out, dictate the type of restraint required. The foal may be restrained for many procedures by raising the head and holding the tail (Fig. 15.8).

To increase the level of restraint, an ear may be held or a 'gypsy twitch' (i.e. grasping a fold of skin on the neck) used. It is inappropriate to use a twitch on a young foal. Sedation with α_2-agonists and butorphanol is useful for carrying out any prolonged or painful procedure. After sedation has taken effect, it is usually possible to lay the foal down.

It may be necessary to restrain foals in lateral recumbency. It is important to have one person holding the head and forelimbs and another on the hindlimbs. Often the foal will struggle less with less restraint. It is sometimes helpful to cover the eye. The lower eye must be protected from trauma.

Further reading

Beech, J. (1985) Neonatal equine disease. *Vet. Clin. North Am.: Equine Pract.* **1**, 1.

Deboer, S. (1992) Transporting ill or injured foals safely. *Equine Vet. Educ.* **4**, 150–153.

Green, S.L. (1994) Hypothermia in the equine neonate. *Equine Vet. Educ.* **6**, 44–46.

Koterba, A.M., Drummond, W.H. & Kosch, P.C. (1990) *Clinical Neonatology.* Lea & Febiger, Philadelphia, PA.

Madigan, J.E. (1991) *Manual of Equine Neonatal Medicine*, 2nd edn. Live Oak Publishing, Woodland, CA.

Rossdale, P.D. (1972) Differential diagnosis and treatment of equine neonatal disease. *Vet. Rec.* **91**, 581–588.

Settle, C.S. & Vaala, W.E. (1990) Nursing care and monitoring techniques for critically ill foals. *Equine Vet. Educ.* **2**, 219–223.

Settle, C.S. & Vaala, W.E. (1991) Management of the critically ill foal: initial respiratory, fluid and nutritional support. *Equine Vet. Educ.* **3**, 49–54.

Vaala, W.E. (1994) Perinatology. *Vet. Clin. North Am.: Equine Pract.* **10**, 1.

Lameness and Orthopaedic Nursing

E. Jones & T. J. Phillips

The approach to all cases of equine lameness should be a systematic progress through the following stages:

(1) Identification of the owner's complaint.
(2) Localisation of the origin of the horse's pain. In some cases this is very easy, e.g. open fractures, but in others it is more difficult, requiring extensive investigation.
(3) Diagnosis of the causative lesion. This may be based on the clinical findings from a physical examination or may require imaging techniques such as radiography, ultrasonography, nuclear scintigraphy or arthroscopy.
(4) Treatment.

The key to understanding equine lameness is to be familiar with the anatomy of the limbs (See Chapter 2).

Lameness diagnosis

Identification of the owner's complaint

Orthopaedic conditions may present as a wide range of problems, e.g. behavioural problems, back pain or poor performance. It is important to establish why an owner is dissatisfied with the horse. Does the lameness explain the owner's complaint? This becomes more difficult to answer when the animal is only displaying a mild degree of lameness.

Localisation of the origin of pain

(see Summary 16.1)

The first stage in an equine lameness examination is

> **Summary 16.1 Assessing lameness**
>
> **Key points on the localisation of the origin of the pain**
>
> - Decide which leg is the problem
> - Use perineural anaesthesia to narrow down which part of the leg is the problem
> - Use synovial structure anaesthesia to decide as accurately as possible which structures are involved
> - Do all the above safely, both for the horse and for the people involved

to find out 'which bit hurts'. It may be possible to decide which structure is painful by eliciting a response to palpation. If not, then a series of questions must be answered.

Which is the lame leg?

This is not always an easy question to answer. However, there are many clues and techniques that can make 'picking a leg' easier. The first stage is to perform a complete examination of the animal, looking for localising signs in each of the four limbs.

The majority of lameness is due to pain. Pain is almost invariably due to *inflammation*. Thus the aim is to look for signs of inflammation:

- Heat
- Pain
- Swelling
- Redness

Physical examination

Examination of the horse in the box (visual)

The horse may be making it very obvious which leg hurts. Is the horse standing normally? Which leg does it spend most time resting? Is the animal continually shifting its weight? Ponies suffering from laminitis often stand leaning back to take weight on to the heel region of the foot. Horses with pain originating from the heels may point one foot out in front of their body or pack bedding under their heels.

Examination at rest (visual/palpation/manipulation)

This involves inspecting the horse, preferably standing square on a level surface. Conformational defects should be noted. Any muscle wastage or swellings may help to localise the region of interest. Then follows systematic palpation and manipulation of each limb in turn. This should identify any areas of heat, pain or swelling. Certain tests also may be performed e.g. the application of hoof testers (Fig. 16.1).

Gait analysis

Examination at walk

If the horse is very lame it may cause further damage to conduct the examination at trot. It is important to look at how the horse places its feet on the floor. Normally a horse should place its foot levelly on the floor; landing heel first may indicate the presence of laminitis. Also it is not uncommon for a horse to place its feet outside edge first; this may indicate a problem with farriery or conformation.

Examination at trot

When the leg that hurts touches the floor, the horse will try to throw as much weight as possible off that leg and to have this limb weight-bearing for the minimum amount of time.

Forelimb

Assuming that the left leg is the lame leg, when this leg is weight-bearing the animal is in pain. It attempts to shorten this phase of the stride by hopping off this leg. This will cause the head to be moved sharply upwards when the lame leg is weight-bearing. Nodding the head down when the right (sound) leg is in contact with the floor helps this reduction in weight-bearing on the lame leg. Factors indicating the presence of a lameness include:

(1) An irregularity in the rhythm of the trot
(2) The position of the head (down on the good leg/up on the lame leg)
(3) Listen to the footfall (louder on the good leg due to more weight being thrown onto it, especially on level concrete).

Hindlimb

The principles remain exactly the same. As the horse moves normally the pelvis rocks, the weight-bearing side being lower than the non-weight-bearing side. If the horse is lame, this rocking will become asymmetrical. The hocks and hips will move in an uneven rhythm and the hip of the lame leg will move further up and down as the horse attempts to keep as much weight as possible off that leg. The stride length is often shorter, with dragging of the toe on the lame leg. If a horse is particularly lame behind, it will also head nod. When the lame leg is on the floor it will throw its weight forward off this limb. This means that at the trot the opposite front leg will be associated with the head moving down.

Tips for detecting lameness

- Take as much time as you need.
- Be consistent in your approach.
- Make sure that the person handling the horse keeps the horse moving forward and active, without moving too quickly.
- Let the horse have enough lead rope so that it can move its head freely.
- Watch it from behind, the side and in front.

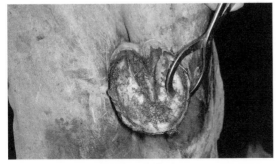

Fig 16.1 Use of hoof testers to assess hoof pain.

Table 16.1 The normal gaits of the horse

- The horse's normal gaits are walk, trot, canter and gallop
- Walking is a four-beat rhythm, as is galloping, whereas trotting is a two-beat diagonal gait and canter is a three-beat gait with both hindlimbs moving together
- Some horses pace rather than trot; pacing is also a two-beat rhythm but involves both legs on one side moving together rather than a diagonal movement

- Watch it on hard and soft ground.
- See the horse on the lunge. This possibly is the easiest time to see subtle lameness because it changes the distribution of weight between the limbs; more weight is carried on the inside leg and the medial aspect of the outside leg. The outside leg has to be moved further and so a lameness of the protraction phase of the stride (swinging the limb forward) also will be accentuated. This also tends to show up bilateral lameness.
- Understand the horse's paces (Table 16.1); most lameness is most easily detected at a trot.

Some gait abnormalities may be associated with neurological disease. This can be manifested by abnormal placing of the feet and lack of 'tracking up', as well as obvious weakness. Proprioceptive (spatial awareness) deficits may be appreciated by placing a horse's feet into abnormal positions and observing whether the horse replaces them immediately. In motion, stumbling and difficulty negotiating obstacles such as slopes or poles may be seen. Horses with neurological disease may show both ataxia (see Chapter 14) and weakness when moving. The tail pull test (where the tail is pulled to one side and then the other as the horse is led forward) can be carried out. A normal horse will resist pulling on the tail, but a neurologically compromised horse cannot and may yield or even come close to collapse.

Grading the lameness

There are various established systems of lameness grading that allow assessment of the severity of lameness and allow quantification of any improvements in the condition. The exact interpretation varies between clinicians, but as long as one is con-

sistent about one's own grading this is perfectly acceptable, such as:

- 0, Sound
- 1, The lameness is subtle and difficult to see but can be heard clearly.
- 2, Head nod visible, moderately lame
- 3, Pronounced head nod
- 4, Horse reluctant to trot
- 5, Non-weight-bearing.

Flexion tests

The principle of flexion tests is to place added stress on selected structures to see if this temporarily increases the lameness (Fig. 16.2). Interpretation of flexion tests is controversial and subjective. The clinician should consider them only as a stage in the examination and not as a definitive decision-maker.

Distal limb flexion

This puts added stress on the interphalangeal joints and the metacarpo/tarsophalangeal (fetlock) joints. This is performed by standing in front of the limb and holding the toe of the hoof. Pull the toe forwards while stopping the upper leg from moving forward with your body. Hold this position for approximately 45 s and then trot the horse away immediately.

Proximal limb flexion

This will put added strain on the carpus and elbow or the hock and stifle. The limb is flexed and supported in the mid-canon region and the lower limb is allowed to relax.

Examination of the hoof

The most common site of lameness in the horse is in the foot. Although the feet should have been assessed in the initial examination, once the lame limb has been identified a closer examination is warranted. It is important to check:

- Is the hoof well balanced?
- Are the heels adequately supported by the shoe?
- When was it last shod?
- Is there any pain with pressure from hoof testers?

If the lame leg has been identified and the degree of lameness quantified but the clinical examination has

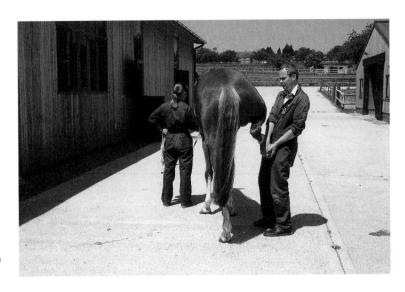

Fig. 16.2 Vet performing a flexion test, which shows how more than one joint is involved.

not provided a diagnosis, only a possible area to investigate, then the next stage is imaging of the area. If the area has not been localised, which often happens, particularly in more chronic cases, then 'nerve blocking' is the next stage. It is the more logical approach rather than randomly radiographing or any other 'fishing exercise' in the hope of finding something potentially significant.

There are risks associated with 'nerve' and 'joint blocking', both to the horse and the personnel. This must be weighed against the risks to personnel of taking unnecessary radiographs, particularly at the high exposures needed for proximal limb views. Also many horses will have boney changes that are not strictly normal but are not painful and therefore are not the cause of the problem. The clinician cannot distinguish between these various abnormalities, or know which to treat, unless you first locate the origin of the pain. Occasionally the procedure may be reversed, e.g. if a fracture is suspected then radiographs are justified first, instead of confirming the site of lameness with diagnostic anaesthesia and risking the fracture being made worse.

Diagnostic regional anaesthesia

The aim of diagnostic regional anaesthesia (nerve blocking) is to identify the site or sites of pain respon-

sible for lameness. To be successful, it is essential that:

(1) The horse is sufficiently lame to assess the effect of local anaesthesia on the gait.
(2) The anatomy is clearly understood so that it is possible to place the local anaesthetic correctly and accurately (Tables 16.2–16.4).

There are two separate techniques.

Perineural anaesthesia

Perineural anaesthesia involves infiltrating local anaesthetic around a sensory nerve. This will block the transmission of pain from the areas supplied by this nerve. If this procedure decreases the level of lameness being shown by the horse, logically the site of pain must be in the area desensitised by the anaesthetic agent. The higher up the limb the injection site, the more of the limb is desensitised. The basic principle involves starting at the most distal point of the limb and working proximally until lameness is abolished. This means that it may take a long time to reach the site of pain. It can be frustrating, but there is no substitute for a complete methodical examination.

Preparation for perineural anaesthesia

(1) Initially brush off the entire limb, so that no dirt or debris falls on the injection site.

CHAPTER 16

Table 16.2 Perineural anaesthesia of the distal limb

Nerve block	Nerves anaesthetised	Injection site	Area desensitised
Palmar/plantar digital	Palmar/plantar digital	Either side of the deep digital flexor tendon at the back of pastern	The deep palmar /plantar foot structures
Abaxial sesamoid	Palmar/plantar	At the base of the sesamoid bones either side of the fetlock	The whole foot and pastern joint
Low 4-point (foreleg)	Palmar	Between suspensory ligament (SL) and deep digital flexor (DDF) tendon	The fetlock and associated structures and the more distal structures
Low 6-point (hindleg)	Palmar metacarpal	5 cm above fetlock	
	Lateral and medial plantar metatarsal	Button of splint bone	
	Lateral and medial dorsal metatarsal	*As for palmar structures*	
	Plantar	Either side of extensor tendon at same level; *As for palmar structures*	
Subcarpal (high 4-point)	Palmar	Between SL and DDF tendon at level of head of splint bone	Palmar cannon bone SL, DDF tendon, superficial digital flexor (SDF) tendon and the distal structures
	Palmar metacarpal	Between SL and head of splint bones	
Subtarsal (high 6-point)	Plantar	*As for palmar structures*	Plantar cannon bone and SL, DDF and SDF tendons and the more distal structures
	Plantar metacarpal		
	Dorsal metatarsal	Subcutaneously around head of splint bones	

(2) The site may or may not need clipping; this will depend on the hairiness of the limb, the vet's preference and the owner's opinion. Generally, clipping enhances the site identification and cleanliness.

(3) Scrub the injection site with a suitable cleansing solution, e.g. chlorhexidine. Four or five scrubs is usually sufficient, until the cotton wool can be wiped over the surface and come away clean. This is not designed to be a sterile procedure so is not essential but it is good practice.

(4) Clean the area with surgical spirit.

(5) Ensure adequate restraint of the horse. Proper restraint is essential, not only to perform the lameness examination but to ensure the safety of staff and patients. Horses undergoing perineural anaesthesia should wear a bit, usually in conjunction with a skin twitch; this is sufficient to allow injection. Further commonly used acceptable restraints are a nose twitch and/or holding up the leg.

If blocking a hindleg, pick up the leg on the same side; if injecting a front leg, pick up the opposite forelimb. There are horses that will not be clipped or injected, and beating them into submission is not acceptable. Occasionally, in the interests of safety, it is necessary to accept that perineural anaesthesia cannot be completed. Finally, always *think about where you choose to stand*; always be on the same side as the vet so that

Table 16.3 Perineural anaesthesia of the upper forelimb

Nerve block	Nerves anaesthetised	Injection site	Area desensitised
Median and ulnar	Median	At the insertion of the pectoral muscle on the forearm	All structures below the elbow (the skin will not be desensitised)
	Ulnar	5 cm proximal to the accessory carpal bone, palmar aspect	
	Medial cutaneous antebrachial	Either side of the cephalic vein, mid-forearm	

Table 16.4 Perineural anaesthesia of the upper hindlimb

Nerve block	Nerves anaesthetised	Injection site	Area desentisised
Tibial and fibular	Tibial	10 cm above hock, medial aspect, cranial to Achilles tendon over deep digital flexor tendon	Hock and all structures below
	Fibular (deep and superficial branches)	In groove between lateral and long digital extensor muscles	

you do not become trapped against the wall if the horse jumps away from the needle. Also, in this position you can pull the horse's head round towards the vet and consequently its quarters away if it decides to take aim!

When perineural anaesthesia has located an area of interest by abolishing the lameness, the next stage of the process may be to perform anaesthesia of synovial structures. Once the perineural injections have worn off and the lameness has returned, the synovial structures (joints, bursas and tendon sheaths) in the area of concern can be anaesthetised selectively.

Intra-articular/intra-thecal anaesthesia

Intra-articular or intra-thecal anaesthesia involves placement of local anaesthetic into a joint cavity, tendon sheath or other cavity, such as a bursa. It is absolutely crucial that the injection of local anaesthetic into any synovial or similar structure be carried out in a sterile manner. In general, perineural anaesthesia is performed first, unless there is suspicion of involvement of a particular synovial structure.

Sepsis of a synovial structure is a career-threatening injury! Although a common procedure in equine practice, the possible consequence of synovial sepsis is potentially catastrophic. It is very important that site preparation is meticulous. If for any reason you have cause to suspect that it is not, repeat the preparation and inform the clinician.

Preparation for the injection of a synovial structure

(1) The area *must* be clipped with a generous margin around the site of injection.
(2) A sterile scrub must be completed: at least 10 scrubs preferably wearing gloves, starting from the injection site and working outwards.
(3) Rinse the area with surgical spirit and allow to dry.
(4) Ensure sterile handling of surgical gloves, syringes, needles and local anaesthetic.
(5) Ensure adequate restraint of the horse.

After synovial structure injection

The exact post-injection protocol will vary between vets; precautions to be considered include:

- Post-injection scrub
- Light bandaging of the area
- Injection of antibiotics

If the lameness is reduced by the injection, then it must be this area that is painful. This technique accurately locates the area of interest.

Diagnostic imaging

The available techniques are:

- Radiography
- Ultrasonography
- Nuclear scintigraphy
- Arthroscopy
- Emerging techniques, e.g. computer-assisted tomography and magnetic resonance imaging (see Chapter 17).

None of the above imaging techniques highlights just the painful lesions; therefore it is necessary to use clinical signs and local anaesthesia techniques to decide which area is generating the lameness.

Arthroscopy

Arthroscopy is particularly useful for investigation and treatment of lameness because horses have relatively large joints, enabling good visualisation and access. Arthroscopy involves the placement of a small rigid endoscope inside a joint and then a video camera is used to project the image onto a monitor, which gives a magnified view of all the structures inside the joint capsule. Arthroscopy can be used to establish a diagnosis and may enable the surgeon to carry out treatment within the joint.

Common indications for arthroscopy

- Removal of fragments associated with chip fractures
- Debridement of damaged cartilage
- Inspection of intra-articular ligaments and menisci.

Advantages of arthroscopy vs. arthrotomy (opening the joint capsule)

- Small incision sites heal more rapidly and so reduce recovery times
- The incidence of joint sepsis is reduced with the smaller size incision

- Surgical time is reduced for the horse due to less time spent closing the joint
- Arthroscopy is less traumatic to the joint and surrounding structures
- The small size of the fibrescope allows areas to be examined that are inaccessible by arthrotomy.

Diseases of the foot and hoof

The old adage 'no foot no horse' highlights the fact that *the most common site of lameness is in the foot*. This justifies considering foot-related lameness in a category of its own because the equine nurse will care for many cases of foot lameness.

Infectious causes of lameness

Horses are particularly at risk of developing tetanus, caused by the bacterium *Clostridium tetani*, which is potentially fatal. *All horses should be vaccinated* but many are not. If the skin or foot has been penetrated and the owner has not had the horse vaccinated recently, then it must receive tetanus cover in the form of tetanus antitoxin.

Subsolar abscess or 'pus in the foot'

This is a common condition that can cause severe lameness. The pain is caused by an inflammatory response to a bacterial infection of the laminae, beneath the hoof horn. The bacteria may enter via a nail hole, a puncture wound or track up the white line. Because the hoof capsule cannot expand, the build-up of fluid and pus causes intense pressure in a very sensitive site.

Clinical signs
- Severe lameness
- Strong digital pulse, due to the intense inflammation
- Pain in response to pressure with hoof testers

Treatment and nursing
The aim of treatment is to relieve the pressure, ideally by cutting down onto the abscess and releasing the pus. The hole in the sole must be large enough to allow further drainage. Once this has been achieved, the area is covered to keep it clean.

Traditionally it is recommended to poultice the wound to aid the drainage of pus. Antibiotics are not given routinely, because their penetration usually is insufficient to provide complete resolution and the problem returns once the antibiotics are withdrawn.

The entire sole may be hot-poulticed to draw out any remaining pus and soothe the bruising that develops due to the pressure. Alternatively, a dry absorbent bandage is applied to keep the area clean. Ideally this is changed twice daily. Wet dressings are rarely beneficial for more than 48 h. It is recommended that when the poultice is changed, the foot should be 'tubbed' (submerged in a warm bucket of water containing Epsom salts). This should continue for 24 h after the pus has stopped. The area is then dry-dressed for a further 48 h, being changed once daily. If the infection tracks up the white line and breaks out at the coronet, the treatment is the same but it will take longer for the infection to resolve. It helps to have a shoe refitted as soon as the horse is comfortable enough to allow it.

Thrush and white line disease

White line disease (separation between the horn and laminae, particularly in the toe region) has been related to anaerobic, keratolytic bacteria and possibly yeast infection, which in turn is related to poorly managed bedding. The alkali and ammonia present in decomposing manure soften the horn. *Thrush* is a common degenerative condition of the central and collateral sulci of the frog, characterised by disintegration of the horn. Various anaerobic organisms are involved in this condition and it is associated with poor foot care, especially in unhygienic moist stables with dirty beds. It can become a problem also in horses continually stabled, e.g. when hospitalised. There is increased incidence of thrush in wet winter weather.

Clinical signs

Lameness only occurs if the infection is severe and extends to involve sensitive tissues. Thrush has a characteristic pungent smell that is associated with black necrotic material collecting around the heels and the frog clefts.

Treatment and nursing

The area should be cleaned and dried thoroughly. Any overgrown tissue is removed. Paring the frog and sole may reveal peeling flaps of loose horn and sometimes subsolar ulcers. Stable management and foot care should be improved, including regular hoof trimming. Frequent scrubbing of the hoof with iodine or hydrogen peroxide is usually effective. The use of a toothbrush to deliver this deep into the frog cleft is helpful. The most important factor in recovery is an improvement in management.

Seedy toe

This term describes a bacterial infection of the white line at the toe, associated with separation of the hoof wall from the underlying tissues. It is often found in horses with chronic laminitis because the white line is already damaged. It is a localised form of white line disease.

Clinical signs

Usually there is a mild lameness but this can become more severe if the infection forms an abscess or extends to the deeper structures.

Treatment and nursing

This entails debridement of the white line affected. In severe cases, antibiotics may be indicated. Poulticing for a short period (~48 h), as described for pus in the foot, may help to draw out the infection. However, the sole should not be made too soft or moist. Regular farriery to keep the toe short, plus good hygiene will help to prevent the return of infection, along with appropriate management of any underlying laminitis.

Sepsis of the lateral cartilage: 'quittor'

This is an unusual bacterial infection of the lateral cartilage of the foot. Infection can be introduced by an injury involving the coronary band or a penetrating wound through the sole. Usually only one of the cartilages is affected. It is a particularly difficult condition to treat because the structures involved are deep within the hoof capsule.

Clinical signs

The intense inflammatory process produces a build-up of pressure on the sensitive laminae and causes severe lameness. The cartilages can be palpated around the outside of the coronary band; pressing on this area causes pain. The infection then breaks out at the coronary band in multiple discharging sinuses.

Treatment and nursing

The necrotic cartilage must be removed surgically and the deficit thoroughly lavaged. Antibiotics and analgesics are indicated. After surgery the area must be kept scrupulously clean and frequent bandage changes are recommended. The coronary band is a difficult area to bandage because the heels are particularly sensitive to pressure and abrasions are easily produced by poor bandaging technique.

Penetrating solar injuries

Penetrating injuries of the sole are commonly caused by standing on a sharp object, e.g. a flint or horseshoe nail. Most are minor, but if vital structures are involved then these injuries can be life threatening. The risk of damage is dependent on:

(1) The site of penetration.
(2) The depth of penetration.
(3) The direction of penetration.

Penetrations in the frog or the mid-third of the foot are potentially the most serious, because of possible involvement of the pedal bone, coffin joint, navicular bursa, digital tendon sheath or navicular bone.

Evaluation of the depth of injury can be achieved by careful probing of the hole. Contrast radiography can provide further information if the wound is still open. If the wound has closed but there is concern that the coffin joint, navicular bursa or digital tendon sheath are involved, a sterile synovial fluid sample should be taken (see later section on joint sepsis). Uncomplicated or superficial penetrations are treated as for pus in the foot. Involvement and infection of the deep structures usually warrant more intensive treatment, often surgery, and carry a poor prognosis.

Traumatic causes of lameness

Fracture of the pedal bone

Fracture of the pedal bone is relatively common in horses and can be a result of turning sharply, acute concussion or kicking a solid object.

Clinical signs

The clinical signs are immediate severe lameness, strong digital pulses, possibly distention (of the coffin joint) and pain on palpation of the coronary band if the fracture is articular, i.e. involves the coffin joint. The response to hoof testers is often not as dramatic as with a subsolar abscess.

Treatment and nursing

The pedal bone is naturally 'splinted' by being encased in the hoof capsule, effectively limiting the movement of the fracture line. This can be supplemented with a bar shoe, with clips around the wall. In some cases, surgical repair is possible using a bone screw across the fracture line. The horse must be box rested for between 3 and 6 months. It is useful to monitor the progress of fracture healing using radiography. The healing process may take up to 18 months to complete.

The fracture line can be difficult to see on radiographs initially, so meticulous foot preparation is essential to remove all dirt and make the fracture easier to visualise.

Careful nursing of horses on prolonged box rest can make the difference between treatment failure and success (see Summary 16.2, p. 317).

Solar bruising

This is a very common cause of lameness.

Clinical signs

Lameness can vary from mild to severe. A pink/red discolouration of the sole, in association with a response to hoof testers, will reveal the area involved.

Treatment and nursing

Remove the shoe and poultice for 48 h. The horse must be rested until it is sound. Adjustments in farriery to alleviate weight-bearing at bruised sites may help in recurrent cases.

Corns

Corns are bruises of the sensitive tissues of the sole at the angle of the bar and hoof wall. The sensitive tissues produce the horn in this area, therefore chronic corns are associated with defective horn growth.

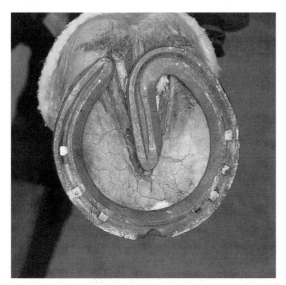

Fig. 16.3 A half-bar shoe fitted to a horse with recurrent corns.

This damaged horn then can allow infection to develop. Corns are often associated with:

- Poor shoeing, either too short or too tight at the heels
- Poor conformation, low collapsing heels

Clinical signs
Lameness can vary. There is localised pain response with hoof testers at the 'seat of corn' plus discolouration of the horn.

Treatment and nursing
Pare out the layer of horn covering the corn to relieve the pressure, address the initiating cause and treat as for bruising. Understanding the principles of good farriery will help to prevent recurrence of the problem (Fig. 16.3).

Laminitis
The term laminitis refers to an inflammation of the sensitive laminae, causing severe pain. This inflammation will occur in many situations, e.g. subsolar abscess or fractured pedal bone. However, the term laminitis is used to describe a diffuse non-septic inflammation, usually in more than one foot.

Clinical signs
The most common presenting signs are a reluctance to move or increased time spent lying down. The horse will attempt to carry all its weight on its heels because this is less painful, resulting in the characteristic leaning back stance and a heel-first foot-fall when walking. There will be marked digital pulses and heat in the feet.

Laminitis is a systemic disease with many causes, including:

- Metabolic disruption, e.g. carbohydrate overload associated with overeating, most common particularly in ponies on lush grass.
- Repetitive concussion, e.g. prolonged trotting on roads.
- Excessive weight-bearing e.g. non-weight-bearing on the contralateral limb due to injury.
- Endotoxic shock causing circulatory disruption, e.g. severe systemic bacterial infection.
- Steroids administered as a treatment for another condition or endogenous steroids, e.g. equine Cushing's disease.

Whatever the cause of laminitis, the pathological process is the same: *inflammation of the laminae permanently weakens the bond between the hoof wall and the pedal bone*. This weakening may be sufficient to allow the pedal bone to move relative to the hoof capsule in response to the normal forces applied to these structures.

The deep digital flexor tendon will pull on the back of the pedal bone and act to flex the coffin joint. The 'detached' hoof capsule rotates in the opposite direction. This will push the toe of the bone towards or through the sole: called pedal bone rotation (Fig. 16.4).

The weight of the body will act to push the pedal bone down within the hoof capsule, causing a condition called 'sinking'.

Both rotation and sinking can be diagnosed on radiographs. If the pedal bone has moved, this cannot be reversed. Treatment must be given rapidly to attempt to prevent this.

Treatment and nursing
(1) Remove the initiating cause.

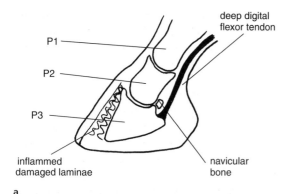

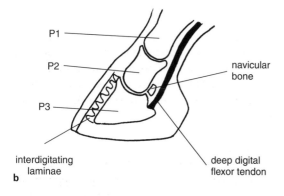

Fig. 16.4 (a) Representation of the normal anatomy of the lateral equine foot. (b) Representation of the anatomy of a laminitic foot.

(2) Use anti-inflammatory drugs to reduce the inflammation and provide pain relief.

(3) Try to prevent movement of the pedal bone by supporting it in the correct position and removing the role of weight-bearing from the hoof wall and thus the strain on the laminae.

(4) Try to restore normal blood flow to the feet using vasoactive drugs.

(5) Possibly sedate the horse to increase the amount of time spent lying down.

In the short term the following will be required:

- Box rest. This will restrict exercise and food intake.
- Reduced level of feeding. This is particularly important if carbohydrate overload is a contributory factor in the laminitis (see Chapter 5).
- Application of frog supports (Fig. 16.5). This will help to take the stress off the laminae and make the horse more comfortable. There are

manufactured frog supports available, which are bandaged onto the sole of the foot. A self-adhesive rolled up bandage such as 'vet wrap' with the cardboard centre removed, which is then positioned under the frog and bandaged in place, is acceptable. The frog support should be thick enough so that all the weight is taken off the hoof wall. Frog supports should be removed regularly and the solar surface examined for any evidence of bruising before the pads are repositioned. If the pads shift, they may do more harm than good! As soon as possible, fit shoes with a frog support, e.g. heartbar shoes.

- Ensure that the animal has a deep bed to encourage it to lie down frequently. A sand or shavings bed is preferable because these will conform to the contours of the feet and provide more support, and greedy ponies are quite likely to eat large amounts of a straw bed.

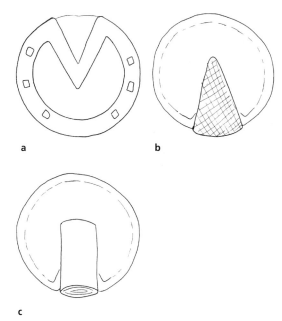

a   b

c

Fig. 16.5 Frog supports. (a) The heartbar shoe. (b) The 'Lily' pad: this can be obtained commercially from Brooks Smithy Ltd, Units 1 and 2, Old Salt Works, Brooks Lane Industrial Estate, Middlewich. Cheshire CH10 0JH (Tel: 01606 737155). Another alternative is styrofoam pads, obtainable from Total Foot Protection Ltd, Bramble Hill Farm, Slinfold, Horsham, West Sussex RH13 7RL (Tel: 01403 791000). (c) A rolled up bandage provides effective emergency frog support (see McDiarmid & Duff, 1996).

Once a horse has had laminitis, the laminae will be permanently weakened and there is greater risk of the condition returning. Long-term careful management is crucial, as follows:

(1) *Management of grazing.* When the grass is growing rapidly it contains the most sugar and is therefore most likely to trigger laminitis. Restrictions of the area and time available for grazing should be considered. Strip grazing using electric fencing is often an acceptable solution.
(2) *Regular farriery.* The hooves of horses that have had laminitis tend to grow more rapidly, therefore the trimming interval may need to be shortened. The toe should be kept short to ease the breakover phase of the stride and reduce the leverage on the laminae. Other adjustments to farriery can be made in conjunction with radiographs, depending on the individual case.

(3) *Specialist farriery.* There are a range of specialist shoes available to help in the management of laminitis; plastic lightweight shoes or heartbar shoes are designed to support the frog.

Navicular syndrome

The navicular region in the heel of the foot is a complex anatomical area. Navicular syndrome is the name given to pain originating from this area. The damaged structures could include the bone itself, the navicular bursa, navicular suspensory ligaments, coffin joint, laminae of the heels or the deep digital flexor tendon.

Clinical signs

Navicular syndrome causes low- to medium-grade lameness, which initially may be intermittent. This is usually a bilateral forelimb problem. It is often associated with poor foot conformation, increasing the concussive forces on the navicular region.

Treatment

Remedial farriery is needed to support the heel region and reduce concussion in this area. Egg bar and bar shoes may prove useful. Surgical and medical management is possible and will depend on the exact combination of structures involved.

Within the spectrum of navicular syndrome, a separate subset of cases can be isolated. These cases are referred to by some clinicians as having 'genuine navicular disease': defined as a degeneration of the navicular bone, which is visible radiographically. Despite this condition being recognised for over 200 years, the condition and its management remain controversial. There are a variety of treatments available, because no single solution is successful in all cases.

Neoplastic causes of lameness

Keratoma

A keratoma is an uncommon condition of the laminae causing an overgrowth of horn, which is a benign tumour. It is usually found towards the toe of the foot.

Clinical signs

A keratoma may or may not cause lameness, with or without deformation of the outline of the hoof. A diagnosis can be made radiographically.

Treatment

If the condition is problematic, surgical excision is the treatment of choice. Recurrence cannot be ruled out.

Diseases of bones

Bone responds to injury in one of three ways, no matter what has happened:

(1) Fracture.
(2) New bone production.
(3) Lysis of existing bone.

All of these changes can be seen radiographically and the combination of signs allows identification of the cause.

Infectious diseases of bone

Infection of the cortex

Infection of cortical bone is a potent stimulus both for the formation of new bone and for lysis of existing bone. This response can be seen on radiographs. Infection is often associated with *sequestrum* formation: a small piece of detached bone removed from its blood supply.

Clinical signs

Infection of a bone surface usually occurs after a deep wound that introduces bacteria onto the surface of the bone. A wound will not heal satisfactorily if there is infected bone involved.

Treatment and nursing

Prolonged antibiotic therapy is unlikely to be sufficient. Surgical debridement of the infected tissues is the treatment of choice.

In the post-operative period, good wound management is very important:

• Keep the wound clean; wear gloves during bandage changes

• Lavage wound using isotonic fluids
• Keep the wound moist, by using either occlusive dressings or hydrocellular gels
• Keep the wound covered if possible.

Osteomyelitis

Osteomyelitis refers to inflammation of the medulla and cortex of bone. The term usually is used to imply an infection. The condition is important in foals where the infection usually is blood-borne. This is rare in adults. Because blood vessels cross the growth plates in young animals, simultaneous seeding of the epiphysis and metaphysis may occur. The same animal may have multiple sites of infection in one bone or more than one bone affected. If the foal is septicaemic, an origin elsewhere in the body should be sought.

Clinical signs

• Fever associated with severe lameness
• Pain on manipulation of the joint.

Treatment

The prognosis for haematological osteomyelitis is very poor. Foals often are presented too late for medical therapy to be effective. Surgical removal of infected bone may be possible if the osteomyelitis is not too close to a joint.

Traumatic conditions of equine bones

Exostoses of the second and fourth metacarpal bone: 'splints'

When a bone is subjected to trauma, either a blow or repetitive concussion, the periosteum will become inflamed. It will produce more bone, called an *exostosis*. This will happen to any bone covered with periosteum. One of the commonest sites is on the splint bones.

Clinical signs

A hard lump appears on the splint bone; if the 'splint' is still actively forming, it will be warm and painful to touch.

Treatment and nursing

Concussion is believed to play an important role in

splint formation, therefore the horse should be rested until it is sound and the lump is non-painful to the touch. Anti-inflammatory medication may be useful. Once the splint has formed, the only treatment is surgical removal. If the horse has become sound at this point, this is cosmetic surgery and the risks of general anaesthesia should be weighed against a cosmetic improvement, especially as there will be remodelling with time anyway.

Some horses may find that warm poulticing of the forming splint may be pain relieving. There are various topical medications that can be applied to reduce inflammation.

Fractures

Fractures of the bones of the equine limb can be split broadly into two categories:

(1) Fractures of the small bones, e.g. carpal, tarsal, sesamoid bones. These bones may suffer a range of fracture types and their therapy depends on the size of the fragment, the angle of the fracture plane and the degree of joint involve-

ment. However, in general, fractures of these bones are not catastrophic and treatment is possible.

(2) Diaphyseal fractures of the long bones of the limb. Because these bones have a weight-bearing role, fracture is a potentially life-threatening injury (see Table 16.5).

Clinical signs

Horses with a fracture usually display a severe lameness and are likely to be distressed and unpredictable. The site of fracture usually can be identified by:

• Deformity
• Pain and lameness
• Presence of crepitus (grating feel of broken bone fragments)
• Loss of function
• Swelling.

It is important to be aware that incomplete undisplaced fractures, which are relatively common in the horse, will not cause pronounced clinical signs.

Table 16.5 Negative factors affecting the prognosis of equine long bone fractures

Factor	Reason for poor prognosis
Fracture site:	
Humerus	Inability of the horse to bear weight
Femur	Lack of sufficiently strong internal fixation implants for the size of the bone
Tibia	Inability to stabilise sufficiently using bandage
Radius	Muscle pull will displace fracture fragments
Open fracture of any long bone	Infection likely to compromise fracture healing
Multiple fracture fragments (comminution)	Risk of displacement and non-union increased
Severe soft-tissue damage	Loss of blood supplies and support structures
Displacement of fracture fragment	Risk of non-union is increased; difficulty of reduction
Size of the horse	The larger the horse, the more weight both the damaged limb and the sound limb will be expected to bear, increasing the chances of implant or splint failure and tendon/ligament strain or laminitis in the opposite limbs
Horse's temperament	A fractious animal is less likely to cope with pain or boredom associated with prolonged box rest sufficiently

Instead, there may be simple lameness. If this is of sudden onset, the possibility of a fracture should be considered.

With any fracture, considerations include:

- Open or closed, i.e. is there an open skin wound?
- Simple or comminuted, i.e. is the bone fragmented into several pieces?
- Complete or incomplete, i.e. is the bone completely broken?
- Soft-tissue damage
- Concurrent injuries.

Economics, insurance and the welfare of the horse are all important issues.

Treatment and nursing
For treatment of the multitude of possible fracture configurations, see the further reading list. The basic principles initially are the same:

- Assess as far as possible the bone affected and the degree of damage
- Consider whether treatment options are possible or if euthanasia is justified
- Stabilise the limb to prevent any further displacement or soft-tissue damage
- Provide sufficient analgesia to allow humane transport to a centre equipped to treat such equine emergencies.

There are many different ways recommended of supporting and stabilising a fractured limb, depending on which bone is fractured in which plane; it is not always possible 'in the field' to know with certainty the exact fracture type (see Chapter 7):

- Ensure that the horse is adequately restrained
- Assist in the stabilisation of the limb
- Put support bandages on the other limbs
- If possible, place a frog support on the opposite limb
- Keep calm; this will help to keep the owners and the horse calm.

Neoplastic causes of bone disease

Primary bone tumours are very rare in horses. They include:

- *Osteochondroma*: abnormal bone and cartilage growth, often on the caudodistal aspect of the radius. Technically this is not neoplastic.
- *Hypertrophic osteopathy/Marie's disease*: abnormal proliferative reaction of the long bones in response to a space-filling abdominal or thoracic mass. The mechanism of this response is unclear.

Metabolic bone disease in the adult horse

Calcium ions have a large number of crucial functions in the body, including nerve impulse transmission and muscle contraction. If the level of calcium ions in the circulation falls it will be replenished from the body's reserves, which are located primarily in bones.

Nutritional secondary hyperparathyroidism/bran disease/big head
This condition occurs when the intestines do not absorb enough calcium, because the diet is either calcium deficient or it contains too much phosphorus, which interferes with calcium uptake.

Clinical signs
As the calcium is removed from the bones, it is replaced by fibrous tissue; this causes the bones to enlarge. In the adult horse this is most noticeable in the bones of the head, hence the name big head. An insidious shifting lameness and generalised bone and joint pain accompany this.

Treatment and nursing
In horses this is a purely dietary problem (in small animals, renal failure may be a factor), so returning the diet to an adequate calcium/phosphorus ratio will cause the symptoms to resolve.

Hopefully this disease is historical due to improved equine nutrition. Bran has a particularly high level of phosphorus and therefore should not form the major part of the food ration.

This condition should not be confused with *suture line exostosis*, which causes firm swelling along the suture lines of the skull. These swellings are due to the proliferative response of the periosteum to trauma. In many cases these are of minimal clinical significance.

Osteoporosis

This is a term used to refer to bones that have reduced mineral density. Although this can occur in chronic malnutrition of aged horses, it is seen more commonly as *osteoporosis of disuse*. If a limb is immobilised for a prolonged period, e.g. in a cast, the lack of stress on that area will trigger increased bone resorption. The bone will become weakened and more susceptible to fracture.

Developmental orthopaedic disease

This term refers to a range of conditions that disrupt the development of the equine limb; they are therefore more commonly associated with foals and youngsters.

Angular limb deformity

This is a common condition in foals and refers to deviation of the limb in the frontal plane, i.e. the leg will bow either inwards (known as a *varus* deformity) or outwards (a *valgus* deformity). The commonest example is carpal valgus, i.e. the limb bends out from below the carpus (Fig. 16.6).

Causes include:

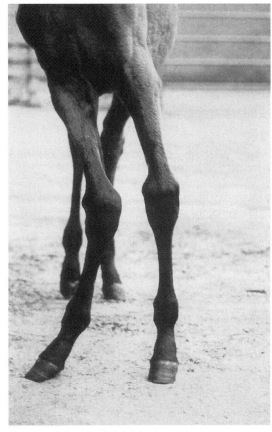

Fig. 16.6 A foal with angular limb deformity.

- A laxity of the ligaments around the joints of the limb. This will improve with age. Restricting exercise and stabilising the limb, either by bandage or by splinting, may help.
- A malformation (wedging) of the small bones of the hock or carpus. Once mineralisation is complete, at about 4 weeks, little can be done.
- A growth asymmetry. This occurs when a particular physis (growth plate) does not grow evenly along its length, resulting in one side of the bone growing more slowly than the other, leading to a wedged epiphysis.

It is possible that in a single limb more than one of the above conditions may be present. If the growth plates are still 'open', i.e. capable of growth, then they can be manipulated in an attempt to compensate for the growth abnormalities. A detailed radio-

graphic study of the limb should be performed to decide exactly which bones are involved and to what degree.

Conservative treatment
- Confine the animal.
- Dietary modification.
- Maintain limb balance by foot trimming and application of lateral or medial hoof extensions.

Many affected foals are growing rapidly and restriction of their intake may stop the growth abnormality from progressing. There is also some evidence that abnormal levels of copper, zinc, calcium and phosphorus in the diet may be contributing factors.

Surgical treatment

Growth acceleration can be induced on the side of the bone that is too short, i.e. the side towards which the limb is bent. The periosteum is stripped from the physis on one side of the bone and then replaced. The release caused by this procedure increases the rate of bone growth on that side. The advantage of this procedure is that it is not possible to overcorrect the lesion.

Growth retardation can be induced by placing surgical implants across the physis on the side that is growing too rapidly. This should be used only in severe cases because it is possible to overcorrect if the implants are not removed when the deviation has been corrected. Treatment must be given early because once the growth plate begins to close the treatment will not work.

Flexural deformities

This condition (also known as contracted tendons) describes limbs that are either too upright in their conformation or, in extreme cases, bent forwards. This is thought to be caused by an imbalance of growth rates between the bones and the tendons of this distal limb. The result is that the tendons are effectively too short for the bones and the joints are not capable of extending. This may affect the distal interphalangeal joint in young foals (2–6 months), producing a 'club foot abnormality' where the foot becomes upright and boxy. Less commonly the fetlock joint can be affected but this is usually in older animals (8–18 months).

Treatment and nursing

Conservative treatment includes physiotherapy, exercise and a reduced plane of nutrition to treat most mild cases of flexural deformity. If the condition is more severe, splints or casts may help to induce muscle and tendon laxity. Toe extension shoes will help force the foal to stretch the tendons. A single high dose of oxytetracycline is known to change the use of calcium by muscle and will help to induce tendon laxity.

Surgically, a distal check ligament desmotomy will help to produce deep digital flexor tendon laxity, thus reversing a club foot deformity.

Physitis

This is a painful condition caused by inflammation of the physis.

Clinical signs

It is commonly seen in foals of 4–8 months of age. The physeal areas are hot, painful and enlarged. The foal will be reluctant to stand and lame on movement. The condition usually affects the distal radius and/or metacarpus/metatarsus. Diagnosis is via radiography and clinical signs.

Treatment

Ensure balanced nutrition, restrict exercise and use low-dose phenylbutazone therapy. Care is needed with the use of phenylbutazone in foals because it can cause gastric ulceration.

Osteochondrosis

See later section on joint disease.

Diseases of muscle in adult horses

Traumatic muscle injuries

Muscle wounds in horses are common because horses are behaviourally inclined to cause damage to themselves or their companions. However, if the basic principles of wound therapy are followed, even large muscle lacerations will heal satisfactorily (see Chapters 7 and 18).

Fibrotic myopathy

This condition occurs mostly in the hindlimb and causes lameness when part of the muscle is scarred to form fibrous bands within the muscle.

Metabolic muscle diseases

Equine rhabdomyolysis syndrome

This condition presents as a generalised muscle pain after exercise (see Chapter 14).

Diseases of joints

Developmental joint disease in the adult horse

- *Osteochondrosis*. This condition arises when the

developing cartilage template laid down during bone growth fails to ossify (turn to bone) correctly.

- *Osteochondritis dissecans (OCD).* This is the name given to the cartilage flap that forms when there is an underlying problem with ossification.
- *Osseous cyst-like lesions (OCLLs).* Aetiology is uncertain. It can be developmental but it may have other causes, e.g. trauma. Subchondral bone cysts (SBC) were thought to be part of the osteochondrosis syndrome, but are now considered separately with a possible traumatic origin. Both OCLLs and SBCs will be encountered similarly by the equine nurse as radiographically detectable cystic lesions in the subchondral bone. The commonest site is the medial femoral condyle of the stifle, but they can occur in other load-bearing areas.

Clinical signs

Osteochondrosis cases often present as young horses; OCLLs and SBCs are also seen in older animals. The joints involved will become distended and flexion may be resented. Diagnosis is possible by radiography in some cases. Some OCD flaps will be formed of cartilage so may be visible only at arthroscopic surgery. Although in the initial phase the lameness may be mild, the constant low level of inflammation of the affected joint will lead to degenerative joint disease if not treated properly.

Treatment

Rest, controlled exercise and dietary restriction may help the inflammation of the joint to subside. Chondroprotective agents (see later section on osteoarthritis) also may help. Removal of cartilage flaps or debridement of the cyst may provide a better prognosis.

Infectious causes of joint disease in the adult horse

Joint sepsis

Joint sepsis is a potentially catastrophic injury and is always an emergency. In the adult, bacteria enter the joint via a traumatic injury that breaches the joint capsule. The bacteria set up an intense inflammatory response. These inflammatory proteins rapidly begin to damage the articular cartilage.

Clinical signs

- Intense pain and lameness will develop, usually within 2 h of injury
- Localised heat around the joint
- Marked effusion of the joint and pain on manipulation

The wound may be obvious but some puncture wounds will reseal. Even if the site of entry is not visible, the above clinical signs always should be treated as possible sepsis. The pain response may not be as severe if the joint is draining fluid because the pressure generated in the joint can be released.

Any wound close to a joint is an emergency and should be examined carefully immediately, with the potential of joint sepsis in mind.

Signs indicating joint involvement

- Clinical signs as above.
- Synovial fluid exiting from the wound.
- Changes in the synovial fluid. Synovial fluid collection, known as *arthrocentesis*, should be carried out in a sterile manner.
- Communication of the wound with the joint. Sterile saline may be injected aseptically at a separate site to distend the joint and assess whether there is communication with the wound. Exploration of the wound should be done carefully because there is a risk of further contamination.

Treatment and nursing

- High-dose broad-spectrum antibiosis.
- Anti-inflammatory therapy.
- Large-volume joint lavage. This will remove the damaging inflammatory proteins and the bacteria. Depending on the horse's temperament and the joint involved, this may be done standing or preferably under general anaesthesia. It is particularly important to inspect the joint arthroscopically if the injury is more than 4 h old because it is often necessary to debride infected tissue.
- Monitor progress, clinical signs and synovial fluid sample results. Anti-inflammatory drugs may mask the pain caused by ongoing sepsis. One

joint flush is often insufficient to resolve the condition; repeated flushes under general anaesthesia are commonly needed at 24–48-h intervals.

These wounds will need to be kept scrupulously clean. They also may be producing large volumes of exudate and bandage changes may need to be frequent. Care must be taken when dealing with these horses because they are initially likely to be in a large degree of discomfort. Any increase in the level of lameness is a potential warning sign and should be noted.

The specialist nursing requirements of horses with *profound lameness, requiring prolonged box rest* and on *high-dose antibiotics* are given in Summary 16.2 and should be revised in these cases.

Septic arthritis in foals: 'joint ill'

The principles for diagnosis and treatment in foals are similar to the adult. However, the pathogenesis does differ. The infection of the joint is more likely to be due to septicaemia than a wound entering the joint. The bacteria in the blood will settle in areas of high capillary density, e.g. the synovial membranes, causing joint sepsis.

More than one joint is commonly affected and the foal is likely to be systemically ill. Common origins of the septicaemia include umbilical infection, pneumonia and enteritis. Any young foal presenting with septic arthritis should be checked for adequate passive transfer of immunoglobulins.

Another difference to the condition in the adult is that there is much more likely to be infection of the bones due to a difference in blood supply (see previous section on bone disease, osteomyelitis).

Traumatic joint disease in the adult horse

Acute arthritis/joint sprain
Inflammation of the joint due to an acute traumatic event.

Clinical signs
- Heat pain and swelling of the joint
- A marked response to flexion test
- Lameness is severe to moderate in the acute phase

- Occasionally collateral ligament or other support structures will rupture, resulting in obvious instability.

Treatment
- Rest the joint.
- Systemic anti-inflammatories, e.g. phenylbutazone or flunixin meglumine. This will provide analgesia and reduce the production of degradative enzymes.
- Intra-articular medication. In the acute phase the profound anti-inflammatory effect of soluble short-acting corticosteroid therapy may be the treatment of choice.

Remember the risks associated with intra-articular injection. Correct preparation of the injection site is a vital nursing role.

Osteoarthritis/degenerative joint disease/arthritis
Osteoarthritis is a common chronic condition in the horse. It is associated with a prolonged low-level inflammation of the joint. Any inflamed joint may progress to develop this condition. The development of osteoarthritis may be linked to repetitive concussion and abnormal conformation in some horses. Once the process of cartilage degradation has begun it becomes self-perpetuating, as the breakdown products of cartilage will stimulate further inflammation in the joint.

Clinical signs
- Chronic low-grade lameness, may 'work out' of the stiffness.
- Often a positive response to flexion.
- Sometimes but not necessarily distention of the joint.

In chronic cases radiographic changes occur, such as periarticular osteophytes, trabecular remodelling and enthesiophyte production.

Treatment
Treatment of osteoarthritis needs to be considered in two groups:

(1) *The treatment of high-motion joints*. These joints are capable of a large degree of movement and the function of the limb will be limited severely if the joint is damaged, e.g. the fetlock. The aim of treating these joints is to reduce inflammation and to protect the remaining cartilage (chondroprotection). Treatment comprises:

(a) Rest.
(b) Systemic non-steroidal anti-inflammatory drugs (NSAIDs).
(c) Intra-articular corticosteroids.
(d) Chondroitin sulphate/glucosamine (oral; as yet unproven).
(e) Hyaluronic acid (intra-articular or intravenous).
(f) Glycosaminoglycans (intravenous, intramuscular or intra-articular).

(2) *The treatment of low-motion joints*: e.g. the lower hock joints. The function of the limb would not be seriously affected if the joint were in a fixed position. The aim of the treatment of these joints is to obliterate the joint space and thus remove the pain. *Joint ankylosis* is the acceleration of the degenerative process to cause the bones to fuse across the joint. This is achieved by increasing the work level of the horse while on phenylbutazone. An acceleration in degradation may be achieved also by injecting an irritant chemical into the joint. *Joint arthrodesis* involves surgically removing the cartilage and obliterating the joint space.

Diseases of the tendons, ligaments and tendon sheaths in the adult horse

Tendonitis/strain of the digital flexor tendons

Damage to the flexor tendons in competition horses is a common injury, the forelimbs being more commonly injured than the hindlimbs and the superficial more commonly than the deep digital flexor tendon.

Clinical signs
The severity of the lameness is proportional to the extent of tendon fibre breakdown and is often mild. There will be heat, pain and swelling of the tendons. Distortion of the outline of the tendons when viewed from the side often is referred to as a 'tendon bow' or 'having a leg'. Ultrasound evaluation will show an increase in cross-sectional area of the tendon and also may show disruption of the fibre pattern associated with fibre tearing.

Treatment
Healing of tendon lesions is slow; the laying down of scar tissue may take many months to complete. This can be monitored ultrasonographically. The scar will never be as strong as the original tissue for two reasons: it consists of a different type of collagen and it is not arranged in the linear pattern of the original tissue. Many techniques have been proposed to attempt to accelerate lesion healing and improve the quality of the scar. These include:

(1) Physiotherapy.
(2) Intra-lesional or intramuscular injection of glycosaminoglycans to provide the building blocks of tendon repair.
(3) Surgery:
   (a) Tendon splitting.
   (b) Superior check ligament desmotomy.
   (c) Firing. This therapy is controversial and produces significant discomfort to the animal undergoing treatment. There is no scientific evidence to support its use but historically it has been popular on the basis of anecdotal recommendation.

Clinicians vary in their opinions as to the value of these therapies. Ultimately the horse must receive a prolonged rest period (often 12 months or more) and a controlled return to work only when the tendon appears to have healed by clinical and ultrasonographic assessment.

Complete rupture of tendons

Extensor tendon
Complete rupture of the extensor tendons of the distal limb is much less serious than damage to the flexor tendon. Most horses will learn to adapt their gait to compensate for this injury. Fibrous repair will occur with time. If associated with a wound, the healing time of that wound may be prolonged.

317

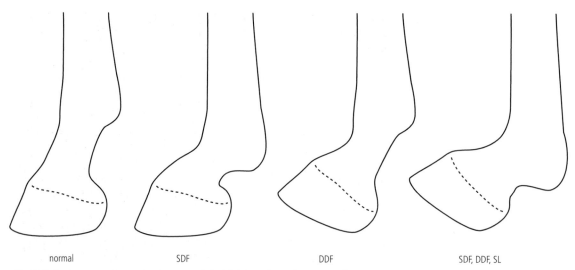

normal   SDF   DDF   SDF, DDF, SL

Fig. 16.7 Tendon rupture: diagram showing posture of distal limb depending on the structure affected.

Superficial digital flexor tendon

This is potentially catastrophic. The fetlock will drop when the injured limb bears weight. Can attempt surgical repair or splinting but recovery is very prolonged, if at all.

Deep digital flexor tendon

This is potentially catastrophic. The toe of the foot comes off the ground when the limb bears weight. Treatment is unlikely to be effective.

Superficial digital flexor, deep digital flexor tendon and suspensory ligament

The toe comes off the ground and the fetlock drops to the ground (see Fig. 16.7).

Gastrocnemius tendon

Dropped hock, unable to bear weight and the prognosis is guarded.

Rupture of the peronius tertius tendon

This condition results in disruption of the reciprocal apparatus, allowing the stifle to be flexed while maintaining the hock in extension (Fig. 16.8). Although there is no surgical option, many of these horses recover after extended box rest.

Luxation of the superficial digital flexor tendon from the point of the hock

The tendon is able to slip off the point of the hock if the fibrous band (retinaculum) is damaged. There is swelling of the point of the hock and the tendon can be seen to subluxate on movement. Some horses are able to return to athletic function after surgical repair of the retinaculum. Others can perform with residual gait deficits after stabilisation of the tendon in its displaced position.

Upward fixation of the patella

This is a mechanical rather than pain-generated lameness. The horse is capable of fixing its leg in extension by hooking the medial patellar ligament over the ridge of the medial trochlea of the femur. The patella is pulled upwards and inwards into this position by the quadriceps muscle and unhooked by the biceps femoris muscle (see Fig. 2.40).

Clinical signs

There are a range of clinical signs associated with differing severity of upward fixation of the patella. In severe cases the stifle (and therefore the hock, due to the reciprocal apparatus) will be locked in extension. The leg will be held stretched out behind the horse (Fig. 16.9). Some horses can become agitated

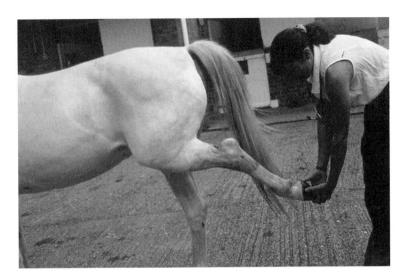

Fig. 16.8 A horse with a ruptured peronius tertius, showing the resultant abnormal limb position.

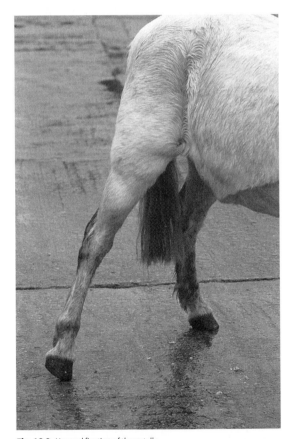

Fig. 16.9 Upward fixation of the patella.

although they are not in pain. The condition may relieve itself within a few moments or it may take considerably longer. In milder cases there may be only a 'catching' of the patella as the horse moves. This can be exaggerated if the horse is halted rapidly from a trot.

Treatment
Mild cases may be associated with a lack of muscle in the hindquarters, particularly in young horses. An increase in fitness level will produce more muscle tone and resolve the problem.

In more serious cases, or those with a congenital component, the medial patellar ligament can be cut, which is usually performed in the standing horse.

Lateral luxation of the patella

This congenital condition, most commonly seen in Shetlands and miniature ponies, presents as an inability to extend the stifle as the patella sits lateral to its correct position. The condition is often bilateral. Surgical correction is possible and the prognosis is fair, particularly if treatment is started early.

Desmitis

Desmitis means a strain of a ligament. There are two

common types in horses: desmitis of the suspensory ligament and desmitis of the inferior check ligament.

Desmitis of the suspensory ligament

Clinical signs

Lameness can vary from quite severe to mild and intermittent. It is not possible to palpate the proximal suspensory ligament because it passes between the splint bones. Distal suspensory injuries, either to the lower body of the ligament or its branches, can result in palpable swelling. Diagnosis is confirmed by ultrasound and radiographic imaging.

Suspensory breakdown can be complete or localised, e.g. to one branch.

Treatment

Controlled walking exercise is necessary until there is ultrasonographic evidence of improvement. The larger the region of damage, the more prolonged this period of controlled exercise should be. Recurrence is a problem.

If there is rupture of the suspensory ligament, prognosis is hopeless unless salvage by fetlock arthrodesis is an option for breeding purposes.

Desmitis of the inferior check ligament

Clinical signs

- Mild to moderate level of lameness.
- Swelling and pain associated with the ligament, medially and laterally between the suspensory ligament and the deep digital flexor tendon in the proximal one-third of the cannon bone.

Treatment

This condition is associated with animals expected to turn sharply and put a lot of strain on the forelimbs, e.g. polo ponies and show jumpers. Rest is the key to resolution but recurrence is frequently a problem.

Septic tenosynovitis

Septic tenosynovitis is a relatively common condition, particularly in the digital flexor tendon sheath due to the frequency of injury to the distal limb. It is a potentially catastrophic injury and always is an emergency although frequently it is not detected

early enough. Nurses need to be aware that wounds at the palmar/plantar aspect of the pastern justify an urgent veterinary examination.

If treatment is delayed, the infection can be impossible to resolve. The inflammatory proteins produced will organise and cause the formation of adhesions between the tendons and the synovial sheath, causing permanent lameness.

The principles of evaluating and treating infection of the tendon sheath are identical to the treatment of joint sepsis. General anaesthesia is recommended because it is very difficult to achieve an adequate flush of a tendon sheath in the standing animal. There also tends to be a higher incidence of complicating soft-tissue trauma, e.g. severed flexor tendons, than in joint sepsis.

Synovitis of the digital flexor tendon sheath

This is the name given to inflammation of the tendon sheath, colloquially called tendinous windgalls (articular windgalls are a distention of the fetlock joint). Although distention of the tendon sheath may not be associated with lameness, it should be treated as a warning sign of a potential problem.

Clinical signs

- Distention of the tendon sheath
- Positive response to flexion
- Lameness may be very mild to moderate
- Some horses with aseptic tenosynovitis (i.e. an inflamed but not infected tendon sheath) will begin work with moderate lameness that will improve with exercise

Assessment

Ultrasound examination of the tendons and the annular ligament is used to exclude any damage to the structures associated with the sheath. An evaluation of conformation and farriery is necessary to check that there are no underlying problems increasing the concussion on the area.

Treatment and nursing

The excess synovial fluid may be drained from the sheath, although this is likely to provide only a temporary resolution unless combined with anti-

Nursing care of orthopaedic patients

Boredom may cause temperamental problems

Many equine orthopaedic patients will require prolonged periods of box rest. During this time they may not feel ill or in pain and they become frustrated. This will be a particular problem with horses that have suffered an injury while competing, because they will be particularly fit. It will be necessary to reduce the plane of nutrition because of the reduction in exercise level. Splitting the daily food intake into multiple small feeds may help. Regular grooming also will help to keep these horses happy. Thought as to which box they are put in can help avoid problems. Some horses are kept amused by having a lot to watch but others find this even more frustrating.

Always ensure that a horse is adequately restrained before walking out

Horses that are normally fairly relaxed may become difficult after a period of confinement. If there is any doubt as to their behaviour, the horse should wear a bit.

Orthopaedic patients are at risk of developing colic

Several factors increase the risk in these patients. Some drugs used as anaesthetic agents will reduce gut motility. Pain also decreases gut motility, as does a lack of exercise. Many horses on box rest have an enforced change in their eating patterns, e.g. reduced grass intake will predispose them to impaction. If possible, frequent short walks to graze in hand will help to minimise these risks. Auscultation of the gut sounds should be done at least once daily with horses on box rest and faecal output should be monitored. Prolonged administration of phenylbutazone also will increase the risk of colic.

Orthopaedic patients are at risk of developing laminitis

When weight-bearing on a limb is compromised, the other legs are under increased strain. One of the problems that this may cause is laminitis. All the feet should be checked daily for warning signs, including increased warmth, digital pulses or bruising on the sole. A deep bed that encourages the horse to lie down will help to reduce this risk, as would the placement of frog supports on patients at risk.

Orthopaedic cases are at risk of developing tendon strain

This is due to the increased weight-bearing on the other legs. The other legs should be support-bandaged. These bandages should include a lot of padding and should be reset daily to check for evidence of bandage rubs and to remove any straw or shavings that may have slipped down the bandage.

Nursing care for foals with orthopaedic conditions (also see Chapter 15)

Foals have very delicate skin

This makes them very susceptible to bandage rubs and pressure sores. They should be checked all over daily for any signs of skin abrasion, particularly around the top and bottom of the bandage and on their heels if glue-on shoes are being used.

Stressed foals are very susceptible to intestinal upsets

Gastric ulceration occurs easily in foals and one should be familiar with the warning signs. Stress also will predispose them to the development of diarrhoea. Owing to the large amount of fluid lost in the faeces, this can become life threatening very quickly. Frequent inspection of the hindquarters, tail and legs for faecal staining is important.

It is not always easy to monitor the food intake of foals before weaning

Watch the foal suckling. Any signs of dehydration, prolonged skin tenting or dry mouth are an emergency. It is also worth regularly checking the mare's udder; if she is running milk or the udder is warm or hard the foal may not be receiving enough milk.

Nursing care for horses in a cast

Cast sores are a potentially serious complication of cast use

It is necessary to be very vigilant in the care of horses with casts. Any subtle changes in behaviour, e.g. not finishing a feed or standing in one corner of the box rather than looking over the door, may mean that a skin sore is developing under the cast (see Chapter 18).

An increase in lameness

This may indicate a problem with the cast.

The cast should be checked at least three times daily

Any cracks or creases in the cast may mean that the cast is about to fail.

Swelling or pain of the limb above the cast

This may indicate that the cast is too tight or causing skin abrasions.

inflammatory therapy. This can be delivered either systemically or intrathecally. Intrathecal corticosteroids and other medications are commonly used. If the sheath has been drained, a pressure bandage will help to prevent the fluid reforming. The horse should be rested after the procedure.

All tendon sheaths in the limb can become inflamed and should be managed in the same manner. Other common sites of synovitis include the *tarsal sheath* ('thoroughpin'), the *carpal sheath* and the *sheaths of the extensor tendons*.

Annular ligament constriction

The annular ligament is a fibrous band that runs between the sesamoid bones at the back of the fetlock. Its function is to hold the deep and superficial digital flexor tendons in position as they pass over the fetlock. If this ligament is damaged it will become thickened. This will cause a constriction of the tendon sheath. A relative constriction syndrome also can occur with swelling of the flexor tendons inside the sheath.

Clinical signs
- Moderate lameness and no improvement with exercise
- Distention of the tendon sheath both proximal and distal to the fetlock

- Characteristic flat outline to the palmar/plantar aspect of the fetlock due to hypertrophy of the ligament

Assessment
Ultrasound evaluation of the tendons, the tendon sheath and the thickness of the annular ligament.

Treatment and nursing
Surgical transection of the ligament will resolve the condition in many cases. During the post-operative period, a firm bandage must be kept in place over the incision site. The horse must return to exercise relatively soon after surgery to prevent adhesions forming in the inflamed tendon sheath.

Further reading

Coumbe, K.M. (1996) *All about Laminitis*. J.A. Allen, London.

McDiarmid, A.M. & Duff, A.J. (1996) A new method of applying frog support for the treatment of laminitis. *Equine. Vet. Educ.* **8**, 165.

Nixon, A.J. (1996) *Equine Fracture Repair*. Saunders, Philadelphia, PA.

Pollitt, C.C. (1995) *Colour Atlas of the Horse's Foot*. Mosby-Wolfe, London.

Ross, M. & Dyson, S.J. (in press) *Diagnosis and Management of Lameness in the Horse*. WB Saunders, Philadelphia, PA.

Williams, G. & Deacon, M. (1999) *No Foot, No Horse*. Kenilworth Press, Buckingham.

CHAPTER 17

Diagnostic Imaging

E. R. J. Cauvin

Imaging techniques have been designed to help us 'look' inside an animal, to detect specific pathology. Each technique has its advantages and drawbacks. The images obtained are always artificial representations as seen by a machine. One must therefore understand how the machine 'sees' in order to use it to its best potential.

Radiography

Radiography is the most widely used imaging modality in horses. Obtaining good-quality radiographs is a difficult art based on a complex science. Images are obtained by the effects of X-rays on a film or reading device.

Definitions
- *X-ray*: high-energy electromagnetic radiation (same family as light)
- *Radiation*: emission of energy by matter
- *Radioactivity*: spontaneous radiation from the nucleus of atoms
- *Radiograph*: image produced by the effects of X-rays on a film or recording device
- *Radiography*: the production of radiographs
- *Radiology*: science relating to the study and use of radiation (not only X-rays)

Nature of X-rays
X-rays are *electromagnetic* radiation, similar to light and radio waves, but with a shorter wavelength (billionth of a metre, 1000 times less than light). Electromagnetic radiation behaves as a stream of particles, or *photons*, that carry energy at the speed of light through a vacuum. It also behaves like a wave (Fig. 17.1) but, unlike sound or water waves, it does not need any medium to spread. Waves are characterised by their *wavelength* (λ), distance between the peaks of each successive oscillation and *frequency* (υ). The energy of the photons is proportional to their frequency, so the shorter the wavelength, the more energetic the radiation.

Production of X-rays—theory
X-rays are produced through the excitation of the electrons of an atom. An atom can be imagined as a central *nucleus*, made of positively charged *protons* and non-charged *neutrons*. *Electrons* gravitate around the nucleus like moons orbiting around a planet. They are negatively charged but much lighter than protons. There is normally the same number of protons and electrons (this number is called the *atomic number Z*).

Electrons normally gravitate within different energy levels, or *orbits* (Fig. 17.2a). If sufficient energy is given to an electron, it can jump to a higher orbit (this is called *excitation*; Fig. 17.2b), or even be expelled from the atom, which loses a negative charge and becomes a positively charged ion (process of *ionisation*) (Fig. 17.2c). The electrons reorganise themselves to stabilise the atom, releasing the excess energy in the form of an X-ray photon. Practically, X-rays are created in X-ray tubes by hitting the atoms of a target with fast (and therefore highly energised) electrons.

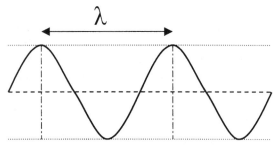

Fig. 17.1 Schematic representation of a wave with wavelength λ.

Design of X-ray machines

The beam of X-rays is produced in an *X-ray tube* (Fig. 17.3) consisting of three main components:

(1) A source of free electrons (cathode)
(2) An electron accelerator (electric field)
(3) A target (anode).

The cathode

Electrons are released from a *tungsten filament* (which can sustain very high temperatures without

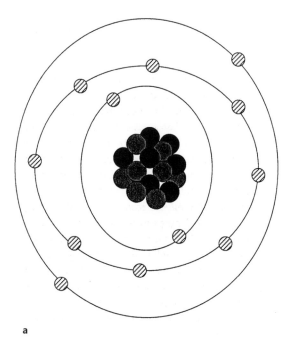

a

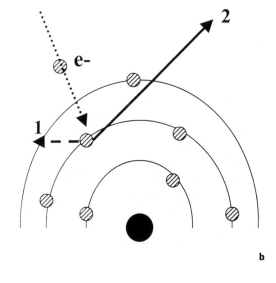

b

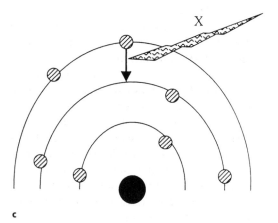

c

Fig. 17.2 (a) Schematic representation of an atom of sodium ($Z = 11$). The nucleus is made up of 11 protons (grey) and 13 neutrons (black). The electrons (shaded) gravitate in energy shells or orbits. (b) A fast electron can 'knock out' one of the electrons, which may jump to a higher orbit via excitation (1) or be ejected via ionisation (2). (c) A higher energy electron jumps in to take its place, releasing energy in the form of an X photon.

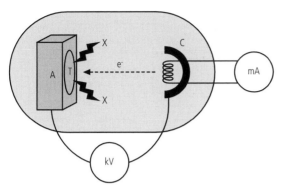

Fig. 17.3 Basic design of an X-ray tube. The cathode (C) consists of a tungsten filament placed in a focusing cup. The electrons are accelerated toward the anode (A) by a strong electric field (kV). The electrons hit the target (T), creating X-rays (X).

melting), heated by applying an electric current (as in a light bulb). The higher the current (measured in milliamperes, mA), the greater the temperature and the more electrons are released (therefore the more X-rays are created). The beam of electrons must be kept narrow to avoid hitting the anode outside the target. A focusing cup is placed around the filament for this purpose. To prevent the electrons from colliding with particles, all the components of the X-ray generator are kept in a vacuum within a sealed glass tube (hence the name *X-ray tube*).

The electric field

In the absence of an electric field, the electrons released would return to their source. A strong electric field is created by applying a *potential difference* (voltage) between the cathode and a positively charged anode, which attracts the electrons. This has three purposes:

(1) The electrons are freed from the cathode.
(2) They are oriented towards the anode, which contains the target atoms.
(3) The huge potential difference (thousands of volts, i.e. kilovolts) accelerates the electrons, giving them tremendous kinetic energy.

The stronger the potential difference (measured in kilovolts, kV), the faster the electrons and thus the more powerful the X-rays produced.

The anode

This is the most complex part of the tube and carries the *target*, i.e. the atoms used to produce X-rays. Only 1% of the energy of the electrons hitting the anode is converted into X-rays, the rest is transformed into *heat*. The target is therefore heated to tremendous temperatures. *Tungsten*, often alloyed with other metals, is used because of its high melting point (3400°C) and its high atomic number (Z = 74), which makes it more efficient at producing X-rays (it has a lot of electrons).

Tube design

There are two basic tube designs to dissipate the heat produced:

(1) *Stationary anode* (Fig. 17.4a): the target is fixed on an anode, usually made of *copper*, which is a good conductor of heat. The heat is dissipated from the anode via a radiator placed outside the tube (using oil as a coolant around the tube). The larger the target area bombarded with electrons, the less heat is produced in a single point and the less the potential damage; but the larger the source of X-rays, the less accurate the image obtained. As a compromise, the target is placed at an *angle*. The *source* of photons is wider, but appears narrower when seen at an angle: this effect is called 'line focus' (Fig. 17.4b). X-rays are produced in all directions, but only those passing through a window placed at the required angle in the tube are used. The rest of the tube is lined with lead, which absorbs the undesirable X-rays. The greater the angle, the smaller the line focus, but if it is too steep then the X-rays have to go through a thicker part of the target and most of them are absorbed. The usual compromise is 17°.

(2) Rotating anode (Fig. 17.5): the anode is disk shaped and rotates rapidly while being bombarded by electrons. A narrower target area can be used as it is constantly replaced by cooler metal as it rotates. Greater mA and kV can therefore be used but the technology is more complex and costly. The anode is mounted on a molybdenum rod, which is a poor conductor and therefore protects the motor and bearings from damage by the heat produced. These tubes are often bulky.

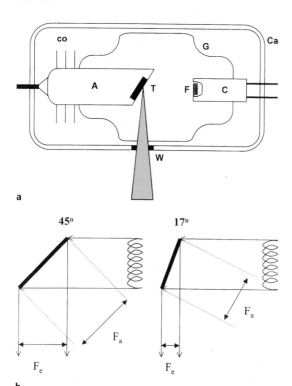

a

b

Fig. 17.4 (a) Basic structure of a stationary anode tube. The glass tube (G) is surrounded by oil coolant (co) encased in a lead-lined protective shield (Ca). C, Cathode with filament (F) in its focusing cup; A, anode; T, target; W, aluminium window. (b) Line focus principle. On the left side, the target is placed at 45°. The effective focal size (Fe) is smaller than the actual focal size (Fa). If using a 17° angle, Fe becomes smaller still in relation to Fa.

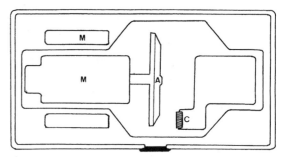

Fig. 17.5 Rotating anode tube. The rotating anode (A) is placed within an induction motor (M). The cathode filaments and focusing cups (C) are similar to fixed anode units.

Tube casing

The glass tube and internal components are placed in a protective casing, commonly lined with lead to absorb radiation. The window is usually made of aluminium. The casing also contains the cooling elements and, in rotating anode tubes, the induction motor which rotates the anode.

Other components of an X-ray machine

- Several *electrical circuits* are required, one to heat the cathode, one to accelerate the electrons toward the target and one to rotate the anode. The more precise and independent these components, the more complex and expensive the technology.
- *Timer*: controlling the exact duration of the X-ray production is paramount because this determines the total number of X-rays that the patient is exposed to. Very short durations are used because the shorter the exposure, the less movement blur occurs. The timer opens the current in the above circuits and cuts it at the end of exposure. Electronic timers equip most modern machines and are accurate to 0.01 s.
- *Filters*: the X-ray beam contains a whole spectrum of rays of varying wavelength. Less energetic photons cannot contribute to the image on the films but can have undesirable effects on the patient. These are filtered out using an aluminium filter over the tube window. The glass and other materials used in the casing of the tube also act as filters.
- The *beam collimator*: collimation is important for safety and radiographic quality. The X-ray cloud produced by the anode is reduced to a beam by the radiolucent window in the tube casing, but remains fairly large. The size of the beam should be reduced to fit the area of interest. This is achieved with lead collimators, which absorb X-rays outside the required area.
- *Light-beam diaphragms*: movable plates of lead are placed in a device permanently attached to the tube. It also contains a light source, so that the size and position of the beam can be visualised and accurately selected.
- *Switch*: the *exposure switch* is used for manual activation of the tube circuits and to produce the pre-set exposure. Pressing the switch activates the tube and then the timer interrupts the current.

Some machines are equipped with a *one-stage switch*, which activates both high tension and filament circuits. If a rotating anode is used, however, it is necessary to start the rotation of the anode before the exposure. Using a *two-stage switch*: the button pressed half-way starts the rotation and heats the filament, then the operator presses the button fully to switch on the high-tension circuit and initiate the production of X-rays. Unless the control box is located behind a shielded screen, the switch must be at the end of a cable at least 2 m long.

Types of X-ray machines

Portable machines

Portable machines (Fig. 17.6a) are designed to be lightweight. They are less powerful (i.e. produce fewer X-rays) and use a low, fixed current (usually 10–60 mA). The exposure times therefore must be increased, affecting image quality. Stationary anode tubes are used. These systems are suitable for ambulatory work but not for radiography of the trunk and proximal limbs of horses. A robust stand should be used to allow for adequate positioning. Unfortunately, many commercially available stands are too flimsy, making it difficult to position the tube and causing movement blur.

Mobile machines

Mobile machines (Fig. 17.6b) are heavier and mounted on a mobile trolley, which may be wheeled around a yard but rarely transported. The technology involved for both circuits and tube (some have rotating anodes) varies. Some units are based on condenser circuits, which allow them to be charged up and used disconnected from the mains. Higher voltages (up to 90 kV) and a wider range of current settings (up to 400 mA) can be used. The design of the head arm is often impractical for horses, especially in older models.

Fixed units

Fixed units (Fig. 17.6c) use more advanced but more cumbersome technology, usually a three-phase generator, a separate control unit and a rotating anode tube, often mounted on an overhead gantry railing.

The installation costs are therefore much greater and a specially designed room must be available. They are best for radiography of the trunk and proximal limbs.

Tube rating

The maximum exposure factors (voltage and current) that can be used depend on the heat that the anode can withstand. Rating charts give the maximum factor combinations that may be used (more voltage may be used by decreasing the current, and vice versa). If this is exceeded, the tube is said to be *'overloaded'* and may be damaged. Modern machines have fail-safe devices to prevent overloading. With use, the anodes become worn and the ratings decrease, so regular checks should be performed on older tubes.

Formation of the radiographic image

Interaction of X-rays with matter

Radiography is based on the ability of X-rays to be absorbed by the materials they pass through. Through absorption and scatter, the X-ray beam is gradually reduced as it goes through tissues. The proportion of X-rays absorbed varies depending on tissue thickness, density and nature. This is called *attenuation* of the beam. Because the body is made up of many different types of materials, the absorption varies within the beam of X-rays, i.e. the part of the beam going through bone is attenuated more than that going through soft tissues or gas-filled organs. The ability of a substance to attenuate the beam is its *radiodensity*. The radiodensity of tissues decreases in the following order:

Metals and positive contrast media (metallic density) > Bone, plaster (mineral density) > Water and soft tissues, including muscle and cartilage (soft-tissue density) > Fat > Air (gas density)

Substances absorbing most X-rays are termed *radiopaque*, and those causing very little attenuation are called *radiolucent*.

Converting X-rays to image

X-rays are used to form an image on X-ray-sensitive films. The homogeneous primary beam generated by

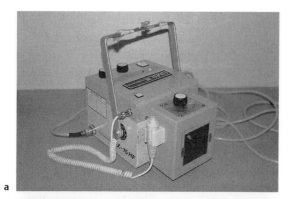

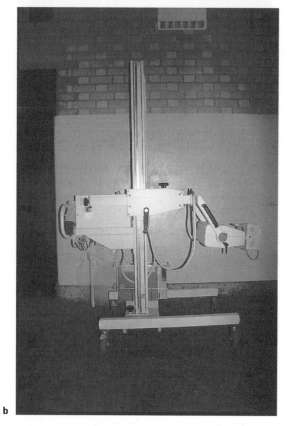

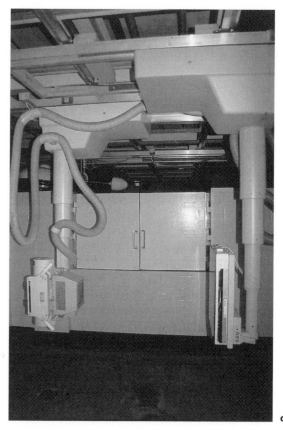

Fig. 17.6 (a) Portable X-ray machine. (b) Mobile X-ray machine. (c) Fixed X-ray machine unit: the tube head is mounted on an overhead gantry unit and linked to a Potter–Bucky mobile grid system.

the X-ray machine passes through the patient and is attenuated by the tissues. The outgoing beam is heterogeneous, forming a virtual image (Fig. 17.7). The films are designed to react to X-rays to create a visible image.

Photographic effect

X-rays react with the silver halides in the emulsion of an X-ray film. Once developed, areas of the film that have received more radiation will appear much more lucent or black than those that have received a lower amount. Their silver halide grains are sensitised by

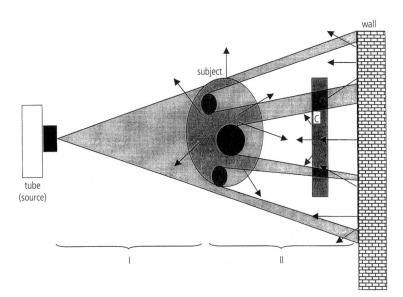

Fig. 17.7 Formation of the virtual image: I, primary beam; II, secondary beam containing a pattern of varying densities or virtual image; C, cassette; arrows indicate scatter and backscatter.

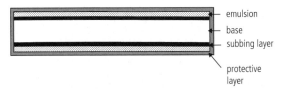

Fig. 17.8 Structure of a double-sided radiographic film.

light and then must be converted to black silver through development.

Structure of radiographic films (Fig. 17.8)
The grains are finely dispersed within a thin coating of gelatine, called the *emulsion*. This layer is stuck, using an adhesive (the *subbing layer*), to a polyester support. This *base* is transparent to light and X-rays but is often tinted green or blue. With the exception of mammography films, which have emulsion on one side only, most films have emulsion on both sides, to double their sensitivity to radiation. An outer layer of harder, clear gelatine, *the supercoat*, protects the emulsion.

Intensifying screens
Only 1 or 2% of the X-ray beam interacts with the film emulsion, so to enhance the image intensifying screens are used to convert X-rays to light and thus increase the signal on the film. *Fluorescent* materials are used. Several points should be noted here:

(1) Certain substances, called *phosphors*, emit light when irradiated by X-rays. Each type of phosphor emits light of a given wavelength. The screen therefore must be chosen to emit the optimal light for a given film (*film–screen combination*). The intensity (the amount, not the wavelength) of light emitted is related to both the intensity of photons (i.e. the number of photons per second) and their energy. Therefore, the more energetic and numerous the X-rays, the brighter the flash of light produced and the more blackening occurs on the film. There are many phosphors available and their properties dictate their cost and efficiency. Traditional intensifying screens contained *calcium tungstate*, which emits blue and ultraviolet light. More modern phosphors, such as barium sulphate, lanthanum and *rare earths*, have since been developed to improve the efficiency of the screens.

(2) Design of phosphors: the screen should convert as many X-rays into light as possible, emit light of the right wavelength for the right film without producing any afterglow (or phosphorescence, i.e. persistent emission of light after irradiation, which would overexpose the film) and must be

329

re-usable. *Rare earth screens* are preferred because of their greater conversion efficiency, making screens *faster*. The *speed* of a screen is a subjective measurement of its efficiency. The faster the screen, the fewer X-rays are required to produce an image on the film. Using larger crystals, which can absorb more X-rays, may also increase the speed. Unfortunately, this also decreases the detail of the image. Most screens emit blue light. Some phosphors emit in the ultraviolet, blue and green spectra and are used with *green-light-sensitive films* called *orthochromatic films*. This allows better selection of contrast for certain films (note that one must use red rather than brown safelights in the darkroom for these films).

(3) Structure of the screens (Fig. 17.9): screens are optimised to produce more light and transfer it to the film. The screen is made of a *plastic or cardboard support*, coated on one side with a layer of a *binding substance* containing millions of *phosphor crystals* (a few microns in diameter). A thin layer of reflective material may be placed between the support and phosphor layers to reflect light and thus increase the amount of light going towards the film. Obviously, it is important that the screen be placed the right way round, with the phosphor layer facing the film. The screen is coated with a hard, protective layer to prevent scratches or damage to the phosphor layer.

(4) The *cassette* (Fig. 17.10): film and screens must be kept in a lightproof container that lets X-rays through (radiolucent). A hard material is used for protection, usually plastic, aluminium or carbon fibre. A lead sheet is placed on the back of the cassette to prevent backscatter (see later). Foam or other padding is used on the back to ensure good screen–film contact. The screens (one on each side, except in single-screen mammography cassettes) are secured. The film is placed directly between the screens.

Film processing

Processing changes the activated silver halide crystals to silver grains and stabilises the emulsion to produce a permanent image. A lot of common mistakes

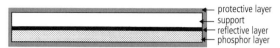

Fig. 17.9 Structure of a screen.

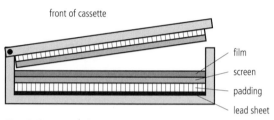

Fig. 17.10 Structure of a cassette.

occur during processing that can markedly decrease the image quality. There are four main stages:

(1) Development
(2) Fixation
(3) Washing
(4) Drying and storage

Development

The films are placed in a developer solution that contains a complex combination of chemicals:

- *Alkaline reducing agents* (a mixture of metol-hydroquinone and phenidone in specific, balanced concentrations) are used to turn the partially transformed (reduced) silver bromide crystals in the emulsion to silver grains by a process of *reduction*.
- *Buffer*: the developer works best in alkaline conditions. The buffer keeps the solution at the adequate pH.
- *Accelerators* catalyse (i.e. promote) the reduction of the crystals to increase the speed. *Restrainers* are also used to protect the non-sensitised crystals from being reduced.
- *Preservatives* (sodium sulphate) are used to prevent deterioration of the solution during storage.

Developer rapidly deteriorates despite the use of preservatives. It should be changed every 4–6 weeks, otherwise the efficiency of the development will decline and become unreliable. Also, chemicals become used up, so that the more the solution is used, the more regularly it must be replaced. Topping up with new solution is not adequate. Special replenisher solutions can be used but the solutions should be replaced regularly.

Development is time and temperature dependent: if the time is too short, the chemicals too weak or the temperature too low, not enough crystals are reduced and insufficient blackening occurs (*underdeveloped film: cloudy, white image*); if these factors are too high, non-activated crystals become reduced and too much blackening occurs (*overdeveloped film: too dark, poor contrast*). It is therefore important to keep as close as possible to the optimal conditions to obtain meaningful images. An exposure factor chart can be relied upon only if processing is standardised. Overdeveloped films appear too dark.

Fixation

The *fixer* is an acidic solution that stops the action of the developer. It also contains chemicals that remove non-reduced silver bromide from the emulsion (clearing it, i.e. making it turn from yellow to clear) and hardens the gelatine to protect it in the long term. Sodium or ammonium thiosulphate, with an acid such as acetic acid or ammonium metabisulphite, are used. The temperature is not so important, but the films should be fixed for approximately 10 min for adequate hardening, unless an automatic processor is used. Like the developer, the fixer solution deteriorates and must be replaced regularly. Under fixed films show cloudy areas.

Washing

The films should be washed between the developer and fixer to avoid carrying too much developer over into the fixer. This would speed up fixer deterioration. More thorough washes in running tap water are used, after fixation, to remove chemicals from the emulsion and it is generally advised to wash the films in water before drying. Poorly washed films show yellow–brown stains of dried chemicals.

Drying and storage

The gelatine-based images remain fragile and are easily scratched or stained. They are difficult to clean, so they should be kept in a dry environment, free of dust. Folding tears the emulsion and should be avoided. The films also will deteriorate at high temperatures and exposure to light will turn them yellow. Special envelopes are the most common method of storage.

Safelights

Safelights are designed to allow the operator to see in the darkroom, without exposing the film emulsion. They produce visible light in a part of the spectrum to which the film is not sensitive. Most films are sensitive to blue and ultraviolet light, so red or amber filters are used. However, with orthochromatic films, which are sensitive to green–ultraviolet light, only red filters must be used.

Manual processing

With the advent of more affordable, less cumbersome automatic processors, manual processing is gradually phased out because it is less reliable, more difficult and time consuming and less clean. If it is used, all parameters should be controlled as well as possible, including room temperature and humidity. *Cleanliness* is paramount, because unprocessed films are very sensitive to dust, scratches, grease and chemical stains. The wet processing area and sink should be separated physically from the film storage area and the workbenches (used to unload and reload the cassettes) to avoid chemical splashes and stains (Fig. 17.11). The temperature of the developer and fixer must be kept constant. It is preferable to use baths in which the temperature can be controlled. Purpose-designed waterbaths with a thermostat and heater are available and are well worth the investment. Otherwise, there should at least be a temperature gauge or thermometer available and some heating device such as thermostatic heaters or immersion coil heaters. The procedure varies between manufacturers. The films are hung on frames and placed in the developer tank, where they should be gently moved up and down. After the required development time (usually 5 min at 20°C), the film is washed in fresh water to prevent transporting developer into the fixer solution. The film is then placed in the fixer, where it should remain for twice the time required to clear the emulsion (5 min is usually adequate). The film is then rinsed in running

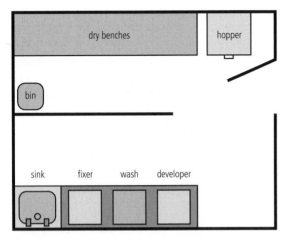

Fig. 17.11 Example of a typical set-up for the dark room. The dry bench and storage area are separated from the wet processing area and sink (a partition may not be necessary).

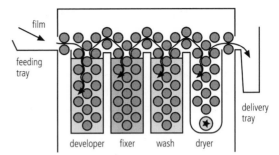

Fig. 17.12 Automatic processor. The number and size of the rollers determine the duration of each cycle.

water and left in a clean waterbath for at least 10 min. The frame is finally hung over a sink to drain and dry the film.

Automatic processors

Inexpensive, lightweight processors are now available, and small, portable processors can even be used from the boot of a car. Most automatic processors must be used in a darkroom, but 'daylight' processors are available: special cassettes are inserted directly into the feeder, then the film is replaced automatically. Processors use the same solutions as above but work at higher temperatures (usually 35°), making processing faster. The films are carried into a tank of developer first, using rollers (Fig. 17.12). The size, number and speed of the latter determine the duration of each step. No wash tank is necessary after development because the solution is squeezed out by sets of rubberised rollers. The film is then carried into a fixer tank, followed by a wash tank in which the water is constantly renewed. The solutions are automatically replenished. After washing, the films are carried through a drying compartment, where hot air is blown before delivery of dry films. Automated processors have many advantages:

- They are clean and faster than manual processing
- They ensure constant processing factors
- They do not require any special training to operate.

Adequate maintenance is paramount, however, with regular cleaning of the machine.

Dark room

X-ray films are handled in a lightproof environment that is only lit by a safelight. It cannot be overemphasised that tidiness and cleanliness are paramount to prevent damage to the films and to optimise image quality. *Storage* of the films is another important item to consider. Films must be kept in a lightproof environment. When the daily throughput of radiographs is small and only one or two sizes of cassettes are used, the films are best kept in their packaging. The boxes must be kept in an area protected from radiation by adequately shielded walls. *Film hoppers* are a more convenient way of storing films: a trapdoor containing compartments for various sizes of films is kept closed, usually by a spring system. These cabinets are light and X-ray proof. In all cases, the dark room should be designed so that the chances of accidentally exposing the films to light are minimal. The door must be fitted with a lock. Care and discipline when using the darkroom are necessary: the door should be locked from inside during film handling and processing, the light turned off and the safelight switched on.

Disposal of chemicals

The chemicals are not environmentally friendly and should be disposed of with care, as recommended by the manufacturers. They should be collected carefully in leak-proof containers that can be transported easily. This can be arranged with the providers. Used or poor-quality films should be discarded.

Other means of recording

Films take up space and deteriorate with time. Radiographs now can be stored in electronic format. Films may be scanned and saved as computer files.

Digital radiography, where X-rays are directly recorded as digital files, is probably going to become the new standard in radiography. Normal X-ray machines can be used in combination with special cassettes and processing equipment. There are many advantages: the images take virtually no space, they do not deteriorate, they are easily archived on computer and they can be retrieved immediately. They also can be processed digitally to alter contrast and greyscale (no need for several views to image bone or soft tissues), filter out the noise and measure angles, distances, radiodensity, etc.

Radiographic quality: primary beam

The radiographer, using the above principles, can dramatically influence the quality of images produced (see Key points 17.1). Some factors inherent to the technique cannot be altered. Others are under the direct control of the operator. Image quality can be altered at three major levels:

(1) The incoming X-ray beam (exposure).
(2) The patient and resulting beam (the virtual image).
(3) The recording system.

Definitions

- The *primary beam* is the beam of X-rays arising from the tube and light beam diaphragm. The amount and nature of the X-rays applied to the patient (also called the *exposure*) are determined by a set of *exposure factors*, namely current (mA), time (s) and voltage (kV).
- *Secondary* beam refers to the X-rays exiting the patient after the primary beam has been attenuated. The aerial or *virtual image* is the variation within this beam, which can be recorded as an image on film.
- *Exposure*: this refers to the amount of X-ray energy

that the patient is exposed to. It is often used to describe the characteristics of the primary beam, i.e. intensity and quality. The term *overexposed* is used when too many photons pass through the subject, causing excessive blackening on the film. This is associated with too 'strong' a primary beam, i.e. too high exposure factors (voltage, current and time). *Underexposed* is the opposite.

Characteristics of the primary beam

Intensity of the beam

The beam may be seen as a volume (a cone with its point at the tube) through which runs a shower of X-ray photons. The *intensity* of the beam is the number of photons passing through a cross-sectional area of the beam per second (Fig. 17.13). This is primarily determined by the number of electrons produced by the cathode (the more electrons are produced, the more X-rays are generated), which is itself determined by the intensity of the current going through the filament, measured in milliamperes. The higher the current, the more X-rays are produced. The total number of photons produced during exposure (the dose) is therefore the intensity of the beam (in mA) multiplied by the duration (in seconds) of the exposure, i.e. mA×s or mAs.

Quality of the beam

The photons within the X-ray beam are produced within a certain range of wavelengths, determined by the potential difference between cathode and anode (which accelerates the electrons) measured in kilovolts. The low-energy photons are absorbed by the tube and filter; the higher ones are most likely to go through the patient and film unhindered. The more energetic the photons, the less likely they are to

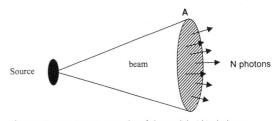

Fig. 17.13 Beam intensity = number of photons (N) within the beam crossing a cross-sectional area (A) during 1 s.

be absorbed by the patient, but the more *scatter* they produce. Therefore, increasing the potential difference (voltage) makes the beam more penetrating but also causes more scatter.

Film focal distance (FFD)

The *FFD* is the distance between the centre of the target (the point of origin of the X-rays or *focal point*) and the X-ray film. The further the film, the fewer X-rays reach it due to the *inverse square law*. This law states that the intensity of photons is inversely proportional to the square of the distance to the focal point. Multiplying the distance by a factor of x results in dividing the exposure by x^2. The reason for this is that X-rays diverge from the source and therefore move further and further away from each other, making the beam less concentrated as the distance increases, e.g.:

- Doubling the distance is equivalent to using a fourfold lower dose (mAs).
- Using an FFD of 1.2 m instead of 1 m decreases the intensity by >30%.

It can be compared to a torch beam. The closer the wall is to the torch beam, the brighter is the beam against the wall. This plays an important role in radiation safety. The greater the distance between yourself and the source of radiation, the lower the dose you will receive.

Key points 17.1

- The current (mA), time and FFD determine the number of X-rays
- The voltage determines their quality (energy)
- The FFD should be checked every time
- Ideally the current should be as high as possible with a short time

---

Radiographic quality: effects of the patient

The primary beam goes through the patient because X-rays penetrate solid matter. When X-rays interact with an object:

(1) They pass straight through unaltered, in which case the photons are not deflected and do not lose energy.

(2) They can be absorbed.
(3) They can be scattered in any direction, so are deflected from their original path.

Scatter formation depends on the X-ray energy (kV) and the amount of tissue (volume and density) but not its nature (bone or soft tissue). The thicker and denser the area of interest, the more scatter is produced. This type of radiation causes many problems: it exits the tissues in all directions, radiating into the patient and around it and creating a significant hazard for the patient and operators. Scattered X-rays reach the cassette in a random fashion, causing even blackening (noise) on the film. It is an inherent limitation of the technique and, in horses, it often precludes the use of radiography to image thickly muscled areas (proximal limb, pelvis, abdomen and neck). Generally, thicknesses below 20 cm (limbs up to knee and hock) or areas composed mostly of gas (head) do not produce significant amounts of scatter.

Virtual image formation

The attenuation of the beam varies between organs and surrounding tissues and within organs. The primary beam is homogeneous but the secondary beam contains a pattern of varying intensities, depending on the nature and thickness of tissues it has traversed, forming an aerial or *virtual image*. This pattern of absorption varies with:

- *The energy of the X-rays* (kV): if the voltage (kV) is increased, more X-rays go through (i.e. penetration is increased), attenuating differences between bone and soft tissues. It also produces increased scatter, so that differences between areas may become swamped by the background blackening of the film. At low voltage, on the other hand, low-energy photons are absorbed and everything remains white. Practically, there are a range of voltage settings for a given area that produce the right level of attenuation or penetration.
- *Beam intensity*: the more X-rays in the primary beam, the more emerge from the patient. The dose (mAs) has no effect on *relative* differences of absorption between two tissues, but it affects the amount of film blackening. If it is too high, the image overall becomes too dark to assess.

Conversely at low settings, not enough X-rays are produced and insufficient blackening occurs in the emulsion to create an adequate image.

- *Atomic number* (Z): if the atomic number is high, then more absorption will occur. Bone absorbs more X-rays than soft tissues, which attenuate more than fat and gases (air). Some areas, such as the limbs, head or chest that contain bones, soft tissues and gas, have a high *inherent contrast*, i.e. strong differences of X-ray attenuation between areas. Conversely, the abdomen, mostly made up of soft tissues and large areas of muscle, has a low inherent contrast. Thus, to obtain more details on the structure of bones, a sufficient voltage must be used to increase the *penetration* of the beam.
- *Tissue density*: the denser the tissue (i.e. the more atoms are present in a given volume), the more likely photons are to interact with them. This is why fat and gas cause less attenuation. At low and medium voltages (<70 kV), relatively smaller differences in density can be seen. Subtle differences between soft tissues are difficult to detect at the higher voltage settings used in horses.
- *Tissue thickness*: the thicker the area of interest, the more atoms to go through, the more attenuation occurs. This must be compensated for by increasing both the intensity of photons over the exposure period (mAs) and their penetrative power (kV). This is a problem where the thickness varies in the area of interest. In the back, the muscle depth over the vertebral bodies is much greater than over the spinous processes. Therefore, the tips of the processes are usually overexposed whereas the bodies are relatively underexposed. *Aluminium wedges* can be used to compensate for the lower thickness over the spinous processes.

Radiographic quality: recording the image

Reducing scatter

Scatter negatively affects image quality by reducing contrast and increasing the radiation hazard. Scatter is formed in the patient (*primary scatter*) but also in all materials encountered by the primary, secondary and scattered beams (*secondary scatter*). In particular, it may arise from the cassette itself, cassette holders,

walls and floor of the X-ray room. This secondary scatter is referred to as *backscatter*.

Scattered radiation may be reduced by:

- Decreasing the voltage below 70 kV: this is often impractical in horses because sufficient energy is required to penetrate thick tissue masses.
- Keeping the size of the primary beam as small as possible by *collimating* to the area of interest: the beam also should be collimated to within the confines of the cassette to decrease backscatter.
- Placing a lead sheet at the back of the cassette: this is necessary and further increases the dose (mAs).
- Having an *air gap* between the patient and the film: because scattered rays are very oblique, the intensity of the scattered beam decreases much more rapidly with distance than that of the primary beam, so increasing the distance between subject and film decreases the proportion of scattered to useful photons. Unfortunately, the resulting magnification is also undesirable.
- Using grids: these reduce the amount of scattered radiation reaching the film.

Grids

Grids are placed between the patient and the cassette to absorb the scatter but not the secondary beam.

Primary beam X-rays reach the cassette at more or less right angles to it, whereas most scattered photons travel obliquely. The latter may be removed, therefore, by placing lead strips parallel to the beam (Fig. 17.14), separated by strips of radiolucent spacer (carbon fibre or aluminium) to let the useful X-rays reach the cassette. The efficiency of the grid depends on the type of grid and the *grid ratio*, i.e. the ratio of the height of the strips to the thickness of the spacers. The higher the lead strips and the narrower the spacers, i.e. the greater the grid ratio, the more scatter is removed. Unfortunately, the lead strips also have a certain thickness and primary photons also are absorbed, so that in a stationary grid the strips are visible on the radiograph. The more *lead strips per centimetre* (usually 20–40) and the thinner they are, the more efficient and less visible the grid is. The more efficient a grid, the more useful radiation is removed. So, when using a grid *the dose (mAs) must*

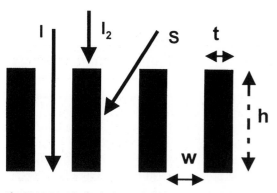

Fig. 17.14 Principle of grids. The primary photons (I) pass through the grid. Both scatter (S) and some primary photons (I₂) are absorbed by the strips. If *h* increases or *w* decreases (grid ratio increases), more S but also I₂ are removed.

be increased to compensate for the loss in proportion of photons. The *grid factor* is a predetermined number by which the dose (mA · s) must be multiplied for a particular grid. It is usually 2.5–3, so the dose must be increased by 2–3 times (thus increasing the radiation hazard).

Parallel grids are made with parallel strips perpendicular to the cassette. However, the primary X-rays are not all perpendicular to the cassette: due to the conical shape of the beam, the further the rays are from the centre, the more oblique they are and, consequently, the more likely they are to be absorbed by the grid. This results in a decrease in image density and a widening of the striped pattern at the edges. This effect is termed *grid cut-off*. To prevent this, the height of the lead strips may be decreased from the centre to the periphery of the grid (pseudofocused grid) (Fig. 17.15a) or the strips may be tilted gradually towards the centre, to match the obliquity of the beam (*focused grid*) (Fig. 17.15b). These are very efficient but only work if the primary beam is absolutely perpendicular to the cassette, centred exactly with the grid, and the FFD is such that the obliquity of the rays is the same as that of the strips. Practically there is a range of FFDs that can be used, and this is usually indicated on the grid as the *focal range*. Grids are difficult to use with horses because the location of the cassette must be assessed subjectively by the operator. The use of a fixed unit with a special cassette holder is ideal for this purpose.

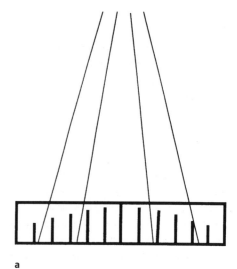

a

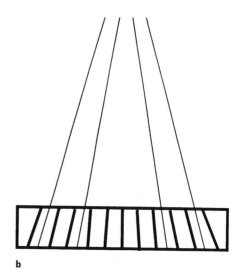

b

Fig. 17.15 (a) Pseudo-focused grid. (b) Focused grid.

To eliminate the visible strips produced by *stationary grids* on the radiograph, one can blur the image of the grid. This is achieved by vibrating the grid during exposure. This system is called a *moving grid* or *Potter-Bucky diaphragm* and is only available in fixed units.

Scattered photons travelling in planes parallel to the strips are not removed so two grids can be placed at right angles to each other (*crossed grids*). This is rarely used because it further increases the dose required.

Film and screens for horses

Depending on the nature, size and number of silver halide crystals, different films show a variable response to the same radiation. Other important factors include:

(1) *Film speed*: a subjective measurement of its efficiency at converting light to an image. The lower the exposure (i.e. number of photons used to expose a given area of the film) required to give it a certain density, the faster the film. For the same exposure, a faster film gives a denser (blacker) image. Speed is a relative measurement, i.e. it can be used only to compare films. It is often difficult to compare the speeds of films from different manufacturers. Film speed is usually quoted as multiples of 100: a 200 film is twice as fast as a 100 film. Typically, mammography films have a speed of 50, high detail films are 100 (for use with small parts and orthopaedics) and fast films are 400–800. The faster the film, the less detailed it is (due to increased grain size). Fast films should be reserved for thick areas or machines with low current (mA), necessitating longer exposures.

(2) *Types of film*: they *must* match the screens used. Most films are double sided, i.e. have emulsion on both sides. This increases speed and contrast because the X-rays going through the cassette can produce twice the reaction. Mammography films are single-sided and used with one screen only. They are therefore slower but provide excellent definition. In equine radiography, the area of interest often dictates the type of film used:

    (a) For thick, well-muscled areas, fast films are necessary to decrease the required exposure.

    (b) If a portable X-ray machine is used, faster films also are required.

    (c) To image the distal limb, detailed films are preferable to detect subtle lesions.

(3) Film–screen combinations: the above description may be extended to the use of films in combination with screens. In particular, some screens are 'faster' than others. With the use of double-sided films and two screens, the speed can be

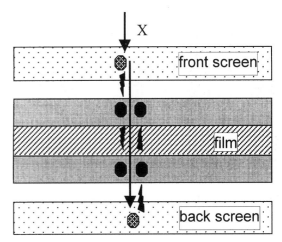

Fig. 17.16 Effect of double screen system. One X-ray can sensitise phosphors in both screens, forming four silver grains.

increased dramatically: each group of photons in a single ray will encounter phosphor crystals in both screens, causing the emission of two flashes of light. Each flash will, in turn, activate chemicals in both emulsions. So one ray can create four times more response than with one screen/one emulsion (Fig. 17.16). One disadvantage is screen *unsharpness* or blurring, caused by diffusion of light through the film base. This is avoided with the use of non-screen films: very sensitive films sensitised directly by the X-rays and used for dental work in humans and small animals.

Unsharpness

Image quality depends on image density and contrast, which itself depends on a combination of subject and film contrasts. A third major factor is sharpness, i.e. how obvious the edges of shadows are on the film, which is affected by movement (*blur*). Especially when radiographing a horse's thicker body parts, there can be a relatively large distance between the patient and the film. Consequently, a small movement can cause significant blurring of the image (Fig. 17.17). This can be reduced by:

- Immobilising the patient: ideally the patient should be anaesthetised, both for safety reasons and to decrease movement. This is rarely practical in horses due to the cost, impracticality and risks associated with general anaesthetics. It is generally recommended to use chemical and other forms of restraint. Deep sedation may result in the patient constantly swaying, so low doses should be used unless the patient is intractable. Certain techniques help to immobilise the subject, e.g. weight-bearing techniques for foot radiography rather than techniques where the limb is held in a block.

- Lower exposure times: this may be achieved with some machines by increasing the current and decreasing the exposure time to obtain the same dose. Although relatively small changes of current lead to the same effect on the film, large variations can lead to alteration in the film response and therefore a different radiodensity, despite preserving the same dose (a phenomenon called *reciprocity failure*). Faster films help to reduce the exposure time, but there must be a compromise between image quality and speed.

In rounded objects, the edges result in a gradual decrease in thickness, corresponding to a fading effect on the film. The edges are therefore not as sharp as in squared objects (Fig. 17.18).

Mottle

This may be due to variations in the size and concentration of crystals in the screen or the film. Generally, larger grains are used in faster devices, so that the image appears grainier. These films also are used with lower exposures, so that mottle may become a significant problem: the image appears grainy or flea-bitten to frankly mottled.

Distortion

A final factor in image quality is distortion of the image on the film. There are two major effects:

(1) *Magnification* (Fig. 17.19): because of the conical shape of the beam, any structure in the patient appears magnified on the film (Fig. 17.19a). Magnification can make it difficult to assess distances but also decreases sharpness (because dots are larger on the film). The greater the FFD (Fig. 17.19b) and the shorter the distance between the subject and the film (Fig. 17.19c), the smaller the magnification. Practically, one should place the cassette as close as possible to the area of interest. Short FFD techniques also should be avoided (a 1-m FFD is generally a good compromise). Occasionally, magnification may be used to separate structures that otherwise would be superimposed, such as the temporomandibular joints in the skull. Although the images on lateral radiographs should not be distinguishable, the further joint from the cassette will appear the larger (Fig. 17.19d). Because detail is best with lower magnification, the joint of interest should be closer to the plate.

(2) *Distortion* (Fig. 17.20): if the film and/or the subject are not perpendicular to the beam, the image is unevenly magnified, causing distortion of the shape. The cassette, therefore, should be as perpendicular to the beam as possible.

Artefacts

Artefacts in radiology are images not directly associated with the subject and there are various causes.

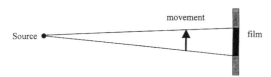

Fig. 17.17 Movement blur: movement during the exposure amounts to each dot in the subject being smeared as a patch on the film.

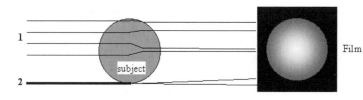

Fig. 17.18 Inherent unsharpness: the edges of round objects are thinner than the centre, causing loss of contrast (1). Further loss of sharpness is due to refraction of the rays at the edges (2).

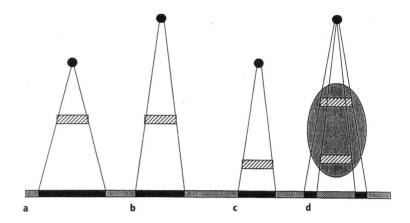

Fig. 17.19 Magnification (a) is decreased by increasing the FFD (b) or decreasing the subject–film distance (c). Two objects of the same size but at different distances from the source are magnified to a different degree (d).

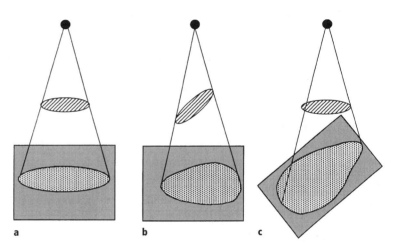

Fig. 17.20 Distortion: no distortion occurs if the subject and film are perpendicular to the beam (a); the image is distorted if the subject (b) or the film (c) are oblique to the beam.

Film faults

These are abnormal images created by poor handling or processing of the films and screens. They are common but should be recognised and avoided. Surface stains or scratches occur over the top of the emulsion. This is recognised by observing the film end-on and looking for any denting or bulging of the film surface. The silver halide grains are extremely sensitive to both light and physical factors, such as pressure and temperature. A small to moderate amount of pressure can sensitise and convert grains to silver, causing black artefacts. High pressure, such as in deep scratches or folding of the film, can displace the grains into the surrounding emulsion and cause focal depletion of silver, i.e. white artefacts.

The various film faults are:

- *Surface marks* (Fig. 17.21a). These superficial marks occur over the top of the image. Rubbing the films against the cassette, the feeding tray of the processor or the benchtop often causes fine surface scratches. Discrete, linear, shallow scratches may be caused by dirty or damaged processor rollers. Stains usually occur during or after processing, including greasy stains and sticky substances but also dirt from the rollers, especially algae, forming green or brown deposits on the film. This can be avoided by regular cleaning of the equipment and adding bleach to the wash tank when the processor is not in use.
- *Pressure marks* (Fig. 17.21b). Roller marks are usually identified as linear or regularly repeating marks in the direction the film travelled through the processor. Any dirt or scratches on the rollers

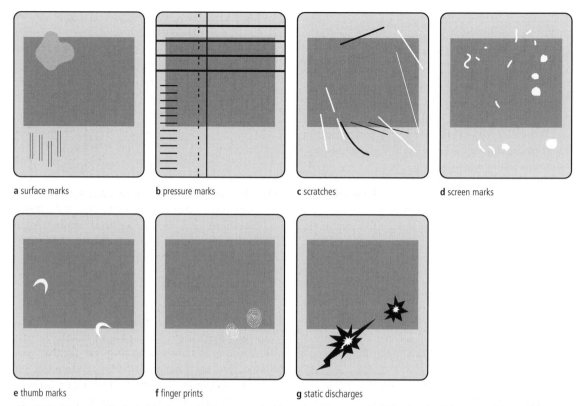

a surface marks   **b** pressure marks   **c** scratches   **d** screen marks

e thumb marks   **f** finger prints   **g** static discharges

Fig. 17.21 Artefacts and film faults: (a) surface marks; (b) pressure marks; (c) scratches; (d) screen marks; (e) thumb marks; (f) finger prints; (g) static discharges.

cause repeating marks, and the rollers being too tight causes transverse black lines. Regular cleaning of the rollers and adequate maintenance usually help to reduce these. Black pressure marks can be caused by excessive pressure when holding the film to load the cassette or processor.

- *Scratches* (Fig. 17.21c). Deep scratches can either sensitise the emulsion, causing black lines, or damage the emulsion, causing white lines.
- *Screen dust* (Fig. 17.21d). This is the most common artefact, caused by dusty screens or films. Any foreign material occurring between the screens and film blocks light emitted by the screens, causing white artefacts. This can dramatically affect image quality. To avoid this, the screens should be cleaned regularly with special antistatic solutions (static electricity attracts dust).
- *Thumb marks* (Fig. 17.21e). These are black or white (white means severe enough to damage the emulsion) crescent-shaped marks, caused by slightly bending the film between the thumb and other fingers when holding it with one hand.
- *Fingerprints* (Fig. 17.21f). Hands are naturally greasy. Grease or fat stop solutions from penetrating the emulsion, causing a local area of underdevelopment and therefore lighter or white fingerprints.
- *Static* (Fig. 17.21g). Static electricity build-up can create small flashes of electricity, the light from which sensitises the film. These are recognised by their odd, complex patterns (sprays and sunbursts) or zigzag appearance. This is reduced by keeping the humidity at around 70% with a humidifier or by boiling a kettle in the room.

Abnormal exposure (fogging)

Any source of radiation or heat can directly affect the film:

- *Scatter*. A halo of scattered, dark-grey radiation is usually visible around the margins of the primary beam. This cannot be avoided but films and cassettes should be stored away from the X-ray tube and in areas protected from X-ray sources.
- *Safelight*. Wrong choice of safelight for a particular film or leaking light filters can cause fogging.
- *Light fogging*. Films may be accidentally exposed to light by opening a box of films, hopper or loaded cassette. When exposed to light, a film will be entirely black after processing. If a pack of films is exposed, light penetrates through the few most superficial films, which are spoiled, but only for a few centimetres into the exposed edges of the more central films. Fogging starting at the corner of a film and fading towards the centre is typical of a cassette that was not closed properly or is damaged and no longer lightproof.
- *Abnormal exposure*. Faulty X-ray machines may deliver an abnormally high exposure, so that the film appears entirely black. Conversely, it may not have been exposed, in which case the film turns out transparent.
- *Processing fog*. Overdevelopment can cause fogging of the film. It can be caused by a high pH (not acidic enough) in the fixer, due usually to developer carried over to the fixer. The film should be washed between the two stages.
- *Other causes of fog*. Ambient ground radiation, excessive heat or films past their sell-by-date may show an overall grey fog, similar to scatter, but it is even over the whole film.

Processing faults

Processing can affect the image density and quality:

(1) *Developer errors*. These are the most common and usually due to chemical exhaustion:
 (a) Underdevelopment, i.e. an image not dark enough (pale grey) and flat (low contrast), can be differentiated from an underexposed film, where the background is black but the image too pale. Typically with faulty or exhausted developer, the image has poor contrast and may have a mottled, patchy appearance.
 (b) Overdevelopment may be due to excess temperature, time or chemical concentration. This causes the film to appear too dark, with low contrast and typically the non-exposed part of the film is uniformly darkened.

(2) *Fixer faults*. These are due to exhausted fixer, causing uneven overdevelopment and poor removal of the pale-yellow emulsion. Under-fixed films appear opaque and the clear areas are grey to pale yellow. Poor washing of the fixer causes the film to become brown, streaky and sticky.

(3) *Chemical splashes*. Developer splashes will cause dark stains (they look like splashes or droplets) whereas fixer causes milky white stains. Other chemicals can damage or sensitise the silver halide, causing varying shades of stains.

Patient artefacts

Some unexpected images may arise from objects superimposed on (i.e. overlying) the patient. Ropes, bandages and other protecting gear usually have a radiodensity similar to or slightly greater than soft tissues. Dirt and mud are heterogeneous and often combine soft-tissue and mineral densities. Streaky effects may result from wet or bloodstained hair, which has a soft-tissue radiodensity but often traps air pockets, causing mixed-density patterns. Air pockets, e.g. air trapped in the clefts of the frog or in open wounds, can create focal radiolucent areas or simply a decrease in radiodensity, which may be difficult to differentiate from fractures or other lesions. These artefacts may be removed using materials to expel the air, such as modelling dough (e.g. Playdoh®) packed in the frog clefts.

Image artefacts

Some images are not real but are due to the interaction of overlapping objects in the patient. A radiograph is a complex shadowgram, where shadows merge, overlap and create convoluted shapes. A typical example is two bones partially overlapping. The overlapping part will appear twice as radiodense and, if narrow enough, may appear as a dense line. Conversely, less radiopaque areas overlapping can create the impression of a black line, e.g. the narrower parts of the tarsal bones in the distal hock.

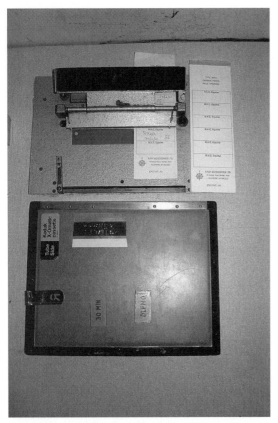

Fig. 17.22 Systems used for primary identification of films: identification camera used on the unexposed corner of a film (top of picture); cassette fitted with lead shield for camera (top left corner); lead-impregnated tape (top centre); R/L metal marker (left); and radiopaque positioning markers (bottom).

Identification of radiographs

It is a legal requirement that radiographs are adequately identified and the minimum requirements for identification include:

- The name of the establishment (veterinary practice)
- The date
- Patient identification, which may be a case number or the animal and/or owner's name
- Other information may be useful to aid interpretation, including left versus right, orientation and, where necessary, identification of the projection.

Methods of identification (Fig. 17.22)

Primary identification

Primary identification means that the information is added before processing and is therefore part of the image. This is the method of choice. Lead markers, blocking the beam (therefore appearing white), may be used for simpler words, especially for left/right or projections. They must be placed in the primary beam to be visible. Lead-impregnated tape is more versatile: writing with a pen removes the lead, showing black writing on the exposed film. Film cameras are the preferred method of identification: a paper insert with the information written on with a dark pen or typed is placed between a special light source and the film. The details appear in white on a black background. To use these, a lead mask must be used in a corner of the cassette where the label is to be placed, so that this part of the film remains unexposed.

Secondary identification

Secondary identification is obtained by writing directly on the developed film, applying sticky labels or punching holes in the film. This is better than no identification but should be avoided whenever possible because the films may not be accepted as evidence in cases of litigation.

Terminology

The correct terminology should be used to label films.

Anatomical directions

For anatomical directions the international terminology is recommended, as indicated in Fig. 17.23. Posterior, anterior, internal and external are no longer acceptable terms.

Projections

The direction of the beam is indicated by first describing the position of the tube in relation to the area of interest and then that of the film (Fig. 17.24). In the head and trunk, *'left to right'* (Fig. 17.24a) and *'right to left lateral radiograph'* are the correct terms but may be referred to as *lateral* on the radiograph. *Dorsoventral* (b_1) and *ventrodorsal* (b_2) projections are straight-

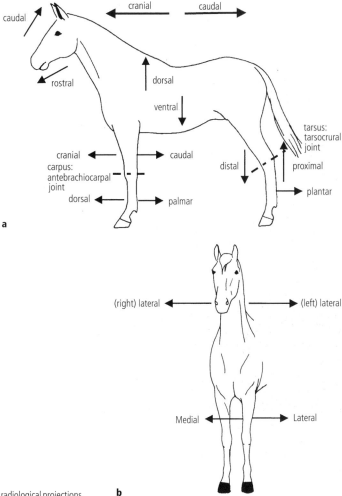

Fig. 17.23 Nomenclature used to describe anatomical and radiological projections.

forward (Fig. 17.24b). Obliques should be described by starting with the closest standard projection and then adding the angle and direction in which the projection is altered (Fig. 17.24c). For instance, a lateral view of the neck with the tube tilted down by 30° would be a *latero-30°-dorsal lateroventral* radiograph (Fig. 17.24d). In the limb, a projection from the side is *lateromedial* (reverse, *mediolateral*). Above the carpus and hock not included, front to back radiographic views should be called *craniocaudal* (reverse, *caudocranial*), whereas below and including those joints one should use *dorsopalmar* (*palmarodorsal*) in the forelimb and *dorsoplantar* (*plantarodorsal*) in the

hindlimb. Obliques are constructed as before but may be more complex. A view from between dorsal and lateral would be a *dorso-x°-lateral palmaromedial* (Fig. 17.24e). An X-ray of the foot obtained by tilting the camera down and placing it in front of the foot, the foot resting on the cassette, is termed a *dorso-x°-proximal palmarodistal* oblique radiograph (Fig. 17.24f). Finally, a radiograph of the point of the hock obtained by flexing the leg, the cassette placed underneath the cannon bone and beam directed from behind the thigh down onto the cassette, would be called a *caudoproximal plantarodistal* projection (even though it is often referred to as a *skyline* view).

343

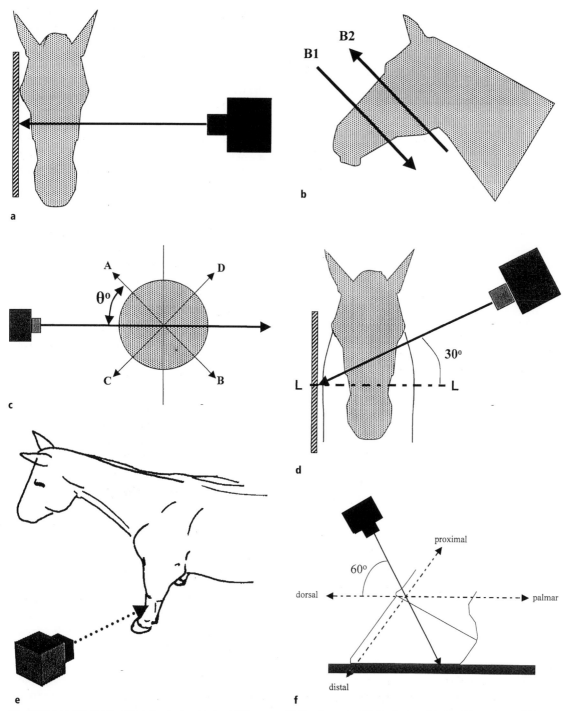

Fig. 17.24 (a) Left to right lateral (lateral) projection of the head. (b) Dorsoventral (b1) and ventrodorsal (b2) projections of the head. (c) Description of oblique projection: A-θ°-C to B-D. Both AB and CD are standard projections. (d) Latero-30°-dorsal lateroventral oblique projection of the head. (e) Dorso-45°-lateral palmaromedial oblique projection of the left forelimb. (f) Dorso-60°-proximal palmarodistal oblique projection of the foot.

Compiling X-ray charts

Technique charts are used to compile the exposure settings for each specific projection. They help to prevent wrongly exposed radiographs and therefore avoid having to repeat exposures. An exposure chart must be compiled for each X-ray machine, because no two units produce exactly the same output. It should be prepared carefully and should record at least the type of film/screen used, the voltage, current, dose and time. One major problem in equine radiography is the major variation in patient size, so different exposure factors should be entered for a set of different sizes (e.g. small, medium and large or approximate weight) and views. Personnel present also should be recorded.

Standardising other factors

As many parameters should be fixed as possible:

- The FFD should be measured and always kept the same (1 m is usually optimal).
- The processing should be standardised.
- The choice of film/screen system should be made for each particular anatomical area, depending on the X-ray machine (faster films are recommended with portable units) and area (slower, more detailed films are better to image the extremities).
- The use of grids should be set for particular views such as back, neck or thorax, and occasionally proximal limb. The same grid should be used for the same area. Some people favour the use of grids for the distal limb, although scatter is not usually a problem at this level, especially with rare-earth screens, but grids impair image quality and require increased exposures.

Choice of exposure factors

A pre-existing chart used for another machine may be used as a base to start with but certain rules of thumb may be helpful:

(1) Altering the dose (mAs) alters the overall film *density* (blackening), not the contrast. The dose should be set to produce an adequate level of brightness, with black background and an acceptable range of greys (*greyscale*) in the image. If the film is generally too pale, or there is marked mottle, or if the voltage should be reduced to improve contrast or decrease scatter, then the dose should be increased.

(2) The voltage settings affect both image density and contrast. Increasing the voltage setting improves the *penetration of the beam* through the tissues. If the bone detail is too low and the tissues too white, the voltage should be increased. If, however, there is low contrast with adequate blackening or too much scatter, the voltage should be reduced. Once the dose is deemed adequate, the voltage should be set to compromise between penetration, contrast and scatter.

(3) Relationship between voltage and dose: as far as the resulting density of the film is concerned, *an increase of 10 kV is comparable to doubling the dose*. So, to improve contrast or penetration but preserve the right level of density, the voltage may be changed and the dose altered accordingly in the opposite direction.

(4) Relationship between exposure factors and tissue thickness (patient size): add 2 kV per extra centimetre between 60 and 70 kV, 3 kV/cm between 80 and 100 kV and 4 kV/cm thereafter.

(5) Individual adjustments: some principles may be used to guess how to alter exposure factors for different patients or anatomical regions:

    (a) Double the dose but use the same voltage for heavily muscled or fat animals.

    (b) Decrease the voltage by 10 kV to examine soft tissues rather than skeleton.

    (c) Increase the voltage by 5 kV for the oblique projections in the carpus and cannon, to compensate for the extra bone thickness.

    (d) Skull: increase the voltage to look at teeth but decrease the voltage and increase the dose to look at sinuses.

    (e) Increase the voltage by 5–10 kV for contrast studies.

    (f) Halve the dose and add 10 kV for the thorax compared with the same thickness in other areas.

Trial exposures

The chart obtained for another machine can be used as a basis but the above principles are applied to optimise the settings. If the results are not satisfactory, trial exposures are made with a set of dose and volt-age values chosen below those of the other chart. Further radiographs are then obtained using the same voltage but twice and four times more dose. Once the right degree of blackness and greyscale have been achieved, the voltage should be adjusted to optimise the picture. All standard projections should be evaluated in this way. Once a basic chart has been compiled, notes should be taken on the quality of the radiographs obtained for several months, in order to adjust the exposures.

Positioning and standard projections

The reader is referred to the further reading list for a detailed description of the various positioning techniques used in horses. The foot will be used as an example of some practical aspects because it is the most common area examined radiographically.

General principles

The details of the examination should be decided before starting, including all the projections required. The animal should be prepared adequately and the coat cleaned in the areas of interest to avoid artefacts. Adequate restraint must be provided. Sedation is recommended in most horses, however calm, because it saves a lot of time, reduces the chances of movement during exposure and repeat radiographs (this is a legal requirement) and makes the procedure safer for the personnel and the equipment. As few people should be present as possible.

The position of the tube in relation to the subject is paramount. The beam should be centred on the most likely location of potential lesions, to decrease the effects of the obliquity of the rays. In particular, to image joints, the rays must be absolutely parallel to the joint space. In the hock, for example, the small distal joints run obliquely (they are more distal, or lower, medially than laterally). So, to obtain a latero-medial projection the beam may be centred on the distal half of the hock and oriented downward by 5–10° (Fig. 17.25a) or kept horizontal but centred on the lateral malleolus (Fig. 17.25b).

The beam should be collimated so that only the area of interest is included in the beam. All four sides of the rectangular beam must be visible on the cas-

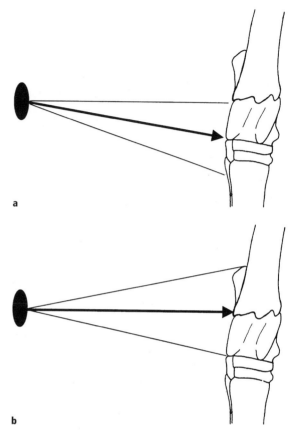

Fig. 17.25 Lateromedial projection of the hock. To obtain a sharp image of the distal joint spaces, which are at an angle to the horizontal, the beam can be centred at their level and tilted distally by 10° (a), or the beam may be centred on the lateral malleolus, using the obliquity of the rays at the periphery of the beam (b).

sette (for safety reasons and to decrease backscatter). Once the beam is adequately set, the cassette is placed behind the subject, as close as possible to it (most horses tolerate the cassette touching the skin) and as perpendicular to the beam as practical to avoid excessive distortion of the image. Finally, the FFD should be checked using a tape measurer or a measuring stick of the appropriate length, because small variations in FFD can dramatically affect the exposure.

Foot radiography

A complete set of standard projections should be obtained to avoid missing subtle lesions. Latero-

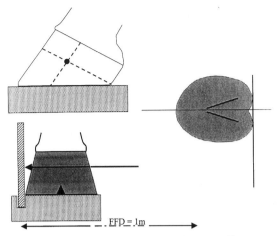

Fig. 17.26 Positioning landmarks for lateromedial projection of foot.

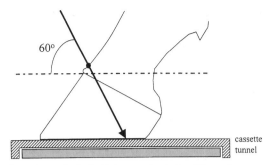

Fig. 17.27 Positioning for 'high coronary' projection of P3, standing technique.

medial and dorsopalmar oblique projections should be included and navicular studies should be added where necessary. The foot should be cleaned. It is usually recommended that the clefts be washed and filled with modelling dough to remove the resulting artefacts. However, many radiologists prefer to leave the clefts unfilled but well cleaned and trimmed.

Lateromedial projection (Fig. 17.26)

The beam should be centred around the middle of the third phalanx, i.e. approximately one-third of the distance from the coronet to the ground and one-third of that between the dorsal hoof wall and the heel. Most tubes cannot be set right down to the ground, so the foot usually must be raised on a block. Wood is best because it is fairly radiolucent; bricks should be avoided. It is best if the horse bears weight on the foot of interest because the sole is then horizontal and a horizontal beam can be used (this also decreases movement). It is often more practical to raise both feet (fore or hind) to the same level and this author prefers the use of two blocks rather than a large one, which often scares the animal. A properly protected assistant (gown and gloves) can pick up the opposite limb in fractious patients, but should stand as far back as possible to keep a safe distance from the beam going through the cassette. This is fairly safe provided that the cassette is adequately shielded with lead and the beam well collimated. It may be difficult to place the tube exactly lateral to the foot. A simple

solution is to place the beam at right angles to a line drawn between the two heel bulbs (provided that the foot is not too imbalanced). The cassette should be placed behind the block and ideally should touch the medial side of the hoof, extending 2–5 cm lower than the sole (a special slot may be used in the block) to take into account the obliquity of the beam.

Dorsopalmar projections

The true dorsopalmar projection is obtained with the foot weight-bearing on a block and using a horizontal beam. This can be a very useful view in selected cases but is rarely necessary for routine radiography of the foot. The more common projection for the third phalanx is a dorso 60° proximal palmarodistal oblique, often termed a *high coronary* view. This projection can be obtained with the foot weight-bearing on a special block under which the cassette can be placed (cassette tunnel) (Fig. 17.27). The tunnel is used to avoid damaging the cassette with the weight of the animal. The major disadvantage of this technique is the fact that the image is distorted. However, movement blur is unlikely and perfect positioning is easily achieved. The tube head is raised and tilted 60° to the horizontal (i.e. 30° to the vertical). For practicality, angles should be premarked on the side of the tube head. The FFD is then checked to ensure that the head is at the appropriate height. It may be helpful to rotate the foot slightly outwards to facilitate placement of the X-ray machine in front of the patient. The beam is centred on the most dorsal point of the coronary band with the tube placed exactly in the dorsopalmar plane of the foot (the central rays of the

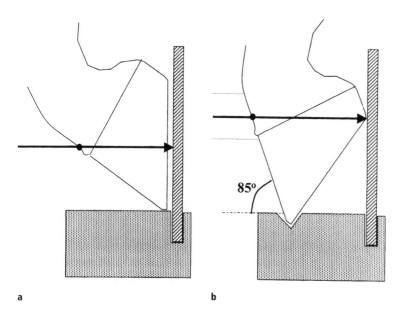

Fig. 17.28 Positioning for horizontal beam techniques: 'upright pedal bone' projection for P3 (a); 'upright pedal view of the navicular bone' (b).

a   b

beam should exit between the bulbs of the heel). It is collimated exactly to the hoof. To avoid distortion, some people prefer using a flexed view (Fig. 17.28a): the foot is placed on a block with the cassette set vertically in a slot behind the foot. The foot rests on the block by the toe and should be flexed so that the sole rests vertically against the cassette. A horizontal beam is used, centred as above. Drawbacks of this technique include:

- Difficulty in positioning the foot.
- A large variation in angle (depending on the length of the sole, the angle to the cassette can vary significantly).
- The likeliness of movement blur.
- The need to hold the limb with a hand close to the primary beam.

For the dorsopalmar projection of the navicular bone, similar techniques are used but a 65° angle to the horizontal is used for the weight-bearing technique, and the dorsal hoof wall should be tilted at an 85° angle to the ground (Fig. 17.28b). The beam is centred 2.5 cm proximal to the coronet and collimated down to just within the sides of the leg so that the lower edge of the beam reaches a few millimetres distal to the coronet.

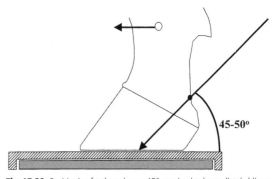

Fig. 17.29 Positioning for the palmaro-45°-proximal palmarodistal oblique projection of the foot ('navicular skyline').

Palmaro 45° proximal palmarodistal oblique projection (Fig. 17.29)

This projection, often referred to as a *skyline* or palmar cortex view of the navicular bone, is probably the most useful radiograph for navicular disease but may be useful also for other conditions affecting the palmar parts of the foot. This must be obtained with the foot weight-bearing on a cassette tunnel. The foot should be placed over the palmar half of the cassette. The tube head is tilted at an angle slightly less steep than that of the dorsal hoof wall of the patient, 45–50° often being adequate. The tube is placed behind the foot, under the chest and the beam is centred in the middle of the fold of the pastern, so that the beam is in the sagittal plane of the foot. In most cases it is difficult to place the tube under the horse. A shorter FFD may be used (the dose should be decreased correspondingly) or the foot may be rotated so that the heels point outwards. Most horses tolerate this with adequate sedation and patience. The foot also should be extended as far back as tolerated by the horse, in order to move the palmar aspect of the fetlock forward (otherwise, it can mask the image of the navicular bone).

Contrast studies

Contrast techniques are used to increase artificially the subject contrast, usually to delineate cavity walls or assess movement through blood vessels or the digestive tract.

Contrast materials

The substances used must have a very different radiodensity from that of the tissues examined. They may be radiolucent, usually air or gases (negative contrast media), or radiodense (positive contrast media):

(1) Air is rarely used deliberately in horses as a negative contrast medium, but the presence of air in tissues, especially wounds, is often useful. Air in a joint or under the skin shows the presence of an open wound. Very rarely, bacterial infections lead to gas accumulation. Gas is naturally present in the trachea and sinuses and this can be used to improve images. For example, fluid in the sinuses decreases contrast and obliterates soft-tissue masses. It may be drained so that lesions are highlighted by air. Air in the trachea can be used to improve the contrast in mediolateral radiographs of the shoulder: the head should be kept low to place the trachea at the level of the scapulohumeral joint.

(2) Positive contrast media have a higher radiodensity than soft tissues. Heavy metallic elements are used, usually barium or iodine:

(a) *Barium sulphate* is non-toxic but can be used only to image the digestive tract. It cannot be removed from joints, lungs or internal organs and can cause severe reactions.

(b) *Soluble iodinated products* are used for internal cavities. Most of these solutions are *ionic* (salts of diatrizoate, metrizoate or iothalamate). They are a lot less costly but can cause some irritation to joints, where they should be diluted with an equal volume of Hartmann's solution. They should not be used for spinal studies (myelography) because they cause severe reactions.

(c) *Non-ionic iodinated substances* have been developed, including metrizamide, iopamidol and iohexol. These are more expensive but safer for myelography.

Special techniques

Digestive tract studies

A *barium meal* consists of mixing barium powder with food. This is ideal to assess the speed and integrity of the passage of food through the pharynx and along the oesophagus in the horse. This is best carried out under fluoroscopy, although one radiograph may be obtained immediately after administration of the meal. To look for damage to the walls and lining of the tract, *barium suspension* (freshly made up from powder) or *paste* is preferable (*barium swallow*). If an oesophageal tear is suspected, barium should be avoided. The advent of endoscopy has rendered these latter studies less common. It must be noted that sedation decreases the oesophageal function and should not be used for barium studies. Contrast studies of the gut distal to the oesophagus are rarely attempted in the horse, apart from occasional barium enemas in foals.

Sinography

Positive contrast media can be injected into a wound to assess the direction of any tracts, their depth and involvement of deeper structures. The simplest method is to use *metal probes*. These must be blunt to avoid puncturing sound tissues, ideally soft (such as lead) to avoid trauma and they should be sterile. The wound should be cleansed and lavaged before introducing the probe. Fluid contrast media also may be injected into a sinus tract through a catheter, although this is often difficult because the fluid escapes, coating the skin and making the radiograph difficult to interpret.

Joints and sheaths

The best way to confirm that a wound has penetrated a synovial cavity is not to inject contrast medium into it, because it often leaks out. Rather, the medium may be injected under some pressure into the joint (*arthrography*), tendon sheath (*tenosynography*) or bursa (*bursography*) to look for any leakage through the wound. Ionic iodinated media (diluted by half with Hartmann's solution), or plain or diluted non-ionic media can be used. Because joints are easily contaminated, the injection site must be prepared *aseptically* as for surgery, especially as the media can cause irritation and increase the risk of infection. Only freshly opened vials or bottles of both diluent and medium should be used.

Fluoroscopy

Fluoroscopy is the use of radiography to obtain real-time, moving images by continuous generation of X-rays. Historically it used high levels of radiation. Modern units use traditional X-ray tubes, but the cassettes are replaced with a fluorescent photomultiplier tube or *image intensifier*. These tubes convert X-rays to light, which is highly amplified so that a small amount of radiation gives out a visible image. This is recorded by a camera and displayed on a TV screen. It may be recorded also on video recorders. Mobile units (C-arms) are generally used: a C-shaped arm is used to hold an X-ray tube at one end and an intensifier directly opposite; this can be adjusted in all directions to aid positioning.

Real-time fluoroscopy is useful to observe movement, especially for angiography (blood vessels are assessed by visualising the flow of contrast medium) or for placement of catheters in blood vessels, e.g. for the treatment of guttural pouch mycosis. A more common application is the intra-operative assessment of surgical procedures. Fluoroscopy is more convenient than serial radiographs to check for bone alignment or plate and screw placement during fracture repair. The increased exposure is justified by decreased time, anaesthetic and infectious risks.

The exposure settings used vary between units, and charts should be compiled as above. Generally, the same voltage as for standard radiographs should be used. The main disadvantages of this method are the very high radiation exposure and the generally low image detail.

Scintigraphy

Gamma scintigraphy ('bone scanning') is a relatively old technique that has regained popularity in the past few years, especially in equine orthopaedics. It involves the detection of gamma radiation emitted by a radioactive isotope administered to the animal. This is linked to a chemical molecule and scintigraphy is used to trace this in the patient's body and assess its behaviour (localisation, dose, rate of elimination, etc.). Unlike other techniques, scintigraphy does not image the anatomy but rather the physiology of the tissues. It will show lesions that are not obvious radiographically.

Radioactivity refers to radiation produced by physical reactions within the nucleus of atoms, called radioactive decay. An unstable nucleus will change itself to attain a more stable structure. In the process, it loses mass and/or energy in the form of particles (alpha radiation and beta particles) and/or electromagnetic radiation (gamma radiation). This results in the formation of a different isotope or a different atom more stable than the initial one. In some cases, the resulting atom is still unstable and may disintegrate again, forming a chain reaction.

Radioactive atoms disintegrate at a rate that is characteristic of the isotope. This rate is measured by the *half-life* of the disintegration, which is the time it takes for half of the nuclei to have undergone the change. The isotopes do not keep radiating: once the nucleus has disintegrated, no more emission occurs, so each photon emitted corresponds to one stabilised isotope. Once all the atoms have been changed, the radioactivity stops. The gradual loss of radioactivity is called *decay*.

Properties of gamma radiation

Gamma radiation is in the same range of wavelengths as X-radiation. The only difference between

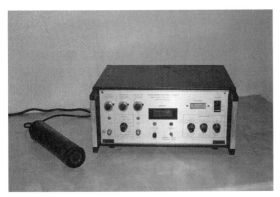

Fig. 17.30 Point probe gamma scintigraphy scanner, with lead-collimated hand-held point probe and counter.

X-rays and gamma photons is the way they are formed: the former in the electron cloud, the latter in the nucleus. The properties are therefore the same as for X-ray photons. The wavelength of the radiation is characteristic of the isotope, so the radiation is pure (made up of all the same photons).

The isotopes used for diagnostic scintigraphy produce radiation that tends to penetrate tissue much better than X-rays and is less likely to be absorbed. However, when the isotopes do interact with the other atoms, they give rise to high-energy electrons that can cause significant damage.

Recording the radiation

The radiation can be recorded on X-ray films, but it is more useful to measure the amount of radiation with more sensitive, quantitative methods. Photomultiplier tubes are used to increase the signal, so that one single ray may be detected. There are two main types of recording devices for medical scintigraphy.

Point probe counters (Fig. 17.30)
These are made of a single photomuliplier tube. A collimator, made of lead or other heavy metal such as tungsten, is placed before the tube so that only the rays arriving in a straight line are recorded. The probe is placed against the patient and therefore measures the radiation arising from the part of the animal's anatomy located exactly in line with the probe. The reading is a single number, corresponding to the amount of radiation at this point. Point

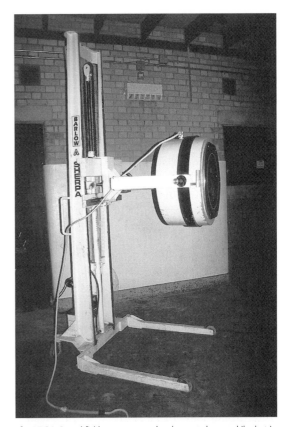

Fig. 17.31 Round-field gamma camera head, mounted on a mobile electric trolley. The cable is linked to a gamma counter and a computerised analysis system.

probes are highly precise but do not provide an anatomical picture (only selected points). The point-by-point examination is time consuming and the long exposure to the operator represents an increased risk. It may be difficult to compare the results between right and left sides because a small variation in the positioning of the probe can result in a large variation in readings. Custom-designed computer software produces graphs comparing right and left sides. This technique is more accurate but less sensitive than camera scans, i.e. it is easier to miss a lesion.

Gamma cameras (Fig. 17.31)
These devices are variously shaped plates (camera head) made of many tubes placed side by side, each with its own collimator. The radiation therefore can be measured for each point over a broad area. A com-

puter is used to form a two-dimensional image: each dot corresponds to a tube, i.e. a point on the horse, and the radiation intensity is translated as either a degree of brightness (the brighter the dot, the higher the radioactivity) or as a colour. Gamma cameras require a much larger radiation dose due to the smaller size of the tubes. Doses 4–8 times higher than for point probe scintigraphy are used, thus increasing the radiation hazard. On the other hand, they provide an anatomical picture that is much easier to interpret. Square field-of-view cameras are more practical than older round-field camera heads, and often have a higher number of tubes, hence a higher definition (detail). However, the most important part of the system is probably the software used to form and analyse the image.

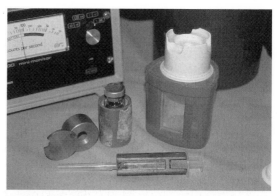

Fig. 17.32 Equipment used for delivery of gamma-emitting radioisotope. The syringe is encased in a tungsten alloy shield. The vial of radioactive solution is shielded in a lead container (left) or purpose-designed eluting jar (right). Note the appropriately calibrated Geiger-Müller counter in the background.

Bone scintigraphy

Principles

Bone scintigraphy consists of injecting a compound that specifically binds to bone in areas of active bone formation. Methylene diphosphonate (MDP) is usually used as a bone seeker because it is soluble in water and blood, it is non-toxic and it is easily eliminated by the kidneys in urine if it has not bound to bone. The isotope used is usually technetium 99m (^{99m}Tc), which emits gamma radiation. Its half-life of 6 h is extremely short, so the radiation hazard is rapidly eliminated. The MDP may be bound to ^{99m}Tc using a kit system, or the labelled tracer may be bought from a radiopharmaceutical provider.

Dispensing of the drug (Fig. 17.32)

The vial of MDP is a concentrated source of radiation. Appropriate training in the handling of radioactive substances is a legal requirement and is strongly advisable to avoid unnecessary exposure. It is recommended that two pairs of gloves be worn because the radioisotope can penetrate the skin and be absorbed. The vial of MDP should be kept in a radiation-proof container. Gamma radiation is not absorbed by Perspex, so the syringe should be shielded in a special, purpose-designed sheath (usually made of lead or a tungsten alloy) and the drug should be drawn into the syringe behind a lead shield. The needle is discarded and a fresh needle should be used to inject the

horse. Any materials coming into contact with the drug should be kept in a special container behind a lead shield. It is safe to handle the vial and contaminated equipment after 72 h. To reduce the exposure, the most important factor is speed, making adequate training even more important.

The drug must be injected intravenously

Any liquid injected subcutaneously causes a loss of isotope and undesirable accumulation of a source of radiation at the injection site in the neck. An intravenous catheter is often used, which can be removed and discarded appropriately after the injection. An examination may be carried out at different time points:

(1) Upon its administration, MDP rapidly spreads with blood to all vascularised tissues. A recording may be taken immediately after injection (first 30 s) to assess the blood flow (vascular phase). Only one recording may be obtained. The camera must be placed next to the area of interest prior to administering the drug.

(2) Between 10 and 30 min, MDP accumulates in the tissues and capillary beds. Recording at this time (pool or soft-tissue phase) allows some assessment of the blood supply to an area (amount of blood delivered, rate of clearance from the tissues). The results from these two phases are often unreliable and difficult to interpret.

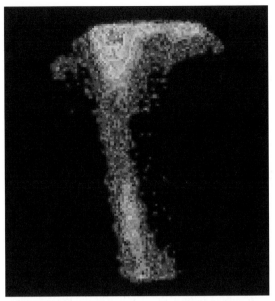

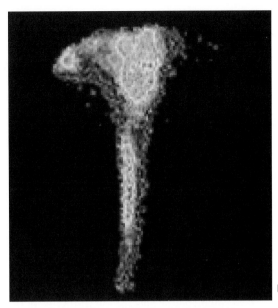

a

b

Fig. 17.33 Gamma scintigram (scan) of a normal tibia (a) and of a radius with a stress fracture (b). Note the 'hot spot' (whiter image) in the middle of the radial shaft.

(3) The third phase (bone phase) occurs once MDP has been cleared from the soft tissues. Only the chemical bound to bone should remain by 4 h. This phase is the most important to detect skeletal problems.

Normal findings

The image obtained does not relate to the anatomy but rather to the metabolic rate of bone. The thicker the bone (e.g. ends of long bones), the more MDP accumulates and the higher the reading. Consequently, one can see the shape of normal bones (Fig. 17.33a). Tissues absorb gamma rays, like X-rays, so bones covered by muscle or fat appear less hot (radioactive) than areas close to the skin, such as bony prominences (tuber coxae of the pelvis, tibial plateau, dorsal processes of the spine). Finally, bone is actively produced in growing horses at the level of growth plates, which produce extremely high readings. It is therefore important to recognise these normal patterns to interpret scans.

Abnormal results

The MDP accumulates where bone is actively formed. Most lesions are associated with inflam-

mation and active bone remodelling, causing an increased uptake of radioisotope. With bone destruction (fractures, infections) there is increased bone deposition around the lesion. These changes translate as discrete areas of high reading, or *hot spots* (Fig. 17.33b). Occasionally, the lesion is inactive or purely destructive, therefore no MDP is taken up, causing a local area with no or low reading (*cold spot*) (e.g. bone cysts and sequestra).

Artefacts

Some normal processes can cause a focal increase of activity. The most common is accumulation of MDP in the bladder, because it is eliminated in urine. Urination within 2 h after injection removes most of the free drug. However, large amounts of MDP may accumulate in the bladder, causing a very large hot spot over the pelvis area. This can interfere with imaging of this area. To prevent this, it is often recommended to administer a diuretic (furosemide) 1 h before the examination is to take place. The horse should be kept in the box until it has passed urine to avoid contaminating the scintigraphy room. It is also preferable to cover the limbs (up to and including the knees and hocks) with bandages, because urine splashes

353

can create hot spots in the distal limbs. Another common artefact is caused by variations in blood flow. Blood determines the delivery of MDP and therefore the amount taken up. As a result, an increase in blood supply, e.g. with inflammation or increased weight-bearing due to a lame opposite limb, can lead to an overall increase of radioactivity. Reduced blood supply, leading to decreased uptake, also occurs in very cold conditions.

Care of the patient

The patient is a significant source of radiation. The radiation emanating from it immediately after injection is very large and then rapidly decreases. The animal therefore should be handled as little and for as short a time as possible. Sedation is generally advisable to facilitate the examination while handling the patient on a loose rope. As for X-rays, the inverse square law applies, so the further from the horse the safer the operators. Because MDP is eliminated in urine, the bed is very radioactive and should not be handled for 72 h. By that stage, decay has decreased the radioactivity of ^{99m}Tc and the risk has become minimal.

Licensing

The risk associated with the handling of ^{99m}Tc is believed to be minimal. However, as for any ionising radiation, the Regulations require that the premises and protocol for the use of radioactive substances be licensed. For scintigraphy, the main risks are associated with dispensing of the drug and with the animal's urine. Therefore, a special controlled area needs to be designed and licensed for dispensing the technetium and discarding the needles, syringes and gloves. The drainage from the box

must be checked and separated from other parts of the stable or building. It is advisable that horses examined by scintigraphy be kept on absorbing litter such as shavings or paper, rather than straw, to prevent pooling of radioactive urine. A special warning sign indicating a potential danger from radiation must, by law, be displayed on all entrances to the scintigraphy room and on the animal's box door for 72 h.

Ultrasonography

Ultrasonography has become the method of choice to image soft tissues in the horse.

Principles

Generation of the ultrasound beam

Ultrasound is basically normal sound waves but at a frequency that we cannot hear. Ultrasound waves can be created by special crystals in a *transducer* (or probe). The crystals can be made to vibrate with an electric current, this vibration inducing a sound wave. In reverse, sound makes the crystals vibrate and create a current (piezoelectric effect) that can be measured (Fig. 17.34). Transducers produce ultrasound beams in pulses and, between each pulse, can analyse sound echoes coming back. Electronic systems then are used to translate the information into an image.

Generation of the ultrasound image

Ultrasound machines work like radar. Ultrasound waves travel through tissues. Whenever a different tissue (with varying sound propagating properties) is encountered, some of the sound is reflected, like

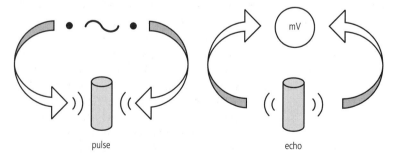

pulse   echo

Fig. 17.34 Piezoelectric principle. A voltage is applied to a piezoelectric crystal, which causes it to vibrate and create a pressure wave or sound pulse. Between pulses, returning echoes make the crystal vibrate, which creates a measurable electric field.

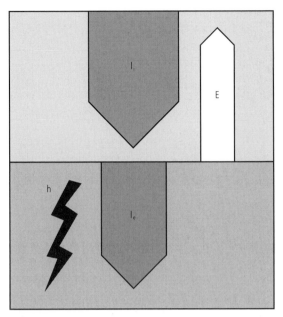

Fig. 17.35 Echo formation. A sound beam with intensity I_i encounters a tissue interface. Some of it is reflected back (E). The remaining beam is attenuated (I_e). Some energy also is lost in the form of heat in the tissues (h).

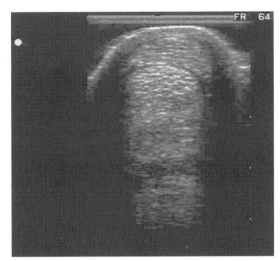

Fig. 17.36 Transverse ultrasonogram of the proximal palmar cannon area of a horse. This B-mode image was obtained using a 7.5-MHz linear array transducer.

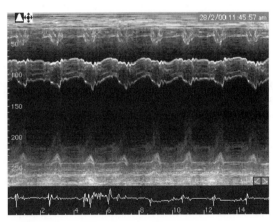

Fig. 17.37 An M-mode ultrasonographic image.

light in a mirror, forming *echoes* (Fig. 17.35). Most of the sound wave continues, but some of it is reflected and some is lost (dissipated as heat or scattered). Its energy thus gradually decreases (*attenuation*). The higher the frequency, the greater the attenuation and therefore the less the sound can penetrate deep into the body.

Returning echoes are converted to electric signals via the piezoelectric effect and are processed by a computer to give the ultrasound image. This information can be *displayed* in several ways:

- *A-mode*: one line of echoes is displayed on an oscilloscope; this is rarely used nowadays.
- *B-mode* (brightness mode or *ultrasound scan*): echoes are represented by dots on a screen. The brightness is related to the intensity (strength) of the echoes. A two-dimensional image is therefore obtained (Fig. 17.36), representing a cross-section through the tissues. This image is displayed in real time.
- *M-mode* (motion mode): a single scan line is obtained with each pulse, but the line obtained

with the next pulse is shown beside it, and so on, to form an image representing the movement of the tissues in the scan line with time (Fig. 17.37).

- *Doppler ultrasonography*: this relies on the Doppler effect, where the frequency of sound is modified by moving structures. This determines the direction and speed of moving materials such as blood. It may be represented by a graph (spectral Doppler) or colours (colour flow imaging).

355

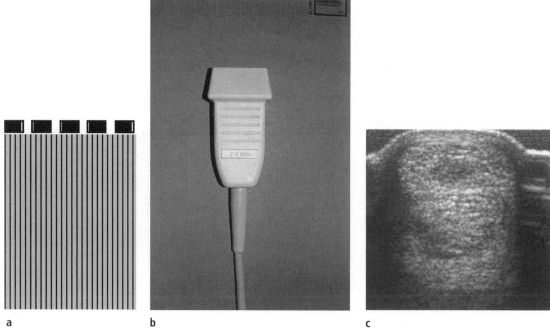

Fig. 17.38 Linear array transducer and resulting image and slide.

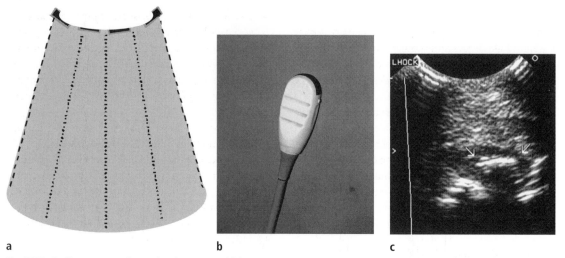

Fig. 17.39 Curvilinear array transducer and resulting image and slide.

Equipment

Types of transducers

- *Linear array*: multiple crystals are aligned along the flat surface of the transducer. This gives a rectangular image on the screen (Fig. 17.38).

- *Curvilinear* or convex: multiple crystals are aligned along a curved line. This produces a pie-shaped image (Fig. 17.39). This system has the advantage of requiring a smaller skin contact area, but image quality in deeper areas is generally inferior to that of linear transducers.

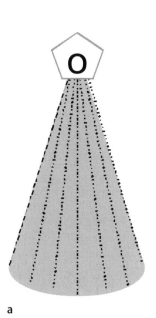
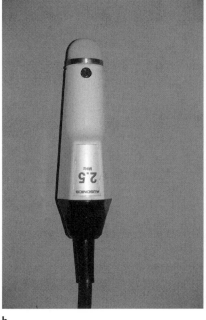
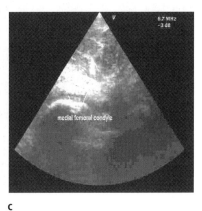

a   b   c

Fig. 17.40 Mechanical sector transducer and resulting image and slide.

- *Mechanical sector*: a single crystal is oscillated back and forth, giving a pie-shaped image (Fig. 17.40). It reduces the skin contact area (ideal for imaging between ribs) but the image is very narrow in superficial areas and poorer quality in deeper fields.
- *Annular array*: a concentric arrangement of ring-shaped elements is oscillated mechanically to give a pie-shaped image. This provides better image quality than the mechanical sector type and uses several frequencies simultaneously. Phased array probes are similar but the elements are steered electronically. These transducers are preferred for colour Doppler but are expensive.

Choice of equipment

There are many models available and the choice should be made carefully depending on the expected workload:

- Most *equine reproduction* work can be carried out satisfactorily with simpler machines and 5–7.5-Mz rectal linear probes. If moved around studs, portability and sturdiness are important.

- *Echocardiography* (ultrasonographic examination of the heart) involves complex technology with sector or similar probes to image between the ribs and Doppler facilities. These are available only in more expensive systems, although there are affordable portable scanners with adequate capabilities.
- For *musculoskeletal* work, most standard tendon examinations can be achieved with any 7.5-Mz transducer. Some clinicians feel that linear systems provide better images close to the skin and for longitudinal scans. More advanced applications, especially those looking at small details (joints), may necessitate more advanced machines with very high resolution.

The choice of transducer depends on operator preference and the area examined. Curvilinear and sector transducers are preferable when the contact area with the skin is small but are less suited for looking at very superficial areas. Transducers of 2–5 MHz are necessary to image deep structures as in the abdomen, thorax, back and pelvis.

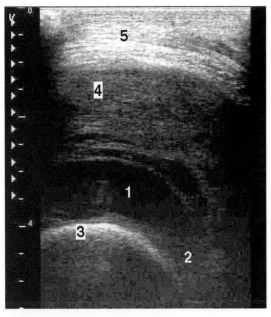

Fig. 17.41 Range of echogenicities encountered on ultrasonograms: 1, anechoic; 2, hypoechoic; 3, hyperechoic; 4 and 5, intermediate echogenicities. The echogenicity increases from 1 to 5.

Improving image quality

Image terminology

The image is composed of grey dots or dashes. The more heterogeneous a tissue, the more dots are formed (echoes) (Fig. 17.41). The brightness of the dots relates not to the true density of the tissue but to how different its physical properties are from surrounding tissues. For example, sound travels through bone, but bone is so much stiffer than soft tissues that most of the sound is reflected. So the interface between the soft tissue and bone is very 'echogenic' and produces a very bright line. No sound is left to produce an image deep to it.

The relevant terminology is as follows:

- Hyperechoic or echogenic: the brightness of the image formed usually describes white area
- Anechoic: a black area on an image where no echos are formed, occurring in even materials such as fluids, gels or cartilage
- Hypoechoic: a grey area imaged where faint echoes are produced, such as blood, loose tissues or muscle

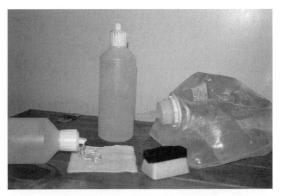

Fig. 17.42 Ultrasound coupling gel in dispensing bag (right) and dispenser bottles (left and top). Note that the thick gel does not drip. Stand-off gel pad (bottom centre).

- Homogeneous: uniform shade of grey
- Heterogeneous: mixture of grey shades

Improving contact

Ultrasound does not travel well through air, hair and hard debris. Ultrasound *coupling gel* usually is used to improve contact between the probe and skin (Fig. 17.42). It must be transparent to sound (*sonolucent*) and stick to both skin and transducer. Very fluid gels are runny, difficult to use and only recommended for rectal work. To examine very superficial structures such as the flexor tendon in the cannon, a '*stand-off*' or 'fluid-offset' containing a sonolucent substance is placed between the transducer and the skin. It moves the superficial structures further away from the transducer and closer to the focal zone, thereby optimising quality. In addition, it produces a better probe to skin contact in rounded or uneven surfaces. These pads are very fragile and expensive.

Ultrasound machine controls

Display screen controls

Brightness and contrast only affect the screen display. They should be set to accommodate the light in the examination area. The room should be kept as dark as possible.

Sensitivity controls

- *Power*: this increases the energy of the beam, creating stronger echoes. Increased power produces a brighter image but too much can mask details. The power control should be set at the lowest level to provide adequate detail.

- *Gain*: this amplifies the returning echoes, increasing the overall brightness of the image. However, it also amplifies noise and can saturate the image. Starting at the lowest setting, it should be increased carefully until the detail is optimal. Excessively high power and gain settings are common errors, leading to saturated images with poor detail.
- *Time gain compensation*: deeper echoes are weaker than superficial ones, because of progressive beam attenuation. The deeper the echoes, the more they need to be amplified to compensate. There are usually several controls for different depths, which should be set so that the brightness of the image is uniform.
- *Focus*: sound beams can be focused and the image is most detailed in the focal zone. The depth of focus always should be set to the area of interest.

Post-processing controls

The above-mentioned controls alter the data before the memory and are called pre-processing; they cannot be altered on a frozen image. Once the image has been collected, it is saved by the computer memory as a data file (displayed when the image is frozen) and then the post-processing controls can be used:

- Greyscale (gamma, dynamic range and compression): the range of greys associated with the intensity of echoes can be modified to change the contrast. An increased number of grey shades shows more subtle differences, improving detail, but decreases the contrast between echoes. It is well worth learning how to use this facility, because different levels of detail and contrast are better for different types of examinations.
- The frame rate: the number of times the image is renewed on the screen per second. Fast frame rates decrease blurring of moving structures but lower frame rates improve image quality by providing more time for the transducer to collect returning echoes.
- Measurement utilities: measuring distances and cross-sectional areas is particularly useful to pro-

vide an objective assessment of individual structures.

- Text utilities: it is paramount that the patient be identified adequately, including identification details, date and area imaged. It is often necessary to compare the evolution of lesions over a long time, which is only possible if each examination is adequately recorded with as much written detail as possible.

Image recording and storage

To keep adequate medical records and monitor the progress of individual patients, representative images should be recorded and stored. Options include:

- Thermal prints
- Video
- Polaroid films
- Radiographic films
- Digital archiving systems

Thermal prints are the most common form of record. They use a video output from the machine. Each printer must be used with adequate thermal paper and be set to obtain quality copies. These prints are fragile and easily damaged by folding, heat, ultrasound gel or water. Video recordings may be useful to record live, moving images such as those in echocardiography. A standard Video Home System (VHS) often gives poor quality images, so it may be worth investing in the better quality SuperVHS. Recently, systems have become available to save the analogue video output of the machine as computer files, which may be stored, archived and optimised on personal computers. These have become affordable but require adequate software and printing equipment, which can increase the cost significantly.

Preparation of the patient

The production of good-quality images relies on good contact between the transducer and skin so that sound is well transmitted from and to the scanner. Air, dirt and grease are poor sound conductors. Hair traps all of the above and is therefore best removed.

Shaving used to be recommended for ultrasonography but this can lead to skin inflammation and infection. Clipping is usually adequate and less time consuming and causes fewer reactions. Very fine blades (no. 40 or more) should be used. They should be kept clean with adequate lubricant/disinfectant and must be sharpened regularly.

The skin should be cleaned to remove dirt and grease. Soap or liquid detergents (washing-up liquid) are better than surgical scrubs for this purpose and tend to cause less reaction. Iodine (as in povidone scrubs) should be avoided because it can decrease sound transmission. Soaking the skin with warm water softens it and improves the image. Alcohol is often used to degrease the skin and may be useful to image through an unclipped coat because it is an excellent sound conductor. It is, however, not necessary in most cases.

Coupling gel is applied liberally to the skin and over the transducer and stand-off pad (Fig. 17.42). Thick gel is generally better. The longer the gel contact time, the better the transmission through the skin. It is therefore advisable to prepare the skin and apply gel before setting up the machine. Between 15 and 20 min should be allowed before starting the examination. If sound transmission remains poor, it may be necessary to soak the skin with wet bandages or gel for several hours.

Vets are frequently requested to scan without clipping. In fine-coated animals, this is possible if the skin and hair are cleaned well and contact gel is allowed to soak in. Contact artefacts are more common though, and the owner/trainer should be informed that subtle pathology might be missed.

After the procedure the area should be washed carefully to remove all gel, which may otherwise irritate the skin.

Care of the equipment

The equipment is expensive and fragile. The scanner is a computer and should be treated as such: shocks, heat and extreme cold can damage it. Transducers are also delicate: the crystals are fragile and involve complex wiring. The cables contain small wires that are easily damaged if overbent or stepped on.

The equipment must be kept clean. Portable units are designed to be sturdy and fairly resistant to water. They can be wiped with damp sponges. No machine is waterproof, however, and heavy water or urine splashes can cause permanent damage. The secret to easy cleaning is to prevent soiling by protecting the machine, e.g. keeping it off the floor. Stand-offs are best soaked and cleaned with warm (not hot) water, avoiding soap. Dry gel can be difficult to remove and can damage the equipment, so it should be removed immediately after use. All gels are water-soluble. Most transducers are watertight but the cable/probe seal often becomes damaged with use, so it is best to clean the probes with a damp cloth rather than dipping them in water.

Emerging imaging techniques

Although the above techniques are used widely in horses, other imaging modalities have been available to human hospitals and some of these are used occasionally for horses. Apart from thermography, other techniques involve major investment and maintenance costs and currently are found only in a few university hospitals around the world.

Thermography

There is a great deal of controversy relating to thermography. This technique is based on the measurement of the surface temperature of the skin using infrared light analysis. Highly sensitive infrared thermography cameras have replaced impractical temperature probes. Inflammation always is associated with an increased blood flow and local increases of temperature. Thermography therefore is useful to detect inflammation. Unfortunately, there are many limitations to the technique. Skin temperature can vary tremendously, depending on the outside temperature and humidity, muscle activity, hair cover, etc. Interpretation therefore can vary. Thermography is a useful adjunct to other techniques but should not be used as a sole diagnostic or even localising technique.

Computed tomography

Computed tomography (CT) is a modified radiography technique used to obtain cross-sectional images. Basically, an X-ray tube rotates 180° around the subject. Special digital recording devices record the X-ray patterns at a number of set positions. Computer technology then combines all the images to recreate a precise cross-section of the body. This procedure is repeated gradually along the subject so that a series of cross-sections are obtained. Special software also may be used to create three-dimensional images. Computed tomography systems have been available to hospitals for over 20 years and may be purchased second-hand at an affordable cost. However, the cost of maintenance is very high and specially trained staff are required to operate and maintain the units.

The advantages of CT are numerous: the spatial representation of organs is very precise, unlike in radiographs where the organs are compressed on the film. Composite shadows are avoided and subtle lesions are less likely to be masked by higher density objects. In horses, the main applications include complex limb fractures and head lesions.

There are many disadvantages of the technique, however, in equine medicine. The tube head and recorders are placed in a ring-shaped construction, through which a human can be placed but only the limbs, head and neck of a horse may fit. General anaesthesia and recumbency are necessary in horses, further increasing the cost of the procedure. The design of the premises also involves major costs, because a special automated table must be designed to advance the relevant part of the animal through the ring during exposure. The radiation involved in CT is much greater than for radiography so the room must be heavily shielded and no personnel allowed in the room during exposure.

Computed tomography is a form of radiography, so the limitations of X-rays for imaging also are encountered. In particular, the resolution of the images for soft tissues is very poor and only obvious lesions are visible. Contrast studies usually are carried out to improve imaging, but this is associated with health risks for the patient.

Magnetic resonance imaging

Magnetic resonance imaging (MRI) has become state of the art in human medicine and is gaining popularity in veterinary medicine. The principles are complex. It uses very powerful magnetic fields around the subject, created by a special set of coil magnets. In such fields, the nuclei of atoms respond to stimulation with radiowaves by producing radiofrequency energy in return, which is analysed by a computer to form images. It is a very accurate and powerful tool: sections in any plane may be obtained and the tissue resolution is much greater than any of the previous techniques, providing very high detail and contrast.

The main disadvantages of MRI currently include extremely high purchase and running costs, both for the equipment and for a magnetically shielded room. The magnets currently available also are very impractical for use in horses, so that only the limbs and head may be easily imaged. The animals must be anaesthetised. Metal such as shoes and nails cannot be placed near strong magnetic fields. However, more practical and even portable systems are currently being developed and it is hoped that MRI technology will become increasingly available to equine hospitals in future.

Further reading

Butler, J.A., Colles, C.M., Dyson, S.J., Kold, S.E. & Poulos, P.W. (2000) *Clinical Radiology of the Horse*, 2nd edn. Blackwell Science, Oxford.

Morgan, J.P., Neves, J. & Baker, T. (1991) *Equine Radiography*. Iowa State University Press, Ames, IA.

Steckel, R.R. (1991) Advanced diagnostic methods. *Vete. Clini. North Am. — Equine Pract.* **7**(2), 1.

CHAPTER 18

General Surgical Nursing

D. Lloyd & B. M. Millar

Tissue injury

Inflammation

Inflammation is the immediate response of tissues to an injury that causes cellular death or disruption. Causes of injury and local inflammation are:

- Mechanical, e.g. abrasion, erosion, contusion, laceration and puncture
- Thermal, e.g. heat, cold, electrical
- Chemical/contact, e.g. acid, alkali, cytotoxic
- Radiation, e.g. radiotherapy.

The signs of inflammation include:

(1) *Heat*. Increased blood flow and cellular metabolism result in a rise in the local temperature of the skin.
(2) *Colour change*. Dilation of blood capillaries can cause redness and damaged capillaries may leak blood into the tissues, causing bruising.
(3) *Swelling*. This is a result of increased tissue fluid (oedema) during the acute phase. During the chronic phase of inflammation, soft-tissue proliferation also may cause fibrous swelling.
(4) *Pain*. Pain is often worse during the acute phase due to nerve tissue damage or increased stimulation of sensory nerve fibres in the inflamed tissues. Different tissues have varying sensory innervations and therefore the pain response to injury can be variable, e.g. a laceration to the muscle may be less painful than if a horse injures a tendon or ligament.
(5) *Discharge*. This may be overproduction of a normal secretion, such as increased tear production in painful eye conditions, or an abnormal secretion, such as serum through the intact skin of a very swollen limb or from a wound. The type and quantity of discharge should be noted because it may give clues to the severity of the inflammation or injury.

Inflammation is a normal process that is essential to allow the tissues to repair. It delivers cells to remove infection and fluid to dilute chemical toxins. Pain prevents overuse of the area until repair has started. As the repairs take place, the increased blood supply provides oxygen and nutrients for this to take place.

Acute inflammation

This is the initial response to an injury. The severity of the acute inflammatory response is related to the severity of the injury. Its characteristics include:

- Oedema
- Heat
- Pain.

For example, a skin wound to the dorsal aspect of the carpus caused by a kick from another horse: the horse is usually lame and there is swelling of the carpus as well as below the wound; there may be heat and a discharge from the site (see Chapter 7 for assessment of injuries).

Chronic inflammation

The acute inflammatory response subsides as the tissues begin to heal. There is less pain and the quantity of discharge will be less because the wound and underlying tissues are healing. Again, taking the horse with a kick to the dorsal carpus as the example, swelling and lameness improve as the wound heals and there is still some heat in the region of the wound.

Treatment of inflammation

Although inflammation is a natural process it is important to control it, particularly the release of inflammatory mediators, and hence help pain control to optimise healing:

(1) Eliminate the cause: it is important to prevent any further injury before repair begins to take place, e.g. by properly cleansing a wound to remove debris.
(2) Anti-inflammatory medication is used extensively to control the excessive effects of inflammation, e.g. tissue destruction. The most potent are steroids but these can have detrimental effects on the rate of tissue healing and the ability to fight off infection, so their use is restricted. Non-steroidal anti-inflammatory drugs (NSAIDs) are commonly used and include:
   (a) Phenylbutazone ('bute')
   (b) Flunixin
   (c) Ketoprofen
   (d) Vedoprofen
   (e) Carprofen
   (f) Meclofenamic acid
   (g) Acetylsalicylic acid
   (h) Ramifenazone
   (i) Eltenac
(3) Painkillers: another useful effect of most NSAIDs is their analgesic properties, although other medicines (e.g. opiates such as butorphanol) are useful.
(4) Hot/cold therapy: in the acute stages cold therapy should be used to reduce swelling. Cold hosing or bandaging cold packs or ice against the inflamed area decreases the skin temperature for several hours. This sort of regime is used frequently to limit the damaging effects of inflammation when a horse sustains a flexor tendon injury.
(5) Immobilisation of the inflamed area will help, particularly with limb injuries.

Wound healing

Wound healing is a series of biological events that result in repair of tissue damage. Apart from bone, the repair tissue is not the same as the original tissue that was damaged. It can be divided into four phases:

(1) *Inflammatory*: the body's initial response to injury, including haemorrhage.
(2) *Debridement*: the influx of the body's natural defence cells such as neutrophils and monocytes to begin the clean-up process. Proper cleansing of the wound helps this. Repair will be improved if the wound is moist and clean with a good blood supply, especially at the wound edges.
(3) *Repair*: this is the epithelialisation stage when the wound contracts and the tissues start to regrow. When the wound is under tension, wound contracture is less and the final scar is liable to be wider. Most wounds heal by granulation tissue being deposited. This has a rich blood supply and provides a surface for epithelial cells to migrate over.
(4) *Maturation* occurs as the granulation tissue matures into scar tissue.

In reality these processes overlap.

Exuberant granulation tissue (EGT)

This is a well-recognised complication of wound healing in the horse, commonly known as 'proud-flesh'. When the granulation tissue is 'proud', i.e. mushrooms out over the edges of a wound, it delays healing and exacerbates scar formation. Once this happens it needs to be removed to allow proper wound repair. This can be done in several ways:

• Applying steroid–antibiotic topical cream and pressure bandaging.

- Surgical resection of excessive granulation tissue, which is simple and effective. Granulation tissue has no nerve supply so no anaesthesia is required. It will bleed profusely, so always start at the bottom and then bandage afterwards.
- Cryosurgery or laser surgery is sometimes used.
- Casting or a supportive bandage helps by immobilising the area.
- Skin grafting may be needed.
- Chemical cautery, e.g. with copper sulphate, is traditionally used but is not recommended because it damages the surrounding healing tissues as well as the EGT.

Exuberant granulation tissue is most common in distal limb wounds, particularly in larger horses rather than ponies. It can be minimised by:

- Good suturing of the wound where possible
- Providing good ventral drainage
- Proper immobilisation
- Controlling infection.

Wound evaluation

Many equine wounds are a result of trauma and contain foreign debris. These are called *contaminated* wounds. *Dirty* wounds are those that are already infected, e.g. with pus or faecal contamination. This includes traumatic wounds more than 5 or 6 h old or containing foreign material. *Clean* wounds are those produced under aseptic conditions with minimal trauma to tissues and not entering respiratory, alimentary, genitourinary tracts or oropharynx. A *clean–contaminated* wound is a surgical wound made under aseptic conditions but entering the respiratory, alimentary or genitourinary tracts or oropharynx.

Clean and clean–contaminated wounds are the easiest to manage. It should be possible to suture these closed provided that they are not under excessive tension. Contaminated wounds can be closed similarly if converted to clean–contaminated wounds with surgical cleaning and debridement. *Dirty infected wounds should never be sutured.*

Practical considerations also include:

- The size of the wound
- The time since the initial injury
- The overall condition of the horse
- The cause of the injury, e.g. if it is a stake wound, the possibility of a foreign body within the wound
- The animal's temperament, which may prevent proper wound repair without heavy sedation or even general anaesthesia
- Available facilities
- Type of horse, e.g. proper cosmetic wound repair may be crucial in a show animal
- Financial constraints.

The immediate management of wounds is covered with first aid (Chapter 7).

Methods of wound closure

(1) *Primary closure*: this is the method of choice used for clean wounds, where they are cleaned, debrided and lavaged immediately. The wound edges are mechanically apposed with staples or sutures. The wound then heals without infection or breakdown. This is known as *first intention healing*. This works well with wounds of the head, neck and body or skin flaps with a good blood supply.

(2) *Delayed primary closure*: where the wound is not closed immediately, but is initially cleaned, debrided and dressed to allow infection to be controlled and swelling to be reduced. Antibiotic and anti-inflammatory treatment will help. The wound edges are then apposed with sutures or staples after further debridement and lavage. It is important that this is performed before granulation tissue forms. This works for severely contaminated wounds.

(3) *Secondary closure*: when wounds are allowed to granulate initially and then are closed surgically after a healthy bed of granulation tissue has formed.

(4) *Second intention healing*: when wounds are not closed surgically but are left to heal by wound contracture and granulation tissue formation. This can work well for large wounds over moveable areas, e.g. the pectorals and gluteals in the horse.

Drainage tubes

These are frequently useful in the horse, particularly when there is a large dead space, i.e. gap in the wound. They provide a route for discharge to drain from an infected area of tissue. A drain should be sutured proximally, traverse the wound and exit through a small incision separate to the wound itself.

Drains used include:

(1) Penrose drains, which are commonly used in horses. They are made of soft flexible rubber and are good for skin wounds. When a wound is cleaned daily the drain should be moved slightly to break any seal between the drain, exudates and the surrounding skin.
(2) Tube drains also are fairly commonly used in horses, although they are more bulky and less flexible. They are most commonly used to drain cavities such as the abdominal or thoracic cavity, with use of valves, bungs or clamps as necessary.
(3) Sump, Penrose sump, closed suction and vacuum suction drains are other options used occasionally in horses.

Drains usually are left in place for 24–48 h but may remain for longer if drainage persists.

Skin grafts

A skin graft is the detachment and relocation of a portion of skin from one site to another, which is used sometimes to reduce a skin deficit in large equine wounds. There are a variety of different techniques used, e.g. pinch grafts, punch grafts and tunnel grafts. The cosmetic result is often disappointing. Although worth considering as an option, many wounds will heal, if given time and good management without resorting to such techniques.

Wound healing can be adversely affected by:

- Anaemia
- Blood loss
- Blood supply and oxygen tension
- Continuing trauma, e.g. self-mutilation by the patient

- Excessive tension on the wound
- Foreign body within a wound
- Haematomas/seromas/synovial fluid
- Hypoproteinaemia
- Infection, including abscesses
- Malnutrition
- Medication, e.g. steroids may slow healing and NSAIDs may help
- Movement, e.g. if edges of a wound are over a high motion joint then healing will be slowed
- Temperature and pH.

Any collection of blood or serum pooling within the tissues will delay healing by mechanically separating the tissue layers. An accumulation of serum is known as a *seroma* and an accumulation of blood is known as a *haematoma*. Blood and serum provide an excellent medium for bacterial growth. An *abscess* is defined as an accumulation of pus surrounded by inflamed or damaged tissue. It is said that the only difference between a seroma and an abscess is a needle, by which it is meant that an attempt to drain a seroma should be avoided. The majority of seromas will resolve on their own, whereas an actual abscess should be lanced if possible to drain the infection. An abscess will be hot, inflamed and painful in comparison to a haematoma or seroma.

A *sinus* is a blind-ended tract or drainage channel and may be the way in which an abscess will discharge. A sinus tract may involve a foreign body and surgical exploration may be required. A *fistula* is an abnormal epithelial-lined tract, e.g. a rectovaginal fistula links the rectum and vagina following trauma at foaling.

For details on obstetrics, see Chapter 4.

Nursing of the colic patient

What is colic?

The term colic refers to abdominal pain and is commonly associated with the alimentary tract. Occasionally thoracic pathology, e.g. pleuritis, or other abdominal problems, e.g. liver disease, which may present like colic (see Chapters 7 and 14, especially Table 14.4)

Medical or surgical

Colic cases are classically categorised as:

(1) Surgical.
(2) Medical.

The most important factor with any case of colic is regular re-evaluation of pertinent clinical signs. There is no single clinical sign that immediately indicates that the horse necessarily requires surgical treatment. Important nursing points to monitor are:

- Cardiovascular signs (heart rate, mucous membrane colour, mucous membrane capillary refill time and hydration state)
- Respiratory rate and depth
- Rectal temperature
- Abdominal auscultation for gut sounds (borborygmi)
- Abdominal distension
- Pain and response to medication
- Appetite, thirst, whether urine and faeces passed.

Additional information can be gathered by the clinician from rectal examination, nasogastric intubation, abdominocentesis (peritoneal tap) and transabdominal ultrasonography.

In 6–10% of cases surgical intervention is required. Such cases may present as sudden-onset severe pain,

frequently with a high pulse (>80 bpm). Others may show mild signs initially, before gradually deteriorating. Surgical conditions often require an exploratory laparotomy before they can be diagnosed and specific terms are used to describe these conditions (see Table 18.1).

Preparation of a colic case for surgery

It is important to prepare a horse for exploratory laparotomy as quickly as possible once a decision has been made to proceed. Important nursing tasks include:

- The horse should be weighed or the weight estimated.
- An intravenous catheter is placed using sterile techniques in either the left or right jugular vein.
- Assessment of cardiovascular function may indicate the horse to be severely dehydrated, so preoperative fluid therapy may be needed, frequently using hypertonic saline (see Chapter 13).
- While the horse is sedated a stomach tube should be passed and left in place after attempts are made to decompress fluid or gas from the stomach. The tube should be left in place during the anaesthetic.
- If time permits or the animal is quiet, then the ventral abdomen can be clipped to decrease the

Table 18.1 Types of colic that may require surgical intervention

Displacements	Non-strangulating	Strangulating/obstructing
	Impactions Infarctions	Intussusception (telescoping of bowel, which can produce a complete or partial obstruction) Volvulus Torsion Incarceration
Left dorsal displacement of the large colon (nephrosplenic entrapment)	Pelvic flexure impaction (more often medical) although other impactions, e.g. ileal impaction, are more likely to need surgery	Pedunculated lipoma (benign fatty tumour) that grows on a stalk within the abdomen and commonly causes small intestinal strangulation or obstruction, especially in older ponies
Right dorsal displacement of the large colon	Caecal impaction (some cases fail to respond to medical treatment.)	Colon torsion

amount of time needed to prepare the horse for abdominal surgery once it has been anaesthetised.

- The shoes should be removed to prevent damage to the horse or theatre facility.

Surgical procedures for colic

Colic surgery can involve replacing or correcting the position of the bowel, removing the cause of any obstruction, e.g. freeing entrapped small intestine or clearing impacted large-colon contents, known as 'dumping the colon'. On other occasions extensive surgery needs to be performed and pieces of small intestine or large intestine have to be resected (removed surgically) and/or an anastomosis (surgical joining together) performed. Bowel anastomosis can be performed either end-to-end (where two ends are joined in a straight line) or side-to-side (the ends of the bowel are closed and then a separate opening is made). In order to speed up intestinal surgery, intestinal stapling devices sometimes are used instead of sutures. Stapling is faster but more expensive. Large quantities of fluids are required for lavage of the abdomen and lavage of the surgical site once the anastomosis has been completed. Surgery can be challenging (Table 18.2) and large quantities of swabs and instruments are used. A swab count and instrument check are essential to make sure none

Table 18.2 Surgical categories

Category of surgery	Types of surgical condition
Clean	Displacement such as left dorsal displacement of the large colon and right dorsal displacement of the large colon, early, simple strangulating obstructions or early strangulating lipomas, all of which are operated on early with little or no vascular compromise to bowel affected
Clean–contaminated	Intestinal biopsies (small incisions into the bowel under a controlled technique)
Contaminated	Pelvic flexure enterotomy, small intestinal resection, jejunocaecostomy and caecal resection
Heavily contaminated	Most other types of large colon surgery and surgery requiring opening of the stomach

are left behind! If surgery is performed early and rapidly after initial colic signs are seen, the chances of a successful outcome are higher.

Post-operative care of the colic patient

Following recovery from anaesthesia the horse requires intensive medical therapy and very close regular monitoring in order to detect complications as soon as they arise. The level of intensive care will depend on the surgical category involved (see Table 18.2). Any case may have complications and all require a dedicated team of vets and nurses working anti-social hours to care for them properly. Optimal post-operative management of the equine abdominal patient is as important to the horse's survival as the surgery itself.

Nursing role in post-operative management of colic patients

Horses with complications or that are particularly ill demand a great deal of nursing care.

Critical care monitoring—a 24-h commitment

Record sheets (see Chapter 8) are essential in systematically recording the physical and laboratory data collected at each examination. The following parameters are valuable for assessing subtle changes in the patient's condition:

- Heart rate, rhythm and pulse quality
- Mucous membrane colour, condition (i.e. tacky, dry) and capillary refill time
- Respiration rate and character
- Packed cell volume
- Circulating white blood cell count
- Rectal temperature
- Evidence of pain
- Appearance of the wound, with or without discharge
- Defaecation, amount and consistency
- Urination: note volume and colour
- Gut sounds
- Nasogastric intubation, with or without reflux
- Abdominal distension
- General demeanour

- Rectal examination
- Ability to move
- Heat and digital pulses in feet.

All drug treatments must be recorded, including the amounts of fluids being administered. The frequency of the checks is dictated by the clinician and can be required hourly in the initial stages of recovery. Foals are especially prone to rapid changes in the above parameters. Normally the horse just recovering from colic surgery would benefit from critical care checks every 2–3 h until its condition stabilises and improves. When its parameters stay within normal limits, the checks could be reduced to every 6 h.

Intravenous catheter care

This is of utmost importance in enabling efficient fluid therapy, drug administration and intravenous access in an emergency. Colic patients that are suffering from endotoxaemia will be more susceptible to thrombophlebitis (inflammation of a vein associated with a thrombus), therefore meticulous care of intravenous catheters is essential. Daily monitoring of catheters includes:

- Vein patency
- Adverse signs (i.e. heat, pain, swelling or exudate at insertion site)
- Catheter patency, heparinise every 6 h
- Check for leaks, clots, missing stay sutures, damage to catheter
- Change giving sets and extension sets if damaged or contaminated
- Wipe injection caps with surgical spirit prior to injecting with drug
- Change injection cap daily.

If any adverse signs are present, remove the catheter immediately.

Note: if the jugular vein shows signs of thrombophlebitis it must no longer be used. Lateral thoracic, cephalic or saphenous veins are the next choice for catheter placement so as to preserve the one remaining patent jugular vein.

Fluid therapy

Because many post-operative colic patients need to have limited oral fluid intake, the daily fluid require-

ment must come from intravenous fluid administration (see Chapter 13):

- Administration of fluids must be documented
- Monitoring during fluid therapy is a 24-h commitment
- Daily serum electrolyte tests may indicate the need for supplementation
- Adjustments in fluid rates should coincide with the patient's progress and haematology findings.

Medication

Medication is essential in preventing and treating post-operative complications uniquely associated with the critically ill colic patient. It is usually started before surgery commences:

(1) Non-steroidal anti-inflammatory drugs (NSAIDs):
   (a) Small doses reduce the effects of endotoxaemia.
   (b) Provide analgesia.
   (c) Reduce inflammation.
   (d) Prevent the depressive effect of endotoxins on gut motility.
   (e) Flunixin meglumine and phenylbutazone are most commonly used.
   (f) Can cause a precipitate in fluid lines.
(2) Antibiotic therapy:
   (a) Prevents and treats infection.
   (b) Injections of aminoglycosides and penicillins are most commonly used.
   (c) Ensures that horse's weight and dose level are calculated.
   (d) Metronidazole is used to treat suspected anaerobic infections.
(3) Other specialist treatments include plasma transfusion for the treatment of endotoxaemia and pro-kinetic agents (to stimulate gut movement) to help reduce ileus.

General nursing duties

Some simple procedures can significantly improve the patient's demeanour:

- Daily grooming
- Periodically rinse out the mouth with fresh water if the horse is being starved for any length of time

- Walk out to encourage interest in surroundings
- Use rugs, sheets and heat lamps to retain body heat
- Have a clean deep-bedded box always available

Visitors from home help to brighten the patient.

Monitor and manage complications
See next section.

Complications following colic surgery

Haemorrhage
During colic surgery, blood pressure (BP) may be considerably lower than normal. A damaged blood vessel not seen or ligated during surgery may cause bleeding on recovery as the BP rises. In most cases haemorrhage stops spontaneously.

Leakage of abdominal fluid
Large quantities of fluid are flushed into the abdomen during abdominal surgery. It is possible to see fluid dripping from the wound post-operatively. The vet should be informed, but unless associated with pain or increased heart rate it is unlikely to be serious.

Ileus
This is when the bowel fails to regain its normal propulsive movement post-operatively and can be due to several factors, including pain, handling at surgery, anastomosis, distension prior to surgery and endotoxaemia. There are often reduced or absent borborygmi. Fluid builds up within the small intestine and eventually accumulates in the stomach with spontaneous nasogastric reflux. Pro-kinetic drugs (to stimulate gut activity) such as metoclopramide or erythromycin may be prescribed. A stomach tube should be passed regularly to check for gastric distension. Occasionally repeat surgery may be required, and sometimes normal gut function never resumes.

Peritonitis
This is a possible complication of all surgeries but is much more common in contaminated and heavily contaminated surgeries.

Endotoxaemia
Large quantities of endotoxin often can be absorbed through strangulated intestine. This is responsible for increases in heart rate together with haemoconcentration and potentially fatal shock. *Laminitis* is a further complication associated with this.

Phlebitis
Long-term intravenous catheterisation, especially in sick horses, increases the risk of damage to the vein used (see Fig. 13.8).

Colitis
Several factors, including antibiotic treatment, changes associated with the 'stress' of abdominal surgery and specific conditions such as large-bowel displacements or large-colon torsion, may cause severe diarrhoea.

Incisional complications (dehiscence and herniation)
A plaque of ventral oedema is commonly seen along the abdominal incision line 48 h post-operatively and this can be substantial in some horses. Heat or discharge from the abdominal incision should be monitored closely, cleaned appropriately with antibacterial cleansing agents, e.g. povidone-iodine scrub, the wound packed with a wound gel. If a purulent discharge is present or there is heat over the wound, then a swab may be submitted for bacterial culture and sensitivity. A belly bandage may be used to support the wound. Ultrasonography is useful to diagnose bowel herniation through the abdominal incision.

Longer term management

Colic patients are usually discharged between 7 and 14 days post-operatively. Owners should be advised to continue a laxative diet (see Chapter 6). Skin staples or sutures are removed by a veterinary surgeon at approximately 14 days. The abdominal incision requires a long time to heal, so horses should be rested from ridden exercise for several months, with initially approximately 1–2 months of box rest and in-hand exercise before turning out into a small restricted paddock. In time, many colic patients will return to full competitive work.

Hernias

A hernia describes a defect in a structure through which an organ or part of an organ can pass and potentially become trapped. Hernias are described as either *internal* or *external*. *Internal* hernias occur within the abdominal cavity and *external* hernias result in internal organs extending beyond the abdominal cavity. Hernias can be described as *reducible* or *nonreducible*, depending on whether the contents within the hernias can be repelled by palpation. If the bowel becomes strangulated or *incarcerated* animals usually show severe colic signs.

Internal hernias

Internal hernias include epiploic foramen herniation, gastrosplenic incarceration and mesenteric rents. There are several well-recognised conditions where intestine or other abdominal organs, such as the spleen or liver, may pass in and out of the hernias in the mesentery or supporting ligaments without clinical signs, but if bowel becomes incarcerated then abdominal surgery should be performed as quickly as possible.

External hernias

Hernias that extended beyond the abdominal space may be enclosed within a sac or out-pouch of the peritoneal lining. If this has torn and the herniated bowel is free in the subcutaneous tissue, it is termed a *ruptured* hernia; this should not be confused with the intestine itself rupturing.

1. Inguinal (scrotal) hernia
This can occur as a *congenital* hernia and most resolve spontaneously as the foal grows. They are often reducible but large hernias may need to be repaired surgically. *Acquired* inguinal hernias occur in stallions and may become incarcerated, requiring emergency surgery. They often require castration at the same time due to irreparable tissue damage.

2. Umbilical hernia
This is most commonly seen in young horses. Spontaneous resolution is common, otherwise rubber rings (used for docking a lamb's tail) can be placed carefully on smaller hernias. Larger umbilical hernias need to be repaired under general anaesthesia.

3. Ventral abdominal hernia
This may occur spontaneously but is usually secondary to previous abdominal surgery (*incisional hernia*).

4. Diaphragmatic hernia
Congenital diaphragmatic hernias occur in foals and they present with breathing difficulties and possibly colic signs. *Acquired* diaphragmatic hernia may result from trauma and also is seen in post-parturient mares following abdominal straining. Midline laparotomy may replace the bowel but repair of the diaphragm is difficult in many cases. Occasionally a thoracotomy may be used to repair the diaphragm in foals.

Ruptures

Although rupture can be used to describe failure in continuity of any structure (e.g. ruptured eyeball, ruptured haematoma, ruptured bowel), it is also used to describe the failure of supporting tendons and ligaments, e.g.:

- Rupture of the pre-pubic tendon (see Chapter 4)
- Rupture of the superficial/deep digital flexor tendon or suspensory ligament (see Chapter 16)
- Rupture of the peroneus tertius muscle (see Chapter 16).

Urogenital system

Conditions involving the urinary tract system have many presentations but owners may notice a change in the colour or volume of the urine, in urinary frequency or a change in the behaviour of their horse while urinating. *If a foal or horse fails to urinate over a prolonged period then the cause of the problem should be investigated immediately.*

Conditions affecting the foal

Ruptured bladder

Most common in colts, a tear in the dorsal part of the bladder occurs either at foaling or soon afterwards and urine leaks into the peritoneal space (*uroperitoneum*). Foals can produce a normal stream of urine, or more commonly no urination may be seen. The foal becomes progressively more *depressed* and the abdomen more distended. Transabdominal ultrasonography demonstrates free fluid within the peritoneal space and a small bladder. The peritoneum absorbs nitrogenous waste products and *potassium* from the urine, causing depression, uraemia, electrolyte disturbances and cardiovascular aberrations. The foal must be stabilised before general anaesthesia is performed. Urine can be drained from the abdomen by abdominocentesis, and a dog urinary catheter is sutured in place to promote drainage from the bladder. Normal saline should be substituted for Hartmann's solution if blood potassium levels are elevated. The bladder is repaired through a midline incision and the urinary catheter left in place for 48 h to allow the bladder to heal. Normal urination should resume soon after the catheter is removed and ultrasonography can confirm a normal bladder.

Patent urachus

The urachus is a tube connected from the bladder through the umbilical cord to the allantoic sac, where urine is excreted from the fetus. Normally at the time of foaling the urachus closes and degenerates. As a result of excessive traction on the cord at the time of foaling, or as a result of infection (see Omphalophlebitis below), the urachus remains patent and urine leaks from the bladder out through the umbilicus. This may be constant or seen when the foal strains for defaecation or urination. In many cases, early treatment is with a cauterising compound such as strong iodine solution (*Lugol's iodine*) or *silver nitrate*. Resection of the urachus and cranial pole of the bladder is performed through a midline incision under general anaesthesia and the bladder is repaired. Post-operative care includes observation for normal urination.

Omphalophlebitis (navel-ill)

Infection of the umbilical remnants may be seen separately or in conjunction with patent urachus. There is swelling and thickening of the umbilicus and the foal usually is pyrexic. Purulent material may be expressed from the umbilicus. *Septicaemia* and *septic arthritis* (joint-ill) are serious complications. Transabdominal ultrasonography of the umbilical region confirms abscessation and can indicate the degree of involvement of the umbilical arteries and vein. Surgical resection of the infected portion is performed under general anaesthesia, broad-spectrum antibiotics are given for extended periods, and in cases of septic arthritis the joints are treated accordingly. Foals are closely monitored post-operatively for joint swelling, lameness and pyrexia.

Ectopic ureter

This is a rare congenital condition where the ureter inserts into the urethra rather than the bladder. There is persistent dribbling of urine from the vulva or penis. Diagnosis is confirmed with positive contrast urography under heavy sedation or general anaethesia. For unilateral cases *nephrectomy* (kidney removal) can be performed through a rib resection.

Conditions affecting adults

There are many medical and surgical conditions that affect the urinary system in adults, with alterations in urinary characteristics being an important clinical feature.

Urolithiasis

This uncommon condition results in the build-up of calculi (mineral salts, usually calcium carbonate) within the kidney, ureter or most commonly the bladder. Horses show signs of dysuria, incontinence and haematuria. Diagnosis can be confirmed by rectal palpation, rectal ultrasonography and endoscopy of the bladder. In mares, the calculi may be removed manually through the urethral sphincter. In stallions or geldings a midline laparotomy and cystotomy is required, unless lithotripsy equipment is available (which uses electrical current to break down the calculi into pieces small enough to be removed).

Pyelonephritis

This is an uncommon chronic infection of one or both kidneys, characterised by multiple abscess formation. If unilateral and long-term antibiotic treatment fails, then nephrectomy can be performed.

Castration (gelding or cutting a colt)

This is probably the commonest surgery performed in the horse. It is a routine procedure performed to turn stallions into manageable geldings by eliminating masculine behaviour, although this is not always successful. It is usually done in horses between 1 and 2 years of age, but can be done at any age.

Before the procedure is performed, the horse should be examined to ensure that both testicles have descended into the scrotum and there is no hernia. If there are any abnormalities, the surgical approach may be changed. Options include:

(1) Castration performed on the standing horse under sedation and local anaesthesia.
(2) Castration under general anaesthesia.

The surgical technique may vary:

- Closed technique: each testis is located and removed, still encased in its tunic.
- Open technique: here the tunic is opened before each testis is removed. This is simpler to perform and often is used for the standing castration.
- Semi-closed: here, each testis is isolated in its parietal tunic but is exteriorised before removal.

The scrotal skin often is left unsutured to allow drainage, and the terms 'closed' or 'open' do not relate to the skin wounds but to the underlying tissues surrounding the testis itself. Even though castration is a commonly performed procedure, there are many potential complications, including:

- Haemorrhage
- Post-operative oedema
- Prolapse of bowel; more likely with an open castration

- Infection, either locally or peritonitis
- Damage to the penis during surgery

Nursing care after surgery includes:

- Ensuring that tetanus prophylaxis is performed (as with any surgery)
- Ensuring wound hygiene by cleaning and hosing to reduce swelling
- Encourage exercise after 24 h to reduce swelling
- Ensuring that antibiotic, analgesic and fly control are adequate

Ovariectomy

Unlike small animal surgery, ovariohysterectomy is virtually never performed in the mare. Unilateral ovariectomy is performed for tumour removal and very occasionally a bilateral ovariectomy is done because of congenital defects or behavioural problems. A hysterectomy is technically very difficult but is reported, e.g. for treatment of pyometra (pus in the uterus).

Fracture fixation

Fractures in horses range from tiny chip fractures to catastrophic injuries of long bones, vertebrae or the pelvis (see Chapters 7 and 16).

Fracture classification

Fractures can be classified in various ways, including:

- Anatomical position of fracture line: e.g. transverse, longitudinal, oblique, comminuted (several fragments).
- Degree of displacement of fragments: such as overriding, distracted or compressed, as with vertebral fractures.
- Complete or incomplete: i.e. whether the whole bone is broken.
- Open or closed: a compound or open fracture is one where there is an open wound exposing the fracture site.
- Complicated: involving damage to other organs or systems, such as a rib fracture penetrating the thorax.

- Pathological: caused by underlying disease, such as a tumour.

Fracture healing

This occurs in three separate stages:

(1) *Inflammatory phase*: injury to the bone causes haemorrhage and an organising clot forms, similar to that described for wound healing.
(2) *Repair phase*: this is variable and dependent on stability at the fracture site; more stable fractures heal quicker with less callus formation, and a bony column is reformed.
(3) *Remodelling phase*: the bone changes shape in response to the forces exerted upon it and differentiates further into the original anatomical structure preceding the fracture.

This is healing by *callus* formation, the callus being the repair tissue formed, made up of fibrous tissue, cartilage and immature woven bone. Sometimes *primary bone healing* can occur, when the fracture ends can be fixed rigidly so that direct bone healing results.

Complications of fracture repair

- Infection, especially if an open wound is present.
- Fracture disease, where, as a result of disuse of the limb, problems such as muscle atrophy and joint stiffness occur.
- The fracture fails to heal, producing a delayed union (practically longer than 4 months for adults and 3 months for foals). This may involve several factors but instability, infection and poor blood supply are the most critical. If fracture healing stops altogether, then a non-union has occurred.
- Growth disturbance, seen in foals.

Many factors must be considered before a fracture is repaired:

- Type and location of the fracture
- Presence of a compound fracture
- Other injuries, i.e. soft-tissue injuries, joint injuries
- Age, breed and weight of the individual
- A good candidate, temperament-wise

- Costs involved
- Time since injury
- Long-term prognosis.

Surgical techniques for fracture repair

Although great advances have been made, there are unfortunately limitations on the type of injuries that are suitable for successful surgical repair (see Chapter 16).

Arthroscopy
Arthroscopy has been a useful innovation to enable effective removal of small chip fractures, particularly from the carpus and fetlock, plus accurate reduction of major displaced articular fractures, e.g. third carpal slab fractures. Arthroscopy also often enables a rapid return to work.

Internal fixation
Internal fixation helps to provide the most stable fixation to allow the bone to repair with little callus formation, although in other cases, e.g. splint bone injuries, the fracture will heal adequately with either external support or even box rest.

All equine internal fixation should follow the principles of the Association for the Study of Internal Fixation (ASIF). Using internal implants and a combination of screws, plates, wires and pins, rigid fixation of a fracture can be achieved.

The most common bone screw used is the cortical bone screw, which requires a pre-drilled hole and the cortical bone to be tapped prior to the screw being placed. Bone screws usually are applied in one of three ways:

(1) *Lag screws* are placed across the fracture line and are applied to provide interfragmentary compression. The screws are placed as perpendicular to the fracture line as possible. The hole in the bone closest to the screw head is drilled as a glide hole (larger than the screw) so that the pressure is applied between the screw head and the bone gripped by the screw on the opposite side of the fracture.
(2) *A neutral screw* is where no compression is applied, commonly used in plating a long

bone; it grips as much bone as possible to provide pressure on the plate or wire under the screw head.

(3) *Loaded screw*: using a loaded drill guide, an eccentric hole can be positioned through the plate so that when the screw head is tightened onto the plate, an interfragmentary compression is produced.

Narrow, wide and low-contact dynamic compression plates

These are the most commonly used plates and are sized by the number of holes. They are easy to contour to the shape of the bone using plate benders. The low-contact dynamic compression plate is made from titanium and requires titanium screws. These are very expensive.

Other options include:

- Cobra-head plates, designed to give more rigid support to the metaphysis. They can be modified for use on the radius and humerus.
- Steinmann pins are most commonly used for transfixation casts and occasionally for long-bone fractures in foals.
- Interlocking nails are a more recent development, which can be used for some long-bone fractures in adult horses.

External skeletal fixators

External skeletal fixators provide a minimally invasive method to stabilise a fracture. They can be used to treat compound fractures where implants over the fracture site are contraindicated or where soft-tissue injury makes placement of a plate very difficult. Transfixation pins are placed both sides of the fracture and then fixed to one or two bars that do not contact the patient. The disadvantage is that most skeletal fixators are too weak to use in horses other than for foals, where the weight of the animal is much less and the recovery from anaesthesia can be fully assisted.

A quiet coordinated recovery from anaesthesia is essential to avoid further injury after fracture repair (see Chapter 20).

Aftercare for the surgical fracture patient

(1) Careful nursing during box rest (see Chapter 16).
(2) Appropriate medication, including analgesia and antibiotics.
(3) Monitoring for complications, which can include:
    (a) An increase in lameness or a severe lameness in the post-operative period, suggesting complications such as sepsis or implant failure.
    (b) Excess load-bearing on other limbs, leading to weight-bearing laminitis, tendon rupture, osteoarthritis and angular limb deformities in foals.
    (c) Implant failure.
    (d) Re-fracture.
    (e) Infection.
    (f) Wound breakdown.

Use of casts

External coadaptation (immobilisation) fibreglass casts are commonly used to:

- Immobilise fractures of the distal limb
- Protect damaged soft-tissue structures, i.e. deep distal limb lacerations, degloving injuries, trauma to ligaments and tendons
- Restrict movement of wounds sutured under tension because these wounds are prone to dehiscence.

Types of cast

- Foot: below coronary band (slipper cast)
- Distal limb: below fetlock
- Half-limb: below carpus/hock
- Full-limb: below proximal radius/tibia.

Further injury and fracture to other limbs may occur when using a full-limb cast and therefore its use should not be undertaken lightly. With the exception of a foot cast and occasionally in an amenable patient, the application of a half-limb and particularly a full-limb cast requires a general anaesthetic.

Materials used

Plaster of Paris is used only for foals and for occasional foot casts because it takes 24 h to obtain full strength and is very heavy. Modern synthetic cast materials are:

- Strong
- Conforming
- Quick setting
- Radiolucent
- Activated by hot water.

Vetcast plus® (3M) is the most commonly used. The roll width of the cast material used depends on the size of the animal. Generally foals require 7.5 cm, ponies 10 cm and adult horses 12.5 cm. Usually three to four rolls are used in an adult thoroughbred for a half-limb cast and seven or eight rolls used in a full-limb cast. All materials required for cast application should be available before you start because the materials harden very quickly.

Cast application

- Wounds and surgical incisions should have an appropriate dressing applied before a length of stockinette is fitted over the length of the limb to be immobilised. This should be twice as long as the cast itself so that it can double back on itself and provide two layers of protection.
- The shoe is removed and the sole pared, cleaned with an antiseptic solution and the sole packed with swabs soaked in strong povidone iodine.
- Wearing gloves, the casting material is soaked in water at 35°C and then applied from the coronary band to just above the level of the desired length of the cast. Particular attention is paid to any boney prominences, such as sesamoid bones, accessory carpal bone, lateral and medial malleoli of the distal tibia and calcaneus. An even tension is used throughout. As successive rolls are applied, more water is squeezed from the roll before its application to encourage fast curing rates so that the whole cast sets at the same time. The stockinette should be folded down to the desired level over the penultimate layer and incorporated under the final layer of cast material.

- The toe and heel of the cast can be made more durable by using a reinforcing cast material, e.g. Hexalite®, or a hoof repair product, such as Technovit®.
- A layer of Elastoplast® is wound around the top of the cast to prevent bedding and debris falling inside.

Nursing cast care

If not monitored closely, a cast can cause the horse serious discomfort and pressure sores if it rubs excessively. If ignored, serious injury can occur to the soft-tissue structures.

Daily monitoring is required at least four times a day and the horse should have strict box rest in a deep-bedded box to prevent cast wear. Rubber floors are ideal under the bedding.

The cast should be checked for:

- Cracks
- Heat
- Wear at the toe
- Blood or fluid discharge seeping through
- Evidence of rubbing at the proximal end
- Unpleasant odour.

Watch the horse to see if:

- It lies down more than usual
- It has increased signs of lameness
- It has an increased temperature

If any of the above signs occur, the veterinary surgeon will need to be informed immediately because the cast will need to be checked and possibly removed.

The most common complications of casting are:

- Pressure sores and movement rubs at the proximal end of the cast and at the heels
- Pressure sores over the bony prominences, i.e sesamoid bones
- Laxity of tendons and ligaments
- Contralateral limb laminitis
- Cast breakage or delamination

Cast removal

The removal of a cast requires an oscillating saw and preferably cast spreaders, unless embryotomy wire

Table 18.3 Robert Jones bandage

Advantages	Disadvantages
• Even support/reduced risk of pressure sores	• Expensive if changed frequently
• Can be changed regularly	• Can become contaminated/wet if copious discharge or stable dirty
• Does not require a general anaesthetic	• Heavy
• Slowly reduce the size of the bandage	• Some flexion possible
	• No significant weight-bearing support given

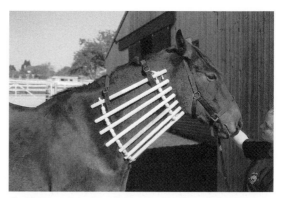

Fig. 18.1 A cradle can be used to prevent a horse from attacking a wound or bandage.

was incorporated into the cast. These saws are not intended to cut through skin, although they can do so, particularly if the horse is not well restrained, or the skin is thin or the padding limited. Cast removal needs to be done carefully. After the cast is removed it may be refitted or, more likely, a bandage applied to avoid 'rebound oedema'.

Robert Jones bandage

A *Robert Jones bandage* is a form of external fixation but it cannot provide as much support as a cast; for instance, in the adult it will not prevent the fetlock joint from sinking (see Chapter 7 for details and Table 18.3).

General rules concerning bandages

- Collect all materials first.
- Unwind a small amount of bandage at a time.
- Bandage firmly enough for it to stay on but not so tight as to impede the blood supply or damage tissues. Apply pressure evenly.
- Secure end of bandage with adhesive tape. Do not use safety pins.
- When bandaging the lower limb, go right down to the hoof to prevent the bandage slipping.
- The bandage roll always should face out when unrolling.
- Cover two-thirds of the previous turn of unrolled bandage.
- Bandages should be kept dry at all times; wet bandages constrict and must be changed.
- Horses in general need to be box-rested while bandaged.

The frequency of bandage changing will depend on the reason for the bandage. A clean dry bandage over a sterile wound can be left in place for 7–14 days. An infected discharging wound may need changing daily.

Occasionally horses will attack a wound and a bandage may prevent this. Occasionally the horse will need to be cross-tied or a cradle fitted (Fig. 18.1) to prevent bandage chewing. If the horse does chew a bandage, it is important to check that there is no specific reason for the discomfort, such as pressure necrosis or gangrene from too tight a bandage or too loose a bandage causing irritation and rubbing.

The basics of bandage application are covered elsewhere (see Chapter 7 and its further reading list).

Subluxation and luxation of joints

- *Subluxation*: partial dislocation of a joint where there is still some contact between the articular ends of the bones.
- *Luxation*: dislocation of a joint so that there is no contact between the bone ends.

Luxation or subluxation of joints is uncommon in the horse but does occur. The cause is traumatic and the force required to cause such an injury is great, so it is usually associated with open wounds.

It is most commonly seen in the fetlock, when the foot is trapped in a hole. It can also happen to the pastern, hock, carpus or rarely other joints.

A complete luxation is obvious, with heat, pain, swelling and loss of function. It may be confused with a fracture. A subluxation may be more subtle and require careful manipulation of the limb to detect.

Dental disease and surgery

In the horse the teeth grow throughout life. Long *incisor* and *molar* teeth replace deciduous teeth, which gradually grow and wear down.

A routine surgical procedure is the removal of *wolf teeth*. These appear on the maxilla just rostral to the first molar cheek teeth. They can vary in size and number; some can be palpated only below the gum margin. Traditionally horse owners consider these teeth to be sensitive and to interfere with the horse when bitted, consequently they are removed under standing sedation using a dental elevator, a Burgess wolf tooth kit and forceps.

Occasionally more serious dental problems occur, such as a fractured tooth or peri-apical abscessation caused by periodontal disease or infundibular necrosis, and removal of a tooth or teeth may be required. Tooth root abscesses in the upper (*maxillary*) arcade may cause a secondary *sinusitis* due to the proximity of the maxillary sinuses. In the rostral maxillary cheek teeth or the lower (*mandibular*) cheek teeth, an abscess causes facial swelling and if left untreated a discharging sinus (often foul smelling) will develop over the tooth.

Removal of equine cheek teeth

With specialist equipment and expertise, some cheek teeth can be removed under standing sedation and perineural anaesthesia. A *stand* or head support, *good light source*, *tooth spreaders*, an assortment of *molar extractors* and *spacers*, together with a great deal of patience, are required.

If the vet is unable to extract the diseased tooth then the tooth must be *repulsed* under general anaesthesia. A *trephine hole* is made over the tooth (radiography or fluoroscopy may be needed to locate the exact tooth root) and a dental punch is located on the tooth root before being repulsed into the mouth using a hammer. The oral cavity is checked intermit-

tently to ensure that the tooth is moving. Intraoperative radiography may be required to check that the entire tooth has been removed and *only* that tooth! After removal, the tooth socket is packed with either *dental impression wax* or *bone cement*. Once set, the packing is checked to make sure that it is securely in place. If the trephine hole is through the maxillary sinuses or into the nasal cavity, then a Foley catheter is secured in place so that the sinus can be flushed with a weak antiseptic solution on a daily basis until nasal discharge decreases.

Post-operative nursing care

The horse is fed soaked hay and wet feeds, the dental plug should be checked on a daily basis and any food trapped between the teeth should be removed and the area flushed. If the plug loosens too quickly it may need to be replaced. Dental plugs in the maxilla prevent communication with the nasal cavity or sinus; if food material impacts in the tooth socket or the plug falls out prematurely it may result in an *oronasal* fistula. This is a serious complication that causes a chronic purulent nasal discharge. The dental plug often will loosen and fall out after several weeks. Granulation tissue plugs the socket and the teeth on either side move to fill the gap. Regular dental checks are required post-operatively to control overgrowth of the opposing tooth.

Nursing for respiratory surgery

On planning for respiratory tract surgery, it is prudent to ensure that all diagnostic radiographs and videos are available for the surgeon. The respiratory tract is a contaminated epithelium and therefore many of the surgeries performed are contaminated and, although preparation and draping is carried out, the surgical incisions are seldom closed completely to promote drainage from the surgical site.

Surgery of the nares and nostrils

Occasionally surgery is performed in this region following wounds, trauma or removal of small tumours or cysts such as an atheroma.

Surgery of the sinuses

Exploratory sinus surgery of either of the maxillary sinuses or frontal sinus is a common surgical technique. A sinus trephine, hammer and chisel or oscillating saw can be used to make a window in the bones of the skull. The respiratory tract is very vascular and surgery performed in the sinuses often causes significant haemorrhage, particularly if surgery involves a tumour or cyst removal from the turbinate regions.

Lavage of the sinuses during surgery with large volumes of weak povidone-iodine solution is often helpful and a 5- or 10-l garden pump used for spraying (see Chapter 7, Fig. 7.10) can be modified easily. Sinuses may require packing, and a roll of absorbent bandage can be packed into the sinus before the skin is partially closed and the bandage left protruding from the wound to be pulled out 2–3 days postoperatively.

Another technique commonly used following surgery to the maxillary or frontal sinuses is the placement of a drainage device such as a Foley catheter either through the nostril or through a trephine hole made in the maxilla or frontal bone. Once the balloon is inflated, the Foley catheter can be secured in place by taping it to the headcollar and again a garden pump is used to flush the sinus daily.

Surgery of the pharynx/larynx

For surgical procedures such as a ventriculectomy, a midline incision is made between the mandibles and routinely the skin incision is left open to drain. A salivary/mucoid discharge often can be quite copious. Horses often are reluctant to eat immediately postoperatively. The wound should be cleaned on a daily basis and a soft paraffin barrier cream applied between the mandibles to the chin and around the operation site to prevent skin scalding from the salivary discharge. These wounds usually take approximately 2–3 weeks to begin to heal by secondary intention.

Laryngoplasty ('the tieback')

This procedure usually is done in right lateral recumbency and the area over the left cranial neck and angle of jaw is clipped and prepared for a sterile surgical technique. After making an incision close to the linguofacial vein, sterile surgical implants (usually braided nylon) are sutured in place to abduct the left arytenoid cartilage. The incision always is closed primarily and subcutaneous seroma formation is quite common. This usually can be expressed through the incision. However, the region should be cleaned copiously because any infection at this site is potentially very serious and the implants may need to be removed and therefore the surgery would be a failure. Following this surgery, horses may have problems such as dysphagia and chronic coughing and are best fed from the floor.

Surgery of the trachea

A temporary or permanent tracheostomy is performed under standing sedation and local analgesia (see Chapter 7).

Surgery of the thorax

Thoracotomy is performed rarely and specialist anaesthetic equipment or pressure ventilation is required (except in foals). Chest drains may be placed prior to closure of the chest.

Placement of surgical chest drains

The most common cause of pleural effusions requiring draining is pleuropneumonia but haemorrhage secondary to trauma and pleural exudates secondary to neoplasia are not uncommon.

Ultrasonography of the thorax will indicate the most suitable place for placement of the chest drain, although this is usually caudal to the elbow in the ventral one-third of the chest cavity.

After clipping and sterile preparation of the area, local anaesthetic is injected in the subcutaneous tissue and intercostal muscles before a stab incision is made in the skin. The chest drain is advanced through the intercostal muscles into the chest and the stilette is removed to allow drainage of the fluid. A suture should be applied to the skin and drain to prevent movement and the horse closely monitored for discomfort associated with placement of the chest drain. The cavity can be drained intermittently with suction and the drain clamped in-between periods or with a continuous one-way drainage system using a commercially available spontaneous pneumothorax aspiration set (from Cook Veterinary Products). Alternatively, to prevent retrograde flow, the collapsible end to the tube can be made from a Penrose drain, latex glove or condom, or a Heimlich valve can be used.

Surgical nursing for conditions of the guttural pouch

Guttural pouches are specifically important because major vessels such as the internal and external carotid arteries and veins and cranial nerves are all located close to the lining of the guttural pouch. Similar to sinus surgery, a mainstay of treatment for guttural pouch conditions is improving the drainage from the pouch or pouches affected. Surgical approaches are from the angle of the jaw and incisions are usually left to heal by secondary intention with routine wound management.

Guttural pouch tympany

This is a rare condition seen in young foals where the ostia act as a one-way valve, air is trapped in the guttural pouch and the foal often has difficulty breathing. This may be unilateral or bilateral and the treatment of choice is to place a Foley catheter via the nostril, through the ostia and into the guttural pouch to relieve the pressure.

Guttural pouch empyema

Similarly, a catheter can be placed into the guttural pouch in any age of horse to treat a build-up of purulent debris in the guttural pouch due to infection such as strangles. Lavage of the guttural pouch on a daily basis promotes resolution of the infection.

Guttural pouch mycosis

This can be potentially fatal in two different circumstances:

(1) A fungal growth occurs within the guttural pouch close to the internal or external carotid artery. A weakness in the arterial wall develops and occasionally ruptures, with haemorrhage filling the guttural pouch, and the horse usually presents with nosebleeds containing bright-red arterial blood. If left untreated, the haemorrhages may become more severe and a fatal haemorrhage can occur. Treatment for guttural pouch mycosis is ligation of the arteries affected. There are various techniques involving balloon catheterisation of the internal or external carotid arteries. This is commonly performed through a deep incision just ventral to the wing of the axis on the side affected and the carotid artery is isolated before a 6F or 8F Foley catheter is used to prevent blood flowing in both directions within the artery. This technique is performed under aseptic conditions and the catheter remains in place permanently.

(2) A fungal plaque develops over a wall of the guttural pouch away from the carotid arteries, causing cranial nerve damage and possibly dysphagia, preventing the animal from eating properly. A Foley catheter placed in the guttural pouch again can be used to deliver antifungal washes into the guttural pouch on a daily basis. Alternatively, a rigid catheter can be passed into the guttural pouch on a regular basis and antifungal powder insufflated into the pouch in order to treat the fungal plaque. In those cases where dysphagia occurs the nerve damage often can be permanent, and prolonged supportive care is difficult to justify.

Neoplasia

The term neoplasia, 'new growth', describes the uncontrolled proliferation of cells. In some cases the proliferation is of a specific type of cell, such as an epithelial or muscle cell. In other instances there can be proliferation of stem cells that are undifferentiated. The rate of growth of a tumour (accumulation of neoplastic cells) depends on the type of cell involved:

(1) *Benign* tumours are usually well differentiated and grow only on their site of origin. Their rate of growth can vary, as can the extent to which a tumour invades the tissue surrounding it.

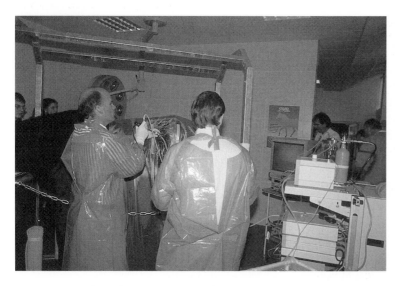

Fig. 18.2 Laparoscopy.

Table 18.4 Classification of tumours

Tissue type	Benign	Malignant
Epithelial tissue		(Carcinomas)
Skin		Squamous cell carcinoma
Glands	Adenoma	Adenocarcinoma
Mucosal lining	Adenoma	Adenocarcinoma
Connective tissue		(Sarcomas)
Bone	Osteoma	Osteosarcoma
Cartilage	Chondroma	Chondrosarcoma
Fibrous tissue	Fibroma	Fibrosarcoma
Fat	Lipoma	Liposarcoma
Smooth muscle	Leiomyoma	Leiomyosarcoma
Striated muscle	Rhabdomyoma	Rhabdomyosarcoma
Vascular tissue	Lymphangioma	Lyphangiosarcoma
White blood cells		Lymphomas (lymphosarcoma)
Plasma cell		Multiple myeloma

Example 18.1   Common equine neoplasms

- *Squamous cell carcinoma*: this may occur anywhere on the skin but it is seen more frequently along the margin of the third eyelid in horses with unpigmented skin around the eyes. It is seen also on the penis of older geldings: if it is small then the tumour can be removed easily, but as the tumour increases in size or spreads locally then the tip of the penis must be resected to prevent further spread.
- *Granulosa cell tumour*: this occurs in the ovary of older mares. Commonly there are changes in either oestrus behaviour or general behaviour. If diagnosed early, the affected ovary can be removed laparoscopically, otherwise larger granulosa cell tumours must be removed through a laparotomy incision under general anaesthesia.
- *Melanomas*
- *Lymphomas*
- *Equine sarcoids*

(1) *Malignant* tumours have the potential to spread to other areas of the body by invading either the blood or lymphatic system. Tumour cells then settle in a distant site before growing to develop metastases. Table 18.4 describes the type of cell a tumour has developed from and also the potential for the tumour to be malignant and spread to other regions. Specific types of tumour have more common areas to which they spread, although the organs that filter blood and lymph are most commonly affected, i.e. local lymph nodes, lungs, liver and spleen. Once metastases have occurred, then total surgical excision usually is impossible.

Example 18.2 Laparoscopy

Laparoscopy (or *keyhole surgery*) can be used to diagnose and treat medical and surgical conditions of both the abdomen and thorax (pleuroscopy). Performed under standing sedation or general anaesthesia, the abdomen is inflated with inert carbon dioxide to improve visualisation by expanding the body cavity. The instruments are inserted into the abdomen through a stab incision in the skin. Laparoscopy is commonly used for the investigation of weight loss, chronic colic, ovariectomy and abdominal rig castration (see Fig. 18.2).

Advantages are:

- Procedures can be done under standing sedation
- Lesions can be visualised
- Post-operative management, including recovery, can be much shorter than that for a large laparotomy incision
  The main disadvantages are:
- There are a limited number of surgical procedures that can be performed
- There is a risk of bowel perforation
- Standing sedation requires a cooperative patient

A laparoscope differs from an arthroscope in its size and length, although camera, light source and monitor equipment are basically the same. Other pieces of equipment needed are trochars and laparoscopic instruments such as Babcock forceps or scissors; bipolar or, better still, tripolar diathermy is very useful.

Common sites for equine tumours

Compared with small animals, tumours in horses are relatively uncommon. Specific neoplasms are more common in young horses but most occur in the older animal (see Summary 18.1) and are seen more often as the population of horses ages (see Chapter 14).

Diagnosis of neoplasia

In some cases a particular type of tumour can be diagnosed on appearance alone, such as with many sarcoids. With others, a biopsy of the tumour may be needed if it can be visualised, palpated or otherwise located. Occasionally diagnosis is difficult and neoplasia can be a possible cause of chronic weight loss in the horse. Where diagnosis is difficult, an investigative technique such as a *laparoscopy* can be used (see Fig. 18.2 and Summary 18.2). Sometimes diagnosis is not possible until post-mortem.

This chapter has given an overview of the basic surgical principles, such as wound repair, and also has concentrated on some of the more technical equine surgical procedures performed on the basis that these are seen more rarely and therefore are more interesting. The size of most major surgical texts is larger than this whole manual, so it is impossible to cover every option in detail. It should be remembered that basic surgical principles are important in any procedure involving the equine nurse.

Further reading

Edwards, G.B. (1991) Equine colic: the decision for surgery. *Equine Vet. Educ.* **3**, 19–23.
Mair, T., Love, S., Schumaker, J. & Watson E. (1998) *Equine Medicine, Surgery and Reproduction*, 1st edn. WB Saunders, London.

CHAPTER 19

Theatre Practice

D. P. McHugh

The equine veterinary nurse should have a thorough understanding of the principles of theatre asepsis because this is the basis of theatre practice. In addition, it is important to have a wide knowledge of the range of equine surgical procedures and the instruments and equipment needed for them, and to provide competent assistance both as a 'scrubbed nurse' or circulating assistant during surgery.

Factors that may affect the development of infection

Sepsis is the presence of pathogenic microorganisms or their toxic products in the blood or tissues of the body. This is commonly called *infection*. Most surgical wound infections occur at the time of surgery not, as is usually thought, during the post-operative period. *Aseptic technique* during surgery aims to provide an operating environment free from microorganisms and spores. The establishment of this is usually a nursing responsibility.

There are four main sources of contamination in the operating theatre:

(1) *Operating theatre and environment.* It is not possible to *sterilise* (eradicate all microorganisms and spores) the buildings themselves. The aim should be to achieve as high a standard of *disinfection* (removal of microorganisms but not spores) as possible and to minimise the introduction of contamination from outside. Many microorganisms are airborne and movement will disperse them. All operating suites should be easy to clean and good ventilation is important.

(2) *Equipment and instruments.* All instruments, implants and equipment in contact with the surgical site must be sterile.

(3) *Personnel.* All theatre staff should wear specific theatre clothing: scrub suits, footwear, hats and masks that are worn only in the designated theatre area. These must be easy to wash/sterilise. In addition, the surgical team should scrub their hands aseptically and wear sterile gloves and gowns.

(4) *Patient.* The equine patient is probably the greatest source of potential contamination to a surgical wound. The source of microorganisms may be:

  (a) *Endogenous:* those that originate from within the animal's body.

  (b) *Exogenous:* those that are found on the skin and coat. This is frequently the most common cause of contamination in a clean surgical wound, partly due to the fact that the entire body is covered in hair and partly due to the environment in which the horse is kept, which may result in contamination of the coat and feet with potentially harmful bacteria, even in the best managed yards. Meticulous pre-operative preparation of the horse is therefore essential.

Microorganisms will enter any wound that is exposed to air, but whether infection follows depends on several variable factors that include:

- *Length of surgery*: the longer a wound is open, the greater the bacterial contamination. Infection rates double for every hour of surgical time.
- *Surgical skill*: the size of the surgical wound, excessive trauma to tissues and damage to vascular supply will increase the risk of infection.
- *Host resistance*, balanced with the *virulence* (disease producing ability) of any microorganism, may affect the likelihood of infection. There may be impaired host resistance due to underlying disease, poor nutritional status or medication such as steroid treatment.
- *Contamination of the wound*: surgical wounds are categorised according to their potential for infection (see Chapter 18).

Sterilisation

All instruments and equipment that are to be used during surgery must be sterilised before use. There are several different sterilisation techniques available. Each method has advantages and disadvantages. No single method is suitable for all types of equipment.

Sterilisation can be divided into two basic types:

(1) Heat sterilisation:
  (a) Autoclave (steam under pressure).
  (b) Dry heat (hot air oven).
(2) Cold sterilisation:
  (a) Ethylene oxide (gas).
  (b) Chemical solutions.
  (c) Irradiation (gamma).

Heat sterilisation

Steam under pressure (autoclave systems)
This is the most widely used and efficient method available and also the most economical, although the initial outlay may be large. Items that may be sterilised in the autoclave include:

- Instruments
- Drapes and gowns
- Swabs
- Most rubber articles
- Some glassware
- Some plastic goods.

Heat-sensitive items, which may be damaged by this method, include fibre-optic endoscopes, some plastic items (especially those designed to be disposable) and some power tools.

Principles of sterilisation using steam under pressure
When water boils at 100°C it is converted to steam and the temperature remains the same however long it is heated. This temperature is insufficient to kill resistant bacteria, spores and viruses. By applying pressure to the chamber, the temperature of the steam is raised to destroy resistant microorganisms and spores, which are killed by coagulation of cell proteins. The higher the temperature (caused by higher pressure), the shorter the time needed to achieve sterilisation. A temperature of 134°C will destroy even the most resistant microorganisms, so an autoclave capable of operating at this temperature is desirable (Table 19.1).

There are three main types of autoclave:

(1) *Vertical pressure cooker*. This is a fairly simple type of autoclave found in many veterinary practices. It operates by initially boiling water in a sealed chamber containing items to be sterilised. It has an air vent at the top, which is closed once the air has been evacuated, and pressure is allowed to build up and the cycle is then timed manually. This type of machine has several disadvantages:
  (a) The maximum temperature/pressure combination is usually 121°C/15 psi, which is insufficient to guarantee destruction of all resistant spores/microorganisms.

Table 19.1 Operating figures for autoclaves

Temperature (°C)	Pressure (kg/cm; psi)	Time (min)
121	1.2; 15	15
126	1.4; 20	10
134	2.0; 30	3.5

(b) Because the air vent is at the top there is a danger that some air will remain trapped under the steam. The temperature here will be lower and therefore sterility cannot be guaranteed.

(c) It is manually operated, so there is room for human error in the sterilising cycle.

(d) There is no drying cycle; designed for unwrapped instruments only.

(2) *Downward displacement autoclave.* This type of machine usually is fully automatic and is becoming the most commonly used machine in veterinary practice. It usually incorporates an electrically operated boiler as a source of steam. Air is driven out more efficiently by downward displacement of steam. There is an air outlet at the bottom and a steam outlet at the top. There may be a choice of programmes, but the 134°C cycle is all that should be necessary and is the best. The main disadvantages are:

(a) The chamber is often of very small capacity and unsuitable for the larger instruments used in equine work.

(b) It is designed for unwrapped instrument sterilisation only, rather than packs, because it has insufficient penetrating ability and drying cycles.

(c) Vacuum-assisted.

(3) *Vacuum-assisted autoclave (porous load).* This works on the same principle as the others but uses a high vacuum pump to evacuate air rapidly from the chamber at the beginning of the cycle. Steam then is pumped rapidly into the chamber and the sterilisation cycle begins very quickly. A second vacuum cycle rapidly withdraws moisture after sterilisation to dry the load. This type of machine is the most versatile and is suitable for all types of instruments, drapes, gowns, swabs, etc. Vacuum-assisted autoclaves are fully automatic, with fail-safe mechanisms (usually warning lights and alarms) that indicate when there is a problem and sterilisation is incomplete. They are usually larger than either of the other types of autoclave. The main disadvantages are:

(a) A separate steam-generating boiler is needed, taking up considerable space.

(b) Cost of purchase and maintenance is quite high.

However, the machine's efficiency and reliability in sterilisation far outweigh those of the other types. It is the only machine designed to sterilise wrapped packs and hence remains the machine of choice.

Autoclave safety and maintenance

All autoclaves should be serviced regularly by a qualified engineer to ensure that they remain in good working order and electrically safe. Automated machines usually will have cut-out systems to prevent danger to users. However, because autoclaves operate at high temperatures and pressures, great care and vigilance should be taken when using them and the operating instructions should be followed at all times.

Monitoring efficiency of sterilisation

(1) *Bowie–Dick indicator tape.* This is a beige-coloured tape commonly used to seal packs for autoclaving. It is impregnated with heat-sensitive chemical stripes that change from beige to brown when a temperature of 121°C is reached. It is a useful way to distinguish packs waiting to go through an autoclave cycle from those that have already gone through a cycle, but is not a reliable stand-alone indicator that sterilisation has been achieved. This is because it does not ensure that the temperature is maintained for the correct time.

(2) *Chemical indicator strips.* These are placed inside each pack and produce a colour change when the correct time, temperature and pressure have been reached. Different types of strip are available for a range of cycles, so it is important to use the correct type or a false result may be achieved.

(3) *Browne's tubes.* These work on the principle of a colour change. A small glass tube is partly filled with an orange–brown liquid, which changes to green when the appropriate temperature/pressure has been reached. Tubes are available that change at 121°C, 126°C and 134°C. The correct tube appropriate to the cycle must be used.

(4) *Spore tests.* Strips of paper impregnated with a species of dried spores (usually *Bacillus stearothermophilus*) are placed inside a load. On completion of the cycle it is placed in the culture medium provided and incubated at the appropriate temperature for up to 72 h. If the sterilisation process has been successful, the spores will be killed and there will be no growth. This system is very reliable but is only suitable as a check on the machine's efficacy because results are not available immediately.

(5) *Thermocouples.* Electrical leads with temperaturesensitive tips (thermocouples) are placed in various parts of the sterilising chamber and the results are recorded on a chart. This is the most efficient method of testing but has to be performed by an engineer and is expensive and time consuming.

(6) *Recording charts.* Many vacuum-assisted autoclaves will have a recording chart or gauge on the outside that reveals details of the entire cycle.

Dry heat (hot air oven)

Microorganisms are more resistant to dry heat than when heated in the presence of moisture, so temperatures of 150–180°C are needed for a prolonged period of time (Table 19.2). This method has been superseded largely by the more reliable method of autoclaving.

The hot air oven is heated by electrical elements and is suitable for glassware, unwrapped instruments and instruments with sharp cutting edges (not blunted by this process). The disadvantages include:

- Units are small so are not ideal for equine use.
- Long sterilising cycle/cooling down period.

Table 19.2 Operating figures for hot air ovens

Temperature (°C)	Time (min)
180	60
160	120
150	180

- Not suitable for drapes, etc. because it will cause charring.

Monitoring efficiency of sterilisation

Spore strip tests and Browne's tubes are available that have been designed for hot air ovens. However, it is difficult to monitor effective sterilisation because this is dependent on the size of the load.

Moist heat (boiling)

This is no longer considered as a method of sterilisation. It cannot be guaranteed to kill all microorganisms and spores because the maximum temperature of 100°C is insufficient to kill resistant spores.

Cold sterilisation

Ethylene oxide

This is a highly effective method of sterilisation that is commonly used in equine veterinary practice. Although its use is currently permitted under the Control of Substances Hazardous to Health (COSHH) regulations, there have been concerns expressed about safety because it is a toxic, inflammable gas that is an irritant to tissues. The only system available ('Anprolene', Anderson Products) for use in veterinary clinics operates at room temperature and does not require a power supply for the sterilisation process. Ethylene oxide inactivates the DNA of cells, thereby preventing cell reproduction.

Ethylene oxide steriliser

The steriliser consists of a rectangular plastic-coated container that is fitted with a ventilation system (for safety and to comply with COSHH regulations). It should be situated away from the main workplace, preferably in a designated room away from people. Items to be sterilised are washed and must be dried before being packed individually and then placed in a plastic liner bag inside the container. A vial of ethylene oxide liquid and the ventilation tubing are placed in the bag that is sealed around the bag using clips provided. The top of the glass vial is snapped from the outside of the liner bag to release the sterilant gas. The door to the steriliser unit is closed and locked, the ventilator is turned on and the contents are left for 12 h to sterilise. At the end of this a pump is switched on to aerate the chamber. The door then may be opened safely and the load removed. The items then should be left to ventilate for a further 24 h prior to use, to allow complete dissipation of the gas. Items that may be sterilised using ethylene oxide include:

- Instruments
- Drapes, etc.
- Fibre-optic equipment, e.g. arthroscopy and endoscopy equipment
- Plastic items
- Battery-operated drills.

Ethylene oxide is an extremely useful method of sterilisation for equine clinics, where fibre-optic and other heat-sensitive equipment is used. It also allows the re-sterilisation of items that are intended to be disposable (such as intestinal and skin staplers and plastic tubing) and that would be damaged by heat.

Disadvantages include:

- Toxicity
- Long duration of cycle
- Container often small; larger ones available
- Although power required only for venting, the vials are relatively expensive.

Testing efficiency of sterilisation
(1) *Indicator tape* similar to Bowie–Dick tape is available with the same disadvantage that colour change does not guarantee effective sterilisation. It is blue with yellow stripes, which turn red after exposure to ethylene oxide gas.
(2) Chemical indicator strips are available that undergo a colour change when sterilisation is complete.
(3) Spore strips similar to those used to test the efficiency of the autoclave are available.

Chemical solutions
This method actually should be classed only as a method of disinfection, although some manufacturers guarantee sterilisation after prolonged immersion (18–24 h). It should be kept as a last resort when other methods are not possible. It is popular for dis-

infection of endoscopic and arthroscopic equipment. Ethylene oxide remains a preferable alternative, but in cases where the equipment has to be used several times in a day it is not practical to use ethylene oxide because it has a 12-h cycle.

There are many different commercial preparations available and not all have the same efficacy. Some preparations are aqueous whereas others are alcohol based. Choice of solution will depend largely on individual preference. A suitable solution will produce rapid and efficient destruction of microorganisms, be harmless to tissue and to the equipment to be soaked and be economical to use.

Gamma irradiation
This is a form of irradiation and, as such, can be carried out only under controlled conditions. Many prepackaged disposable items are sterilised by this method, e.g. suture materials, surgical gloves and drapes and many plastic items, but it is not feasible for a veterinary, clinic.

Packing supplies for sterilisation

There are many different materials and methods available for packing supplies for sterilisation. Choice will depend on:

- Method of sterilisation (autoclave/ethylene oxide) and size of machine/container.
- Personal preference.
- Cost.
- Packaging material must be resistant to damage when handled or sterilised and protect the equipment from damage.
- Steam and gas must be able to penetrate the wrapping to allow sterilisation and must be evacuated easily from the pack once the process is complete.
- Microorganisms must not be able to penetrate from the outer surface of the wrap to the inner.

Nylon film

Advantages
- Packs can be made into many sizes and sealed with Bowie–Dick tape
- Ready-made bags are available but expensive

- Transparent, so can identify items readily
- Strong

Disadvantages
- Intended to be re-useable, but unseen perforations may lead to contamination
- Can be difficult to remove sterilised items from the pack without contaminating them

Seal-and-peel pouches
Disposable bags, consisting of a paper back and a clear plasticised front with a fold-over seal, are available in a wide range of sizes.

Advantages
- Suitable for use in an autoclave or with ethylene oxide and have a colour indicator strip to test efficacy of sterilisation
- Relatively inexpensive
- The careful wrapping decreases the risk of damage to the item inside and contamination during opening

Disadvantage
They are not that strong and the paper tears easily.

Paper
Paper sheets commonly are used for wrapping instrument packs.

Advantages
- Relatively inexpensive
- Large sheets can be cut to appropriate size
- Many are highly water repellant
- Ideal as any outer layer for wrapped instrument packs
- May be re-used
- Can be used with autoclave and ethylene oxide

Disadvantages
- If using in an autoclave, a drying cycle is needed
- May tear during handling and storage

Linen/cotton sheets
These are frequently used for wrapping instrument and drape packs.

Advantages
- Conforming and strong
- Re-useable
- May be used in autoclave or with ethylene oxide

Disadvantage
They are permeable to moisture and therefore present a threat to asepsis, so a double layer of linen is usually covered by a waterproof, paper-based wrap to maintain asepsis.

Metal drums
Metal drums with steam vents in the side that are closed after autoclaving are used frequently in veterinary practices, especially with small pressure-cooker-type machines.

Advantages
- Suitable for instruments and drapes
- Re-useable: initial cost may be high but will last many years
- Strong and not easily damaged
- Waterproof once vents are closed; items inside are well protected

Disadvantages
- Frequently multi-use, therefore a degree of environmental contamination each time lid is opened
- Risk of contamination of items as they are removed from the drum

Boxes and cartons
These are available for use with autoclaves and ethylene oxide.

Advantages
- Provide protection for enclosed items; particularly useful for delicate or heavy instruments
- Ideal for specialised kits such as orthopaedic packs
- Suitable for use in autoclaves or ethylene oxide
- Re-useable

Disadvantages
- May be bulky
- If using an autoclave, a drying cycle is needed

Labelling packs for sterilisation

All packs/instruments should be clearly labelled:

- Identification of pack/instruments
- Date of packing
- Initials of packer
- Evidence of sterilisation: indicator tape or stickers.

Storage after sterilisation

Sterile instruments and packs should be stored separately from non-sterile equipment, ideally in closed cupboards that are dust-free, dry and well ventilated. Cupboards or containers for storage should be well labelled for ease of use. Packs should be handled as little as possible to minimise damage to wrapping materials and therefore contamination of packs. The length of time for which packs may be stored safely after sterilisation is debatable. A sealed pack should remain sterile for a limitless period but may become damaged as a result of handling. It is therefore recommended that any unused packs should be re-sterilised after 6–8 weeks.

The operating theatre

The operating theatre suite consists of several defined areas, each with specific requirements.

Induction/recovery box

Features

- Padded walls (usually PVC-covered) that are slightly compressable and non-slip flooring (often rubberised) to minimise risk of injury during anaesthetic induction/recovery
- Rounded corners and curved borders of floor and walls; no projections that might lead to injury
- Easily cleanable
- Source of heat and light
- Doors from outside and doors leading to theatre
- Large clinics may have two or more boxes to allow efficient throughput of cases
- Some means of monitoring horse during recovery, e.g. CCTV camera or spy-hole
- Overhead hoist to move horse to table, preferably mechanical and electrical (see Chapter 20).

Preparation area

Ideally there should be a preparation area where the horse can be positioned and clipped and the skin prepared for surgery. With the horse anaesthetised, this requires a mobile table that can be pushed into theatre.

Operating theatre

Many practices will have just one operating theatre, but larger clinics may have two: one for elective surgery such as orthopaedic work and the other for general or 'contaminated' surgery such as colic, airway and dental surgery. The standard of asepsis should be the same in both theatres. Arguably, greater care has to be taken in the 'contaminated surgery' theatre, because undoubtedly there will be a greater concentration of pathogenic microorganisms there.

Size

The theatre has to be large enough to accommodate a horse positioned on the table in dorsal or lateral recumbency and to allow room for bulky surgical equipment such as an arthroscopy monitoring trolley, suction and fluid pumps, anaesthetic machine, anaesthetic monitoring equipment, instrument trolleys and a surgical team (Fig. 19.1). There should be room also to allow intra-operative radiography/imaging. A horse positioned in lateral recumbency will take up approximately twice the space of a horse in dorsal recumbency. A theatre that is too small will compromise both asepsis and general working conditions.

Other requirements

- Wide doorway into theatre: essential with a mobile table (and to remove carcases).
- Easily cleanable: walls and floors should be made of impervious, non-staining material. Floors should be hard-wearing and non-slip. Marble or terrazo stone is probably the material of choice. Industrial vinyl or rubberised floors are used, but may be damaged by equipment. Walls and ceiling should be painted with a light-coloured waterproof paint. Tiles are expensive,

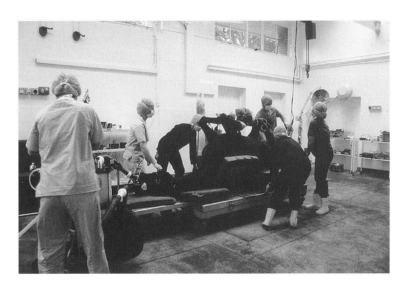

Fig. 19.1 Equine theatre in use.

easily damaged and tend to harbour dirt and bacteria in cracks and crevices. The corners and edges of walls should be coved to facilitate cleaning. Drains, although considered as a potential source of bacteria, are essential in an equine operating theatre if a good standard of asepsis is to be maintained. Liberal use of water and disinfectant will dilute and destroy harmful microorganisms. Flushing systems are sometimes used.

- There should be as little shelving and furniture in the theatre as possible.
- There should be a good supply of electric sockets around the room, either recessed into the wall or with protective covers.
- Other fixtures: X-ray viewer flush with the wall; rings in the wall for limb positioning; medical gas and air supply for power tools.
- Good lighting is essential. Where possible, advantage should be taken of natural daylight. Ideally lighting should be concealed within the ceiling to facilitate cleaning. One or more moveable overhead theatre spot-lights will be necessary to illuminate the surgical site.
- Some form of heating will be necessary. The ambient temperature should be 15–20°C. Panel heating within the walls is ideal but expensive. Modern wall-mounted radiators are the most realistic method of heating. Fan heaters should be avoided because they cause air and dust movement.

- Some system of ventilation or air-conditioning may be desirable.
- Windows should not open because this would be an obvious threat to asepsis.
- A wall clock is needed for anaesthetic monitoring and timing of surgery.
- A dry-wipe board is useful for recording details such as swab numbers and sutures used.
- Emergency lighting should be available in case the power fails.

The operating table

This is likely to be one of the most expensive pieces of equipment to be purchased.

Ideal requirements
- Adjustable to allow the horse to be placed in any desired position and height
- Easily moveable to any position in the room
- Easily cleanable, maintained and rust-proof
- Battery- or mains-operated hydraulics
- Easy to use limb-supports and positioning aids.

Types of table
(1) *Fixed hydraulic*: not very versatile because positioning of horse, equipment and surgeon may be restricted.

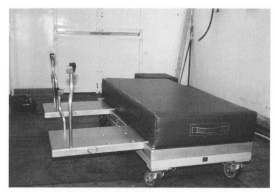

Fig. 19.2 Kimsey operating table with padding.

(2) *Mobile*: most versatile. It is important that it is light and easily moved by two or three people, e.g. 'Haico', 'Kimsey' and 'Shanks' (Fig. 19.2).

(3) *Inflatable*: restrictive for positioning of horse, equipment and access for surgeon. It is too unstable for most surgery and the table will tilt as weight positions alter. A tendency to leaks increases instability.

Whatever type of table is used, attention must be paid to providing good padding to minimise the risk of post-operative myopathy (see Chapter 20).

Area for washing and sterilising equipment

There should be a separate room where used instruments and equipment are washed, packed and sterilised. This should be close to the operating theatre but separate from the sterile storage area. It should include a washing machine and tumble drier, sterilisation equipment and possibly an ultrasonic instrument cleaner.

Sterile storage area

Sterile supplies should be stored in closed cupboards close to and accessible from the theatre.

Scrubbing-up area

There should be a scrubbing-up area adjacent to the theatre. If there are two theatres, this ideally should be situated between the two rooms and with access via swing doors. It should be large enough to lay out a trolley with gloves and gowns for the surgical team.

Changing rooms

Should be situated at the entrance to the theatre. It is a good idea to have a red line delineating the sterile area and notices displayed to indicate these areas. Theatre footwear should be at the entrance to theatre, beyond the red line.

The layout of rooms within the theare suite is important for the sake of asepsis. There should be a one-way traffic system so that the surgical team and sterile supplies enter through one door and unscrubbed personnel enter and leave through a separate doorway.

Maintenance and cleaning of operating theatre

There should be a routine cleaning programme in the operating suite if a high standard of asepsis is to be established and maintained:

- At the beginning of each day, all surfaces and equipment should be damp-dusted using a dilute solution of disinfectant.
- Between cases, the operating room and preparation room floors and the operating table will need to be washed using an appropriate disinfectant. Floors can be dried quickly using a rubber 'squeegy'. All equipment used will need to be washed or wiped over.
- At the end of the day all rooms of the theatre should be washed. The operating table, padding and accessories such as limb supports should be washed, along with any other equipment used. Surfaces should be wiped over.
- On a regular basis, depending on caseload, there should be a more thorough cleaning session where all equipment is removed from each room and the floors and walls are scrubbed with a suitable disinfectant with detergent properties. This must remove organic matter and inactivate a wide range of bacteria, including *Pseudomonas* spp. All equipment should be cleaned meticulously.

• Cleaning utensils used in theatre should not be used elsewhere. Mop heads that may be removed and washed in the washing machine should be used, and buckets always should be emptied, rinsed out and dried.

Surgical team preparation

Personnel are a major source of contamination within the operating theatre suite, so steps should be taken to minimise this. Anyone entering the theatre area should change from their ordinary clothes into designated theate attire before entering. This usually consists of a simple *two-piece 'scrub suit'* or a *one-piece boiler suit* made of cotton or polyester that is easily laundered or sterilised if desired. A clean suit should be worn each day and changed between cases, if dirty. *Theatre footwear* needs to be easy to clean and for equine surgery wellingtons (traditionally white) are probably the best choice, although clogs are preferred by some surgeons. All footwear should be wiped over with disinfectant at the end of the day or washed more thoroughly if severely soiled, e.g. after colic surgery.

Various types of disposable headwear and masks to filter expired air from the nose and mouth are available. Masks are effective for relatively short periods only and so ideally should be changed between cases.

Scrubbing-up

Those directly involved with the surgery take further steps towards asepsis. Pre-operative scrubbing-up is a systematic washing and scrubbing of the hands, arms and elbows. Because it is not possible to sterilise the skin, the aim of the scrubbing routine is to eliminate as many microorganisms from the surface of the hands and arms as possible, prior to putting on a sterile surgical gown and gloves. Research has shown that significant numbers of common skin bacteria continue to be removed after 5 min of scrubbing but at 10 min no greater benefit ensues. Thus it is logical to adopt a scrubbing technique that takes 5–10 min, allowing time for rinsing in-between stages.

A suggested approach is as follows:

(1) Remove jewellery/watch and make sure nails are short.

(2) Adjust the water supply (which should be elbow- or foot-operated) to a safe flow and temperature. Once the scrubbing routine has begun, the hands should not touch the taps, sink or soap dispenser. If they are inadvertently touched, the last stage of the procedure should be repeated.

(3) Wash the hands thoroughly using either a plain soap or surgical scrub solution and clean under fingernails with a non-sterile nail pick.

(4) After hand washing, the arms are washed up to and including the elbows. Always keep the hands above the elbows so that water drains down towards the unscrubbed arms to avoid recontamination. The aim of this is to remove organic matter and grease from the skin.

(5) Rinse the hands and then the arms by allowing water to wash away the soap from the hands to the elbows (avoid the temptation to use the opposite hand to assist with rinsing because this could lead to recontamination).

(6) Repeat this procedure, once again beginning with the hands, using a surgical scrub solution, e.g. chlorhexidine or povidone iodine. Use minimal water to produce a lather because the bactericidal properties of the scrub solution are dependent on the contact time with the skin. Excessive amounts of water will rinse away the scrub solution before it has destroyed sufficient bacteria.

(7) Rinse off the scrub solution from the hands but leave the arms coated.

(8) Take a sterile scrubbing brush and systematically scrub the hands. Scrub the palms of the hand, wrist and four surfaces of each finger and thumb, nails and nailbed. Either rinse the brush and use it on the other hand, or discard it and take a second brush. It is best to avoid scrubbing the backs of the hands and arms as the skin here tends to be sensitive and scrubbing with a brush may damage the skin, which in turn increases surface microorganisms. Some of the commercially available disposable scrub brushes have very soft bristles and a sponge back, which may

be less traumatic to this sensitive skin and so allow scrubbing of this area without leading to excoriation. If a brush is used on the arms, then both hands and arms should be rinsed during stage 7.

(9) The final stage is a repeat of stage 6. Wash the hands and arms in surgical scrub solution, but this time finish just a few centimetres below the elbow so that there is no danger of contact with a previously unscrubbed area.

(10) Rinse the hands and arms as before and then turn off the taps using elbows or foot.

(11) Allow excess water to drip from the elbows before leaving the sink.

(12) Take a sterile handtowel, holding it at arm's length so that it does not touch your scrub suit. Use a different section to dry each hand and each arm and then discard the towel.

It is a good idea to check the clock at the start and again before the final stage to ensure that the procedure has taken the allotted time.

Surgical scrub solutions

These are detergent solutions with antiseptic properties. Two agents commonly used are:

(1) *Chlorhexidine* ('Hibiscrub', 'Nolvasan')
  (a) Broad spectrum of antimicrobial activity.
  (b) Viricidal, fungicidal and sporicidal properties.
  (c) Effective in the presence of organic matter.
  (d) Long residual activity.
  (e) Causes irritation to tissues in only a small number of cases.
  (f) Relatively low toxicity to tissues.

(2) *Povidone iodine* ('Pevidine', 'Betadine')
  (a) Broad spectrum of antimicrobial activity.
  (b) Viricidal and fungicidal.
  (c) Efficacy impaired by organic matter.
  (d) Relatively short duration of action.
  (e) May cause eczema in some individuals.

Newer compounds are available but have not been shown to be superior.

Putting on a surgical gown

Gowns may be disposable or re-useable:

- *Disposable gowns*: usually paper based, water repellent, conforming, pre-sterilised and comfortable. They are more expensive than re-useable gowns but the cost is saved in not needing to wash and re-sterilise them, so they are widely used.
- *Re-useable gowns*: usually linen/cotton or, more recently, waterproofed polyesters. A major disadvantage is that fabric gowns will allow fluids to penetrate rapidly. There are also the disadvantages of laundering time, cost and the quality deteriorating over time.

There are two different designs of surgical gown: back-tying or side-tying. The technique for putting on both types is basically similar, but with a slight variation for each:

(1) The sterile gown (folded inside out) is taken from either its sterile pack or a sterile trolley on which it is placed. It should be picked up by the shoulders, held at arm's length and allowed to unfold.

(2) One hand should slide into each sleeve. No attempt should be made to adjust the gown because this will lead to contamination of the hands or outside of the gown (remember that the hands, although clean, are *not* sterile, whereas the gown is). An unscrubbed assistant should pull the back of the gown over the shoulders by touching only the inside surface of the gown and secure the ties at the back.

(3) In the case of a *back-tying* gown, the unscrubbed assistant then takes the ends of the waist ties and secures them at the back (Fig. 19.3). The back of the gown now must be considered non-sterile and must not come into contact with any part of the sterile surgical field. In the case of a *side-tying* gown, the waist ties are held together at the front of the gown by a piece of card. The scrubbed person pulls the card away from the shorter tie (with hands remaining within the cuffed sleeves) and passes the card with the longer tie attached to it to the unscrubbed assistant. This is then taken around the back to the opposite side. The

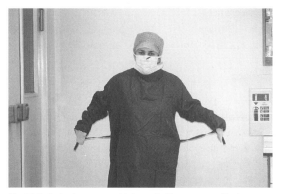

Fig. 19.3 Back-tying gown: waist ties are held out, an unscrubbed assistant takes the ends and secures the ties at the back.

scrubbed person then pulls the tape, so that the paper card comes away. The gown then is tied at the waist by the scrubbed person (Fig. 19.4). This type of gown is preferable because it allows all-round protection from contamination and therefore more freedom of movement around the surgical site. Most disposable surgical gowns are of this type.

Putting on surgical gloves

There are two methods of gloving that are commonly used.

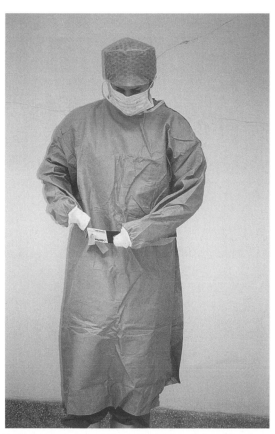

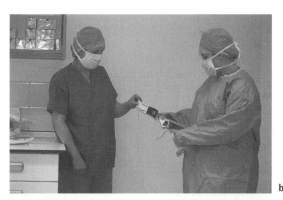

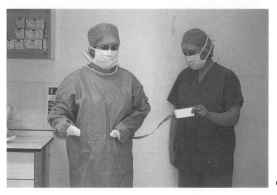

Fig. 19.4 Side-tying gown: (a) the scrubbed person pulls the card away from the shorter tie at the front; (b) the card attached to the waist tie is passed to the unscrubbed assistant; (c) the tie is passed around the back of the scrubbed person, who then pulls the tie away from the card and secures the ties at the waist.

Closed gloving

The hands remain within the sleeves during gloving. This technique minimises the risk of contaminating the outside of the gloves, because the outside of the gloves should not contact the skin (Fig. 19.5):

(1) Hands remain within the sleeves of the gown. The glove packet is turned so that the fingers point towards the body (the right glove now will be on the left, and vice versa).
(2) The glove is picked up at the rim of the cuff.
(3) The hand is turned over so that the glove lies on the palmar surface with the fingers pointing towards the body.
(4) The rim of the glove is lifted up with the opposite hand and the cuff then is pulled over the fingers and over the dorsal surface of the wrist.
(5) The glove then is pulled on as the fingers are pushed forwards.

Open gloving

This technique (Fig. 19.6) has the disadvantage that because the hands are exposed through the cuffs the gloves are quite easily contaminated by skin contact:

(1) The glove pack is opened so that the fingers are pointing away from the body.
(2) With the left hand the right glove is picked up at the cuff, holding only the folded-back inner surface of the cuff, and pulled onto the right hand.
(3) The rim of the cuff is hooked over the thumb.
(4) The gloved fingers of the right hand then are placed under the cuff of the left glove, which is pulled onto the left hand holding only the outer surface of the glove.
(5) The rim of the left glove is hooked over the thumb while the cuff of the gown is adjusted.

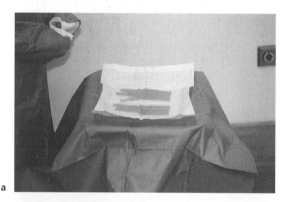
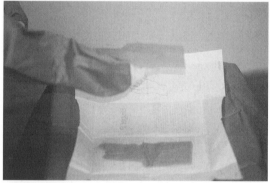
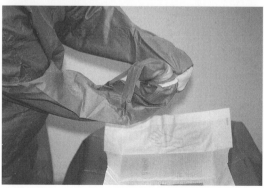
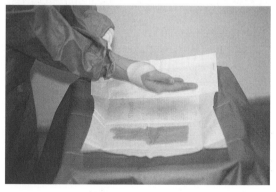

Fig. 19.5 Closed gloving: (a) hands remain within the cuffed sleeve and the glove packet is turned round so that the fingers point towards the body (right glove now on left); (b) the right glove is picked up at the rim and the hand turned over so that the glove lies on the palmar surface; (c) the rim of the glove is lifted with the opposite hand and the cuff is pulled over the fingers; (d) the glove is pulled on as the fingers are pushed forwards.

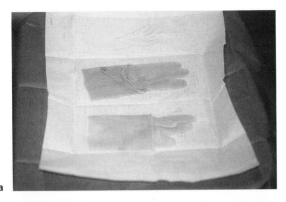

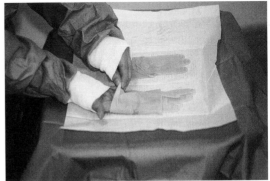

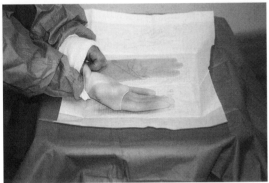

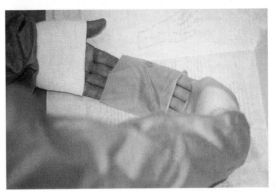

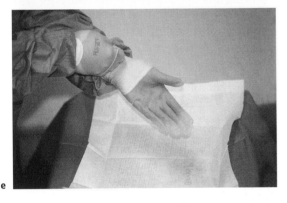

Fig. 19.6 Open gloving: (a) the glove packet is opened with the fingers pointing away from the body; (b) with the left hand, the right glove is picked up at the cuff, holding the inner surface only; it is then pulled onto the right hand; (c) the rim of the cuff is hooked over the thumb; (d) the gloved fingers of the right hand are placed under the cuff of the left glove, which is pulled onto the left hand; (e) the cuff of the glove is then pulled over the cuff of the gown using the right hand; this is then repeated for the right glove.

(6) The cuff of the glove then is pulled over the cuff of the gown using the right hand.

(7) The procedure is repeated for the right hand.

Conduct during surgery

The theatre nurse has two main roles:

(1) Scrubbed nurse.

(2) Circulating nurse.

Scrubbed nurse

Duties include:

- Helping to prepare theatre, instruments and equipment for surgery
- Scrubbing-up to assist with surgery
- Assisting with draping the patient
- Passing instruments, swabs and sutures

- Assisting with surgery: retracting tissue, cutting sutures, swabbing surgical site, irrigating wound
- Being responsible for all equipment, swabs and sutures.

The role of the scrubbed nurse requires organisation if mistakes are not to be made. The nurse should aim to anticipate the needs of the surgeon, so a knowledge of the surgical procedure is important:

(1) It is essential to know *exactly* what instruments and equipment are on the trolley, so that they can be accounted for at the end of surgery.
(2) All swabs, sutures, needles and other kit must be counted before surgery starts and again before the wound is closed to prevent items being left within the surgical cavity.
(3) Instruments should be passed to the surgeon so that he/she can use them easily, i.e. the right way round.
(4) Instruments always should be returned to the same trolley position so that they can be located readily. They should be removed from the surgical site, where they could easily be dropped or hidden from view.
(5) The nurse should keep a constant check on the swab count and never use more than one swab at a time.
(6) Swabs should be applied firmly to a wound but not wiped across it because this may damage tissue and disturb blood clots.
(7) All tissues should be handled gently to avoid trauma.

Preparing an instrument trolley

Instrument trolleys should be laid up immediately prior to surgery and then a sterile drape placed over the top to prevent contamination. Trolleys can be laid up using sterile cheatle forceps or by a scrubbed nurse. All equipment and instruments, drapes, suture materials, saline and other kit required for the surgery should be placed on the trolley. Lists with requirements for different operations may be useful.

Circulating nurse

Duties include:

- Helping to prepare theatre, equipment and instruments for surgery
- Tying the surgical team into gowns
- Helping to position the horse on the table
- Preparing the surgical site
- Connecting equipment, e.g. power tools, arthroscopy equipment
- Opening packs, e.g. sutures
- Counting swabs with scrubbed nurse
- Assisting the anaesthetist
- Ensuring that sterility is maintained: watching for slipping drapes, etc.
- Preparing post-operative dressings
- Being available at all times
- Recording items added to the instrument trolley
- Helping to clear theatre on completion of surgery.

Pre-operative preparation of the patient (see Chapter 20)

Clipping

Clipping the surgical site is necessary for most procedures.

Clipping prior to anaesthesia

Advantages
- Improves asepsis: loose hairs are shed before surgery; allows an initial washing of surgical site prior to anaesthesia
- Saves anaesthetic time
- Improves theatre efficiency: less time clipping and scrubbing the skin.

Disadvantage
Restraint of the horse may be difficult: it may require sedation.

Clipping after induction of anaesthesia

Advantages
- Takes less time because there is no movement
- No restraint necessary and it is safer
- Desirable with fractious animals or painful/inaccessable sites.

Disadvantages

- Decreases asepsis: small loose hairs are almost impossible to remove even with a vacuum cleaner
- Increases anaesthetic time
- Decreases theatre efficiency: more time clipping and scrubbing the skin.

Preparation of the skin (Fig. 19.7)

With a horse the skin and coat are major wound contamination risk areas. It is impossible to remove all the bacteria, so the aim is to decrease significantly the number of microorganisms present without damaging the skin itself.

Surgical scrub solutions such as chlorhexidine and povidone iodine are ideal for the preparation of the patient's skin. An antiseptic solution (aqueous- or alcohol-based) then usually is applied to provide residual antibacterial activity. Different skin preparation techniques are used in different theatres, including the following approach:

(1) The horse is positioned for surgery.
(2) Using lint-free swabs, the surgical site is washed using chlorhexidine and a little warm water, beginning at the proposed incision site and working towards the periphery. On reaching the edge or if soiling is severe, the swab is discarded and a fresh one taken. Surgical gloves should be worn to prevent contamination of the patient's skin from the nurse's hands. It is not necessary at this stage to wear sterile gloves (Fig. 19.7a).
(3) Continue this procedure until the area is clean, discarding swabs as they become discoloured.
(4) A solution of 70% alcohol then can be sprayed over the site to remove detergent and any surface grease. It should not be used on open wounds (Fig. 19.7b).
(5) A dry swab may be wiped over the site to assess the efficacy of scrubbing. If there is any discolouration on the swab, the scrubbing is repeated (Fig. 19.7c).
(6) When the area is clean (there is no discolouration of the swab), a solution of chlorhexidine (5% concentrate) and 70% alcohol is sprayed over the site (Fig. 19.7d).
(7) The final stage of skin preparation is performed some minutes later by a member of the surgical team, using the same chlorhexidine/alcohol solution applied using a sterile swab on a pair of sponge-holding forceps (Fig. 19.7e).

Preparation of eyes and mucous membranes

The solutions commonly used for preparation of the skin are likely to be irritant to the eye or other mucous membranes. A very dilute aqueous solution of povidone iodine (0.1–0.2%) is recommended to irrigate the eye and may be used also on oral and other mucous membranes. Other scrub solutions have been shown to be more irritant.

The skin around the eye is extremely sensitive, so it is important that clipper blades are in good order and great care is taken when clipping around the eye. Application of a KY jelly may help to prevent hair being introduced to the eye or a wound during clipping. Skin around the eye should be washed gently using a 1% aqueous solution of povidone iodine.

Other preparations prior to surgery

- Cover feet and tail (e.g. rectal sleeves)
- When limb is the surgical site, cover foot with surgical glove
- Application of Esmarch's bandage if surgery of lower limb (rubber bandage used to exsanguinate limb and so provide bloodless surgical field) (see Fig. 19.8)
- If appropriate, suture the sheath and place a urinary catheter to minimise the risk of contamination by urine
- Cover any wounds unconnected with surgery.

Positioning for surgery

Horses usually will be positioned in *dorsal recumbency* (on their back) or in right or left *lateral recumbency* (right or left side down). Exact positioning on the table will vary with different procedures and with the surgeon's and anaesthetist's preferences. Limb supports that attach to the operating table or rings in the wall are used frequently to position limbs for surgery. With some tables, the sides

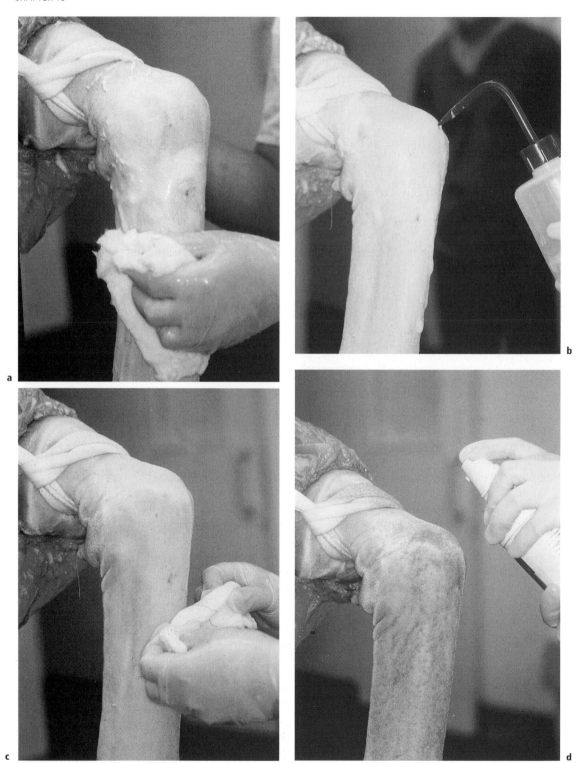

Fig. 19.7 Preparation of the skin of a hind fetlock.

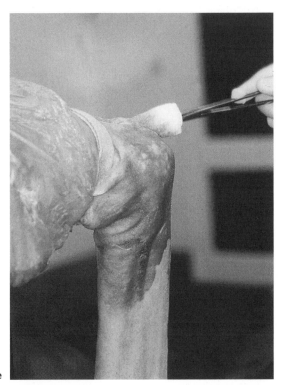

e

Fig. 19.7 *Continued*

may be lifted to form a U shape to support the horse in dorsal recumbency. Air- or foam-filled wedges also can be helpful to aid positioning.

Draping the patient

Regarding asepsis, one of the major problems with the horse as a surgical candidate (compared with (humans) is that the entire body is covered with hair that is usually heavily soiled, even in a well-groomed horse. Drapes, therefore, play a very important role in providing a barrier between the animal and the surgical site. To be effective, they must cover the entire animal, leaving only the surgical site exposed.

Drapes may be divided into two main types:

(1) Disposable.
(2) Re-useable.

Disposable drapes
For equine work disposable drapes are the best choice.

Advantages
- Originally designed for the human market but size and type are ideal for all equine work; some are now purpose-made, e.g. colic drapes
- Waterproof: cost does reflect the quality, but inexpensively priced, good-quality drapes are available

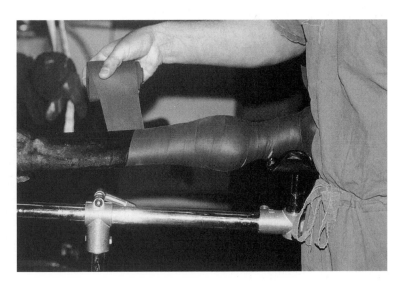

Fig. 19.8 Application of an Esmarch's bandage to the distal limb.

- Pre-sterilised
- Conforming
- Optimum quality every time
- No launderering time or cost.

Disadvantages
- Large stocks may be needed
- Cheap brands tend to be less water resilient, tear easily and are non-conforming.

Re-useable drapes

Re-usable drapes can be made to suit individual preferences. The disadvantages are:

- Porous: bacterial strike-through is a real threat
- Laundering time and cost
- Quality is variable.

Plastic drapes (e.g. '*Buster*') are available in a variety of sizes. These are simply sheets of plastic that may be used alone or underneath linen drapes as a waterproof layer. They can be a useful compromise but are non-conforming, have a tendency to slip and tear and are relatively expensive in comparison with most large disposable drapes.

Instruments and equipment

It is beyond the scope of this book to provide a comprehensive guide to all the instruments and equipment used in equine surgery and instrument suppliers' catalogues. The veterinary nurse should become familiar with the more commonly used instruments in equine surgery.

Surgical instruments are expensive and should be well-maintained and handled correctly. *Stainless steel* is the material of choice for most surgical instruments: it is expensive, but resists corrosion, is very strong and has a pleasing appearance. *Chromium-plated carbon steel* is often used for veterinary instruments because it is less expensive but it tends to be damaged by chemicals and saline and sharp edges also tend to blunt quickly. *Tungsten carbide* is often used for cutting edges and gripping surfaces in good quality instruments. It is very hard and resistant to wear and, although it is more expensive than stainless steel,

its quality justifies the expense. Instruments with tungsten carbide inserts usually have gold-coloured handles.

General surgical instruments

Scalpels

Scalpels are ideal for dividing tissue with least trauma. Re-useable handles with disposable blades are normally used, although some surgeons prefer a fixed scalpel for some procedures (Fig. 19.9). Several different-sized handles are commonly used in equine surgery:

- Size 3 handle, suitable for blade sizes 20, 21, 22, 23 and 24
- Size 4 handle, suitable for blade sizes 10, 11, 12 and 15
- Size 7 handle (longer and slimmer), suitable for blade sizes 10, 11, 12 and 15.

A folding scalpel handle designed for use in castrations is also available. This carries the same blades as a size 4 handle. Use of disposable blades ensures consistent sharpness.

Dissecting forceps

These are commonly referred to as 'dressing forceps', 'thumb forceps' or 'rat-toothed forceps':

- Used to lift and retract tissue
- May have plain or toothed jaws
- Jaws opposed by gripping two sides together
- Fine, plain forceps used for holding delicate tissue such as viscera.

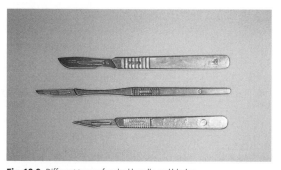

Fig. 19.9 Different types of scalpel handle and blades.

- Toothed forceps generally used for holding denser tissues
- Should be held like a pencil

Scissors

Scissors are available in a variety of shapes and lengths (see Fig. 19.10):

- Mayo scissors are commonly used for routine dissection
- Metzenbaum scissors (finer and longer) are used for delicate dissection
- Paynes scissors are designed for removal of sutures
- Scissors are held correctly with the ring finger and thumb inserted in the rings of the scissors and the index finger on the shaft to guide the scissors.

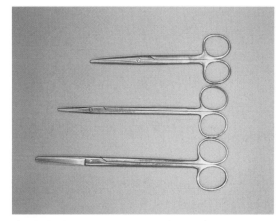

Fig. 19.10 Scissors. From top: Mayo; Metzenbaum; Carless suture scissors.

Artery forceps

These are commonly referred to as 'haemostats' or 'clips' and are used for clamping blood vessels:

- May be straight or have curved jaws
- Enormous variety available, such as Spencer Wells, Dunhills, Criles, Kochers, Halstead
- Most have transverse striations on jaws to facilitate gripping
- Should be held like scissors

Tissue forceps

These are designed for tissue retraction (Fig. 19.11):

- Used to grip without excessive trauma to tissue
- Allis and Babcock are most popular types used
- Have ringed arms and a ratchet grip like the artery forceps

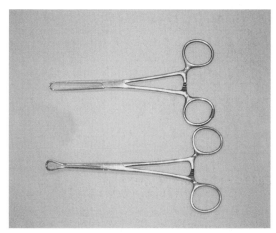

Fig. 19.11 Tissue forceps. From top: Allis; Babcock.

Retractors

Retractors are used to retract tissue and so facilitate visibility of the surgical field:

- May be hand-held, such as Langenbeck or Senn
- May be self-retaining, e.g. Gelpi, Wests, Travers, Gossett, Finochettio

Needle-holders

These are used for holding suture needles during suturing and to aid knot-tying (Fig. 19.12):

- Mayo-Hegar needle-holders resemble a long-handled pair of artery forceps. They have a ratchet but no scissor edge.
- McPhail's needle-holders have a spring ratchet so that by squeezing them together the jaws open and release the needle.
- Mathieu's needle-holders are similar to McPhail's but have tungsten carbide inserts, a much finer tip and superior ratchet action.
- Olsen-Hegar needle-holders resemble Mayo-Hegar needleholders but have a longer jaw and a scissor edge along the shaft. Although the scissor edge is useful, it has the disadvantage of inadvertently cutting suture material as material passes through the jaws.

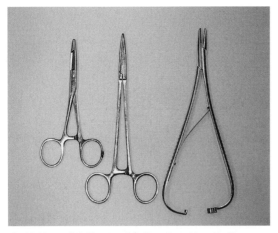

Fig. 19.12 Needle-holders. From left: Olsen–Hegar; Mayo; Mathieu.

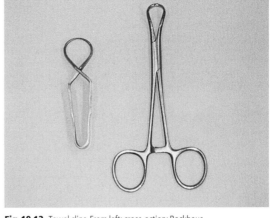

Fig. 19.13 Towel clips. From left: cross-action; Backhaus.

- Gillies needle-holders are commonly used by vets but are not ideal. Their main disadvantage is that they have no ratchet, so the needle has to be held still by gripping, which allows considerable movement of the needle. They have a scissor edge to cut sutures.

Towel clips

These are used to attach drapes and equipment to the surgical site (Fig. 19.13):

- Backhaus and Mayo clips have a ringed handle and curved, fang-like jaws
- Grays cross-action clips have a strong gripping action, which is traumatic to the skin.

Sponge-holding forceps

These are used to hold swabs and for skin preparation prior to surgery. The most common type is Rampley.

General orthopaedic instruments

Osteotome, chisel and gouge (Fig. 19.14)

- Available in several sizes
- Used to divide or shape bone or cartilage
- An osteotome has an edge that is tapered evenly on both sides
- A chisel has one tapered side only, giving the appearance of a step

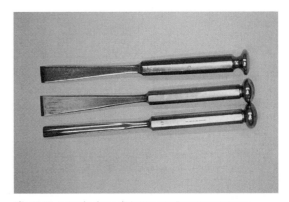

Fig. 19.14 General orthopaedic instruments. From top: osteotome; chisel; gouge.

- A gouge has a groove in its shaft to allow bone or cartilage to be scooped out.

Mallet

- Used to tap bone staples into place
- Used with osteotome, chisel or gouge to remove bone.

Curette

- Has a sharp-edged oval-shaped cup to remove tissue
- Volkmann scoop is commonly used: has cups of different sizes at each end of shaft, tends to bend easily and handle is uncomfortable to grip.

Periosteal elevators
- Used to lift periosteum and soft tissue from bone
- Variety of types available.

Bone rongeurs and cutters
- Rongeurs are used to remove tiny fragments of bone or cartilage
- Bone cutters are designed to cut larger pieces of bone, e.g. dorsal spinous processes (Fig. 19.15).

Bone-holding forceps (Fig. 19.16)
These are designed to grip and hold bone fragments in place during reduction and repair of fractures.

Retractors
- General retractors often used in orthopaedic work
- Gelpi retractors are particularlty useful (Fig. 19.17)
- Hohmann retractors are designed to retract muscle, tendons and ligaments (Fig. 19.18).

Bone rasps
These are useful to produce a smooth edge when pieces of bone are removed, e.g. following amputation of part of a splint bone.

Wire cutter and forceps
Wire cutters and twisting forceps are used for applying cerclage wires, e.g. for repair of a fractured mandible.

Drills
Air- and battery-driven bone drills are an essential item in an equine clinic performing orthopaedic surgery. Hand drills have little place except for minor procedures where little drilling is required, e.g. drilling holes in the hoof wall.

Air drills
- Expensive initial outlay
- Require a supply of medical air, either cylinder or piped supply into theatre
- Specifically designed for surgery
- Easily sterilised.

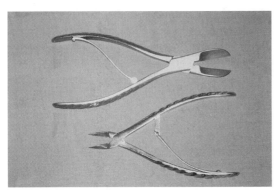

Fig. 19.15 Bone cutters.

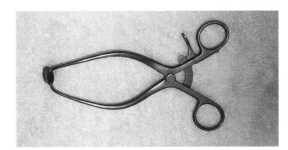

Fig. 19.17 Gelpi retractor.

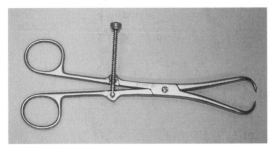

Fig. 19.16 Bone-holding forceps.

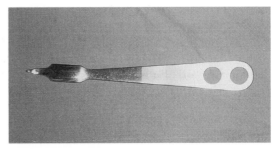

Fig. 19.18 Hohmann retractor.

Battery drills

- Relatively inexpensive
- No air supply needed
- Speed may be too slow for some procedures
- Not specifically designed for surgery and may be cumbersome to use
- Sterilisation can be a probem because they are plastic coated
- Battery may go flat during use; recharge after each use.

Oscillating saw/burr

- Air supply needed
- Useful for osteotomies, sinus flap surgery, hoof wall and sole resection, removal of dorsal spinous processes
- Care needed to ensure safe use.

Instruments for fracture repair

The equine nurse should be familiar with the different internal fixation techniques that are used in equine orthopaedic surgery and the equipment required. Methods of internal fixation may include:

- Lag screw fixation: the most common method used
- Bone plate and screw fixation
- Cerclage wire
- Intramedullary pins.

There are a range of different sizes of both screws and plates. Choice will depend largely on the site of injury and the size of the fragments. Many clinics will stock only instrumentation of the most commonly used size: 4.5- and 5.5-mm screws.

For fracture repair a *general instrument set* is needed (see Summary 19.1) plus the following sets of instruments.

General orthopaedic instruments

- Osteotomes
- Long-handled curettes
- Mallet
- Hohmann retractor
- Ferris Smith rongeurs

Summary 19.1

General instrument set

- Scalpel, handle size 3 (×1)
- Toothed dissecting forceps:
  fine (×1)
  heavy (×2)
- Plain dissecting forceps (×1)
- Scissors, Mayo (×2)
- Scissors, Metzenbaum (×1)
- Artery forceps (×10)
- Allis tissue forceps (×4)
- Suture scissors (×1)
- Needle-holders (×2)
- Retractors:
  Langenbeck (×2)
  Gelpi (×2)
- Towel-holding forceps (×15)
- Bowl/kidney dish (×2)
- Swabs (3 × 5)
- Scalpel blades (few of each size used)

- Wireholding and cutting forceps
- Bone-holding forceps: reduction forceps/condylar clamps.

Association for the study of internal fixation (ASIF) equipment

A 4.5-mm set (Fig. 19.19)
- Drill bit, 4.5-mm (×2)
- Drill bit, 3.2-mm (×2)
- Tap, 4.5-mm (×2)
- Tap sleeve/drill guide, 4.5-mm (×1)
- Drill insert, 3.2-mm (×1)
- Tap handle (×1)
- Countersink, 4.5/5.5-mm (×1)
- Depth gauge, large (×1)
- Large screwdriver (×1)
- Cortex screws, 4.5-mm, length 14–105 mm (5 of each).

A 5.5-mm set
- Drill bit, 5.5-mm (×2)
- Drill bit, 4.0-mm (×2)
- Tap, 5.5-mm (×2)

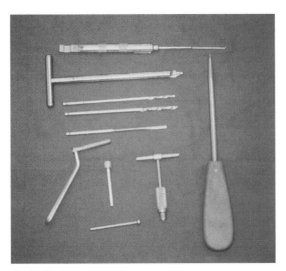

Fig. 19.19 ASIF instruments, 4.5-mm set.

- Tap handle (×1)
- Tap sleeve/drill guide, 5.5-mm (×1)
- Drill insert, 4.0-mm (×1)
- Depth gauge, large (×1)
- Countersink, 4.5/5.5-mm (×1)
- Large screwdriver (×1)
- Cortex screws, 5.5-mm, length 24–100 mm (5 of each)

A 3.5-mm set
- Drill bit, 3.5-mm (×2)
- Drill bit, 2.5-mm (×2)
- Tap, 3.5-mm (×2)
- Tap handle (×1)
- Tap sleeve/drill guide, 3.5-mm (×1)
- Drill insert, 2.5-mm (×1)
- Depth gauge, small (×1)
- Countersink, 3.5-mm (×1)
- Small screwdriver (×1)
- Cortex screws, 3.5-mm, length 8–50 mm (5 of each)

A 2.7-mm set
- Drill bit, 2.7-mm (×2)
- Drill bit, 2.00-mm (×2)
- Tap, 2.7-mm (×2)
- Tap handle (×1)
- Tap sleeve/drill guide, 2.7-mm (×1)
- Drill insert, 2.00-mm (×1)

- Countersink, 2.7-mm (×1)
- Small screwdriver (×1)
- Cortex screws, 2.7-mm, length 6–45 mm (5 of each)

Plate fixation
- Selection of narrow 4.5-mm dynamic compression plates (DCPs), from 4-hole to 18-hole
- Selection of broad 4.5-mm DCPs, from 8-hole to 18-hole
- Loaded/neutral drill guide, 4.5-mm (×1)
- Tension device (×1)
- Plate bending press (×1)
- Bending irons (×1)

Plates and loaded/neutral drill guides are also available for 3.5-mm and 2.7-mm screws. Most equine practices will not stock these because they are not commonly used in equine surgery. Usually they can be borrowed from an associated small animal clinic if necessary.

Also required are:

- Air drill/battery drill
- Oscillating saw
- Monofilament wire: 0.6-mm, 0.8-mm, 1.2-mm

Equipment for arthroscopy

Arthroscopic procedures are among the most common orthopaedic procedures performed on horses. The nurse needs to be familiar with both the instruments and the electrical components of this type of equipment.

Arthroscopy instruments (Figs 19.20–19.24)
- Arthroscopic cannula
- Conical obturator
- Hook probe
- McIlwraith elevator
- Osteotome, 4-mm
- 1-mm Bruns curette straight
- 2-mm Bruns curette straight
- 4-mm Bruns curette straight
- 6-mm Bruns curette straight
- 2-mm Bruns curette curved
- 4-mm Bruns curette curved
- 2-mm Ferris Smith rongeurs straight
- 3-mm Ferris Smith rongeurs straight

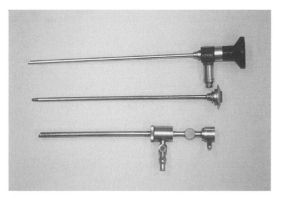

Fig. 19.20 From top: arthroscope; arthroscopic cannula; conical obturator.

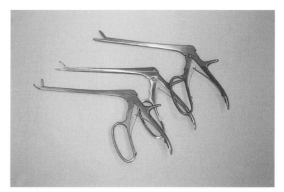

Fig. 19.22 Ferris Smith rongeurs.

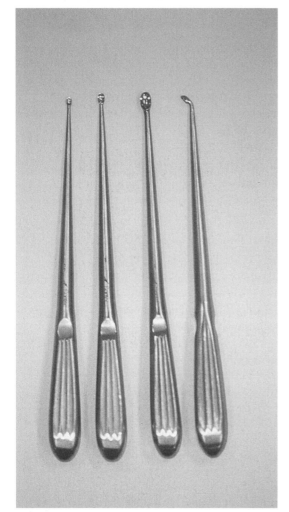

Fig. 19.21 Bruns curettes.

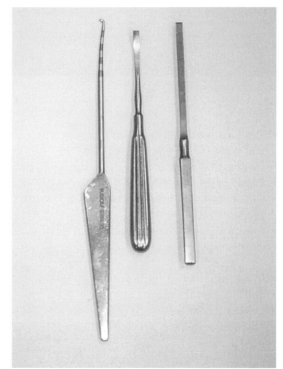

Fig. 19.23 From left: Hook probe; McIlwraith elevator; osteotome.

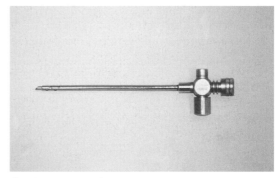

Fig. 19.24 Egress cannula.

- 4-mm Ferris Smith rongeurs straight
- 6-mm Ferris Smith rongeurs straight
- 3-mm Ferris Smith rongeurs angled up
- 3-mm Ferris Smith rongeurs angled down
- Egress cannula

Fibre-optic equipment (Fig. 19.25)
- Arthroscope 4-mm 30 lens
- Light cable
- Camera

Motorised power tools
- Handset
- Probes for handset: burr, synovial resectors
- Power unit for handset: with footswitch

Arthroscopy monitoring units (Fig. 19.26)
- Television monitor
- Light source: xenon/halogen
- Video camera unit
- Video recorder

Additional equipment
- Fluid pump and delivery system (see Fig. 19.27)
- Suction apparatus (see Fig. 19.28)

General instruments
- Scalpel handle and size 11 blade
- Rat-toothed forceps
- Needleholders
- Suture scissors

Equipment for laparoscopy

For *laparoscopy*, similar monitoring equipment is required as for arthroscopy. Instrumentation is very similar in design but much longer in length. A supply of carbon dioxide will be needed to visualise structures rather than fluid.

Instruments for other procedures

Colic surgery
- General instrument set (see Summary 19.1)
- Fluid irrigation
- Sterile towels
- Bowel clamps
- Mechanical stapling device (for bowel resection)
- Viscera retainer
- Sterile hose connection for flushing large bowel

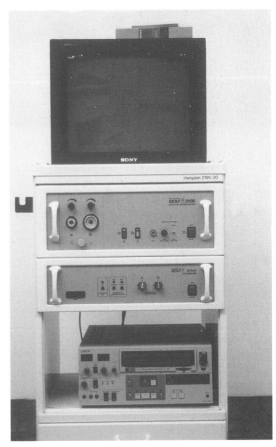

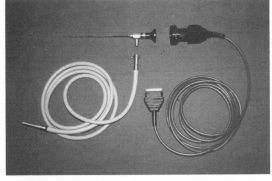

Fig. 19.25 Arthroscopy fibre-optic equipment: arthroscope, light cable and camera.

Fig. 19.26 Arthroscopy monitoring unit.

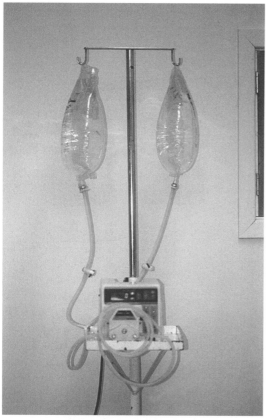

Fig. 19.27 Fluid pump and delivery system.

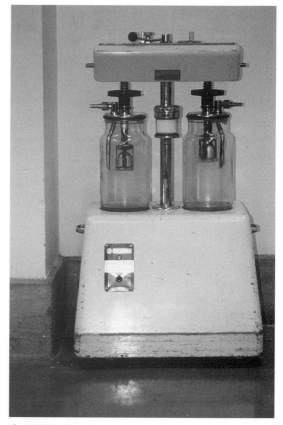

Fig. 19.28 Suction apparatus.

- Collection tub for evacuated bowel contents
- In addition: viscera tray attachment for operating table, to allow bowel to be laid out and examined

Dental/sinus surgery
- Mouth gag
- Oscillating saw
- Dental punches
- Horsley's trephine
- Long dental forceps
- Dental rasps
- Osteotome and mallet
- Curettes

Castration
- Scalpel handle and blade
- Toothed dissecting forceps
- Scissors

- Long artery forceps, e.g. Roberts
- Emasculators

Ophthalmic surgery
- Scalpel handle size 7, blades 11 and 15
- Fine dissecting forceps
- Fine scissors
- Corneal scissors
- Capsule forceps
- Castroviejo needle-holders
- Eyelid speculum
- Irrigating cannula
- Ophthalmic swabs

Care and maintenance of surgical instruments

New instruments should be lubricated with an instrument lubricant spray before sterilisation.

Cleaning after use

- All sharps, such as needles and blades, should be removed and disposed of safely
- Clean as soon as possible after use to prevent saline, blood and chemicals causing damage to metal
- Soak in cold water or proprietary solution to remove gross debris; open joints/dismantle where appropriate
- Wash items individually using warm running water and brush, paying attention to joints/ratchets and moveable parts
- Avoid using abrasive agents or wire brushes, which might damage metal
- Rinse under running water and lay out to dry
- When dry, lubricate with water-soluble instrument lubricant
- Re-assemble instrument set, inspecting each instrument individually for cleanliness and damage

Ultrasonic cleaners

- Benchtop models available; may be suitable for equine use
- Most effective method of cleaning instruments
- Work by production of sinusoidal energy waves with vibration frequency of 20 000/s
- Instruments should have excess debris rinsed off prior to placement in the cleaner; water and a commercial cleaning agent are added and the machine switched on for a variable amount of time, approximately 15 min
- Instruments then are removed, rinsed and examined as before, prior to re-packing

Cleaning of compressed air machines

- Air-driven and electrical equipment never should be immmersed in water or ultrasonically cleaned.
- The handpiece should be detached from the air hose and wiped over thoroughly with a soft cloth and proprietary cleaning agent, paying particular attention to the triggers and couplings. It is then rinsed without immersing totally in water. The air hose can be cleaned in the same way. The instrument then should be lubricated using the manufacturer's recommended solution, re-

connected to the air supply and the trigger pressed for approximately 20 s so that oil is dissipated. Excess oil then is wiped off and the machine packed for sterilisation.
- Most air machines may be autoclaved safely but the manufacturer's recommendations always should be followed.
- Ethylene oxide is suitable for all air- and battery-driven equipment and there is usually less risk of damage to the equipment.

Care of arthroscopy and laparoscopy equipment

- Instruments should be washed in the usual fashion.
- The arthroscope/laparoscope, camera, light cable and power tools should be handled with great care because they are very easily damaged.
- Each item should be disassembled and washed by hand under running warm water immediately after use.
- Care should be taken to avoid soaking the connecting plugs (even though many are designed to be immersible).
- Dry each item carefully and inspect for damage.
- Pack for sterilisation.
- Arthroscopy/laparoscopy instruments may be autoclaved safely.
- Camera, light cable, power tools and arthroscope/laparoscope should be sterilised using ethylene oxide whenever possible but, because this is a 12-h process, between cases it will be necessary to use a chemical solution to soak them and then they must be rinsed with sterile water prior to use.

Suture materials

Suture material may be:

(1) Absorbable or non-absorbable.
(2) Natural or synthetic.
(3) Monofilament or multifilament.

Choice will depend on many factors. No material fulfils all requirements. Some desirable characteristics of suture material are:

- High tensile strength

- Good knot security: ties easily, without tendency to slip
- Minimal tissue reaction

Common absorbable suture material

Catgut
- Made from the submucosa of sheep small intestine
- Produces significant tissue reaction
- Largely superseded by newer synthetic absorbable materials
- Absorbed by phagocytosis and enzyme degradation
- Absorption rate affected by blood supply, infection and tissue pH
- 'Chromic' catgut treated with chromic salts to try to decrease tissue reaction and increase strength
- Loses tensile strength rapidly
- Handles well

Polyglactin 910 ('Vicryl', Ethicon)
- Copolymer of lactide and glycolide
- Absorbed by hydrolysis
- Commonly used in equine surgery
- Some tissue reaction
- Coated to improve handling
- Loses 50% strength in 14 days and totally absorbed in 60–90 days
- Has considerable tissue drag
- Braided multifilament
- Commonly used for abdominal closure: size 8 (metric)

Polyglycolic acid ('Dexon', Davis & Geck)
- Polyester made from hydroxyacetic acid
- Absorbed by hydrolysis
- Braided, may be coated or uncoated
- Loses 30% strength in 7 days and 80% in 14 days
- Poor knot security
- Considerable tissue drag

Polydioxanone ('PDS', Ethicon)
- Monofilament
- Absorbed by hydrolysis
- Tissue reaction minimal
- Synthetic

- Loses 30% strength in 14 days and only minimally absorbed at 90 days
- Tissue drag minimal
- Ideal in infected sites
- Springiness affects handling

Polyglyconate ('Maxon', Davis & Geck)
- Similar properties to polydioxanone
- Synthetic
- Monofilament

Polyglecaprone ('Monocryl', Ethicon)
- Newer material
- Monofilament
- Synthetic
- Handles well
- Tissue reaction minimal
- Absorbed by hydrolysis
- Only 30% tensile strength left at 14 days
- Tissue drag minimal
- Useful in gastrointestinal and urogenital tracts and muscosa

Common non-absorbable suture material

Non-absorbable suture material maintains strength for longer than 60 days and becomes encapsulated within fibrous tissue. It is used where prolonged mechanical support is needed and the main indications for use are:

- Skin sutures
- Slow-healing tissue

Polypropylene ('Prolene', Ethicon)
- Inert
- Monofilament
- Great tensile strength
- Reasonable handling properties
- May stretch and snap if crushed by instruments
- Variable knot security
- Little tissue drag

Polyamide ('Ethilon', Ethicon; 'Supramid')
- Monofilament or multifilament
- Monofilament: little tissue drag or reaction; poor handling characteristics; poor knot security

- Multifilament: braided and sheathed; should not be buried; capillarity; some tissue drag

Polyesters ('Ethibond' and 'Mersilene', Ethicon)
- Braided
- Good handling charcteristics
- Retain tensile strength
- Some coated to improve handling
- Poor knot-tying characteristics
- Some show capillarity

Stainless steel

- Rarely used nowadays
- Monofilament/multifilament
- Inert
- Strong
- Poor handling and knot-tying characteristics
- Useful in slow-healing tissue, e.g. linea alba break-down after colic surgery

Silk
- Braided usually
- Good handling and knot-tying characteristics
- Good tensile strength
- Risk of capillarity
- Less popular than used to be

Linen
Linen has been largely superseded by newer products.

Sizes of suture material

Sizes of suture material can be confusing. In the UK and Europe metric sizes now tend to be used whereas in the USA US Pharmacopeia (USP) sizes are used (Table 19.3).

Alternatives to sutures

Staples
Metal staples for use in the skin or other tissues are now used routinely in equine surgery.

Skin staples
- Quick and easy to insert
- Inert

Table 19.3 Sizes of suture material

Metric	USP (non-absorbable and synthetic absorbable)	Catgut
0.2	10/0	
0.3	9/0	
0.4	8/0	
0.5	7/0	8/0
0.7	6/0	7/0
1	5/0	6/0
1.5	4/0	5/0
2	3/0	4/0
3	2/0	3/0
3.5	0	2/0
4	1	0
5	2	1
6	3 and 4	2
7	5	3
8	6	4

- Easy to remove
- Cause little tissue reaction
- Stapling guns are designed to be disposable but may be sterilised using ethylene oxide

Gastrointestinal stapling devices
- Designed for human use but adapted for equine alimentary tract
- Expensive
- Disposable, but can be cleaned and gas sterilised
- Time saving
- Inert
- Linear cutter: for anastomosis
- Permit resection of areas of bowel that would be inaccessible to routine surgery

Ligaclips
- Metal clips used as ligatures
- Time saving where large blood supply to be ligated, e.g. mesentery with colics
- Inert
- Expensive

Packaging of suture materials

Individual packets
- Method of choice: better sepsis

- Pre-sterilised
- Variety of needle shapes and sizes
- Relatively expensive
- Large stock may be needed
- Synthetic absorbable materials all packaged this way

Cassettes
- Multi-use cassettes commonly used in equine practice
- Threat to asepsis because contamination is likely over time
- Inexpensive
- Variable quality
- Used for polyamides, catgut and stainless-steel wire

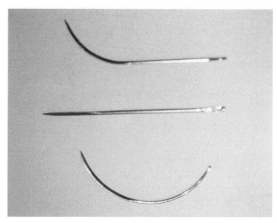

Fig. 19.29 Suture needles: different longitudinal shapes..

Suture needles

Swaged needles
- These are needles that are attached to the suture needle and therefore do not need threading
- Most pre-packaged sutures have swaged needles
- Also known as 'atraumatic' needles because trauma to tissue is minimised by the smooth junction between the suture and needle
- Needle in perfect condition each time
- Variety of shapes and sizes of needle for all types of suture material

Eyed needles
- Require threading
- Variable quality
- Blunt and bend readily
- Tend to be used for skin

Needle shape
(1) Longitudinal shape (Fig. 19.29).
(2) Cross-sectional shape:
   (a) *Round bodied*. No cutting edge; designed to go through delicate structures such as mucosa.
   (b) *Modified point*. The *taper-cut* needle has a cutting tip and a round body. This allows penetration of denser tissue without increasing tissue trauma. The *trocar point* needle has a strong cutting tip and a robust round body. The *Mayo* needle is a variation of this. It has a large eye and a trocar tip with a dense half-circle-round body.
   (c) *Cutting needle*. Used in dense tissue, e.g. skin. Cross-sectional appearance is usually triangular.
   (d) *Micro-point*. Very fine needle with a sharp cutting edge, e.g. for ophthalmological work.

Special equipment

Diathermy

- Used for cutting and coagulation of tissues using high-frequency alternating currents, producing local heat at the site of application
- Used to control haemorrhage
- Reduces amount of ligatures needed and decreases surgery time
- Probe may be applied either directly to tissues or to a haemostat applied to the tissue
- The lead and handpiece may be autoclaved readily
- A contact plate is placed under the patient and connected to the machine to provide grounding to the current; insufficient earthing will result in a direct contact burn to the patient
- The machine is operated using a footswitch
- Machines should be serviced regularly

Cryosurgery

- Cryosurgery destroys tissue by application of extreme cold.
- Liquid nitrogen is used as the refrigerant agent.
- A small flask container is available, which is filled with liquid nitrogen and variable sized probes or a spray are used to apply it to the horse, e.g. for sarcoid removal.
- Great care must be taken when using liquid nitrogen: wear gloves and protective goggles when using or filling cannister; avoid splashing clothes, skin or touching metal probes used for freezing.
- After use the pressure in the cannister is allowed to fall, and when thawed the probes and flask can be washed in a proprietary detergent. The probes then can be autoclaved or gas sterilised.

Suction apparatus

- Used for aspiration of fluids and blood from body cavities and surgical wounds

- For equine work, where there may be considerable volumes of fluid, a machine with two fluid collection bottles is desirable
- The bottles should be autoclavable
- The machine should be serviced regularly

Hazards in the operating theatre

There are many potential hazards in the operating theatre (see Chapter 9).

Reading list

Auer, J.A. & Stick, J.A. (1999) *Equine Surgery*, 2nd edn. WB Saunders, London.

Lane, D. & Cooper, B. (1999) *Veterinary Nursing*. Butterworth-Heinemann, Oxford.

McIlwraith, C.W. (1990) *Diagnostic and Surgical Arthroscopy in the Horse*. Lea & Febiger, Philadelphia, PA.

McIlwraith, C.W. & Turner, S. (1988) *Equine Surgery: Advanced Techniques*. Lea & Febiger, Philadelphia, PA.

Nixon, A. (1996) *Equine Fracture Repair*, 1st edn. WB Saunders, London.

Tracy, D.L. (2000) *Small Animal Surgical Nursing*, 3rd edn. Mosby, London.

Anaesthesia

J. C. Murrell & C. B. Johnson

Equine anaesthesia for complex surgical procedures is now more common. It remains challenging because the peri-operative mortality rate in horses is significantly higher compared with humans and small animals.

Standing chemical restraint of the horse

Sedation of horses is routine for many husbandry and veterinary procedures when other methods of restraint are unsuccessful (see Chapter 1). The medicines used have been classified traditionally as tranquillisers, sedatives or hypnotics. It is more useful to classify the different drugs on the basis of pharmacological mechanism of action. Using this system, drugs in the same class have similar properties and side effects (Table 20.1).

Local anaesthetic agents and techniques in horses

In horses, patient cooperation limits the usefulness of local anaesthesia alone. However these techniques can be a useful adjunct to general anaesthesia and sedation (Table 20.2).

Mechanism of action of local anaesthetic agents

Local anaesthetic agents block the transmission of action potentials along nerve fibres. The mechanism involves the blockade of sodium channels, preventing depolarisation of the nerve membrane. Duration of action is determined by protein binding and vasoactivity. Protein binding increases duration of action. Agents that vasodilate local blood vessels have a shorter duration of action, because this increases removal and metabolism of the drug. Adrenaline commonly is added to local anaesthetic preparations to produce vasoconstriction. This improves the quality and duration of anaesthesia by reducing systemic absorption and metabolism of the local anaesthetic agent. The use of local anaesthetic solutions containing adrenaline for epidural administration is controversial.

Different types of local anaesthetic block

- Topical analgesia: direct application of local anaesthetic agents to the skin or mucous membranes, e.g. to facilitate ophthalmic examination.
- Intrasynovial anaesthesia: a form of topical analgesia where the agent is injected into synovial structures.

Table 20.1 Agents commonly used for chemical restraint in horses

Class of agent	Mechanism of action	Clinical effects	Side effects	Metabolism
α_2-Agonists (e.g. detomidine, romifidine, xylazine)	• Activation of α_2 adrenoceptors in the CNS • Analgesia is mediated by action at central and peripheral adrenoceptors	• Potent sedation • Muscle relaxation • Analgesia	• Initial hypertension followed by severe hypotension • Bradycardia • Respiratory system depression • Hypothermia • Sweating • Hyperglycaemia • Increased urination • May cause abortion • Ataxia	Liver metabolism and renal excretion
Phenothiazines (e.g. acepromazine maleate)	• Dopamine antagonist • Inhibition of catecholamine activity in the CNS	• Calming • Anti-emetic • Anti-arrhythmic • Antihistamine	• Hypotension due to blockade of peripheral α_1-receptors and a direct vasodilator effect • Hypothermia • Penile protrusion • Use reduced doses in foals and animals with liver dysfunction/ cardiovascular compromise	Liver metabolism and renal excretion
Benzodiazepines (e.g. diazepam, midazolam)	• Potentiate the action of inhibitory neurotransmitters, particularly GABA in the CNS • Specific benzodiazepine receptors adjacent to the GABA receptor complex	• Not sedative • Calming • Hypnosis • Muscle relaxation • Anticonvulsant action • Useful for sedation of young foals	• Minimal cardiovascular or respiratory side effects	Liver metabolism and renal excretion
Opioids	• Act at opioid receptor sites in CNS and other tissues • Act as agonists, antagonists or a combination of both	• Analgesia • Synergistic effect when used in combination with other classes of drugs	• Increased locomotor activity • Respiratory depression • Miosis • Reduced gastrointestinal motility • Euphoria	Liver metabolism and renal excretion

• Infiltration analgesia: direct infiltration into tissue to affect local nerve endings. The technique is used for minor surgical procedures in the standing horse, e.g. wound repair.

• Regional analgesia: the blockade of specific sensory nerves. Small volumes of agent are targeted at specific anatomical sites. A good knowledge of anatomy is essential. Distal limb nerve blocks are examples of regional analgesia.

• Spinal analgesia: the injection of a local anaesthetic agent into some part of the spinal canal. During subarachnoid or intrathecal injection the agent is delivered into the cerebrospinal fluid. This technique is used rarely in horses. Local anaesthetic may be injected into the epidural space, where the needle enters the spinal canal but does not penetrate the meninges. This more commonly is used in horses, e.g. for urogenital surgery.

Systemic and toxic effects of local anaesthetics

Local anaesthetic agents can have systemic ill effects

Table 20.2 Pharmacology of the local anaesthetic agents commonly used in horses

Local anaesthetic agent	Class of agent	Clinical pharmacology	Comments
Lignocaine hydrochloride	Amide	• Rapid onset of action • Duration of action 90–180 min • 2% Solution used for infiltration and local nerve blocks • 4% Solution used in topical preparations	• Preparation containing adrenaline available • Can be irritant to tissue • Multiple nerve blocks may result in tissue swelling
Mepivacaine hydrochloride	Amide	• Rapid onset of action • Duration of action longer than lignocaine because of less vasodilator action • 2% Solution used for infiltration and local nerve blocks	• Commonly used in clinical practice, particularly for nerve blocks of the distal limb • Less irritant to tissue than lignocaine • Less effective topically than lignocaine • Preparation containing adrenaline available
Bupivacaine hydrochloride	Amide	• Slow onset of action • Prolonged duration of action 180–500 min • More potent than lignocaine and mepivacaine, used at concentrations of 0.124%–0.75%	• Preparation containing adrenaline available

when they are absorbed in high concentration. This can result from inadvertent intravascular injection or absorption from tissues. Accurate placement of peripheral nerve blocks minimises the dose of local anaesthetic agent required. Care should be taken during infiltration analgesia to avoid the injection of large volumes of agent. More potent local anaesthetic agents such as bupivicaine can be diluted to reduce the risk of inadvertent overdose.

Effect on the central nervous system
High concentrations of local anaesthetic drugs cause seizures. At lower concentrations, agents cause sedation and have an anticonvulsant action.

Effect on the cardiovascular system
Lignocaine is used clinically for the treatment of ventricular arrhythmias. At high concentrations all local anaesthetic agents depress myocardial function.

Local toxic effects
Large doses cause local tissue and nerve damage. This may result in delayed wound healing.

Analgesia for the equine surgical patient

During general anaesthesia the animal is unconscious and incapable of experiencing pain. Peri-operative analgesia (i.e. before and after surgery) is a critical component of any anaesthetic regime. If inadequate, it can prolong recovery and produce more long-term pain.

Administration of analgesic drugs before the start of surgery, termed pre-emptive analgesia, is recommended. Pre-emptive analgesia contributes to balanced anaesthesia and reduces post-operative pain.

Recognition of pain in horses

Analgesic drug administration should be appropriate for the degree and type of pain experienced by the animal, but recognising pain in horses can be difficult, particularly in more stoical breeds, e.g. cobs. Pain scoring systems to aid decisions about peri-operative analgesic currently are not well developed in horses, but recognising signs of discomfort e.g. behaviour changes, is an important part of nursing.

Classes of analgesics

- Opioids
- Non-steroidal anti-inflammatory drugs (NSAIDs)
- Local anaesthetic agents
- α_2-agonists
- Ketamine

Opioids

(1) Actions of the opioids:
    (a) Analgesia.
    (b) Sedation.
(2) Mechanism of action:
    (a) Opioid analgesic agents produce their effects by action at endogenous opioid receptors.
(3) Clinical use:
    (a) Butorphanol is commonly used to provide analgesia and sedation, particularly in combination with other medication. In comparison with morphine, it has weak analgesic efficacy.
    (b) Opioid agonists are schedule 2 controlled medicines and subject to restrictions regarding purchase, storage and record keeping.
(4) Metabolism:
    (a) Liver metabolism.
(5) Side effects:
    (a) Opioid agonists can produce central nervous system (CNS) excitement and increased locomotor activity in horses, which can manifest as box walking and restlessness. Until recently, these side effects have limited the use of potent opioids in this species.
    (b) Ileus.
    (c) Respiratory depression, unlikely with routine clinical use.

Non-steroidal anti-inflammatory drugs (NSAIDs)

(1) Actions of NSAIDs:
    (a) Analgesia.
    (b) Anti-inflammatory.
    (c) Antipyretic.
    (d) Anti-endotoxic.
(2) Mechanism of action:
    (a) Peripheral action to inhibit the production of tissue prostaglandins by inhibition of the enzyme cyclooxygenase, which mediates inflammation.
    (b) Central nervous system action mediating analgesia.
(3) Clinical use:
    (a) All NSAIDs have similar side effects. Avoid concurrent administration of more than one agent.
    (b) Do not use in animals less than 6 weeks of age; reduced liver metabolism increases the risk of toxicity.
    (c) Care in animals with disease predisposing to gastrointestinal ulceration; particularly foals.
(4) Metabolism:
    (a) Liver metabolism.
(5) Side effects:
    (a) Gastrointestinal ulceration is the most significant side effect.
    (b) Renal toxicity.
    (c) Hepatotoxicity.
    (d) Blood dyscrasias.

Phenylbutazone

- Available as intravenous injection, oral powder or oral paste
- Highly protein bound, avoid administration during anaesthesia
- Oral preparations bind to hay, delaying absorption from the gastrointestinal tract
- Oral preparations licensed for long-term use to treat musculoskeletal disorders

Flunixin meglumine

- Available as intravenous injection, oral granules or paste
- Commonly used to treat endotoxaemia
- Licensed for short-term use (3–5 days)

Carprofen

- Available as intravenous injection and oral granules
- Licensed for short-term use

Ketoprofen

- Available as intravenous injection
- Licensed for short-term use

Meclofenamic acid

- Available as oral granules
- Licensed for long-term use in the treatment of musculoskeletal disorders

Local anaesthetic agents

See section on local anaesthetic agents and techniques above. Local anaesthetic agents can provide good peri-operative analgesia, particularly if long-acting drugs such as bupivacaine are used. Care should be taken with the intraoperative administration of distal limb nerve blocks to avoid blockade of motor nerves. This may contribute to an uncoordinated and poor recovery from anaesthesia.

α_2-Agonists
- See Table 20.1 for pharmacology and clinical use
- α_2-agonists are used primarily for their potent sedative action
- The agents also have an analgesic action, mediated by an effect on adrenoceptors located in the CNS

Ketamine
Ketamine is principally used as an anaesthetic agent in equine anaesthesia. It has a potent analgesic action.

Pre-operative preparation of the patient

General anaesthesia must be preceded by appropriate preparation of the patient. Elective surgical cases ideally should arrive at the clinic at least 1 day before surgery. This allows time for the animal to calm down after transport and to be evaluated thoroughly.

Clinical examination of the horse prior to anaesthesia

History
A complete history always should be obtained before anaesthesia:

- History of previous anaesthesia
- Known adverse drug reactions or allergy
- Current drug therapy
- Careful attention should be paid to history relating to chronic lung infection or evidence of chronic obstructive pulmonary disease
- Careful questioning relating to exertional rhabdomyolysis, because such horses may be at greater risk of developing post-anaesthetic myopathy
- Stable management and behaviour.

Physical examination
A complete physical examination should be performed before general anaesthesia, with particular emphasis on the cardiovascular and respiratory systems, plus checking for any pre-existing lameness or other injuries. If no abnormalities are detected on a thorough routine clinical examination, it is not necessary to perform further laboratory screening tests to establish normality.

Assessment of anaesthetic risk
Anaesthetic risk relates to the skill of the anaesthetist, the facilities available and the pre-operative physical state of the animal. The American Society of Anaesthesiologists (ASA) has devised a system to classify anaesthetic risk. Termed the ASA system, it has been adopted widely by vets. It is useful because it aids the identification of high-risk cases. The assignment is made after a complete history and physical examination. If the case is an emergency, an 'E' is added to the allocated number:

I   Healthy patient
II   Mild systemic disease, no functional limitation
III   Severe systemic disease, definite functional limitation
IV   Severe systemic disease that is a constant threat to life
V   Moribund patient unlikely to survive 24 h with or without operation.

Preparation of the horse for surgery

Bodyweight
Anaesthetic doses are calculated on the basis of bodyweight. A weigh scale is the only method to obtain an accurate weight. The scales should be located in close proximity to the surgical facilities. Formulae to estimate weight based on girth width and the height of the horse or weigh bands are available. Both are relatively inaccurate.

Starving
Starvation for 12 h before anaesthesia will reduce the volume of the gastrointestinal system. The pres-

sure imposed by the weight of a full abdomen compromises diaphragmatic movement and contributes to hypoventilation, particularly when the horse is positioned in dorsal recumbency.

Removal of water

It is not necessary to remove water. Clear fluids are rapidly absorbed from the stomach and deprivation of water may result in dehydration.

Removal of shoes

Removing the shoes and cleaning the feet before the horse enters the induction area reduces contamination of the surgical facilities. The shoes may cause trauma to the horse or personnel during induction and may damage the floor of the induction area. When shoe removal is not possible, boots or bandages can be placed over the shoes before induction and the shoes removed during surgery.

Grooming

Grooming and placing a tail bandage prior to anaesthesia reduces contamination of the surgical facilities.

Mouth cleansing

The mouth is rinsed out before anaesthesia to remove food debris. This prevents food being pushed down the trachea during intubation.

Other preparation

Ideally, clip the surgical site before induction to minimise anaesthesia time.

Premedication

Premedication is the administration of an appropriate medication prior to anaesthesia to facilitate induction, maintenance and recovery. It is an integral part of any anaesthetic regime.

The aims of premedication are to:

- Calm the patient
- Provide analgesia and muscle relaxation
- Decrease anaesthetic requirements
- Minimise side effects of general anaesthetic agents

- Promote a smooth recovery
- Continue therapeutic regimes through anaesthesia, e.g. the treatment of chronic diseases such as chronic obstructive pulmonary disease (COPD).

Routes of administration

Intramuscular

Intramuscular administration leads to quick and reliable absorption. It is the common route for pre-anaesthetic drugs but not for the administration of anaesthesia induction agents.

Intravenous

Direct administration into the circulation produces the fastest onset and most reliable effect. Administration of anaesthesia induction agents intravenously should be via an intravenous catheter. Medicines for premedication are also used for chemical restraint in horses.

Phenothiazines (e.g. acepromazine maleate)

Acepromazine maleate is an important component of premedication regimes in horses (see Table 20.1). Premedication with acepromazine maleate may be significant in reducing equine anaesthetic mortality, possibly due to an anti-arrhythmic action. Its recommended dose range for premedication is wide and its sedative effect in horses is very variable but increasing the dose does not generally increase sedation. Low doses are less likely to produce significant side effects, particularly hypotension. Acepromazine maleate has a long duration of action and also smoothes recovery from anaesthesia.

Opioid drugs

Opioids are not used routinely as part of the premedication regime for horses. This is due to concerns about opioid-induced excitement in horses. In combination with other sedative agents such as a phenothiazine, excitement is unlikely to occur. Neuroleptanalgesia refers specifically to the combination of a neuroleptic or tranquillising drug such as acepromazine and an opioid drug. Administration of an opioid agent as a premedicant will provide peri-operative analgesia and contribute to a balanced anaesthetic technique (see earlier section on analgesia).

α_2-Agonists

α_2-Agonists may be administered as a premedicant with some intravenous induction techniques (see Table 20.1). In these cases the α_2-agonist provides sedation, particularly prior to induction regimes incorporating glyceryl guaiacolate ether (GGE). Following intravenous administration, it may take 5 min before maximum sedative effects are achieved. Sedation is less effective if the horse is stimulated during this period. The agents should be used cautiously in animals with cardiovascular compromise.

Anticholinergic compounds

There is no rationale for the routine premedication of horses with anticholinergic agents, unlike with small animals.

General anaesthesia of the horse

General anaesthesia can be divided into three phases:

- Induction
- Maintenance
- Recovery.

General anaesthesia in theatre conditions

Facilities recommended for general anaesthesia include:

- Padded area for induction and recovery adjacent to the surgical theatre
- Equipment to move the horse between the induction or recovery area and theatre
- Large animal anaesthetic machine, oxygen supply and rebreathing circuit.

Field anaesthesia

Generally only short minor surgical procedures are performed under field conditions. Anaesthesia is induced and maintained using intravenous techniques. The area chosen for induction of anaesthesia should be open, with no walls or fences on which the horse can injure itself during induction or recovery. The ground should be flat and free of objects that might injure the horse.

Physiological effects

Anaesthesia produces major physiological changes in the horse. Normal homeostatic mechanisms designed to ensure optimal function of the body systems are depressed. It is important to provide adequate support of organ function during anaesthesia to prevent complications in the peri-operative period. This can be achieved only with knowledge of the physiological changes that occur during anaesthesia.

Central nervous system

- General anaesthetic agents cause reversible depression of the CNS.
- Consequently, central homeostatic mechanisms to control the cardiovascular and respiratory system are depressed.
- The precise mechanism by which drugs cause general anaesthesia is unknown.

Respiratory system

- Depth and rate of respiration are usually increased in response to an increase in arterial carbon dioxide concentration. This response is reduced during general anaesthesia.
- Hypoxia (i.e. diminished blood oxygen) occurs during general anaesthesia.
- Arterial oxygen concentration is lower than expected compared with alveolar oxygen concentration. This is particularly significant in horses. It results primarily from a mismatch in ventilation and perfusion of the lungs. Consequently, areas of the lung that are well ventilated are poorly perfused and oxygen transfer from the alveoli to the pulmonary blood supply is reduced. The reasons for inequalities in ventilation and perfusion have not been established fully. A reduction in functional residual capacity and atelectasis (collapse or failure of part of the lung to expand) during

anaesthesia are thought to be contributing factors. It is particularly severe in large horses positioned in dorsal recumbency.

Cardiovascular system

- Anaesthetic drugs usually depress myocardial activity. This is particularly true of volatile anaesthetic agents. Ketamine, benzodiazepines and opioids have less significant effects on the cardiovascular system.
- Venous return is reduced by agents that cause vasodilation.
- As a consequence, cardiac output is commonly reduced.

Renal function

- Renal blood flow and glomerular filtration rate are reduced.
- Antidiuretic hormone (ADH) secretion is increased during anaesthesia, causing retention of sodium and water for the first 24 h following anaesthesia.

Liver function

- Anaesthesia decreases blood flow to the liver.
- Consequently, the metabolism of drugs by the liver is reduced, prolonging the action of many anaesthetic agents.

Induction of anaesthesia

Padded boxes reduce the risk of injury to the horse during induction (see Chapter 19). Some boxes incorporate a crush door that forms part of the wall of the induction box and can be folded out at a 90° angle (Fig. 20.1). During induction the horse is positioned between the door and the wall of the box, thus providing greater control as the horse assumes recumbency. The door is folded back into the wall of the box during recovery.

Some equine hospitals use tilt tables for induction of anaesthesia. The horse is sedated and positioned adjacent and parallel to the table, orientated vertically (Fig. 20.2). Bellybands placed under the horse are tightened to provide support as anaesthesia is induced. When the horse is anaesthetised, the table is rotated to a horizontal position.

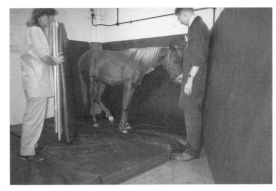

Fig. 20.1 Induction of anaesthesia using a crush door.

A padded box is required for recovery from anaesthesia.

A jugular intravenous catheter should be placed securely prior to induction of general anaesthesia. The administration of anaesthetic drugs through the catheter prevents inadvertent perivascular injection. It reduces trauma to the jugular vein due to repeated venepuncture and provides rapid intravenous access.

The headcollar worn during induction should be padded over the cheek pieces and poll to prevent trauma to the facial nerve and bony prominences of the face.

Restraint during induction of anaesthesia depends on the induction technique, temperament of the horse and anaesthetist's preference. Usually at least one person restrains the head by a rope attached to the head collar. A smoother induction often is achieved when the restraint is minimal and the horse is allowed to assume recumbency freely and slowly.

Maintenance of anaesthesia

General anaesthesia usually is maintained with inhalational agents. Total intravenous techniques are currently best suited to procedures of less than 1 h duration. It is important that the horse is maintained at an adequate depth of anaesthesia for the surgical procedure. Safety is paramount; a horse that moves during anaesthesia is potentially dangerous. Depth of anaesthesia is balanced by the need to keep

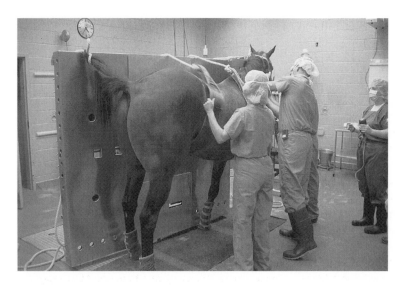

Fig. 20.2 Induction of anaesthesia using a tilt table.

cardiovascular and respiratory function within physiologically acceptable limits. This can be difficult to achieve. Continuous monitoring of the horse is important throughout the maintenance phase of anaesthesia.

Positioning of the horse during anaesthesia

Careful positioning of the horse during anaesthesia is vital to reduce the risk of post-operative myopathy and neuropathy. This is the responsibility of the anaesthetist.

Positioning in lateral recumbency

- Lower forelimb is pulled forward so that the triceps muscle is not compressed by the full weight of the body and upper limb.
- Padding is placed between the limbs so that the upper limb is supported.
- The limbs should not be in full flexion or extension.
- The neck and head should be raised slightly to reduce nasal engorgement.

Positioning in dorsal recumbency

- Square positioning on the table so that weight distribution is uniform between the different muscle groups.
- The legs should be relaxed and slightly flexed.
- Neck should be straight but not overextended,

to prevent stretching of the recurrent laryngeal nerves.
- Head is slightly elevated and care must be taken to avoid compression of the jugular veins.

Components of an anaesthetic machine

The modern anaesthetic machine is designed to deliver a precise, variable mixture of anaesthetic agent and oxygen to the patient. Most inhalant anaesthetic agents are volatile liquids, vaporised for delivery. Oxygen and nitrous oxide are gases at normal temperatures and pressures.

Gas supply

- Gases are stored as liquids or compressed gases.
- The supply may be from large cylinders stored remote from the anaesthetic machine or small-volume cylinders attached directly to the anaesthetic machine. These cylinders attach to hanger yokes on the machine; the yokes are pin coded to prevent attachment of the wrong type of cylinder.
- A universal colour-coding system is used to identify different gas cylinders. Pipelines for supply of gases from a remote source are similarly coded. In the UK the following colour-coding system for cylinders has been adopted:

Oxygen	Black body, white shoulders
Nitrous oxide	Blue
Carbon dioxide	Grey

Pressure / contents gauge

The pressure gauge indicates the pressure of gas in the cylinder when the valve is open. In oxygen cylinders this is an indication of the volume of gas remaining in the cylinder. This does not apply to nitrous oxide cylinders. Nitrous oxide is stored as a liquid in equilibrium with gas. The pressure is maintained constant until all the liquid evaporates, when the pressure falls rapidly. The only satisfactory way of keeping a check on the contents of nitrous oxide cylinders is by weighing them and then calculating the weight. The weight of the empty cylinder is known as the tare weight and is always stamped on the top.

Pressure regulators

Pressures in gas cylinders are high and must be reduced by regulators to provide a constant flow of gas to the flowmeters at a lower pressure:

- This protects the delicate flowmeters and allows the rate of gas administration to be regulated more finely.
- The regulators maintain a constant pressure of oxygen despite a gradual fall in pressure as the cylinder empties.

Flowmeters

Flowmeters measure, indicate and control precisely the rate of gas flow to the common gas outlet. Gas enters the flowmeter through a needle valve and passes through a tapered tube exiting at the top. An indicator rises in the tube as the flow rate increases.

Vaporisers

These vaporise a liquid anaesthetic agent and add a controlled amount of the vapour to the gases delivered to the patient. There are a number of different types of calibrated vaporisers commonly used in equine anaesthesia.

Calibrated vaporisers

Temperature-, level- and flow-compensated vaporisers are most common. They deliver an anaesthetic concentration that is similar to the dial setting, provided that the gas flow through the vaporiser and the temperature are within the ranges specified for the model. The vaporiser comprises a bypass and vaporisation chamber. Increasing the dial setting increases the proportion of gas that flows through the vaporisation chamber. Tilting a vaporiser may contaminate the bypass chamber with inhalant agent. If this occurs, the vaporiser should be dried out before it is used. A bimetallic strip mechanism maintains a constant concentration despite changes in temperature.

Vaporisers are agent-specific. Newer models have a keyed filling system to prevent the vaporiser from being filled with the wrong agent. This system also reduces environmental contamination during filling.

Common gas outlet

This connects the anaesthesia machine to breathing system connectors, ventilators or oxygen supply devices.

Oxygen flush

The flush device activates oxygen flow to the common gas outlet bypassing the vaporiser and flowmeter. It can be used to deliver oxygen in an emergency situation or to flush inhalant from breathing systems before the patient is disconnected from the circuit.

Low oxygen warning devices

These are a useful safety mechanism. Falling oxygen supplies curtail the delivery of nitrous oxide and simultaneously sound an alarm.

Anaesthetic circuits for equine anaesthesia

Anaesthetic circuits fulfil the following functions:

- Connect the anaesthetic machine to the endotracheal tube or face mask
- Deliver inhalant anaesthetics
- Supply oxygen
- Provide a mechanism for controlled ventilation

Anaesthetic circuits can be classified as rebreathing or non-rebreathing. Rebreathing circuits are used to anaesthetise adult horses. *Circle* and *to-and-fro* systems are the two rebreathing circuits commonly used in horses.

Rebreathing circuits incorporate an absorbent agent, soda lime, to absorb carbon dioxide. This allows the circuits to be used with low flow rates of anaesthetic gases. Soda lime is a mixture of 90% calcium hydroxide and 5% sodium hydroxide, with 5% silicate and water to prevent powdering. The reaction with carbon dioxide is exothermic and produces a significant amount of water.

Commercial soda lime preparations contain an indicator dye, which changes colour as the soda lime becomes exhausted due to the change in pH. This indicates when the soda lime needs to be changed.

In theory when a stable plane of anaesthesia has been reached, rebreathing circuits can be run as a completely closed system. In this state the oxygen flow rate into the circuit is equal to the metabolic oxygen consumption of the horse and the concentration of anaesthetic agent in the circuit remains constant. In practice, this state is rarely achieved and the circuits are run as low-flow systems. The expiratory valve must be kept partially open to prevent a build-up of gas.

A disadvantage of rebreathing circuits is the time delay to change the circuit concentration of volatile agent. This is due to the large circuit volume. To change the concentration more quickly, the fresh gas flow rate is increased and the expiratory valve is opened. Nitrous oxide should be used cautiously in rebreathing circuits. There is a danger that nitrous oxide will accumulate unless the fresh gas flow rates are high and the expiratory valve is open.

Advantages of rebreathing circuits
- Low fresh gas flow rates
- Low volatile agent consumption rate
- Expired moisture and heat conserved
- Less atmospheric pollution.

Disadvantages of rebreathing circuits
- Care with nitrous oxide
- Slow rate of change of anaesthetic concentration in the circuit
- Soda lime must be changed regularly
- Cumbersome
- Expensive to purchase.

Circle circuit (Fig. 20.3)

Circle systems are available for small and large animals. The large-animal systems are suitable for horses of >100 kg bodyweight. Foals of <100 kg bodyweight should be placed on a small-animal circle that has a lower circuit volume and presents less resistance to ventilation. The canister of soda lime is remote from the animal, so that inhalation of soda lime dust is unlikely. The vertical positioning of the soda lime canister prevents channelling and so apparatus dead space does not increase as the soda lime is exhausted.

To-and-fro circuit (Fig. 20.4)

These circuits are rarely used for equine anaesthesia. The canister of soda lime is close to the horse's head,

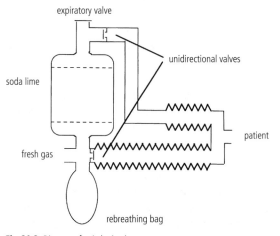

Fig. 20.3 Diagram of a circle circuit.

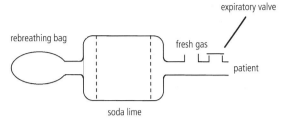

Fig. 20.4 Diagram of a to-and-fro circuit.

expiratory valve

rebreathing bag

fresh gas

patient

soda lime

resulting in inhalation of soda lime dust, and the circuit is bulky and inconvenient for head and neck surgery.

Orotracheal intubation (see Table 20.3)

It is not practical to maintain anaesthesia with inhalational agents using a facemask in adult horses. Instead the horse is intubated with an orotracheal (via the mouth) tube (see How to . . . 20.1). The tube provides a secure airway for delivery of anaesthetic gases from the anaesthetic machine and circuit to the patient. Occasionally, nasotracheal (via the nose) intubation may be required to provide surgical access to the mouth. A 20–25-mm internal diameter tube is suitable for most adult horses. The tubes must be cleaned carefully and hung up to dry after use. Prior to use, the cuff must be checked for leaks.

Inhalant anaesthetic agents

Halothane and isoflurane are the volatile anaesthetic agents currently in common use in equine anaesthesia (see Table 20.4). Nitrous oxide is used additionally in some centres.

Minimum alveolar concentration (MAC)
- Measure of anaesthetic potency of inhalant agents
- Allows the potency of different agents to be compared

The MAC is the minimum alveolar concentration of the agent that produces immobility in 50% of patients exposed to a supramaximal noxious stimulus. The lower the MAC value, the more potent the anaesthetic agent.

How to . . . 20.1

Orotracheal intubation of a horse

- The endotracheal tube is lubricated to reduce trauma to soft tissue during intubation.
- Following induction of anaesthesia, the mouth is opened with a gag.
- The tongue is pulled to the side of the mouth and the tube slid between the dental arcades to the back of the pharynx. The end of the tube must disarticulate the soft palate to allow communication between the oropharynx and the larynx.
- Extension of the head and neck allows the tube to be advanced through the larynx into the trachea.
- It is important to inflate the cuff of the tube to ensure a seal in the trachea and prevent the horse breathing around the tube.
- Overinflation of the cuff may produce necrosis of the trachea or occlusion of the lumen of the tube.

A 20–25-mm internal diameter endotracheal tube is suitable for most adult thoroughbred horses.

Blood gas partition coefficient
- Relative solubility of the inhalant agent in blood and alveolar gas
- Affects the speed of recovery from anaesthesia with the inhalant agent

Blood solubility determines the time delay between changes in concentration of the inhalant agent in the lungs, causing a change in concentration of the agent in the CNS. Increased blood solubility is associated with a more prolonged recovery from anaesthesia.

The volatile inhalant agents all cause dose-related depression of the cardiovascular and respiratory system. No one volatile anaesthetic agent appears superior in terms of peri-operative mortality.

Everyone should be aware of the dangers associated with inhaling anaesthetic gases. An anaesthetic gas scavenging system must be fitted or absorptive filters used to minimise exposure to gases.

Table 20.3 Advantages and disadvantages of inhalational and intravenous anaesthesia in horses

	Inhalational anaesthesia	Intravenous anaesthesia
Advantages	• Rapid recovery from anaesthesia • The horse is intubated and 100% oxygen delivered, supporting the respiratory system • Reduced risk of anaesthetic overdose compared with intravenous anaesthesia	• Rapid induction of general anaesthesia • Requires minimal equipment • Can provide excellent cardiovascular stability compared with inhalant techniques
Disadvantages	• Not suitable to induce anaesthesia in routine clinical equine practice • Requires an anaesthetic machine and circuit • System to scavenge waste anaesthetic gases is needed	• Unless there is a specific antagonist, once the drug is administered removal is dependent on metabolism. Adverse side effects may be persistent; overdose can cause prolonged recovery, particularly in animals with reduced liver function • Repeated doses may result in accumulation, increasing the risk of overdose and prolonged recovery • Some intravenous agents cause excitement during induction and recovery

Table 20.4 Pharmacology and clinical use of inhalant anaesthetic agents in horses

Inhalant agent	Physical properties	MAC	Clinical use	Side effects
Halothane	• Volatile liquid • Colourless • Non-flammable • Non-explosive • Decomposed by light; stored in coloured bottles	0.9%	• In common use • Intermediate blood solubility reflected by relatively slow recovery from anaesthesia • Degree of liver metabolism	• Severe myocardial depression causing hypotension • Cardiac arrhythmias • Muscle tremors in recovery • Risk of liver toxicity
Isoflurane	• Volatile liquid • Colourless • Non-flammable • Non-explosive • Pungent smell • Stable in light	1.3%	• In common use • Lower blood solubility than halothane; more rapid recovery from anaesthesia • Less potent than halothane • No liver metabolism	• Severe respiratory depression • Vasodilation of peripheral blood vessels, producing hypotension
Nitrous oxide	• Colourless gas at standard pressure • Stored as a liquid in nitrous oxide cylinders	205%	• Limited use in equine anaesthesia • Weak anaesthetic agent • To prevent hypoxia, cannot be administered at concentrations >60% • Risk of accumulation when used in rebreathing circuits at low gas flow rates	• Minimal cardiovascular depression • Minimal respiratory depression • Accumulates in gas-filled viscera and body cavities • To prevent diffusion hypoxia, oxygen is supplemented when nitrous oxide administration is stopped

Intravenous anaesthesia (see Table 20.3)

Indications for intravenous anaesthesia

- Induction of general anaesthesia
- Maintenance of general anaesthesia

Intravenous anaesthetic agents always should be administered through an intravenous catheter.

Intravenous drugs used to induce and maintain anaesthesia in horses (Table 20.5)

- α_2-Agonists
- Ketamine
- Thiopentone
- Glyceryl guaiacolate ether (GGE)
- Benzodiazepines
- Propofol
- Etorphine/acepromazine (large-animal immobilon®).

Table 20.5 Pharmacology and clinical use of commonly used intravenous anaesthetic agents in horses

Drug	Mechanism of action	Pharmacology and metabolism	Side effects
Ketamine (10% injectable preparation)	• Dissociative agent • Alters CNS response to sensory input with minimal depression of the brainstem	• Minimal cervical vertebral stenosis (CVS) effects • May cause breath-holding • Nystagmus, blinking and lacrimation common immediately following administration • Liver metabolism; recovery determined by redistribution following a single dose • Repeated doses result in accumulation and prolonged recovery	• Potential to cause CNS excitement during induction and recovery • Poor muscle relaxation • Slow onset of anaesthesia
Thiopentone Unstable in solution. Dry powder preparation that is reconstituted with water to make a 10% solution.	• Potentiates GABA-mediated CNS depression	• Rapid onset of anaesthesia with short duration of action • Highly protein bound in the plasma; hypoproteinaemia increases efficacy • Dose-dependent cardiovascular and respiratory depression • Rapid redistribution to body organs and skeletal muscle followed by slower transfer to body fat • Prolonged liver metabolism; repeated doses saturate body fat, prolonging recovery	• Hypoventilation and apnoea immediately following bolus administration • Hypotension • Strongly alkaline solution (perivascular injection) produces severe tissue necrosis
GGE (15% solution)	• Used in combination with thiopentone or ketamine • Centrally acting muscle relaxant causes immobility without concurrent paralysis of respiratory muscles • Sedative and hypnotic properties	• Minimal cardiovascular and respiratory effects • High doses will induce recumbency • Liver metabolism and urinary excretion • Prolonged infusions may result in drug accumulation and prolonged recovery	• Haemolysis at high concentrations • Perivascular injection produces tissue necrosis
Benzodiazepines (10 mg/2 ml vials)		Commonly incorporated with α_2-agonist and ketamine combinations	• Produces excitement in unsedated healthy adult horses • Produces more profound sedation in sick horses

The drugs are used in a variety of combinations to induce and maintain anaesthesia. Choice of technique depends on the experience of the anaesthetist, the horse's temperament, the ASA category and the reason for anaesthesia.

Total intravenous anaesthesia or 'triple drip'

Anaesthesia can be maintained by a total intravenous technique using a combination of an α_2-agonist, GGE and ketamine given by continuous infusion. This is termed the 'triple drip'. Currently the technique is used to maintain anaesthesia for up to 1 h duration. The regime provides good cardiovascular and respiratory system stability and recovery is excellent.

The technique commonly is used to maintain anaesthesia in field conditions or in a situation where an anaesthetic machine cannot be used, e.g. a horse stuck in a horsebox accident. Compared with techniques involving repeat doses of an α_2-agonist and ketamine, it provides a more constant depth of anaesthesia and a smoother recovery.

Propofol

Propofol has been used alone or in combination with ketamine to maintain anaesthesia. Currently it does not have a licence for use in the horse.

Etorphine/acepromazine (large-animal immobilon®)

This preparation no longer has a licence for veterinary use. It is hazardous and its use is not recommended.

Monitoring during anaesthesia

Regular monitoring allows early identification and treatment of problems. Monitoring of anaesthetic depth is intimately involved with monitoring the cardiovascular and respiratory systems.

Anaesthetic record

A written record of every equine anaesthetic includes information relating to the patient, the anaesthetic drugs administered and intraoperative monitoring.

It is important for the following reasons:

- A visual record of cardiovascular and respiratory variables allows changes to be identified more easily and quickly
- An archive resource is particularly useful if an animal is re-anaesthetised; the records provide accurate epidemiological data for the clinic
- It is a legal document recording the standard of care

Monitoring the depth of anaesthesia

Depth of anaesthesia is difficult to assess in horses. The clinical appearance of the horse and changes in physiological variables are evaluated. Cardiovascular and respiratory system changes are dose related with most anaesthetic agents.

The eye

- The palpebral reflex is elicited by gently running a finger along the free margin of the upper eyelid. It is usually retained during surgical anaesthesia.
- The corneal reflex is closure of the eyelids in response to pressure on the cornea. It is not used routinely to assess depth of anaesthesia.
- Lacrimation and rapid nystagmus are associated with a lightening of anaesthesia.

The eye reflexes must be interpreted with knowledge of the anaesthetic agents administered, e.g. with inhalational agents the palpebral reflex is usually reduced but not abolished and the eye rotates medially and ventrally. Following administration of ketamine, the palpebral reflex is maintained and lacrimation is common. This should not be misinterpreted as inadequate anaesthesia.

Muscle tone

Movement means inadequate anaesthesia. Changes in muscle tone provide a crude indication of depth of anaesthesia. A tightening of the muscles in the neck, resulting in slight head movement, occurs with inadequate anaesthesia. This usually precedes limb movement. Intraoperative limb movement must be treated immediately with the rapid administration of an intravenous anaesthetic agent.

Physiological variables

Cardiovascular and respiratory variables are a poor guide to depth of anaesthesia with the exception of blood pressure. Changes in blood pressure are dose related to the administration of inhalational agents. A rise in blood pressure usually accompanies a decrease in depth of anaesthesia.

Monitoring the cardiovascular and respiratory system

Maintenance of adequate cardiovascular and respiratory system function is a key aim of equine anaesthesia. Anaesthetic agents cause a dose-related depression of both systems. Monitoring allows appropriate support to be given.

Cardiovascular system

(1) *Manual palpation of peripheral pulse rate and quality.* Peripheral pulse quality reflects peripheral perfusion. Pulse quality is assessed by the ease with which the pulse can be abolished by manual pressure. Pulse pressure is the difference between the systolic and diastolic blood pressure. If the difference is large, the pulse strength will be good; this does not reflect arterial blood pressure.

(2) *Mucous membrane colour and capillary refill time.* These are crude measures of cardiovascular function. During halothane anaesthesia the mucous membranes usually become paler, with prolongation of capillary refill time as depth of anaesthesia increases. Mucous membrane colour may provide information relating to the respiratory system. Severe hypercapnia causes brick red mucous membranes; cyanosis indicates severe hypoxia.

(3) *Electrocardiography.* Electrocardiography records the electrical activity of the heart. It is useful in the diagnosis of cardiac arrhythmias.

(4) *Blood pressure.* Arterial blood pressure measurement is the most important component of cardiovascular system monitoring in horses. Blood pressure can be measured using indirect or direct methods.

Direct methods

These require invasive cannulation of a peripheral artery. The facial artery is used when the horse is positioned in dorsal recumbency; the transverse facial artery or metatarsal artery is used for horses in lateral recumbency. An anaeroid manometer or pressure transducer and oscilloscope then are used for blood pressure measurement.

Indirect methods

Indirect methods use oscillometric devices. These measure the magnitude of arterial pulsations in an air-filled cuff. The cuff is placed around the base of the tail or the distal extremity of a limb. Indirect methods are less accurate than direct methods, particularly if blood pressure is low.

Respiratory system

(1) *Respiratory rate and pattern.* Tidal volume can be assessed crudely by chest movement and collapse of the rebreathing bag during inspiration. Anaesthetic agents cause respiratory depression and hypoventilation. Ketamine produces a pattern of breath-holding with alternate short periods of rapid shallow breathing and apnoea. Isoflurane is particularly depressant to the respiratory system.

(2) *Arterial blood gas analysis.* Arterial blood gas analysis provides information on respiratory system and metabolic function. Arterial carbon dioxide, oxygen concentration and pH are the most useful indicators of respiratory function. Carbon dioxide concentration indicates the adequacy of alveolar ventilation. Increases in concentration indicate hypoventilation; decreases in concentration suggest excessive alveolar ventilation. Blood gas analysis measures the concentration of oxygen dissolved in the blood. A reduction in arterial oxygen concentration commonly occurs during anaesthesia.

(3) *Pulse oximetry.* Pulse oximeters are relatively cheap and simple to use. They measure the pulse rate and provide information about the adequacy of arterial oxygenation and peripheral perfusion. In horses, pulse oximeters tend to underestimate haemoglobin saturation but can be useful clinically to detect changes in satura-

tion. They have a number of limitations, which must be understood to enable the information to be interpreted accurately.

(4) *Capnometry*. Capnometry measures the concentration of carbon dioxide in a sample of gas drawn from the end of the endotracheal tube. This indirectly reflects arterial carbon dioxide concentration. End tidal concentration is lower than arterial concentration and the difference is variable, limiting the usefulness of capnometry. It is still useful for measuring trends, particularly in horses being ventilated, and provides information that cannot be ascertained from simple clinical measurement. An inspired reading of >0 mmHg carbon dioxide indicates that the breathing system is not extracting all the carbon dioxide and requires immediate investigation.

(5) *Temperature*. Adult horses rarely become hypothermic during anaesthesia. Monitoring of body temperature is more critical in foals, particularly during long procedures. Measuring body temperature with a nasopharyngeal or oesophageal probe is more accurate than a rectal thermometer.

(6) *Acid–base analysis*. Blood gas analysers measure the acid–base status of the horse, in addition to the partial pressures of respiratory gases. This is useful in the evaluation and treatment of acid–base disturbances.

Recovery from anaesthesia

Horses should be placed in a padded box for recovery from anaesthesia to reduce the risk of injury. The aim is for a smooth and quiet recovery. The quality of recovery can vary, depending on a number of factors:

- Temperament of the horse
- Anaesthetic agents administered
- Speed of recovery
- Design of the recovery box
- External stimulation by noise and light
- Surgical procedure performed and peri-operative pain

During recovery from anaesthesia there is a reduction in support and monitoring, despite depression of the CNS by anaesthetic drugs. Careful observation

during recovery is important, although sometimes little can be done as a horse struggles to stand.

Goals of recovery

- Quiet
- Controlled return to standing
- Minimal exertion or stress.

Recovery boxes

In most equine hospitals the induction box is used for recovery from anaesthesia. A recovery area with the following properties can help to reduce the incidence of complications:

- Recovery boxes should be approximately 3 m square, ideally with a human escape hatch and an observation window.
- Adequate padding of the walls and floor reduces trauma when the horse is recumbent and during attempts to stand. The flooring should provide a secure footing.
- Facility to provide oxygen supplementation.
- A 'crash box' containing drugs for cardiopulmonary resuscitation, tracheostomy kit and endotracheal and nasopharyngeal tubes located close to the box.

Positioning the horse in the recovery box

Positioning in the recovery box should ensure that there is adequate space around the horse to allow movement into sternal recumbency and assume a standing position. Horses positioned in lateral recumbency during anaesthesia are usually placed in the same lateral recumbency during recovery. The lower forelimb is pulled forward. If limb surgery has been performed, the operated limb is best positioned uppermost.

Extubation

Extubation does not need to be delayed until the horse is actively swallowing. The cuff of the endotracheal tube must be deflated to prevent trauma to the trachea and larynx as the tube is removed. The head and neck are slightly extended and the tube gently withdrawn following the arc of the head. The mouth gag then can be removed. Some anaesthetists routinely recover horses with the endotracheal tube *in situ*. This may be indicated following airway or cervical orthopaedic surgery, to ensure a clear airway. In this case the tube is firmly secured to the headcollar and the mouth gag is removed. To check that there is no respiratory obstruction following extubation, a hand is placed close to both nostrils to confirm airflow during expiration. Respiratory obstruction must be treated immediately. A nasal tube should be used if there is any respiratory difficulty.

Sedation during recovery

Some horses may attempt to stand too early in the recovery period. Such attempts are usually uncoordinated and increase the risk of traumatic injury. Sedation with an α_2-agonist will delay recovery from anaesthesia and is widely used, particularly in orthopaedic cases.

Assisted recoveries

Assisting the horse to a standing position during anaesthesia can decrease the incidence of complications but cases must be selected carefully. Human safety is paramount.

Temporary restraint can be achieved by extending the head and neck. This is useful in semiconscious animals and small foals to maintain lateral recumbency.

Head and tail ropes can help horses to a standing position. One rope is attached to the headcollar and another is tied to the tail. The ropes are threaded through secure rings placed high on the walls of the recovery box. Pulling on the tail rope as the horse attempts to stand provides support to prevent falling. It is important not to exert too much pressure on the head rope because some head movement is required for balance.

Recovery score

It is useful to score the quality of recovery from anaesthesia and to record this. A simple descriptive scale has been devised:

- Score 5: no ataxia, no struggling, stood up at first attempt as if fully conscious
- Score 4: slight ataxia and struggling, stood at first or second attempt, no serious instability
- Score 3: some staggering and ataxia, a few unsuccessful attempts to stand, ataxic immediately after standing up
- Score 2: excitement, paddling when recumbent, several attempts to stand, severe ataxia once standing, may fall, danger of self-inflicted injury
- Score 1: excitement when recumbent, persistent unsuccessful attempts to stand, severe ataxia and falls once standing, aimless walking, high risk of self-inflicted injury
- Score 0: very violent ('wall of death'), self-inflicted injury, prolonged struggling or unable to stand 2 h after the end of anaesthesia

Considerations in sedating and anaesthetising foals

Foals commonly require sedation and anaesthesia for diagnostic or surgical procedures. The technique depends on the age of the foal and the reason for anaesthesia. There are significant differences in physiology compared with adult animals. They are greatest in foals less than 4 weeks of age (see Chapter 15). In particular:

- Blood loss, hypovolaemia and the cardiovascular side effects of anaesthetic agents are less well tolerated.
- Foals are less capable of maintaining increased respiratory efforts in response to hypercapnia and hypoxia.

Hypothermia

Hypothermia is a risk due to increased body surface area to volume ratio. Preventative measures include:

- Monitor body temperature during anaesthesia and recovery
- Place the foal on a heat pad

- Wrap the foal in insulating material in areas away from the surgical site
- Raise the ambient temperature
- Warm intravenous fluids and fluids used for abdominal lavage

Energy stores

Foals have limited energy stores, so hypoglycaemia can result from short periods of starvation. In foals up to 1 month of age, muzzling for 15–30 min prior to induction of anaesthesia will allow the stomach to empty without producing concurrent hypoglycaemia. Blood glucose levels should be checked during long procedures.

Drug metabolism and elimination

The enzyme systems in the liver that metabolise most anaesthetic drugs are immature. So drug metabolism is prolonged, resulting in an extended recovery from anaesthesia. Hence, intravenous drug doses and frequency of administration should be reduced.

General anaesthesia of foals

There are some differences in techniques used to anaesthetise foals.

Induction
Commonly anaesthesia is induced in foals of less than 4 weeks old or foals categorised as ASA 4 or 5 using an inhalant agent. Isoflurane is administered by face mask with a small animal non-rebreathing circuit to produce recumbency. A nasotracheal tube is placed and administration of isoflurane is continued until anaesthesia is sufficient to allow orotracheal intubation. Induction of anaesthesia with inhalant agents in foals may be associated with increased mortality. Use of intravenous techniques should be considered where possible. Incorporation of benzodiazepines into sedative and induction techniques is useful because of minimal cardiovascular and respiratory side effects.

Maintenance
Endotracheal tubes ranging in size from 10 to 20 mm internal diameter should be available. The tube must not extend beyond the level of the 5th rib to prevent bronchial intubation. Foals of >100 kg bodyweight can be maintained using a large-animal circle or Mapelson A circuit. Smaller foals are maintained on small-animal circle systems, which present less resistance to ventilation.

Anaesthesia is best maintained using inhalant agents, with isoflurane as the agent of choice because recovery from anaesthesia is rapid.

Recovery
The aim is for a quick recovery to allow the foal to be reunited with the mare. Prevention of hypothermia in the recovery period is important. Techniques used during maintenance of anaesthesia are applied.

The mare

Mares commonly become distressed following separation from their foals during anaesthesia, hence it is usually necessary to sedate the mare. The presence of the mare during induction of anaesthesia may have a calming effect on some foals. Care is required when the mare is reunited with the foal.

Anaesthetic complications and emergencies

The results of a large multi-institutional prospective study of peri-operative fatalities (CEPEF) in equine anaesthesia demonstrate a mortality rate of 0.9% at 7 days post-operatively, excluding colic cases. There is a high mortality rate compared with anaesthesia of other species. Complications can be classed as intraoperative or peri-operative, according to when they occur. A significant number of complications contributing to the high mortality rate occur during the immediate peri-operative period.

Intraoperative anaesthetic complications

Hypoxaemia
This is reduced arterial oxygen concentration and is best diagnosed using arterial blood gas analysis. Cyanosis only occurs when hypoxaemia is severe. Altered respiratory and cardiovascular physiology

during anaesthesia contributes to hypoxaemia. It is particularly common in large horses maintained on inhalant agents positioned in dorsal recumbency. Oxygen delivery to the tissue is determined by haemoglobin saturation. Haemoglobin saturation falls rapidly when arterial oxygen concentration is <60 mmHg.

Causes of intraoperative hypoxaemia
- Low inspired oxygen concentration due to anaesthetic equipment failure
- Hypoventilation due to respiratory depression caused by anaesthetic agents
- Ventilation perfusion mismatch, especially in horses in dorsal recumbency
- Lung atelectasis (collapse)

Treatment of intraoperative hypoxaemia
- Ensure that the inspired oxygen concentration is 100%
- Check that there is no respiratory obstruction
- Minimise respiratory depression caused by anaesthetic agents
- Assist or control ventilation with intermittent positive pressure ventilation (IPPV)
- Maximise cardiac output with fluid therapy and administration of positive inotropes

Hypercapnia
This is increased arterial carbon dioxide concentration and again is diagnosed with arterial blood gas analysis. This results from respiratory depression caused by anaesthetic agents. Hypercapnia stimulates the sympathetic nervous system and cardiac arrhythmias can occur when it is severe. A degree of hypercapnia is permissible, but when it rises over 75 mmHg it justifies treatment.

Treatment of intraoperative hypercapnia
- Minimise respiratory depression
- Initiate IPPV

Hypotension
This is low blood pressure diagnosed by intraoperative monitoring techniques. Mean arterial blood pressure is maintained at >70 mmHg to minimise the risk of post-anaesthetic myopathy.

Causes of intraoperative hypotension
- Myocardial depression caused by anaesthetic agents, particularly inhalant agents
- Hypovolaemia
- Acid–base and electrolyte disorders resulting in depression of the myocardium
- Cardiac arrhythmias
- Pre-existing disease, such as shock

Treatment of hypotension
- Minimise cardiovascular depression caused by anaesthetic agents
- Support the cardiovascular system with fluid therapy; consider hypertonic saline
- Administer positive inotropes (dobutamine or dopamine)

Positive inotropes can increase blood pressure by a direct effect on the myocardium. They are used in conjunction with other treatments for hypotension but they do not address the underlying cause.

Dobutamine is commonly used. It has a rapid onset and short duration of action. It is administered to effect by intravenous infusion. Overdose can cause tachycardia and cardiac arrhythmias.

Inadequate anaesthesia
Inadequate anaesthesia resulting in movement is dangerous. It commonly occurs when there is a sudden increase in surgical stimulation. It is managed with the immediate administration of an intravenous anaesthetic agent concurrent with a reduction in surgical stimulation.

Cardiac arrhythmias
- Detection with manual monitoring of the pulse and auscultation of the heart
- Diagnosis of the type of arrhythmia by electrocardiography

An irregular heartbeat (i.e. an arrhythmia) may cause the heart to stop, so should be assessed carefully.

Controlled ventilation
Controlled ventilation is needed for cases of hypoventilation or apnoea. During controlled ventilation the respiratory rate and tidal volume or peak

433

inspiratory pressure are predetermined. This is achieved by IPPV, which can be performed manually by squeezing the rebreathing bag or automatically by using a large-animal ventilator. Administration of a neuromuscular blocking agent is not a requirement for IPPV.

Intermittent positive pressure ventilation commonly causes hypotension. Application of positive pressure to the chest during inspiration decreases venous return, which decreases cardiac output. Aggressive support of the cardiovascular system is needed.

Peri-operative complications

Monitoring throughout the peri-operative period is vital in the early detection and treatment of complications.

Hypoxaemia
Most horses become hypoxaemic when they start to breathe room air in recovery. This may be reduced by insufflation of 15 l/min of oxygen via a nasopharyngeal tube. The oxygen is delivered by pipeline from an oxygen source remote to the recovery box. Assisted ventilation with a demand valve will lower carbon dioxide and improve oxygenation but requires intubation.

Respiratory obstruction
Following extubation it is vital to check that the horse has a clear airway. Partial upper airway obstruction is a common cause of respiratory obstruction following extubation. It contributes to hypoxaemia by increasing airway resistance, causing hypoventilation. Inspiratory efforts against a partially obstructed upper airway may produce pulmonary oedema.

Causes of respiratory obstruction
(1) *Nasal cavity engorgement.* This is the most common cause of partial upper airway obstruction following anaesthesia. It occurs in horses placed in dorsal recumbency for long periods or if the head has been positioned in a dependent position. Topical administration of 5 ml of 0.15% phenylephrine into each nostril 10–15 min before termination of anaesthesia can reduce nasal

oedema before the horse is extubated. Nasal engorgement causing upper airway obstruction is treated by placement of a nasopharyngeal tube to provide a clear airway.
(2) *Laryngeal dysfunction.* Trauma to the pharynx and larynx during intubation can produce upper airway oedema. Laryngeal paralysis has been described as a complication of anaesthesia.
(3) *Displacement of the soft palate.* Dorsal displacement of the soft palate following extubation is relatively common. Stimulating the horse to swallow or raising the head on a foam pad usually returns the palate to a normal position.

Management of respiratory obstruction
• Immediate treatment required
• Establish a clear airway by placement of an orotracheal or nasotracheal tube
• A tracheotomy must be performed if this is not possible
• Insufflate oxygen at 15 l/min via the tracheotomy or endotracheal tube

Pulmonary oedema
This is a relatively rare complication. Treatment consists of oxygen therapy, diuresis and administration of NSAIDs.

Musculoskeletal system injury
Limb fractures and other injuries can occur during recovery. Injuries are more likely to occur when the horse attempts to stand prematurely and is consequently less coordinated.

Post-anaesthetic myopathy
Post-anaesthetic myopathy is thought to result from inadequate perfusion of muscle tissue, producing ischaemic muscle damage. Maintaining good blood pressure and consequently blood flow to the muscles, plus careful positioning and padding of the anaesthetised horse, are important. It is a relatively common problem.

There is a wide spectrum of clinical signs, depending on severity. Mildly affected horses show stiffness and pain on walking. Severely affected horses are unable to stand and have severe muscle pain. On palpation the affected muscle groups are hard and swollen.

Serum biochemistry demonstrates elevated levels of lactate, creatine kinase and aspartate aminotransferase (AST), reflecting the muscle damage. Changes in these values can be used to monitor the condition.

Nursing horses with post-anaesthetic myopathy
(1) Prevent further muscle damage:
    (a) Restrict exercise if the horse is able to stand.
    (b) Change position regularly if recumbent.
    (c) Ensure that there is adequate padding under bony points to prevent pressure sores.
    (d) Provide physiotherapy to promote blood flow to the limbs and affected muscles.
    (e) Sling if attempting to stand unsuccessfully.
(2) Provide adequate analgesia.
(3) Prevent self-trauma.
(4) Promote repair of muscle tissue:
    (a) Acepromazine may improve blood flow to muscle tissue by its vasodilator action.
(5) Provide supportive treatment:
    (a) Fluid therapy.
    (b) Provide adequate feed that the horse can eat.

Nervous system

Post-anaesthetic neuropathy
Post-anaesthetic lameness may be caused by nerve damage. Lameness solely due to nerve damage is not associated with pain or hardness and swelling of the muscles (cf. myopathy). Neuropathies result from trauma, excessive pressure or stretching of nerve fibres. Superficial nerves, e.g. radial, femoral and facial, are more vulnerable to trauma. Neuropathies are not painful and usually resolve without treatment over a number of days, unless they cause recumbency.

Haemorrhagic myelopathy
Spinal cord damage is a rare complication following anaesthesia, however a syndrome called haemorrhagic myelopathy is recognised. Treatment is unlikely to be successful.

Gastrointestinal and respiratory system
Oesophageal and gastrointestinal motility are depressed by anaesthetic drugs. Horses allowed access to feed early in the recovery period may develop signs of oesophageal obstruction or colic.

Displacement of viscera during movement of the horse under anaesthesia or surgical manipulation of the gastrointestinal tract may produce signs of colic post-operatively.

Diarrhoea, *pleuritis* and *pneumonia* are rare complications following the stress of anaesthesia and surgery.

Cardiopulmonary resuscitation (CPR)

Cardiac arrest occurs when the heart no longer has any output and cardiopulmonary function fails to provide oxygen and metabolic substrate to central nervous and cardiac tissue. Clinical signs that may occur with cardiac arrest include:

- No palpable pulse
- No heart sounds
- Apnoea or terminal gasping ventilation
- Cyanosis or pale mucous membrane colour
- Altered capillary refill time
- Central eye position
- Pupillary dilation
- Absent palpebral and corneal reflexes

There are three main objectives of CPR:

(1) Maintain oxygen delivery to vital tissues
(2) Prevent the development of metabolic changes that cause irreversible tissue damage
(3) Restore normal myocardial activity

Cardiopulmonary resuscitation is a team effort, with everyone knowing their own role.

A 'crash box' containing all the drugs and equipment required for resuscitation must be located close to the theatre. It must be checked regularly and updated. The principles and techniques used in equine CPR are similar to those used in small animals and humans. This is termed the ABC system:

A Airway
B Breathing
C Circulation
D Drugs
E Electrical defibrillation
F Follow-up

To perform effective CPR the horse is immediately positioned in right lateral recumbency.

Airway

- If the animal is not intubated already, then intubate immediately with a suitable endotracheal tube.
- Check that the endotracheal tube is not occluded.
- Check the anaesthetic circuit and oxygen supply.

Breathing

- Check that the animal is apnoeic and that IPPV is required.
- Switch off the vaporiser.
- Perform IPPV with 100% oxygen.

Circulation

- Blood circulation is achieved manually by cardiac massage.
- This is performed externally by compression of the left side of the rib cage over the heart. Compression must be applied aggressively using the knees and the force of the body to be effective. It is an exhausting procedure but can work, especially in smaller ponies.

Drugs

(1) A dose chart for resuscitative drugs in the crash box is useful. This should include dose rates based on bodyweight in millilitres so that the appropriate dose can be administered quickly.

(2) Syringes preloaded with commonly used drugs and clearly labelled as to their contents save time during resuscitation but they must be replaced regularly:

    (a) Adrenaline: the principal drug used in resuscitation. It is a peripheral vasoconstrictor that increases myocardial and cerebral perfusion.

    (b) Atropine: an anticholinergic agent used primarily to treat vagally mediated brady-arrhythmias.

    (c) Lignocaine: an anti-arrhythmic agent.

    (d) Dobutamine: a positive inotrope that provides support of myocardial function during the post-resuscitation period.

Routes of drug administration for CPR

(1) Intravenous. Drugs administered into a peripheral vein are followed by a bolus of saline. This encourages delivery to the myocardium.

(2) Intratracheal. An effective route to deliver resuscitative drugs. The drug is absorbed into the pulmonary circulation.

Electrical defibrillation

This is unlikely to be available or of use in the horse.

Follow-up

Monitoring following successful CPR is vital. Support of cardiovascular, respiratory and renal function is required to treat the consequences of the cardiac arrest.

Humane destruction of the horse

This is potentially a very emotive issue, but one with which equine nurses will be involved. Euthanasia (defined as a good death) provokes strong emotions that, together with the issues of equine welfare and human safety, can make this a stressful procedure.

It is important for the clinician to obtain informed consent from the owners and insurers before proceeding and there are situations when this can be extremely difficult.

Traditionally euthanasia was performed in the horse by shooting using a free bullet. The advantages of this method are:

- When performed correctly, death is very rapid
- The carcase can be disposed of easily
- It is cheap

The disadvantages are:

- It is aesthetically unpleasant to some people
- It is potentially dangerous
- A knowledge of firearms and a licence are required

Alternatively euthanasia may be performed using intravenous anaesthetic agents, which many owners find less distressing. Prior placement of a large-diameter jugular catheter facilitates the procedure. The intravenous agents used are:

- Quinalbarbitone sodium and cinchocaine hydrochloride (Somulose®)
- Thiopentone as a bolus, followed by suxamethonium
- Pentobarbitone

Carcase disposal must be considered carefully following lethal injection. The options are usually cremation/incineration or burial with appropriate permission.

Further information
- *Farewell: Making the Right Decision*; booklet published by the Humane Slaughter Association, The Old School House, Brewhouse Hill, Wheathampstead, Herts AL4 8AN. E-mail: *info@hsa.org.uk*

- *Euthanasia in Horses—a Practical Guide to the Methods and Techniques*; a combined booklet and video presentation in hard cover, which is for sale from Leahurst (CPD Unit), Department of Veterinary Clinical Science, Leahurst, Neston CH64 7 TE.

Further reading

Taylor, P.M. & Clarke, K.W. (1999) *Handbook of Equine Anaesthesia*. WB Saunders, London.

Appendix: National Poisons Information Services Centres

This is a subscription based service available to members of the Veterinary profession only, not to the general public. For annual subscription rates, please contract the London Centre.

The Regional Drug & Poisons
  Information Service
The Royal Hospitals
Belfast
BT12 6BA

Belfast
Tel: 01232 240503
Fax: 01232 248030

West Midlands Poisons Unit
The City Hospital NHS Trust
Dudley Road
Birmingham
B18 7QH

Birmingham
Tel: 0121 507 5588/89
Fax: 0121 507 5580

Welsh National Poisons Unit
Ward West 5
Llandough Hospital
Penarth
Cardiff
CF6 2XX

Cardiff
Tel: 01222 709901
Fax: 01222 704357

Scottish Poisons
  Information Bureau
Royal Infirmary of Edinburgh
  NHS Trust
1 Lauriston Place
Edinburgh
EH3 9YW

Edinburgh
Tel: 0131 536 2300
Fax: 0131 536 2304

V. P. I. S.
Medicines Information
General Infirmary
Great George St.
Leeds
LSI 3EX

Leeds
Tel: 0113 245 0530
Fax: 0113 244 5849

V. P. I. S.
Medical Toxicology
  Unit
Guys & St Thomas'
  Hospital Trust
Avonley Road
London
SE14 5ER

London
Tel: 0207 635 9195
Fax: 0207 771 5309
Email: vpis@gstt.sthames.nhs.uk

Drug & Poisons
  Information
  Service
Regional Drug &
  Therapeutics
  Centre
Wolfson Unit
Claremont Place
Newcastle-upon-Tyne
NE1 4LP

Newcastle-upon-
  Tyne
Tel: 0191 232 1525
  (office hours)
Tel: 0191 232 5131
  (out of hours)
Fax: 0191 261 5733

Index